# Death
# to
# Dust

*What Happens to
Dead Bodies?*

# Death
# to
# Dust

## *What Happens to*
## *Dead Bodies?*

Kenneth V. Iserson, M.D.

**Galen Press, Ltd.**
Tucson, AZ

This publication is designed to present a comprehensive overview of the subject matter. It is not intended as a substitute for professional, legal, or medical advice and is sold with the understanding that neither the author nor the publisher is engaged in rendering such service through this book. If legal advice or other expert assistance is required, the services of a competent professional person should be sought.

All original art by David Vandenberg, Tucson, AZ.
Copyright © 1994 by Galen Press, Ltd.

Galen Press, Ltd.
P.O. Box 64400
Tucson, AZ 85728-4400


Library of Congress Cataloging-in-Publication Data

Iserson, Kenneth V.
     Death to dust : what happens to dead bodies? / Kenneth V. Iserson,
        p.   cm.
     Includes bibliographical references and index.
     ISBN 1-883620-07-4
        1. Death.   2. Death (Biology)   3. Cremation.   4. Embalming.
     5. Funeral rites and ceremonies.   I. Title.
     QP87.I83     1993
     306.9--dc20                                          93-39463
                                                          CIP



Special bulk purchase discounts are available for educational use, sales promotions, premiums, or fund-raising. For details, contact:

Special Sales Director
Galen Press, Ltd.
PO Box 64400-201
Tucson, AZ 85728-4400

10  9  8  7  6  5  4  3  2  1
Printed in the United States of America

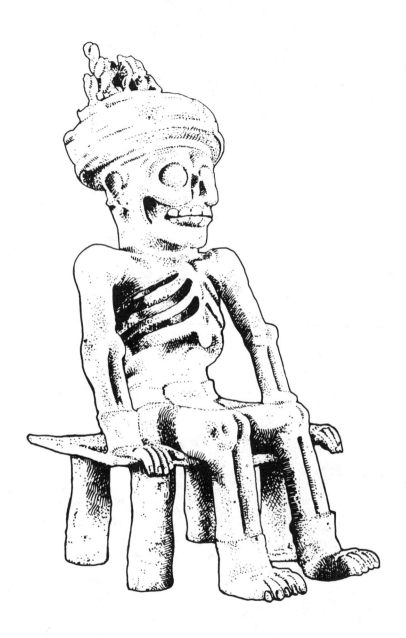

# TABLE OF CONTENTS

# Table of Contents

# Table of Contents

# Table of Contents

# Table of Contents

# Table of Contents

## Table of Contents

# Table of Contents

# Table of Contents

# LIST OF TABLES

# LIST OF ILLUSTRATIONS

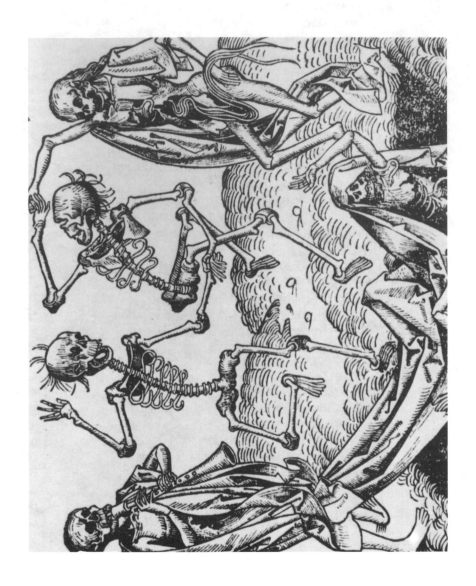

xviii

# ACKNOWLEDGEMENTS

Only one name appears as the author of this book. Any project of this magnitude, however, requires the assistance and support of multiple willing individuals. I am grateful for their help.

At every stage of production, my wife, Mary Lou Iserson, contributed enormously. She acted as in-house editor (sometimes offering cruel and unusual suggestions), reference checker, and a source for new ideas. Without her assistance, this book would not have been published.

Three individuals suffered through the early gestational pains of birthing this book. Don Witzke, Ph.D., now of the University of Kentucky Medical School at Lexington, and Alan Reeter, MSEE, president of Medfilms Inc., willingly read through early drafts of each chapter, giving me excellent advice on ways to solidify and clarify text. Hannah Fisher, RN, MLS, an unbelievably knowledgeable reference librarian at the University of Arizona Health Sciences Library was a valuable resource in locating and verifying many of the bizarre and obscure citations. She also "volunteered" the services of her son, Robert Fisher, MLS, who can only be described as a walking encyclopedia.

Throughout the book's preparation, the entire University of Arizona Health Sciences Library reference staff helped beyond measure. Of special note are Nga T. Nguyen, Marilyn Hope-Balcerzak, and Fred Heidenreich.

Many people contributed by supplying information or written material, and through interviews. Among these are funeral professionals Paul Parker, Howard Belkoff, Alex Ghia, and Larry A. McGee; anatomist Grant Dahmer; pathologists Anna Graham, M.D. and Richard Froede, M.D.; Emmitt Watson, historian of the Neptune Society Columbarium in San Francisco; clinical psychologist Judith Becker, Ph.D.; Daniel D. Stockdreher, M.P.H. from UNOS and Michael R. Merritt from the Donor Network of Arizona; Mike Perry, Ph.D. from the cryonics community; sociologist Kathryn Coe, Ph.D.; southwestern folklorist James "Big Jim" Griffith, Ph.D.; and linguist-classicist David Soren, Ph.D.

I also have to thank the many people who kindly reviewed the prepublication edition of this book and offered their valuable suggestions. These include Diane Leach, Kyle Nash, Evelyn Silvert, Walter Kaniefski, M.D., Douglas Lindsey, M.D., DPH, Sue Clemans, RN, Bruce White, D.O.,

J.D., John Lantos, M.D., Mary Mahowald, Ph.D., Lawrence S. Iserson, William M. Sherk, Nan Davis, Steve Bridge (Alcor), Deborah Mathieu, Ph.D., Ardell and Marion Taylor, and Carol Stocking, Ph.D.

Much of the credit for this book goes to Patti Cassidy, who edited the manuscript while teaching me the rules of English usage I consistently tried to ignore. David Vandenberg's wonderful drawings indicate his world-class status as an artist and add immeasurably to the text. Not to be outdone is the cover by Robert Howard, a renowned book-cover artist.

Finally, thanks goes to the wonderful professionals at Galen Press, Ltd., who believed in *Death to Dust's* importance, and without whom this book would not have been possible. If I inadvertently omitted anyone, I truly regret it. The list above, however, attests to the wonderful participation I received while compiling this book. I hope you enjoy reading it as much as they did.

# 1: DYING TO KNOW: INTRODUCTION

## A. WHY THIS BOOK?

Being dead is a mutilating experience. What happens to corpses is, for the most part, unspoken and sometimes considered unspeakable. Post-death activities have long been enveloped by a mystical shroud. This alone, I believe, has deterred many people from donating organs and tissues after death. I wrote this book to provide professionals and the public with a full picture of what does, used to, and can happen to the body after death. With that information in mind, they can make a reasoned decision about whether to donate their own or a relative's organs and tissues to help those in need.

The Bible says, "As one dies, so dies the other. They all have the same breath, and man has no advantage over the beasts...all are from the dust, and all turn to dust again."[1] Whether we believe that death is a part of life, the end of life, or the start of a new life, we must acknowledge the fact that everyone eventually dies. In the United States alone, more than two million people die each year—about one person out of every hundred and twenty.[2] In personal terms, this means that most of us will have to deal with the deaths of friends and relatives during our lifetime.

This book, though, is not about death. Rather, it is about the unseen after-death activities that go on within our living world. The act of dying is universal and personal, but it is only the first act in a complex social play.

What do we do with our dead?

Societies around the world and over time have found a myriad of ways to dispose of their dead. As Habenstein and Lamers say in *The History of American Funeral Directing*:

> Assume that we are confronted with the dead body of a man. What disposition shall we make of it? Shall we lay it in a boat that is set adrift? Shall we take the heart from it and bury it in one place and the rest of the body in another? Shall we expose it to wild animals? Burn it on a pyre? Push it into a pit to rot with other bodies? Boil it until the flesh falls off the bones, and throw the flesh away and treasure the bones? Such questions provoke others which may not be consciously articulated, such as: "What do men generally think this body is?" And, "What do they think is the proper way of dealing with it?"[3]

Who should know the answers to these questions?

Physicians? My experience is that they have only a partial understanding of even the procedures that are medically related to dead bodies, such as autopsy, anatomical dissection and organ donation. They have no better information about other aspects of corpse disposal than does the general public.

Morticians? Their knowledge also centers only around their own practices.

Perhaps the only people who really know what happens to the dead are a few anthropologists specializing in corpses.

It is always disturbing when important areas of human existence are hidden away from public view. For centuries the taboo subject was sex. William Butler Yeats had the right idea when he wrote, "I am still of the opinion that only two topics can be of the least interest to a serious and studious mood—sex and the dead."[4] The new taboo topic is death—or more particularly the dead.

Not many years ago the National Funeral Directors Association placed a series of newspaper advertisements throughout the country. To grab the audience, they titled these ads, "What Subject Bugs People More Than Sex?" The answer, of course, was death.

Then why doesn't everyone know more about what happens to dead bodies? One answer is that the funeral industry itself helps us hide death. Until one hundred years ago, people in Western cultures had largely come to terms with the dead, only to have their perceptions subverted by modern medical institutions and a funeral industry that hid the dead, orchestrated funeral rites, and depersonalized the process of parting from loved ones.

A fear of the dead and the belief that corpses pollute the living are ancient beliefs, common among nearly all people. The *Sacred Book of the Persians* regarded the corpse as taboo, since it was supposed to be saturated with danger for mortals. Biblical priests (*Kohanim*) were not allowed to touch the dead, and biblical injunctions against those handling the dead were severe, saying "Whosoever is unclean by the dead shall be put outside the camp, that they defile not the camp in the midst whereof the Lord dwells."[5] The ancient Roman high priests (*pontiffs*) performed funerals from behind curtains, never even seeing the dead.[6] Among the Shuswap Indians of British Columbia and the Thompson River Indians, those touching the corpse had to sleep on thorny branches for a year. Even today in the Fiji Islands, anyone touching someone who has died a natural death cannot touch food with his hands for several days; if he has dug a chief's grave, he is considered unclean for a year. In southern China, those who handle the dead are social pariahs and in India, as long as a Hindu body remains in the house, neither members of the household nor neighbors can eat, drink or work.[7]

In present day America, the dying are sent off to hospitals and corpses are disguised to appear alive during the funeral. Reminders of death are not appreciated, perhaps because "All men think all men mortal but themselves."[8] One grave marker amplified this, saying:

> Remember me as you draw nigh
> As you are now, so once was I.
> As I am now, so must you be,
> Prepare for death and follow me.[9]

An American colonial epitaph reinforced that thought:

> All ye who read with little care,
> Who walk away and leave me here,
> Should not forget that you must die
> And be entombed, as well as I.[10]

As a society we are generally ignorant of what goes on after death. Many Americans have never attended a funeral or burial, let alone seen an autopsy, attended a wake, or participated in other rites for the dead. It is not because they cannot, it is because of a committed stance towards ignoring the whole issue. Acknowledging the dead would mean accepting one's own mortality.

When modern people do acknowledge the dead, it is often with an avowed inattention and unconcern. They often treat funerals and burials as disagreeable events to be handled as quickly and perfunctorily as possible. Ceremonies are abbreviated, cemeteries have manicured landscapes, and drive-through visitation at some funeral homes now limits involvement even further. Yet as Leon Kass said,

> One of the most unsettling—yet for the thoughtful man, also interesting—things about confronting cadavers, dead bodies, or the question of organ transplantation is that we are by practice forced to decide who or what we think we are...How to treat dead bodies may seem to be a trivial moral question...But...few are as illuminating of our self-conception and self-understanding.[11]

If the intentional ignorance of society's treatment of corpses merely led to the manipulation of grieving survivors by the "death industry," it would be unfortunate, but not catastrophic. This disregard and misunderstanding, however, have caused the living to suffer and die as well.

Relatives of the deceased, in order not to "mutilate" the body, have repeatedly resisted donating their deceased relative's organs or tissues—unwittingly causing thousands of potential recipients to die. Likewise, medical professionals have also been blocked from practicing, teaching, and experimenting on dead bodies—and unknown numbers of live patients have been used for these purposes instead.

Elisabeth Kübler-Ross, in her ground-breaking book, *On Death and Dying*,[12] began removing the stigma from discussing death. Many books, articles, conferences, and educational courses subsequently appeared to help people measure, discuss and rationalize their attitudes and fears about death. This allowed the public to feel proud of their openness about the topic. It is not clear, however, if this self-congratulatory attitude is appropriate. Geoffrey Gorer suggests, "Death has become more and more 'unmentionable' *as a natural process*...The natural processes of corruption and decay have become disgusting...the art of the embalmers is an art of complete denial."[13] And Enright asks pointedly whether death is "a dirty little secret, a thing of shame, the last taboo in an otherwise totally uninhibited world?"[14] As Ariès says, "When people started fearing death in earnest, they stopped talking about it, starting with clergymen and doctors; death was becoming too serious."[15]

Richard Selzer, a surgeon and author, perfectly described this situation in relation to a similarly necessary and poorly understood medical procedure, the autopsy:

> SHE: Is he dead, then?
>
> HE: I am sorry.
>
> SHE: Oh, God.
>
> HE: I should like to ask...because of the circumstances of your husband's death, it would be very helpful...to do...an autopsy.
>
> SHE: Autopsy? No, no, not that. I don't want him cut up.

Better to have agreed, madam. We use the trocar [a *very* large hollow needle] on all, autopsied or merely embalmed. You have not heard of the suction trocar? Permit me to introduce you to the instrument.[16] (For your own introduction, see Chapter 5, *Beauty in Death*. See a trocar illustrated on p. 198.)

Information about treatment of the body after death has been hard to obtain, though the material is there. It is on medical library shelves and in professional funeral manuals, scholarly books and academic articles. But it has been, for the most part, kept out of mainstream literature. Fiction writers have accessed bits and pieces to spice up horror stories and other macabre tales, but no one source has provided a comprehensive picture.

For the most part, this book is about rituals as action—what happens—rather than rituals as symbols—what they mean. In many cultures, rituals associated with death act as a kind of cultural cement. Two death rituals, classed as *funerary rites* and *rites of disposal*, are closely associated in some cultures; in others they are widely separated in nature and time. This book discusses both types of rituals, although it is heavily weighted towards rites of disposal—the aspect least known or understood. The meaning of these rites, though, isn't always clear, at least to outsiders. As Lewis says, "In ritual as in art, he who devises or creates or performs is also spectator of what he does; and he who beholds it is also active in the sense that he interprets the performance. The value of ritual lies partly in this ambiguity of the active and passive for creator, performer and beholder."[17]

## B. HOW IS THIS BOOK ORGANIZED?

In accordance with this book's title, the text progresses from death to dust, more or less. The book begins by describing how physicians know a person is dead, how people are pronounced dead, when mistakes have been made, and the natural decomposition of corpses. *I'm Dead—Now What?* discusses the difference between brain and heart-lung criteria for determining death, and the often confusing distinction between those in a persistent vegetative state and the dead. This chapter also contains important details about death certificates and obituaries.

Even after people die, they can still contribute to the living. *Help for the Living: Organ, Tissue and Whole-Body Donation* describes how the dead can aid the living with the gift of wholeness—restoring them to a funtioning, intact body. The need for transplantable organs and tissues is enormous, and growing. The dearth of donations relates, in part, to a lack of knowledge about what actually occurs to the donated body. This chapter describes what organs and tissues are needed, how they are taken (surgically, as in an operation), and how donor bodies can still have funerals and viewings. Medical schools, of course, also need entire bodies for anatomical dissection. This chapter discusses that need and their method of use as well as researchers' uses of anatomical cadavers.

The next stop in this journey of discovery is with the pathologist. *My Body and the Pathologist: The Autopsy* discusses both the routine hospital autopsy and the arcane world of the medical examiner (e.g., *Quincy*). How and on whom are autopsies performed? What special techniques do pathologists and medical examiners use? Can the pathologist really determine an accurate time of death? What do pathologists really do at the scene of major disasters? How do individuals get copies of autopsy reports? This chapter sheds a little light into the morgue.

Most of the world is amazed, if not disgusted, by the (primarily) American practice of embalming the dead. While embalming predates the Egyptian mummies, the practice was rarely used in other civilizations. Today it is a common and accepted custom in the United States. *Beauty in Death* takes the mystery out of embalming. Information about embalming is most difficult to obtain, since the funeral industry has made a concerted effort to conceal this process from the public. After reading this chapter, you will know why. It also describes the people who comprise the funeral industry, special restoration techniques embalmers use, the limited legal requirements for embalming, religious attitudes toward the process, and the cost.

Cremation is an ancient method of corpse disposal and an integral part of some religions. Even though this approach to corpse disposal is becoming more popular in the United States and around the world, much confusion and myth surrounds it. *The Eternal Flame* describes not only the process, but also the mystical, religious, legal, and psychological aspects of cremation. It answers questions that arise about what can happen to the "ashes" after cremation and dispels some common myths. This chapter also describes alternative methods people have used to dispose of cremated remains—some of which are distinctly unpalatable.

*Souls on Ice* describes the cryonic suspension of whole bodies and dead heads. It explores the questions: Is this relatively rare procedure a scam or a realistic option? Do reputable scientists believe there is any chance that cryonauts can be revived in the future? Will such bodies be subjects for future research or will they simply be allowed to thaw? Who is undergoing cryonic preservation now and how much does it cost?

Dead bodies do not always find final dispositions in graves or as cremated remains. With so many dead since the dawn of time, some inevitably end up in unusual places. *Wayward Bodies* describes what happens to bodies exposed to the environment, those buried at sea, robbed from their graves, or those taken for archaeological study. There is also speculation about what will happen to dead bodies in space. Bodies can also be "wayward" because people die in distant places. Methods of transporting bodies and cremated remains, and the rules to follow for a smooth passage, are also discussed in this chapter.

Corpses, or their parts, have been used as food, decorations, public warnings to criminals, war trophies, religious fetishes, and as sex objects. Reality can often be stranger than fiction. *Nightmares* describes the reality behind many horror stories and movies.

The pomp and circumstance surrounding funerary rites, especially those of famous people, have always drawn the public's attention. *Going Out In Style* describes the way corpses are used in ceremonies, how they once were the "life of the party" at wakes, and some strange things that have happened to some corpses just because they were famous.

*Black Tie Affairs* discusses the part of the death ritual with which Westerners are most familiar, the funeral. There are, however, unusual aspects to the funeral with which many are not familiar, including United States government regulations, customized rituals, casket choices, memorial services, and the costs. This chapter also touches on burial rites, such as they are, in times of crisis and on the battlefield.

The final disposition for most bodies in the United States and Canada is burial. From *Earth to Earth* discusses both burial and "unburial" (exhumation). What, though, are mausoleums, catacombs, crypts, sarcophagi, vaults, grave liners, memorial parks, and memorial societies? How permanent are cemeteries and who oversees the burial? Finally, how much does all of this cost?

After burial or cremation the body may be gone, but some questions remain. *A Hand from the Grave* takes a look at the environmental impact of different corpse-disposal methods, optimal methods for preserving corpses, the question of who owns the body, the use of advance directives (living wills, etc.) to determe what will happen to the body, a sample instruction sheet to leave with relatives, and a chart comparing the costs of various body disposition methods.

The balance of the book contains maxims and poetry about the dead, notes and references, a glossary of words about the dead, and appendices containing some of the laws and rules concerning the dead and death.

## C. HOW CAN YOU USE THE KNOWLEDGE IN THIS BOOK?

With the information in this book, readers should be able to make informed choices concerning arrangements for disposal of their own or a relative's body. They should also have a better understanding of organ and tissue donations. I hope this book clarifies that the "mutilation" of a body that accompanies organ donation is minimal when compared to what occurs in embalming, natural decomposition, and other rites and practices involving corpses that have taken place over the ages. Although we try to hide it, being dead is a mutilating experience.

While death is universal, so that although dying can be tragic, the postmortem treatment of dead bodies is mundane. With this understanding, our society will be able to proceed toward a more rational and healthy attitude about the various options available for dealing with the dead.

Richard Selzer's fictionalized widow, however, couldn't cope:

> HE: I am afraid, madam, that we have reached an impasse. You prefer neither cremation nor embalming. You are repelled alike by anatomical dissection and the moist relentment of putrefaction. Why don't you admit that you are ashamed of death? You think it is a disgrace to be dead.
>
> SHE: That's it. Yes. A disgrace. That's it exactly.
>
> HE: Exactly, yes.[18]

Now, as Shakespeare said, "Let's talk of graves, of worms and epitaphs."[19]

## D. REFERENCES

1. *Ecclesiastes* 3:19-20.
2. Haub CV: Populations & Population Movements: Demography. In: *1993 Book of the Year*. Chicago: Encyclopaedia Britannica, 1993, p 251.
3. Habenstein RW, Lamers WM: *The History of American Funeral Directing*. Milwaukee, WI: National Funeral Directors Assoc., 1985 (Revision), pp 3-4.
4. Yeats WB: *The Letters of W. B. Yeats*. As quoted in: Bartlett J: *Bartlett's Familiar Quotations*. 14th ed. Boston: Little, Brown & Co., 1968, p 885.
5. *Numbers* 5:2.
6. Bendann E: *Death Customs: An Analytical Study of Burial Rites*. New York: Alfred A Knopf, 1930, p 84.
7. Ibid., p 86.
8. Walker GA: *Gatherings From Grave Yards*. London: Longman & Co, 1839. Reprinted by Arno Press. New York, 1977, p 190.
9. Epitaph found in Wolfpits, CT, dated 1830. Quoted in: Jones B: *Design for Death*. Indianapolis: Bobbs-Merrill Co, 1967, p 148.
10. Portion of an epitaph. Quoted in: Coffin MM: *Death in Early America: The History and Folklore of Customs and Superstitions of Early Medicine, Funerals, Burials, and Mourning*. Nashville: Thomas Nelson, 1976, p 172.
11. Kass LR: Thinking about the body. *Hastings Center Report*. 1985;15:20-30.
12. Kübler-Ross E: *On Death and Dying*. New York: MacMillan, 1969.
13. Gorer G: *Death, Grief, and Mourning in Contemporary Britain*. London: The Cresset Press, 1965, p 172.
14. Enright DJ: *The Oxford Book of Death*. Oxford: Oxford Univ Press, 1983.
15. Ariès P: *The Hour of Our Death*. New York: Oxford Univ Press, 1981, p 406.
16. Selzer R: *Mortal Lessons: Notes on the Art of Surgery*. New York: Simon & Schuster, 1987, p 130.
17. Lewis G: *Day of Shining Red: An Essay on Understanding Ritual*. Cambridge: Cambridge Univ Press, 1982, p 38.
18. Selzer, *Mortal Lessons*, p 139.
19. Shakespeare W: *The Tragedy of King Richard II*. Act 3, scene 2, line 145.

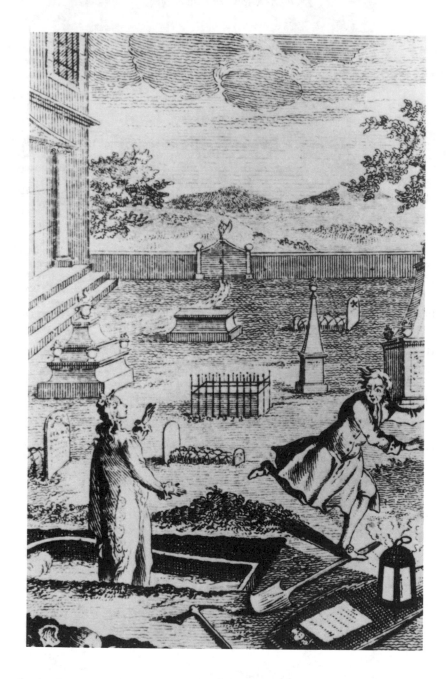

A would-be body snatcher discovering a premature burial. Originally published by J.B.
Winslow: *The Uncertainty of the Signs of Death,* London, 1746. (Reproduced with permission.
National Library of Medicine.)

# 2: I'M DEAD—NOW WHAT?

A. Why do people die?
B. What is death?
C. What is death by brain criteria?
D. How is death by brain criteria determined?
E. Is persistent vegetative state the same as death by brain criteria?
F. Who can pronounce me dead?
G. What is a death certificate, who can sign it, and what does it cost?
H. How will they know I'm really dead?
I. When have physicians erred in pronouncing death?
J. Are there real cases of premature burials?
K. What precautions have been taken to prevent premature burial?
L. Who was buried alive intentionally?
M. What can happen to my body when I die?
N. What will happen to my body when I die?
O. How does my name get in the newspaper?
P. References.

*What is the difference between brain criteria and heart-lung criteria for determining death? How do those in a persistent vegetative state differ from the dead? What do I need to know about death certificates and obituaries?*

## A. WHY DO PEOPLE DIE?

In most discussions of death, one metaphysical question naturally arises, why do people die?

One answer is provided by traditional Fijian lore:

When the first man, the father of the human race, was being buried, a god passed by the grave and inquired what it meant, for he had never seen a grave before. Upon receiving the information from those about the place of interment that they had just buried their father, he said: "Do not bury him, dig up the body again." "No," they replied, "we cannot do that. He has been dead for four days and smells." "Not so," entreated the god, "dig him up and I promise you that he will live again." But they refused to carry out the divine injunction. Then the god declared, "By disobeying me, you have sealed your own fate. Had you dug up your ancestor, you would have found him alive, and you yourselves when you passed from this world should have been buried as bananas are for four days, after which you shall have been dug up, not rotten, but ripe. But now, as a punishment for your disobedience, you shall die and rot."[1]

The Navajo have a more practical answer.

According to legend, when they emerged into this world, the question naturally arose, "would they live forever or die?" Coyote came along and decided the question by throwing a stone into the water. If it floated, they would live, if it sank they would die. It sank and the Navaho became angry, but Coyote rationalized (in a very traditional Navaho way) that "If we all live and continue to increase as we have done in the past, the earth will be too small to hold us, and there will be no room for the cornfields. It is better that each of us should live but a limited time on this earth, then leave and make room for the children." The people realized the wisdom of his words and resigned themselves to their fate. [2]

According to Judaic tradition, before man's creation, God said:

The celestials are not propagated, but they are immortal; the beings on earth are propagated, but they die. I will create man to be the union of the two, so that when he sins, when he behaves like a beast, death shall overtake him; but if he refrains from sin, he shall live forever.[3]

After Adam committed the sin of disobedience, God delivered the whole animal world to the Angel of Death.[4] As one of the punishments for worshipping idols, God then caused the bodies of dead men to decay.[5]

Scientists not only ask why we die, but why do we die when we do, at about 70 to 80 years of age in Western societies? Although the relatively rapid turnover of human lives spurs genetic diversity in a changing environment, other organisms, such as some trees, live a thousand years or more.

## B. WHAT IS DEATH?

Death is the end of life and has traditionally been said to occur when the heart stops. Biologically, however, death is not a discrete event, but is a gradual process that ends with the irreversible loss of function of the entire organism. As Morrison said, "There is no magic moment at which 'everything' disappears. Death is no more a single, clearly delimited, momentary phenomenon than is infancy, adolescence, or middle age."[6] And Horan adds, "Unlike the legal profession, the medical profession looks upon death as a continuing process and not an 'instant' or 'moment' in time as the law believes."[7]

Even though a person may be "dead" because his heart stops working, some muscle, skin and bone cells may live on for many days. So, while the entire person as a functioning organism is dead, parts of the biologic organism live on for varying periods of time. The amount of time these cells and tissues live depends on their ability to survive without oxygen and other nutrients, and with an increasing amount of metabolic waste products building up within them. Richard Selzer described these last living parts as "outposts where clusters of cells yet shine, besieged, little lights blinking in the advancing darkness. Doomed soldiers, they battle on. Until Death has secured the premises all to itself."[8]

Then when *is* a person "dead?"

Clearly it is not when *every* body cell has succumbed, but rather when the individual lacks "the features that humans must possess to be regarded as living persons rather than dead persons."[9] Those features necessary to still be considered among the living vary among societies, in different circumstances, and over time. The 22nd World Medical Assembly pointed out that "clinical interest lies not in the state of preservation of isolated cells but in the fate of a person. The point of death of the different cells and organs is not as important as the certainty that the process has become

13

irreversible."[10]

Defining death as occurring when the heart stops beating became confusing when cardiopulmonary resuscitation (CPR) began to be used to revive people whose hearts had stopped.

This definition is now even more inadequate since cardiac surgeons intentionally stop patients' hearts in surgery or remove them during transplants. These patients are not dead, but rather are expected to recover and lead normal lives after surgery. In these surgeries heart-lung machines maintain the person's circulation. This may suggest that cessation of circulation rather than heart stoppage defines death, yet both are simply mechanisms, rather than definitions, of death.

A newer and often more emotionally difficult concept is death by brain criteria, more commonly known as "brain death." In brain death, the heart often functions normally and circulation continues. This definition relies not on the absence of heart activity or circulation, but on the inability of the whole organism, the person, to continue to function and independently regulate itself. The brain no longer works even though all other organs and tissues in the body may function normally for a limited period of time.

Many individuals with severe brain injuries die when their swollen brains press on the brainstem's respiratory center and their breathing stops. Similarly, the brain's breathing mechanism is often permanently damaged after it is deprived of oxygen for a prolonged period, such as during cardiac arrest, strangulation, or drowning. As the famous physiologist John Scott Haldane said, the "machinery is wrecked." Artificial ventilators (sometimes called "respirators") may keep the body "breathing," but in doing so they eliminate the primary traditional sign of death. While these ventilators have saved hundreds of thousands of lives, it was apparent soon after their development that physicians no longer knew when to pronounce their patients dead.

In 1957, Pope Pius XII questioned whether doctors might be "continuing the resuscitation process, despite the fact that the soul may already have left the body," and if "death had already occurred after grave trauma to the brain, which has provoked deep unconsciousness and central breathing paralysis, the fatal consequences of which have been retarded by artificial respiration." Unfortunately, he declined to answer his own questions, saying that this "did not fall within the competence of the Church."[11]

By defining "brain death," society is obliged to address the larger question, what is the relationship between a human being and his body? This question, often posed as "mind-body dualism," has occupied philosophers, religious experts and physicians throughout the ages.

Two contradictory answers to this question are provided by the "corporealists" who see man as *nothing but body,* and "dualists" who view

14

the *body as purely incidental* to pure will and reason (and who believe in personhood, consciousness and autonomy). [12] No theoretical resolution exists between these views. Western societies, though, have pragmatically sided with the dualists, leading to the concept of death by brain criteria – "brain death."

In the future, people may be allowed to specify under what conditions they wish to be pronounced dead: whether they want their heart to have irreversibly stopped, their entire brain to have ceased functioning, or the part of the brain that defines their identity (neocortex) to have died. Some states, such as Arizona, already allow people to specify in advance directives if they do not wish to be kept alive in persistent vegetative states; the rest of the options may soon be available elsewhere. Then each individual will be able to define death for himself.

## C. WHAT IS DEATH BY BRAIN CRITERIA?

In death by brain criteria the body is physiologically decapitated. In an anatomic decapitation, the head is actually lopped off, but the heart continues to beat for some time, spraying blood from the severed neck arteries. Yet despite the continued pumping of the heart, there is no question that the person is irreversibly dead. Even in ancient times, the Talmud said "the death throes of a decapitated man are not signs of life any more than are the twitchings of a lizard's amputated tail." [13] Likewise, in death by brain criteria, all brain function ceases. The person is dead, even though the head remains attached to the body.

The term "death by brain criteria" can be somewhat ambiguous, since it refers to at least three distinct *types* of brain malfunction: (1) death by *whole brain criteria*, in which the brainstem has ceased functioning; (2) *cerebral death*, in which the brain itself has ceased functioning, but the lowest centers in the cerebellum (back of the brain) and brainstem still function; and (3) *neocortical death*, in which there is a lack of function in the "thinking" part of the brain. Neocortical death is not recognized in the United States, Britain, Canada, and most other countries that recognize death by brain criteria.

The most widely accepted and only legal definition of death by brain criteria in the United States, Britain, Canada, and most other Western countries, is "death by whole brain criteria." Death by whole brain criteria refers to the complete loss of function in the *upper brain* and the *brainstem*.

The upper brain (neocortex) contains thoughts, perceives pain and pleasure, and controls voluntary actions; it is the person.

The brainstem, on the other hand, is a developmentally older organ. It controls basic biological functions without which the upper brain does not work. Found at the base of the brain, the brainstem directly controls wakefulness (reticular activating system), breathing (respiratory center), and

15

blood pressure (vasomotor center). Passing through the brainstem are all of the brain's pathways to the rest of the body for movement, all receptors for conscious sensation, and all controls for integrating body functions (sympathetics and parasympathetics). It is a densely packed highway of nerves. Even minor damage to this area often results in death. *No matter what condition the upper brain is in, once the brainstem is inoperative, the whole brain is dead.*

The most common causes of "death by brain criteria" are (1) injuries or masses (lumps or swelling) in the upper part (supratentorial) of the brain, including blood clots, direct injuries, strokes, tumors or infections; (2) similar injuries or masses in the lower part of the brain (infratentorial) that directly injure the brainstem; and (3) metabolic or chemical disorders such as a persistent lack of oxygen (anoxia), lack of blood flow (ischemia), absence of glucose (sugar), or the presence of intrinsic or extrinsic poisons, that destroy the brain cells' functions. [14]

Most Christian scholars strongly support the concept of death by brain criteria, based on the doctrine that the soul departs the body at the moment of death. [15] Most Jews likewise accept the concept of death by brain criteria, as do many non-Christian religious groups. [16] Yet religions, such as Taoism, Confucianism, Zen-Buddism, and Shintoism which stress the integration of mind and body have difficulty accepting death by brain criteria. Fewer than one-fourth of all Japanese, for example, favor national "brain death" criteria. [17]

By the late 1960s, many totally unresponsive patients were being kept on ventilators in intensive care units until their hearts stopped. At autopsy, pathologists found that these patients had "respirator brains" which had become soft, dark green, or totally liquified after the cells had died days or weeks before. [18] French neurologists recognized that these patients had been in a state beyond coma (coma dépassé). Obviously, new guidelines for declaring death were needed. Experts began to devise these new criteria.

## D. HOW IS DEATH BY BRAIN CRITERIA DETERMINED?

With confusion rampant about how to declare death by brain criteria, medical groups around the world began disseminating their own standards. In 1968, the 22nd World Medical Assembly, Sydney, Australia (Appendix A) and the Ad Hoc Committee of the Harvard Medical School (Appendix B) published their standards for diagnosing death by brain criteria and identified a "brain-death syndrome." [19] In 1979 the Conference of Royal Colleges and Faculties of the United Kingdom equated brainstem death with death, and in 1981 in the United States, the President's Commission for the Study of Ethical Problems in Medicine and Biomedical and Behavioral Research published guidelines very similar to those from the United Kingdom and proposed a model statute, the "Uniform Determination of

Death Act," which has become law in many states (Appendix C).

In most cases, physicians make the diagnosis of death by brain criteria on purely clinical grounds. Not every brain cell need be dead, and in fact all cells are usually not dead when examined by positron emission (PET) scanning. Rather, the physician attempts to establish the fact that there is irreversible loss of brainstem function. This is usually done by physicians specializing in neurology, neurosurgery, or critical care medicine who are neither the patient's primary physicians nor members of a transplant team. They normally follow these steps:

1. determine the cause of coma;
2. decide that irremediable structural brain damage has occurred;
3. eliminate reversible causes of coma such as an extremely low body temperature, drug intoxication or a severe chemical imbalance; and
4. demonstrate that all brainstem reflexes, including breathing, are absent.

The reflexes physicians look for are those that tell whether the vital connections in the brainstem are still intact. They test a patient's ability to breathe on his own by first supplying the patient with 100 percent oxygen for several minutes, while he is still connected to a ventilator. They then continue the oxygen but remove the ventilator just long enough to see if an increase in the body's chemicals (carbon dioxide) will stimulate breathing. This is normally tested twice.

Next, they test other reflexes corresponding to connections between various nerves (cranial nerves) originating in the brainstem: coughing or gagging in response to suctioning the airway, constriction of the pupil in response to light, blinking in response to touching the cornea, grimacing or movement in response to pressure above the eye, and moving the eyes when the head is rotated (doll's eyes phenomenon) or the ears are flushed with ice water.

No patient who failed all of these tests to determine brain activity has *ever* regained consciousness. In the rare cases in which individuals have been mistakenly declared dead by brain criteria, some of these procedural safeguards were not followed.

When patients are kept on ventilators despite being dead, their hearts stop within hours to days. Stiller has suggested that these bodies be called honestly, "life-supported cadavers." [20] What do third-party payers and the auditors of medical performance think about paying for dead "patients?" Is it fraud to bill for keeping these cadavers functioning in intensive care units? These questions have yet to be answered.

In France, the diagnosis of death by brain criteria requires not only that the Harvard criteria be met (generally described above and fully described in

17

Appendix B), but also that the patient have a demonstrated loss of the ability to regulate temperature and blood pressure. In Austria, Germany and many Scandinavian countries, not only must the Harvard criteria be met, but a bilateral carotid angiogram (a dye study showing blood flow into the brain) or a nuclear medicine scan must also show that blood is no longer flowing to the brain. [21] While most patients declared dead by any one of these methods will be dead by all, it is possible that in some cases patients declared "dead" in one country will not be considered dead in another. [22]

Physicians can only tenuously apply death-by-brain-criteria guidelines to children, especially those younger than two years old. The criteria for this age group are still being formalized. Physicians specializing in the care of very young children with brain injuries will normally help make a determination of death by brain criteria.

A unique and confusing group who seem not to fit the guidelines are infants born with very little brain substance and with no skin or bone covering what brain tissue does exist – *anencephalics*. These infants are not dead by brain criteria since their brainstems function, but they will normally not live more than a week without external support (ventilators) and can never interact meaningfully with their environment. Many of their parents wish for them to be transplant donors, but this is not currently possible in the United States. Laws must be changed to make this group a separate entity not requiring death by brain criteria before donation. Some countries in Europe already allow this, [23] feeling, as does ethicist Paul Ramsey, that "such an infant has not been born alive...and no more enters the human community to claim our care and protection than a patient remains in the human community when death by brain criteria...is only disguised behind the heart-lung machine." [24]

## E. IS PERSISTENT VEGETATIVE STATE THE SAME AS DEATH BY BRAIN CRITERIA?

No. Individuals (philosophers continue to debate whether they are "persons") in persistent or permanent vegetative states (PVS) are *not dead*. Their brains still function at a very rudimentary level, they have sleep-wake cycles, and they normally can breathe without assistance. Humans are dead only when their brains have stopped working ("death by brain criteria") or their hearts and lungs have permanently failed ("cardiorespiratory arrest"). It is estimated that there are now 10,000 to 25,000 PVS individuals in the United States.

People go into PVS after sustaining injuries to the brain resulting from a lack of oxygen, a lack of sugar, or similar events. First, the person normally goes into a coma. If he neither dies nor wakes up, he lapses into a "vegetative state." Usually only young, injured individuals awaken from even this simple vegetative state; older or oxygen-deprived individuals (the more common situation) usually do not awaken. After one to three months, the condition is called a "persistent vegetative state." After three months if the brain damage was not from trauma, and after six months (adults) to one year (children) after trauma, it becomes exceedingly rare for anyone to emerge from this state. Some indeterminate time later they are declared to be in a "permanent vegetative state."

What those in PVS *are* is hard to define. Are they still "persons" even though they can no longer interact with or experience their environment? They cannot feel pain, must normally be fed through tubes surgically implanted in their stomachs, cannot receive communications of any kind, and cannot express themselves in any way – their thinking, feeling brain is gone. They will not get better, but they can live with support for many decades. The enormous expense for many of these patients' care is paid by government medical programs. In the recent case of Nancy Beth Cruzan, a young woman in PVS for more than seven years who was finally allowed to die after a prolonged court battle, the state of Missouri paid $130,000 annually for her medical care. [25] Some state statutes recognize the hopelessness of the PVS situation by allowing withdrawal of life support, including artificially supplied nutrition and hydration.

Several biomedical philosophers have suggested a death by brain criteria statute that would include PVS. Hans-Martin Sass, for example, recently developed a model statute that describes the optional use of heart-lung, whole brain, or PVS (higher-brain) standards (Appendix D).

## F. WHO CAN PRONOUNCE ME DEAD?

In all countries, physicians licensed in that jurisdiction can pronounce a person dead. The timeless definition of death remains, "a person is dead when a physician says so." [26] Other professionals also have the legal authority to declare a person dead in some United States jurisdictions and elsewhere. Where a physician is necessary to pronounce death and a person dies unattended, some localities require that the body be transported to an emergency department so that a physician there can pronounce death.

Only relatively recently have physicians been active in most death pronouncements, though. In nineteenth-century Europe, for example, physicians were reluctant to verify death. An 1818 medical compendium noted that, "doctors are rarely called in to certify death. This important responsibility is left to mercenaries or individuals who have no knowledge whatsoever of the human anatomy. When a doctor cannot save a man's life, he avoids being in his home after he has died, and all practitioners seem totally convinced of the axiom of the great philosopher that it is not seemly for a doctor to visit the dead." [27]

It appears that Australian jurists want to return to that situation. An Australian court has ruled that a physician cannot charge for pronouncing a person dead, since a corpse is not a patient. This also has implications for Australian ambulance services, hospitals, and physicians who attempt to resuscitate patients in cardiopulmonary arrest (the heart and lungs have stopped).[28] If they fail, they may not be reimbursed.

In some states, licensed nurses, police officers, and ambulance personnel may pronounce a person dead in the absence of a physician. On board ships in international waters, the captain is usually the final authority on deciding whether a passenger or crewperson is dead, although he normally defers to the most qualified medical person on the ship.

It should be noted that unless the determination of death by an authorized person (usually a physician) is in error by objective criteria, family members, courts and legislatures (except indirectly by passing death by brain criteria statutes) have nothing to say in the matter. Once death has been declared, even the most outspoken patient advocates accept the fact that the family cannot demand continued treatment. [29]

## G.  WHAT IS A DEATH CERTIFICATE, WHO CAN SIGN IT, AND WHAT DOES IT COST?

A death certificate is the official document declaring a person dead.

Death certificates serve two societal purposes: they prevent murder cover-ups and they provide public health statistics. Death registration was first required in the United Kingdom in 1874. Before then it was not even necessary for a physician to view the corpse. In the United States, Britain, and most industrialized countries, physicians must now sign a death certificate listing the presumed cause of death. Otherwise a medical examiner (forensic pathologist) will intervene with an autopsy to decide on the cause of death. This serves to identify those deaths that need police investigation.

People use death certificates in multiple ways. Survivors need death certificates to obtain burial permits, make life insurance claims, settle estates, and obtain death benefits. [30] Families have also found them useful in researching their genealogy. Biostatisticians and epidemiologists pore over death certificate data to discover public health patterns, such as among minorities of a particular age, or as with clusters of cancers that may reveal unknown toxic dumps.

In the United States, there are three types of death certificates: a standard certificate, one for fetal or stillborn deaths, and one for medicolegal cases. They are all based on the international form agreed to in 1948.[31] This form lists the "underlying causes" of death, meaning either the disease or injury which led directly to death (e.g., heart attack, AIDS, stroke), or the circumstances of the injury which produced the fatal injury (e.g., gunshot wound to the chest). Other significant conditions that do not directly contribute to death, such as chronic lung disease, diabetes, or heart disease are often listed separately.

After the physician has completed the death certificate (with or without using an autopsy), it passes to the funeral director, local and state government offices, and finally the United States Center for Health Statistics (Table 2.1).

Funeral directors often struggle to obtain a physician's signature on a death certificate. In an age of managed care groups and multispecialty clinics their problem is not only to snag the busy practitioner for his or her signature, but also to identify the correct physician initially. Survivors cannot bury or otherwise dispose of a corpse until a licensed physician signs a permanent death certificate or a medical examiner signs a temporary death certificate (in which they list the cause of death as "pending" when further laboratory tests are needed to help determine the actual cause of death). Except in unusual cases, disposition of the remains need not wait for the final autopsy reports which may take weeks to complete. [32]

After the death certificate has been signed, local authorities usually issue a Certificate of Disposition of Remains, also known as a burial or cremation permit. Crematories and cemeteries require this form before they will cremate or bury a body. In some places the form is combined with a transportation permit that allows the movement or shipment of a body. The need for regulation of death certificates was made evident in 1866 when F. I. A. Boole, the inspector for the Board of Health of New York and Brooklyn, sold blank burial certificates enabling murderers to conceal their crimes. [33]

Public health policies depend heavily on the mortality data from death certificates to provide the only source of information about the causes of death and illnesses preceding death. A recent example of using these data comes from Italy. When Italy's Del Lazio Epidemiological Observatory reviewed 44,000 death certificates, they found that diseases divided neatly along class lines. The poor died of lung tumors, cirrhosis of the liver, respiratory diseases, and "preventable deaths" (appendicitis, childbirth complications, juvenile hypertension, and acute respiratory infections). Well-to-do women had higher rates of breast cancer. They also found, though, that heart disease, strokes and some cancers did not vary by income. These findings will have a significant impact on how they fund their health care system.[34]

Yet the accuracy of United States death certificates is questionable, with up to 29 percent erring both as to the cause of death and the deceased's age.[35-39] About the same number incorrectly state whether an autopsy was done.[40] Less significant discrepancies occur in listing the deceased's marital status, race, and place of birth. Death certificates of minority groups have the most errors.[41] U.S. practitioners do not appear to think that it is important to accurately complete death certificates. [42]

## TABLE 2.1: Life History of Death Certificates

| RESPONSIBLE PERSON OR AGENCY | DEATH CERTIFICATE | FETAL DEATH CERTIFICATE (Stillbirth) |
|---|---|---|
| **Physician, Other Professional Attendant or Hospital Authority** | 1. Completes medical certification and signs certificate.<br><br>2. Returns certificate to funeral director. | 1. Completes or reviews medical items on certificate.<br><br>2. Certifies to the cause of fetal death and signs certificate.<br>3. Returns certificate to funeral director.<br>4. In absence of funeral director, files certificate. |
| **Funeral Director** | 1. Obtains personal facts about deceased.<br>2. Takes certificate to physician for medical certification.<br>3. Delivers completed certificate to local office of district where death occurred and obtains burial permit. | 1. Obtains the facts about fetal death.<br>2. Takes certificate to physician for entry of causes of death.<br>3. Delivers completed certificate to local office of district where death occurred and obtains burial permit. |
| **Local Office (Registrar or City or County Health Department)** | 1. Verifies completeness and accuracy of certificate.<br>2. Makes copy, ledger entry, or index for local use.<br>3. Issues burial permit to funeral director and verifies return of permit from cemetery attendant.<br>4. Sends certificate to State Registrar. | |

**TABLE 2.1: (continued)**

City and county health departments use certificates in allocating medical and nursing services, following up on infectious diseases, planning programs, measuring effectiveness of services, and conducting research studies.

**State Registrar, Bureau of Vital Statistics**
1. Queries incomplete or inconsistent information.
2. Maintains files for permanent reference and as the source of certified copies.
3. Develops vital statistics for use in planning, evaluating, and administering State and local health activities and for research studies.
4. Compiles health-related statistics for State and civil divisions of State for use by the health department and other agencies and groups interested in the fields of medical science, public health, demography, and social welfare.
5. Prepares copies of death and fetal death certificates or records for transmission to the National Center for Health Statistics.

**Public Health Service National Center for Health Statistics**
1. Prepares and publishes national statistics of deaths and fetal deaths; and constructs the official U.S. life tables and related actuarial tables.
2. Conducts health and social-research studies based on vital records and on sampling surveys linked to records.
3. Conducts research and methodological studies in vital statistics methods including the technical, administrative, and legal aspects of vital records registration and administration.
4. Maintains a continuing technical assistance program to improve the quality and usefulness of vital statistics.

Adapted from: The U.S. National Center for Health Statistics, Public Health Service: *Physicians' Handbook on Medical Certification: Death, Fetal Death, Birth.* Washington, DC: Govt Printing Office, 1967.[Publication No 593-B]

Many certificates are meaningless simply because physicians complete them without knowing the real cause of death. (Listing "cardiopulmonary arrest" means nothing–everyone's heart and lungs eventually stop, the important point is *why?* An autopsy is often needed to determine this.) Other certificates are obscured to protect a family's reputation or income, with listings such as "pneumonia" for an AIDS death or "accidental" for a suicide. In San Francisco, even before the AIDS epidemic, one researcher found that socially unacceptable causes of death frequently went misreported, the most common being alcoholic cirrhosis of the liver, alcoholism, syphilis, homicide and suicide. [43] Disguising deaths from alcoholism, AIDS and other stigmatizing causes of death on death certificates is widespread. [44-46] This practice appears to be exacerbated where medical examiners' autopsy reports are part of the public record. [47] For this reason some states may eliminate the cause of death from publicly recorded death certificates. [48]

A similar problem with the accuracy of death certificates has been reported in Britain. The Royal College of Physicians of London claims that only twenty percent of British death certificates incorrectly list the cause of death. In one instance, for example, the number of reported suicides at Beachy Head (a favorite spot to commit suicide by jumping into the sea) diminished by one-third simply with a change in coroners. [49]

Physicians who complete death certificates in good faith are not liable to criminal action, even if the cause of death is later found to be different from that recorded. Fraudulent completion which obscures a crime or is used to defraud an insurance company is, however, a felony.

False death certificates are especially distasteful to victims of this fraud who are still alive and whose "death" causes officials to freeze their assets, cancel credit, revoke licenses, and generally disrupt their lives. [50]

Death aboard a ship is an entirely different situation. Aboard British ships, the captain registers any crew or passenger death in the ship's log. The information contained in the log at least equals that on a death certificate. On arrival at a British port, the captain must report this to harbor authorities who then investigate the circumstances of the death.

Death certificates and other standard legal papers surrounding death normally cost between $1 and $5 each. Additional official copies cost the same amount. The funeral director usually obtains these forms and itemizes their costs on his bill. Where a body must be shipped to a non-English-speaking country, the forms must often also be translated, necessitating an additional cost.

## H.  HOW WILL THEY KNOW I'M REALLY DEAD?

Since ancient times, people have worried that they would be declared dead when they were, in fact, still alive. To prevent this, ancient Thracians,

Greeks, and Romans waited three or more days for putrefaction to begin before they buried or cremated their dead.[51] In addition, the Romans, before consigning a body to a funeral pyre, would call out a person's name three times to see if he responded, and cut off a finger to see if the stump bled.[52,53] Ancient Celts and Jews also watched their "dead" bodies over a period of time to be certain that they were deceased. While the Celts watched at home, the Jews kept bodies in unsealed sepulchres or caves, returning on each of three days. That was the tradition being followed at Easter, when mourners visited the sepulchre to find Jesus alive.[54]

Shakespeare recorded two of the most famous ancient methods for determining death, the feather and the mirror. In *Henry IV, Part II*, the Prince of Wales says:

> ...By his gates of breath
> There lies a downy feather which stirs not:
> Did he suspire, that light and weightless down
> Perforce must move.[55]

In *King Lear*, the king says to his entourage:

> Lend me a looking-glass;
> If that her breath will mist or stain the stone,
> Why, then she lives.[56]

In fourteenth-century England, precautions were often taken to prevent premature burials. Many aristocrats left written instructions not to bury their bodies until the presence of decomposition made it clear that they were dead. John, Duke of Lancaster, took this to an extreme in 1397 when he left instructions that his body "not be buried for forty days, during which I charge my executors that there be no searing or embalming my corpse."[57] The fear of being buried alive continued through eighteenth- and nineteenth-century England. Lord Chesterfield wrote in 1769, "All I desire, for my own burial, is not to be buried alive; but how or where, I think, must be entirely indifferent to every rational creature."[58] In 1808, Mrs. Elizabeth Thomas of Islington, London, directed her doctor to pierce her heart with a long metal pin to assure that she was dead. He did. She was.[59]

An English invention of 1790 involved painting the words "I am dead" with silver nitrate on a clear pane of glass. The words stayed invisible until air expressed from the decomposing corpse contained enough hydrogen sulfide gas to convert the message into its visible silver sulfide form. It took some time for enough sulfide gas to form to make the message visible.[60]

Another early scientific method to determine death was proposed by Johannes Crève (1769-1853), who suggested that physicians expose a muscle of the apparently deceased person and apply a silver and zinc arc to form an electrical circuit. If a contraction occurred, the person might still be alive.[61]

Today we recognize that muscle contractions can still be activated for a period after death. Many people have seen this demonstrated with frog legs in science class.

An "old wives' tale" described a common method used to see if a person was really dead in early America:

> Touch the flame of a candle to the tip of one of the great toes of the supposed corpse. A blister will raise. If life is gone, the blister will be full of air and will burst noisily when the flame is applied a few seconds more. If there is still life, the blister will not burst. [62]

That the method is *not* accurate can be seen by the second degree burn blisters that are "burst" when additional heat is applied in living people.

In rural villages of Italy and Portugal, it was once the practice to stick pins under a corpse's nails to cause enough pain so that anyone not really dead would awaken.

In the early nineteenth century, Dr. Josat won first prize from the Académie de France for inventing a clawed forceps for pinching a corpse's nipples to assure that a person was dead. John Snart, in his 1817 text, *Thesaurus of Horror*, suggested several other methods for assuring that a corpse was truly dead:

> ...keeping the corpse warm under close watch for at least a week, with no indecent experiments for twenty-four hours except holding a looking-glass to the mouth or brushing the soles of the feet with strong pickle [strong acid]; or electricity; or warm baths; or pasting tissue-paper over the mouth and nose; or blowing Scotch snuff up the nose; or pouring volatile tincture of ammonia down the throat with a funnel. If none of these seem conclusive, cut the jugulars, or separate the carotid arteries, divide the medulla, or pierce the heart. [63]

Despite these precautions, all early medical experts agreed that except for destroying the body, the onset of putrefaction was the only certain sign of death. When Dr. Maze reconfirmed this in 1890, he won the prestigious *Prix Dusgate* award.[64]

Many premature burials are thought to have been the result of *thanatomimesis*, or death feigning. It has been said that "a good swooner and a hasty undertaker make a bad combination." [65]To prevent this, in 1896 the Association for the Prevention of Premature Burial was founded. Its members arranged with medical experts to perform certain tests, specified by the Association, to assure that their members were really dead. [66]

In the early twentieth century, Anthony de Chionski, a retired Polish parson living near Dresden invented an apparatus to check whether a person was dead (and to kill him if he wasn't). His device was a body-sized vacuum chamber from which air was incrementally removed. If the body moved during the process, operators opened the chamber and checked for signs of life. If they saw no movement, all of the air was removed and the corpse was assuredly dead.

Inexperienced people may have difficulty determining when a person is really dead because of the strange but normal events often preceding death. As death approaches, a person frequently gasps for breath and may repeatedly stop breathing for as long as thirty seconds. The dying are commonly in shock or very cold, making it difficult for observers to feel a pulse at the wrist, ankle, or temple – even though the heart has not stopped.

There is less excuse for a physician to make a mistake. The physician has several ways to assess death at the bedside: a stethoscope can assess cardiac activity better than taking pulses; the physician can feel a carotid or femoral pulse; and an ophthalmoscope can show whether blood in the vessels in the eye has broken into the stationary segments ("boxcars") that signal absence of cardiac activity. [67] If necessary, physicians can confirm their diagnoses with electrocardiograms and other sophisticated devices.

Yet except in the very recent past, medical education has appeared to be relatively indifferent to the problem of diagnosing death. As evidence, Arnold's 1968 review of physical diagnosis texts found only one that discussed this problem. It was a 1926 text, Charles L. Greene's *Medical Diagnosis for the Student and Practitioner,* and listed the following "signs of life:"

1. A deep red or purple color in the finger tips will become evident gradually if a firm ligature be applied to the digit. If applied to the wrist, prominence of the veins on the dorsum of the hand indicates life. The ligature must not be so tight as to completely cut off the circulation.
2. Several hours after a supposed death, blood will flow persistently from a cut artery. A small artery should be chosen, not mere wet cupping or haphazard puncture.
3. If a needle thrust into the tissues and left for a time becomes oxidized, life is present.
4. If any cloud repeatedly appears upon an ice-cold mirror held close to the mouth, there is respiration, but its absence does not alone suffice to prove death.
5. If a powerful vesicant produces redness or blisters, there is life.
6. If a body fails to take approximately the temperature of its environment 48 hours after apparent death, there is life.
7. Pupillary response to light shows life, its absence does not prove death. Several hours after death, it is affected neither by atropin nor eserin [sic].
8. Persistence of the red in, and visibility of the arteries of the optic

27

disc are signs of life, as is also persistent clearness of the media six to eight hours after apparent death.

9. A sensitive cornea is a sign of life, absence of the corneal reflex is not a sign of death.

10. Presence of electric excitability in all muscles 24 hours after apparent death indicates life. (Usually lost in from 3-6 hours, but retained from 10-15 hours in certain cases.) [68]

"Actually," said Arnold in the *Journal of the American Medical Association*, "very little is known of the accuracy of the several methods of diagnosing death either in the 19th century or the 20th century. Except for the electrocardiogram and the electroencephalogram, it appears that medicine has acquired no new tools for determining the functional state of organs critically important to the diagnosis of death." [69] The only significant additions to these tests have been cerebral blood flow studies, which are rarely performed. Many of the tests listed in 1926 are still the foundation for making a diagnosis of death.

The British medical journal *Lancet* in 1884 spoke about the misdiagnosis of death in words that still ring true today: "It is not so much the undue haste as inexcusable carelessness that must be blamed for the premature burying of persons who are not really dead." [70]

## I. WHEN HAVE PHYSICIANS ERRED IN PRONOUNCING DEATH?

None of the above methods was fool-proof. Mistakes were made, even by such noted physicians as Andreas Vesalius, a sixteenth-century Flemish physician to the Holy Roman emperor Charles V, a professor of surgery in Padua, and the greatest anatomist of all time. In 1564 he began an autopsy on a Spanish grandee that he had mistakenly pronounced dead. Once Vesalius opened the chest, it was clear that the heart was still beating. He was brought before the Tribunal of the Inquisition which first sentenced him to a cruel death. After intervention by the King, they booted him out of Spain. As penance, the surgeon had to make a pilgrimage to the Holy Sepulchre in Jerusalem – little comfort to his poor patient who inevitably died.[71] Vesalius was shipwrecked en route to the Holy Land and died of exposure.[72]

An American physician also died because of an erroneous postmortem examination. According to Dr. Franz Hartmann, in his book on premature burials:

In May, 1864, a man died very suddenly at an hospital in the State of New York, and as the doctors could not explain the cause of the death they resolved upon a *post-mortem* examination, but when they made the first cut with the knife, the supposed dead man jumped up and grasped the doctor's throat. The doctor was terrified, and died of apoplexy on the spot, but the "dead man" recovered fully.[73]

Physicians knew from numerous accounts of premature burials that they could not rely on their observations of pulse or breathing to determine death at least as early as the eighteenth century.[74]

Jean Bruhier-d'Ablaincourt, a Paris physician, collected histories in 1742 of seventy-two people mistakenly certified as dead, and in 1842, de Fontenelle recorded forty-six cases in which people had been incorrectly declared dead or had actually been buried prematurely.[75,76] Carré wrote in 1845 that there had been forty-six cases of persons who had been declared dead and recovered while awaiting burial.[77]

M. Josat, a nineteenth-century French physician, compiled a list of the time "apparent death" lasted before patients recovered, based on his own practice:

| | |
|---|---|
| 2 to 8 hours | 30 cases |
| 8 to 15 hours | 58 cases |
| 15 to 20 hours | 47 cases |
| 20 to 36 hours | 20 cases |
| 36 to 42 hours | 7 cases |

These patients suffered, in decreasing frequency, from a lack of oxygen (asphyxia), hysteria, apoplexy, narcotic overdose, and concussion. Those with concussions recovered in the shortest time.[78]

At particular risk of a too-early declaration of death were women in labor. A law in parts of Europe, stemming from Roman times, required surgeons to perform a caesarean section on any woman who died in labor without delivering the child. Before the days of antisepsis and antibiotics these operations were inevitably fatal to women not already dead. Several records exist of surgeons performing the operation on women in labor who had not (yet) died. One eminent Parisian obstetrician, having made the mistake once, vowed never again to do this procedure.[79]

A disturbing paragraph in Charles Berg's *The Confessions of an Undertaker* suggests that even in the early twentieth century, not all the bodies undertakers received were, in fact, dead.

> Upon making the incision in the artery for injection, should there be an unusual flow of blood, it might indicate a possible resumption of the heart action, in which case the artery should be immediately ligated and a physician sent for. [Hopefully not the same one who pronounced the patient dead.] However, such cases are exceedingly rare.[80]

A well-reported case in Accrington, England was that of a Mrs. Holden, who on January 16, 1905, was declared dead and sent to the undertaker. While she was there, the undertaker noted a slight movement of the body and helped to revive her. She survived. [81]

Two cases of premature declaration of death were reprinted from United States newspapers in *The Burial Reformer*. The first, was about Louis Viel, a Des Moines, Iowa, man, whose heart was "pinched" by the pathologist while undergoing an autopsy at Mercy Hospital. "Instantly the organ began to throb at a natural rate." The incisions were closed and Mr. Viel survived to leave the hospital. (Could this have been an early, albeit inadvertent, case of open-chest cardiac resuscitation?) The second case was of a five-year-old Custer, South Dakota girl who had died of typhoid fever and had lain in her casket for viewing for 36 hours. A physician-relative attending her funeral believed that she still looked alive (there was no embalming). He began to treat the child and "half an hour later the stethoscope indicated a return of a strong heart action." The child survived. [82]

Similar events still occur. An Associated Press dispatch from Washington, D.C., appearing in the *Kansas City Star* (Nov 3, 1967, p. 1) and other papers, reported the case of a soldier pronounced dead after an explosion near Chu Lai, Vietnam, July 16, 1967, after a 45-minute resuscitation attempt. An Army embalmer detected signs of life several hours later, and the soldier was returned to a hospital. He was reported to have made a limited recovery three months later. [83]

Similarly, in 1979, Belgian physicians reported the case of a previously healthy 65-year-old man who collapsed on the street and was sent to the morgue after attempts at resuscitation failed. The morgue attendant noticed that his "dead" patient had begun breathing. An emergency medical team responded and eventually the man awoke. He died a few days later from overwhelming pneumonia. [84] Every experienced emergency medical clinician has seen instances in which spontaneous breathing and even heartbeats have returned after resuscitation efforts had apparently failed. Why this occurs is unknown, and virtually all of these patients quickly die (permanently) despite further supportive measures.

This apparently happened on February 1, 1992, when 75-year-old Emma Hellen Brady was pronounced dead in a St. Petersburg, Florida hospital after suffering a heart attack. Resuscitation measures appeared to have failed and she was put into a body bag. However, when her family arrived an hour later, they found her breathing. She was awake and able to speak with them, but remained in critical condition. [85]

On November 1, 1992, a similar event happened. Roberta Jones, a 68-year-old Seattle, Washington, woman suffering from colon cancer was pronounced dead by emergency medical technicians after her cold body (90°F) was found without a detectable heartbeat. She had no pulse and was not breathing. Her body was taken to the Columbia Funeral Home where an employee noticed that the "corpse" was breathing. She was immediately taken to Harborview Medical Center where she died less than two days later.[86]

And again, on June 15, 1993, forty-year-old New York City school teacher Nancy Vitale was pronounced dead, first by an ambulance crew and then by an investigator with the medical examiner's office. Only about two hours later, before the body was moved, did anyone notice life signs. The claim was that the woman was so cold that no pulse, blood pressure, heart beat, or breathing could be detected. (A caveat in emergency and wilderness medicine is that a patient is not dead until they are warm and dead.) The next day she was recovering at the Coney Island Hospital. [87]

## J.  ARE THERE REAL CASES OF PREMATURE BURIALS?

Yes. In fact, some of the first human bodies that were buried may actually have been accidental live burials. Basevi, in his book *The Burial of the Dead*, suggests that the earliest prehistoric cave "burials" may actually have been accidents resulting from hunters leaving ill or wounded compatriots in caves, with the entrances sealed against wild animals. They hoped that once the victims regained strength they would push away the obstructions and follow them. Occasionally, though, the people died in the caves.[88]

Edgar Allan Poe's stories of premature burial still haunt the minds of those who are familiar with his macabre tales. Many of his stories are passed on in folklore as truth. Some well-documented examples, however, demonstrate that the real stories are at least as macabre as fiction.

Puckle relates the curious case of a woman depicted on her tombstone in Rye, Sussex, England, sitting upright in her coffin.

> She was subject to attacks of syncope [fainting], and was supposed on one occasion to be dead. Wrapped in a shroud, her body was placed in a coffin in the old Flushing Inn which is still standing. Thus she lay till the morning of the day appointed for her burial. The oven was being heated for the baking of the funeral repast when she awoke, climbed out of her coffin and walked downstairs, where she was found by the horrified cook, standing before the kitchen fire, complaining that she 'felt the cold.' She lived for some years after this extraordinary experience. [89]

In the late sixteenth century, mourners carried the body of Matthew Wall to his grave in Braughing, England. Only when one of the pallbearers tripped and the bearers dropped the coffin did the "corpse" revive. He lived for several more years, until 1595, celebrating his "resurrection" every year.[90]

In the first decade of the seventeenth century, Marjorie Elphinstone

31

died and was buried in Ardtannies, Scotland. When grave robbers attempted to steal the jewelry from her body, they were surprised by a groan from Marjorie. They fled from the grave in fear and she walked home, outliving her husband by six years.

Margaret Halcrow Erskine, of Chirnside, Scotland, "died" in 1674 and was buried shallowly so the sexton could go back and steal her jewelry, a not uncommon occurrence at that time. While the sexton was trying to cut off her finger to remove a ring, she awoke. Not only did she go on to live a full life, but she also produced two relatively famous sons, Ralph and Ebenezer Erskine, founders of the original Secession Church of Berwickshire. No one knows what became of the sexton.

Premature burials continued into the eighteenth century, and at the beginning of the nineteenth century, a sensation-mongering press alleged that there were "many ugly secrets locked up underground." [91] Between 1700 and 1900, several hundred articles, books and essays described the fallibility of the diagnosis of death, including Poe's *Premature Burial*. [92] Among those was *The Burial Reformer*, which published such fearful writings as this poem by Percy Russell:

### PREMATURE BURIAL
To die is natural; but the living death
Of those who waken into consciousness,
Though for a moment only, ay, or less,
To find a coffin stifling their last breath,
Surpasses every horror underneath
The sun of Heaven, and should surely check
Haste in the living to remove the wreck
Of what was just before, the soul's fair sheath,
How many have been smothered in their shroud!
How many have sustained this awful woe!
Humanity would shudder could we know
How many cried to God in anguish loud,
Accusing those whose haste a wrong had wrought
Beyond the worst that ever devil thought. [93]

There may have been some basis for these claims. Collapse and apparent death were not uncommon during epidemics of plague, cholera, and smallpox. [94] William Tebb compiled, from contemporary medical sources, 219 instances of narrow escape from premature burial, 149 cases of actual premature burial, 10 cases in which bodies were accidentally dissected before death, and 2 cases in which embalming was started on the undead.

One tragic case was reported from Edisto Island, South Carolina. In the 1850s, a young girl visiting the island died of diphtheria. Fearing a spread of the deadly disease, the family quickly interred the body in a local family's mausoleum. When one of that family's sons died during the Civil War, the tomb was reopened and a tiny skeleton was found on the floor just behind the door. [95]

Dr. Brouardel, director of the Paris morgue, published the following missive on October 1, 1867: "I exhumed at eight p.m. Philomèle Jonetre, aged twenty-four, buried at five p.m. in a grave six feet deep. Several persons heard her tap distinctly against the lid of the coffin. These blows appeared to me to have left visible marks, but I did not hear them myself...Ammonia and other restoratives were applied...She was not dead, but like a candle, the flames of which had been extinguished, though the wick continues to glow. No definite sounds of the heart, but the eyelids moved in my presence." She was finally pronounced really dead the next day. [96]

In 1877, the prestigious *British Medical Journal* published an account of the following case of premature burial:

> A correspondent at Naples states that the Appeals Court has had before it a case not likely to inspire confidence in the minds of those who look forward with horror to the possibility of being buried alive. It appeared from the evidence that some time ago, a woman was interred with all the usual formalities, it being believed that she was dead, while she was only in a trance. Some days afterwards, when the grave in which she had been placed was opened for the reception of another body, it was found that the clothes which covered the unfortunate woman were torn to pieces, and that she had even broken her limbs in attempting to extricate herself from the living tomb. The Court, after hearing the case, sentenced the doctor who had signed the certificate of decease, and the Major who had authorized the interment each to three month's imprisonment for involuntary manslaughter. [97]

A case was also published the same year (1877) in *Lancet*:

> An inhabitant of Mount Jory, Paramatta, was believed to be dead. His supposed remains were about to be committed, when a mourning relative startled the bystanders by exclaiming, "I must see my father once more; something tells me he is not dead!" The coffin was thereupon opened and found to contain a living inmate, who justified the presentiment of his son by slowly recovering. [98]

In 1896, T.M. Montgomery, who supervised the disinterment and moving of the remains at the Fort Randall Cemetery, reported that "nearly 2 percent of those exhumed were no doubt victims of suspended animation." He based this on evidence of victims such as the soldier, supposedly dead from a lightning strike, who had attempted to push his coffin lid open.[99] About the same time, Dr. Alexander Wilder wrote of a 35-year-old man who "died" of scarlet fever. When the body was disinterred two months later, "The coffin was found to have the glass front shattered, the bottom kicked out and the sides sprung. The body lay face downwards, the arms were bent and in the clenched fists were handfuls of hair."[100]

The most recent case only came very close to being prematurely buried. In 1993, a 24-year-old South African man, Sipho William Mdletshe, spent two days in a metal box in a mortuary after being declared dead following a traffic accident. During that time, he says he drifted in and out of consciousness. When he finally realized what had happened, he screamed for help and mortuary workers released him. Unfortunately, his fiance then rejected him, considering him a zombie.[101]

## K. WHAT PRECAUTIONS HAVE BEEN TAKEN TO PREVENT PREMATURE BURIAL?

Public apprehension about premature burials increased after the publication of lurid newspaper reports, Edgar Allan Poe's macabre short stories, and a book on the subject by poetess Friederike Kempner in which European royalty (including Kaiser Wilhelm I) showed a strong interest.

As a result, "waiting mortuaries" were established so that decay could occur before burial. At the beginning of the twentieth century, Munich, Germany, had ten such waiting mortuaries, including one reserved for Jewish bodies. William Tebb, an early twentieth-century writer on premature burials described these temporary sepulchres:

> In an immense room, closed by large glass doors, through which the interior can be seen from the outside, are ranged in three rows twenty sarcophagi, fixed in a sloping position. The slabs upon which they rest are supplied with a zinc trench, filled with an antiseptic fluid...From the moment of its arrival at the mortuary the coffin is uncovered, and placed on one of the slabs. The body is raised, and reclines upon a cushion, and the whole is covered by a profusion of flowers, usually allowing only the head of the corpse to be seen...Many families have their dead photographed like this...There is a room for the rich and another for the poor, adjoining each other. Nothing distinguishes them, except perhaps the quality of the flowers.[102]

Each corpse was fitted with a ring on one finger connected to a bell, so that any movement would ring the bell and alert the ever-present caretaker. In fact, the caretakers were not upset to hear a bell ring; it was a common occurrence, but rarely did it signify a live body. Rather, the distention of the corpse due to the build-up of putrefactive gases was the most common cause of bell ringing. As Tebb described:

> At the head of each coffin a rod is fixed, from which falls a cord having a metal ring at its extremity. This cord communicates with a system of bells, and the least pressure on the rope sets it in motion...This frequently happens; the warning bell is so sensitive that the least shade of the corpse sets it in motion. But the guardian is not at all flustered; various causes may agitate the bell, and the waking of a corpse is a very rare occurrence. Nevertheless, the caretaker goes to ascertain the cause of the alarm, and, having assured himself that the corpse preserves all the signs of death, he readjusts the cord, and returns to continue his sleep. [103]

Few corpses revived in these waiting mortuaries and they were soon abandoned. One five-year-old child who did awaken there, was found by attendants "playing with the white roses which had been placed on its shroud." When a mortuary aide brought the child home, however, the child's mother, in mourning, collapsed and died "of fright." [104]

Some people's wills specified the tests they wanted used to make sure they were actually dead. These included making surgical incisions into or applying boiling liquids to various parts of their bodies, touching their bodies with red hot irons, or decapitating them. One lady in Kent, England, for example, specified "that my body shall be stabbed to the heart to make sure that life is extinct." [105] In 1813, the French physician Foderé recommended opening the deceased's left chest to feel whether the heart was still beating. Even if it was beating, the patient was sure to die from infection, if not a collapsed lung. [106]

Francis Douce, an antique dealer, offered Sir Anthony Carlisle, the best-known English surgeon at the time, £200 in 1834 "either to sever my head or extract my heart from my body, so as to prevent any possibility of the return of vitality." [107] Less elaborate preparations included being buried with a gun, poison or a knife with which to kill oneself in case a person awoke to find that he or she had been prematurely buried. [108]

An 1861 publication announced that because of her fear of being buried alive, "the late Lady Burton, widow of Sir Richard Burton [noted explorer], provided that her heart was to be pierced with a needle and her body be submitted to a postmortem examination, and, afterward, embalmed (not stuffed) by competent experts." [109]

The screams of a young Belgian girl who came out of a trance-like state as the earth fell on her coffin so upset Count Karnicé-Karnicki, Chamberlain to the Czar and Doctor of the Law Faculty of the University of Louvain, that he invented a coffin which allowed a person accidentally buried alive to summon help through a system of flags and bells. [110] Patented in 1897, his hermetically sealed coffin had a tube, about 3.5 inches in diameter extending to a box on the surface. The tube was attached to a spring-loaded ball sitting on the corpse's chest. Any movement of the chest would release the spring, opening the box lid and admitting light and air into the coffin. To signal for help, a flag would spring up, a bell would ring for a half-hour and a lamp would burn after sunset. It is not clear if any of these were actually built. Similar "life-signalling" coffins following the Count's lead were patented in the United States. None of these inventions caught on, even though one of the inventors was named appropriately, Albert *Fearnaught*.[111] (See illustration, p. 37.)

Into the twentieth century people were still leaving instructions meant to prevent premature burials. *The Burial Reformer* noted that Miss Louisa Franes Stains, of Lynsore, St. Edmund's Road, Ipswich, who died on January 3, 1906, "left instructions in her will that she was to be cremated, but if this were not possible the main artery of her throat was to be severed before burial." In the same issue, they reported that Mrs. Harriet Proter Telford, of Clarence Square, Brighton, "directed that her coffin and shell should not be closed for seven days after her death, and that two gentlewomen should be employed to guard her body after death, and see to the arrangements in connection with her funeral." They were each paid £6.[112]

The fear of being buried alive should have vanished with the introduction of arterial embalming in the 1880s and 1890s. Embalming a corpse includes removing the blood and injecting lethal chemicals. Once the chemicals are injected into bodies, people are dead, whether or not they had been originally. Addressing the 1910 National Funeral Directors Association convention in Portland, Oregon, the city attorney joked, "there is consolation in the thought that when a man's undertaker is finished with him he can be reasonably sure he is not in a trance."[113] Yet at the onset of the twentieth century, Hallam repeated a limerick of unkown origin current at that time:

> There was a young man at Nunhead
> Who awoke in his coffin of lead;
> "It is cosy enough"
> He remarked, in a huff,
> "But I wasn't aware I was dead."[114]

A fear of premature burial may have been one reason for the early acceptance of embalming in the United States.[115] According to one embalming manual, the chemical reaction between the embalming fluid and the tissues of the cadaver are said to simulate life signs, such as gasps and muscular contractions. "The practitioner is reassured," it says, "that these will go away as the injection proceeds."[116]

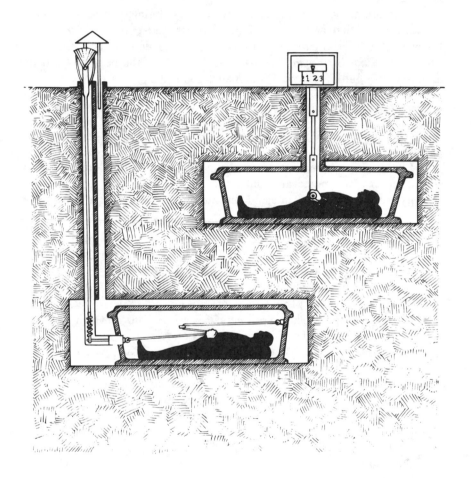

Two devices designed to summon help for premature burials.

An early example of death by embalming occurred in 1837, when Cardinal Somaglia was taken ill, passed out and was thought to be dead. Immediately, preparations were made to embalm this very important church official before the body could putrefy. When the surgeon-embalmer cut into the chest to instill embalming materials, however, he could see the cardinal's heart still beating. Worse, at that point the cardinal awoke from his stupor and wisely pushed the knife away from his chest. Unfortunately, the chest incision killed him. [117]

Cremation, the common alternative to embalming, leaves no doubt in anyone's mind that at the end of the process, the person is *really* dead. Likewise, the Parsee custom of using vultures to devour their dead (see Chapter 9, *What is stripping the flesh?*) only works if the person is actually deceased. The birds *really know* when a person is dead.

## L. WHO WAS BURIED ALIVE INTENTIONALLY?

Not only have premature burials occurred accidentally, but live burial has been used as a method of execution and for religious purposes.

Live burial was once used as a method of execution. Roman vestal virgins, and some medieval monks and nuns who broke their vows of chastity, were intentionally interred alive. Plutarch described the process for vestal virgins:

> ...a narrow room is constructed, to which a descent is made by stairs; here they prepare a bed, and light a lamp, and leave a small quantity of victuals, such as bread, water, a pail of milk, and some oil; so that body which had been consecrated and devoted to the most sacred service of religion might not be said to perish by such a death as famine. The culprit herself is put in a litter, which they cover over, and tie her down with cords on it, so that nothing she utters may be heard. They then take her to the Forum...When they come to the place of execution, the officers loose the cords, and then the high priest, lifting his hands to heaven, pronounces certain prayers to himself before the act; then he brings out the prisoner, being still covered, and placing her upon the steps that lead down to the cell, turns away his face...the stairs are drawn up after she has gone down, and a quantity of earth is heaped up over the entrance to the cell...This is the punishment of those who break their vow of virginity. [118]

Medieval monks and nuns who broke their vows of chastity were often walled into small niches, just barely large enough for their bodies. They also were given a pittance of food and water, and the grim benediction *Vade in Pacem* (Depart in peace).[119]

Some people were ceremonially buried alive to serve the dead in the next life. This happened throughout the world, especially in strictly hierarchical societies. In Africa, for example, two live slaves, a man and a woman, were buried with each dead Wadoe headman. The man was given a bill-hook to use to cut wood for fuel in the next life, the woman cradled the dead chief's head in her lap. [120] In 1849, an observer at the funeral of King Thien Tri of Cochin, China, reported that along with rich and plentiful grave goods, all of his childless wives were entombed with his body so they could prepare his daily meals and provide for him. [121]The living were not only sacrificed to dead men. In Ecuador, near Quito, researchers found at least one grave where eight women were buried alive with a dead woman. In the non-hierarchical societies of the Amazon basin, favorite children were often buried alive with their parent. [122]

Haitian "zombies" were reportedly intentional live burials produced by tetrodotoxin, a fish poison that produces a death-like state in which there is no apparent response to stimulation. Those knowledgeable in voodoo supposedly administered this essentially tasteless drug to the victim's food. The victim then succumbed, had a funeral, and was buried. If just the right dose was given, the victim could later be removed from the grave and restored to a functional (and terror-producing) state. [123]Shakespeare, if not actually aware of such a potion, thought it possible when in *Romeo and Juliet,* Juliet receives a potion to put her into a sleep so that "No warmth or breath shall testify thou liv'st." [124]

The parish register of Malpas, Cheshire, England noted in 1625 that one man, though not quite completely buried alive, came as close as possible to burying himself:

> Richard Dawson being sick of the plague and perceiving he must die at that time, arose out of his bed and made his grave, and caused his nephew John Dawson to cast some straw into the grave which was not far from the house, and went and laid down in the said grave, and caused clothes to be laid upon and so departed out of this world; this he did because he was a strong man and heavier than his said nephew and another wench were able to bury. [125]

## M. WHAT CAN HAPPEN TO MY BODY WHEN I DIE?

Most commonly, a dead body is either buried (often with prior embalming in the United States and Canada), cremated or exposed to the elements. Bodies are occasionally mummified or cryogenically fixed and, rarely, they are cannibalized. Body parts are often removed for transplantation or study. The differences in what happens to corpses are usually dictated by religious or social custom, and sometimes vary by age, sex, social rank, behavior in life, the circumstances of death, and current societal stability.

Primarily, it is custom that dictates how survivors will dispose of a corpse. For example, at the end of the nineteenth century, twelve concurrent methods of body disposal were used by different tribal groups in the relatively small area of New South Wales. They included six different earth burials, exposure to the air, surface burial, tree burial, smoking, eating, and burning.[126] Different methods of disposing of the dead, especially among the same ethnic group, may signify social differences, an amalgamation of various cultural practices into a single group, or moral taboos. The Angoni in central Africa, for example, cremated the bodies of their chiefs but buried commoners in caves. The difference stemmed from the fact that their hereditary line of chiefs originated from another tribe which customarily cremated its dead. They continued this ritual even after becoming part of a culture that normally used burial. [127] In another example of differences in corpse disposition based on social status, the Minnetaree Indians once buried bad and quarrelsome men but laid the bodies of good men on scaffolds. Similarly, they normally used tree burials for young men, women and children, but earth burial for the very old and men who had violated marital taboos.[128]

Modern corpse disposal usually follows one of several courses that Evelyn Waugh succinctly described in *The Loved One:*

> Now, Mr. Barlow, what had you in mind? Embalmment of course, and after that incineration or not, according to taste. Our crematory is based on scientific principles, the heat is so intense that all inessentials are volatilized. Some people did not like the thought that ashes of the casket and clothing were mixed with the Loved One's. Normal disposal is by inhumement, entombment, inurnment or immurement, but many people just lately prefer insarcophagusment. That is *very* individual. The casket is placed inside a sealed sarcophagus, marble or bronze, and rests permanently above ground in a niche in the mausoleum, with or without a personal stained-glass window above. That, of course, is for those with whom price is not a primary consideration. [129]

In the United States, nearly 65% of funerals include open caskets, 16% have closed caskets, 14% are cremated and 5% have other dispositions. [130]

Burial is a world-wide phenomenon. Humans are the only animal known to bury their dead in a systematic way. The practice may have existed since 50,000 B.C. and presumably originated not from health concerns, but rather from an inability to accept death as the end of existence. In some primitive societies, bodies were buried with arms and legs tightly bound before *rigor mortis* set in so the dead would be inhibited from harming the living. Many funeral practices were also designed to allow the dead to move on to the domain of the dead, rather than remaining among the living. Most religions that anticipate an afterlife prefer burial so that the physical body can be joined with the spirit.

Tree burials vary in type, but often include putting an entire coffin or sack containing the corpse into the branches of a tree.[131] An unusual custom among the Warramunga tribe of Australia is for survivors not to enclose the tree-buried body, so that the mother of the deceased and other female relatives can rub the putrid juices dripping from the corpse on themselves as a sign of sorrow.[132]

Cremation is also a world-wide custom, being the primary form of corpse disposition for several religions. It is an ancient practice that has waxed and waned in popularity over the millennia. Its use in Western countries has been on the increase since the mid-twentieth century.

## N. WHAT WILL HAPPEN TO MY BODY WHEN I DIE?

Any corpse that is neither destroyed nor frozen undergoes putrefaction and autolysis. As a modern scientist said of postmortem putrefaction:

> The decomposition process is generally subdivided into five stages: fresh, bloat, active decay, post or advanced decay, and dry or skeletal remains. The overall process can be viewed as a two-act play with an intermission between acts. The first act includes the first three stages of decomposition and is an accelerated performance in which maggots take top billing. The intermission is marked by a rapid decrease in corpse biomass resulting from loss of seepage fluids and dispersal of postfeeding maggots. The second act is comprised of the last two stages of decomposition and is prolonged in duration.[133]

The ancients thought that a corpse's natural putrefaction was caused by the stone coffin "eating" the corpse. To this day, massive bronze and copper caskets are called sarcophagi from the Greek, *sarco* (flesh) and *phagus* (eater).[134] Yet the putrefactive process actually follows a path laid down by anatomic and physiologic changes in the corpse.

Once the heart stops beating, the blood begins to settle in the parts of the body that are the closest to the ground, usually the buttocks and back when a corpse is supine. The skin, normally pink-colored by the oxygen-laden blood in the capillaries, becomes pale as the blood drains out into the larger veins. Within minutes to hours after death, the skin is discolored by *livor mortis*, or what embalmers call "postmortem stain," the purple-red discoloration from blood accumulating in the lowermost (dependent) blood vessels. *Livor mortis* is usually most pronounced eight to twelve hours after death.[135] The skin, no longer under muscular control, succumbs to gravity, forming new shapes and accentuating prominent bones still further. The body cools.

41

At the moment of death, the muscles relax completely—called primary flaccidity. The muscles then stiffen, perhaps due to coagulation of muscle proteins or a shift in the muscle's energy containers (ATP-ADP), into a condition known as *rigor mortis*. All of the body's muscles are affected. *Rigor* begins, within two to six hours of death, beginning with the eyelids, neck and jaw.[136] Over the next four to six hours it spreads to the other muscles, including those in the internal organs, such as the heart.[137] The onset of *rigor mortis* is quicker in a cold environment and if the person had performed hard physical work just before death.[138] Its onset also varies with the age, sex, physical condition and muscular build of the individual.[139] After being in this rigid condition for 24 to 84 hours, the muscles relax and secondary laxity (flaccidity) develops, usually in the same order as it began.[140] The length of time *rigor mortis* lasts depends on multiple factors, particularly the ambient temperature. During this period, the body gradually cools, in a process called *algor mortis*.[141]

In the absence of embalming or relatively rapid cremation, the body then putrefies.

The first sign of putrefaction is a greenish skin discoloration appearing on the right lower abdomen about the second or third day after death. This coloration then spreads over the abdomen, chest and upper thighs and is usually accompanied by a putrid odor. Both color and smell are produced by sulphur-containing intestinal gas and a breakdown product of red blood cells. The ancient Greeks and the Etruscans paid homage to this well-recognized stage of decomposition by each coloring a prominent god aquamarine, considered the color of rotting flesh.[142]

Bacteria normally residing in the body, especially the colon, play an important part in digestion of food during life. They also contribute mightily to decomposition after death—the process of putrefaction. The smell, rather than the sight, is the most distinctive thing about a putrefying body.

Under normal conditions, the intestinal bacteria in a corpse produce large amounts of foul-smelling gas that flows into the blood vessels and tissues. It is this gas that bloats the body, turns the skin from green to purple to black, makes the tongue and eyes protrude, and often pushes the intestines out through the vagina and rectum. The gas also causes large amounts of foul-smelling blood-stained fluid to exude from the nose, mouth and other body orifices. Two of the chemicals produced during putrefaction are aptly named putrescine (1,4-diaminobutane) and cadaverine (1,5-pentanediamine). If a person dies from an overwhelming bacterial infection, marked changes from putrefaction can occur within as little as 9 to 12 hours after death.[143]

By seven days after death, most of the body is discolored and giant blood-tinged putrid blisters begin to appear. The skin loosens and any pressure causes the top layer to come off in large sheets (skin slip). As the internal organs and the fatty tissues decay, they produce large quantities of foul-smelling gas. By the second week after death, the abdomen, scrotum, breasts and tongue swell; the eyes bulge out. A bloody fluid seeps out the mouth and nose. After three to four weeks, the hair, nails and teeth loosen and the grossly swollen internal organs begin to rupture and eventually liquefy. The internal organs decompose at different rates, with the resistant uterus and prostate often intact after twelve months, giving pathologists one way to determine an unidentified corpse's sex.

Richard Selzer poetically described the process in *Mortal Lessons:*

> There is to be a feast. The rich table has been set. The board groans. The guests have already arrived, numberless bacteria that had, in life, dwelt in saprophytic harmony with their host. Their turn now! Charged, they press against the membrane barriers, break through the new softness, sweep across plains of tissue, devouring, belching gas—a gas that puffs eyelids, cheeks, abdomen into bladders of murderous vapor. The slimmest man takes on the bloat of corpulence. Your swollen belly bursts with a ripping sound, followed by a long mean hiss.
>
> And they are large! Blisters appear upon the skin, enlarge, coalesce, blast, leaving brownish puddles in the declivities. You are becoming gravy...Gray sprays of fungus sprout in the resulting marinade, and there lacks only a mushroom growing from the nose.[144]

Aside from the action of microbes, the breakdown of cells (autolysis) helps destroy the body unless the corpse is kept at or below 32°F. Cells die (necrosis) through the progressive destruction of their various parts. First, the cellular fluid (cytoplasm) and the energy-releasing mechanism (mitochondria) swell. Various products, including calcium, begin to coalesce in the mitochondria as other mechanisms within the cell dissolve. Next, loss of energy causes the cell to lose its connections with neighboring cells (tissue destruction), and further lose control over the fluid within its outer barrier, similar to an over-filled water balloon. The cell controller (nucleus) fails and the packs of destructive acids (enzymes) within the cell break loose. These enzymes complete the work of destroying the cell.

A modern sociologist summed up decomposition beautifully, saying, "The physicality of a human corpse is undeniable. It is a carcass, with a predisposition to decay, to become noisome, obnoxious to the senses, and harrowing to the emotions. Disposal of such perishable remains is imperative."[145]

## O. HOW DOES MY NAME GET IN THE NEWSPAPER?

The ancient Greeks, who recognized the difference between humans and their mortal remains, preserved a person's memory through speeches and symbolic acts after the body was dispatched in flames.[146] Modern man relies on the written word—the death notice and obituary, to begin this process.

Funeral homes place a death notice, actually a form of advertising, when they handle a death. While some papers run death notices for free, most charge for the advertising service of mentioning the funeral home.[147] "A death notice, more often than not unaccompanied by an obituary, is the brief, stark, final punctuation of a person's life."[148]

Some newspapers, probably to avoid practical jokers, refuse to take death notices from anyone other than funeral directors. "One of the things that worries us most is fake death notices," said one newspaperman. "Fake notices seem to occur most often in the spring when there's a full moon, when high school graduation is just around the corner, and quite often seem to involve principals of high schools and other favorite characters." Some newspapers have code numbers that funeral directors use when calling in death notices.[149] If a body is donated to a medical school, however, it is up to the family to arrange the death notice. The medical school's mortician can assist in doing this.

Common mistakes funeral directors make in placing death notices include submitting inaccurate information, missing newspaper deadlines, failing to inform relatives that a notice has been placed, misspelling names, and omitting or giving incorrect information regarding visitations, flowers, or donations.

Unlike a death notice, an obituary is a news item written by the newspaper staff about a notable person, informing the community that he or she has died. It reaches a wider circle than can be personally contacted. The obituary, also called a necrologue or necrology, may, if one is lucky, be written by a necrologist or necrographer—a professional obituary writer. In 1856, W.H. Smyth noted that "The truth of history has been greatly corrupted by necrological laudatory essays."[150] Yet Roger Bacon wrote that he considered what was written about him more important than any funerary rites, saying "I bequeath my soul to God....My body to be buried obscurely. For my name and memory, I leave it to men's charitable speeches, and to foreign nations, and the next age."[151]

Newspapers generally print obituaries for people who lived or were known within their circulation area. They also run the obituaries of nationally known or influential people. They try not to err, since it can be very embarrassing. Just such an error occurred when the South African *Daily Dispatch* ran the 1993 obituary of Ray Mali, a former cabinet minister in Ciskei. "It's a rare thing to read about your death in the paper," said Mali, "I am alive." A person named Ray Mali had actually died in a car crash. The paper mistakenly assumed it was the famous man.[152] The same error occurred in the case of 40-year-old actress Margaret Klenck, who once played a character named Edwina Lewis on *One Life to Live*. When a 42-year-old actress whose real name was Edwina Lewis died, both *The New York Times* and *Variety* carried Klenck's obituary. Said she about the two publications pronouncing her dead, "It means I'm dead on both coasts."[153] Even more embarrassing for the media were the November 1993 news bulletins that Britain's Queen Mother was dead which were carried on many leading Australian television stations. She was not dead, and rival stations gleefully broadcast footage of her alive and well while noting the other stations' errors.[154]

Unless a person is a major celebrity or the manner of death itself is noteworthy, obituaries rarely describe much about the circumstances of death. This is true whether the obituary is one paragraph or several pages long. Very famous people, however, such as presidents, popes, popular politicians, and media or sports figures often have their deaths reported in detail. In the past, such phrases as "died after a long illness" connoted cancer and "sudden death" meant heart attack. Today, the combination of a young age and the words "lingering" or "protracted illness" usually means AIDS. In a few cases, prominent individuals have allowed their deaths to be used as rallying cries to make people aware of their disease, such as AIDS, ALS (still known as Lou Gehrig's Disease), and different types of cancer.

Suicide can be a touchy subject in obituaries, since it is still a societal, if not a legal, taboo. Unless the circumstances are unmistakably clear, the word suicide is avoided. Instead, either nothing is said about the mechanism of death, or it may simply be labelled "an accident."

At one time obituaries simply eulogized the deceased. Today's obituaries may include both the positive and negative aspects of one's life, especially if the deceased had gained any prominence. They are written as mini-biographies and long obituaries are often written well in advance of a person's death. People do not, however, have a chance to read these advance obituaries. They are normally under very tight security.

The obituary publicly marks the end of a life. Yet the person can still contribute to society through organ and tissue donation, the topic of the next chapter.

## P. REFERENCES

1. Fijian Legend. As related in: Bendann E: *Death Customs: An Analytical Study of Burial Rites.* New York: Alfred A Knopf, 1930, pp 25-26.
2. Matthews W: Navaho Legends. *Memoirs of the American Folk-Lore Society.* 1897;5:77-78.
3. Ginzberg L: *The Legends of the Jews,* vol 1. Philadelphia, PA: Jewish Publication Society of America, 1937, p 50.

4. Ibid., p 40.
5. Ibid., p 123.
6. Morrison RS: Death: Process or event? *Science.* 1971;172:694-98.
7. Horan DJ, Mall D: *Death, Dying and Euthanasia.* Fredrick, MD: Univ Publications of America, 1980, p 27.
8. Selzer R: *Mortal Lessons: Notes on the Art of Surgery.* New York: Simon & Schuster, 1987, pp 136-37.
9. Gervais KG: *Redefining Death.* New Haven, CT: Yale Univ Press, 1986, p 5.
10. 22nd World Medical Assembly. Sydney, Australia: 1968.
11. Sass HM: Ethical arguments for accepting death by brain criteria. In: Land W, ed: *Ethics, Justice, and Commerce in Organ Replacement Therapy.* Heidelberg: Springer, 1991, pp 249-58.
12. Kass LR: Thinking about the body. *Hastings Center Report.* 1985;15:20-30.
13. *Babalonian Talmud,* tractate *Chullin* 21A: Mishna *Oholoth* 1:6.
14. Cooper DKC, DeVilliers JC, Smith LS, et al: Medical, legal and administrative aspects of cadaveric organ donation in the RSA. *S Afr Med J.* 1982;62:933-38.
15. Sass, Ethical Arguments, p 249-58.
16. Sass HM: Criteria for death: Self-determination and public policy. *J Medicine and Philosophy.* 1992;17:445-54.
17. Sass, Ethical Arguments, p 249-58.
18. Eckert WG: Timing of death and injuries. *Medico-Legal Insights.* From: *Inform Letter.* Fall 1991.
19. Beecher KH: A definition of irreversible coma: Report of the Harvard Medical School to examine the definition of death by brain criteria. *JAMA.* 1968;205:337-40.
20. Stiller CR: Ethics of transplantation. *Transplantation Proc.* 1985;17 (suppl):131-38.
21. Lutrin CL: Radionuclide evaluation of death by brain criteria. *West J Med.* 1992;157(1):61-62.
22. Van Till-d'Aulnis de Bournouill A: How dead can you be? *Medicine, Science, and the Law.* 1975;15(2):133-46.
23. Holzgreve W, Beller FK: Anencephalic infants as organ donors. *Clin Obstet Gynecol.* 1992;35:821-36.
24. Ramsey P: *Ethics at The Edges of Life: Medical and Legal Intersections.* New Haven, CT: Yale Univ Press, 1980, p 213.
25. Angell M: Prisoners of technology: The case of Nancy Cruzan. *New Engl J Med.* 1990;322:1226-28.
26. Ludwig J: *Current Methods of Autopsy Practice.* Philadelphia, PA: W B Saunders, 1972, p 271.
27. *Dictionnaire des sciences médicales en soixante tomes.* Paris: 1818. Cited in Ariès P: *The Hour of Our Death.* New York: Oxford Univ Press, 1981, p 401.
28. Brahams D: Legal status of dead 'patients'. *Lancet.* 1992;339:173+.
29. Annas GJ: *The Rights of Patients.* 2nd ed. Carbondale, IL: Southern Illinois Univ Press, 1989, p 228.
30. Ludwig, *Current Methods of Autopsy Practice,* p 265.
31. *International Form of Medical Certificate of Cause of Death.* Designed by the Sixth Decennial International Revision Conference. Paris, France: 1948.
32. Grollman EA, ed: *Concerning Death: A Practical Guide for the Living.* Boston: Beacon Press, 1974, p 182.
33. Duffey J: *A History of Public Health in New York City, 1866-1966.* vol 2. New York: Russell Sage Foundation, 1974, pp 1-3.
34.
    Rich disease, poor disease. *World Press Review.* May 1993, p 45. (Abstracted from DeBac M: *Corriere della Sera.* Milan, Italy.)
35. American Medical Association (AMA) Council on Ethical and Judicial Affairs: *Confidentiality of HIV Status on Autopsy Reports.* Presented to the AMA House of Delegates. Chicago, IL: June 1992.
36. Kircher T, Nelson J, Burdo H: The autopsy as a measure of accuracy of the death certificate. *New Engl J Med.* 1985;313:1263-69.
37. Kircher T, Anderson RE: Cause of death: proper completion of the death certificate.

*JAMA.* 1987;258:349-52.
38. Wallace RB, Woolson RF: *The Epidemiologic Study of the Elderly.* New York: Oxford Univ Press, 1992, p 263-64.
39. Hunt LW, Silverstein MD, Reed CE, O'Connell EJ, O'Fallon WM, Yunginger JW: Accuracy of the death certificate in a population-based study of asthmatic patients. *JAMA.* 1993;269(15):1947-52.
40. Hanzlick R, Parrish RG: The failure of death certificates to record the performance of autopsies. *JAMA.* 1993;269(1):27.
41. Wallace, Woolson, *Epidemiologic Study of the Elderly,* p 263-64.
42. Hanzlick R: Improving accuracy of death certificates (Letter). *JAMA.* 1993;269(22):2850.
43. Sox ED, Holota M: Underlying causes of death, cardiovascular disease: San Francisco experience in the Pan American Health Organization International Mortality Study. 1966. Reported in: Ludwig, *Current Methods of Autopsy Practice,* p 270.
44. National Center for Health Statistics: Data line. *Public Health Rep.* 1990;105:209-10.
45. King MD: AIDS on the death certificate: the final stigma. *Br Med J.* 1989;298:734-36.
46. Maxwell JD: Accuracy of death certification for alcoholic liver disease. *Br J Addict.* 1986;81:168-69.
47. AMA Council on Ethical and Judicial Affairs, *Confidentiality of HIV Status on Autopsy Reports,* June 1992.
48. Proposed rule would remove cause of death from death certificates. *Forum.* 1992;58(6):11.
49. Gordon R: *Great Medical Disasters.* New York: Dorset Press, 1983, pp 156-57.
50. Polson CJ, Brittain RP, Marshall TK: *The Disposal of the Dead.* 2nd ed. Springfield, IL: Charles C Thomas, 1962, p 68.
51. Herodotus: *History.* Book 5, section 8.
52. Pallis CA: Death. In: *The New Encyclopaedia Britannica.* vol 16 (Macropaedia). Chicago: Encyclopaedia Britannica, 1987, p 1032.
53. Turner AW: *Houses for the Dead.* New York: David McKay, 1976, p vii.
54. Curl JS: *The Victorian Celebration of Death.* Detroit: Partridge Press, 1972, p 31.
55. Shakespeare W: *King Henry IV, Part II.* Act 4, scene 5, lines 31-34.
56. Shakespeare W: *King Lear.* Act 5, scene 3, lines 262-64.
57. Gittings C: *Death, Burial and the Individual in Early Modern England.* London: Croom & Helm, 1984, p 30.
58. Ibid., p 205.
59. Ibid.
60. Harken DE: Pacemakers, past-makers, and the paced: An informal history from A to Z. *Biomedical Instrumentation & Technology.* July/Aug 1991, pp 299-302.
61. Senior JE: Electricity—pure physick of the skies: Part 2. *Biomedical Technology Today.* July/Aug 1991, pp 130-36.
62. Coffin MM: *Death In Early America: The History and Folklore of Customs and Superstitions of Early Medicine, Funerals, Burials, and Mourning.* Nashville: Thomas Nelson, 1976, p 106.
63. Snart J: *Thesaurus of Horror.* London: 1817.
64. Shneidman ES, ed: *Death: Current Perspectives.* Palo Alto, CA: Mayfield Pub, 1976, p 227.
65. Kastenbaum R: Psychological Death. In: Pearson L, ed: *Death and Dying.* Cleveland, OH: Case Western Reserve Univ Press, 1969, pp 3-8.
66. Puckle, BS: *Funeral Customs—Their Origin and Development.* London: T Werner Laurie, 1926, p 22.
67. Ludwig, *Current Methods of Autopsy Practice,* p 12.
68. Greene CL: *Medical Diagnosis for the Student and Practitioner.* 1926. As quoted in: Arnold JD, Zimmerman TF, Martin DC: Public attitudes and the diagnosis of death. *JAMA.* 1968;206:1949-54.
69. Arnold JD, Zimmerman TF, Martin DC: Public attitudes and the diagnosis of death. *JAMA.* 1968;206:1949-54.
70. *Lancet.* 1884;2:329.
71. Pallis, Death, p 1032.
72. Guttmacher AF: Bootlegging bodies—A history of body-snatching. *Bull Soc Med Hist*

*Chicago.* 1935;4(4):353-402.
73. Hartmann F: *Buried Alive: An Examination Into the Occult Causes of Apparent Death, Trance, and Catalepsy.* Boston: 1895, p 80.
74. Mant AK: The Medical Definition of Death. In: Toynbee, et al: *Man's Concern with Death.* London: Hodder & Stroughton, 1968, p 277.
75. Bruhier-d'Ablaincourt JJ: Dissertation sur l'incertitude des signes de la mort et de l'abus des enterrements et des embauments précipités. Paris: 1742. Quoted in: Shneidman, *Death: Current Perspectives,* p 221.
76. de Fontenelle J: Recherchés médico-légales sur l'incertitude des signes de la mort, etc. Paris: 1834. Quoted in: Shneidman, *Death: Current Perspectives,* p 221.
77. Carré: De la mort apparente, Paris: 1845. Quoted in: Shneidman, *Death: Current Perspectives,* p 221.
78. Josat M. Cited in: Tebb W, Vollum EP, Hadwen WR: *Premature Burial and How It May Be Prevented, With Special Reference to Trance, Catalepsy, and Other Forms of Suspended Animation.* 2nd ed. London: Swan Sonnenshein, 1905, p 249.
79. Peu P: *Prx Obstetr. 11 c 11.2.* Quoted in: Shneidman, *Death: Current Perspectives,* p 222.
80. Berg CW: *The Confessions of an Undertaker.* Wichita, KS: McCormick-Armstrong Press, 1920, p 51.
81. Curl, *The Victorian Celebration of Death,* p 178.
82. Hallam A, ed: *The Burial Reformer.* January 1906, p 32.
83. Arnold, Zimmerman, Martin *JAMA,* 1968.
84. Mullie A, Miranda D: A premature referral to the mortuary—cerebral recovery with barbiturate therapy. *Acta Anaesth Belg.* 1979;30:145-48.
85. Beveridge S: Family finds former Valley woman declared dead to be alive. *Observer Reporter.* Washington, PA: February 1, 1992.
86. Woman revives after being declared dead. *Prodigy News Service,* November 2, 1992; and, Woman declared dead Sunday dies. *Prodigy News Service.* November 3, 1992.
87. Quick recovery. *USA Today.* June 17, 1993, p 3A.
88. Basevi WHF: *The Burial of the Dead.* London: George Rutledge & Sons, 1920, pp 16-18.
89. Puckle, *Funeral Customs,* p 24.
90. Gittings, *Death, Burial and the Individual,* p 108.
91. Pallis, Death, p 1032.
92. Arnold, Zimmerman, Martin, *JAMA,* 1968.
93. Russell P: "Premature Burial." In: Hallam, *Burial Reformer,* January 1906, p 33.
94. Pallis, Death, p 1032.
95. Coffin, *Death in Early America,* p 106.
96. Brouardel: *Death and Sudden Death.* Paris, October 1, 1867. Cited in: Puckle, *Funeral Customs,* p 23-24.
97. Buried Alive. *Br Med J.* 1877;2:819.
98. Real and apparent death. *Lancet.* 1887;1:233+.
99. Arnold, Zimmerman, Martin, *JAMA,* 1968.
100. Wilder A: Quoted in: Arnold, Zimmerman, Martin, *JAMA,* 1968.
101. "Dead" man freed after 2 days in a box. *Arizona Daily Star.* March 22, 1993.
102. Tebb, Vollum, Hadwen, *Premature Burial,* p 344.
103. Ibid., 346-47.
104. Ibid, 348-49.
105. Puckle, *Funeral Customs,* p 22.
106. Foderé FE: *Traité de médecine légale.* 2nd ed. Paris, France: 1813;2:366.
107. *Gentleman's Magazine.* August 1844. Cited in: Litten J: *The English Way of Death.* London: Robert Hale, 1991, p 166.
108. Curl, *Victorian Celebration of Death,* p 30.
109. Welby H: *Mysteries of Life, Death, and Futurity.* (pamphlet) 1861.
110. Arnold, Zimmerman, Martin, *JAMA,* 1968.
111. Habenstein RW, Lamers WM: *The History of American Funeral Directing.* 2nd ed. Milwaukee, WI: National Funeral Directors Assn, 1981, pp 180-83.
112. Hallam, *Burial Reformer,* January 1906, p 32.
113. Farrell JJ: *Inventing the American Way of Death, 1830-1920.* Philadelphia, PA: Temple Univ Press, 1980, p 163.

# I'm Dead—Now What?

114. Hallam, *The Burial Reformer*, January, 1906.
115. Farrell, *Inventing the American Way of Death,* p 163.
116. Arnold, Zimmerman, Martin, *JAMA,* 1968.
117. *Journal de Rouen.* France: August 5, 1837.
118. Plutarch: *Numa Pompilius.* In: Hutchins RM ed: *Great Books of the Western World.* Chicago: Encyclopaedia Britannica, 1952, p 54-55.
119. Tegg W: *The Last Act: Being the Funeral Rites of Nations and Individuals.* London: William Tegg & Co, 1876, p 312.
120. Basevi, *Burial of the Dead,* pp 127-129.
121. Ibid., 134.
122. Coe, K: Personal communication. October 21, 1993.
123. Davis W: *Passage of Darkness: The Ethnobiology of the Haitian Zombie.* Durham, NC: Univ of North Carolina Press, 1988.
124. Shakespeare W: *Romeo and Juliet.* Act 4, scene 1, line 98.
125. Quoted in: Gittings, *Death, Burial and the Individual,* p 9.
126. Fraser, John: *The Aborigines of New South Wales.* Sydney, Australia: Potter, 1892. (Published by authority of the New South Wales Commissioners to the World Columbia Exposition, 1893.)
127. Basevi, *Burial of the Dead,* p 165.
128. Ibid., p 168.
129. Waugh E: *Loved One: An Anglo-American Tragedy.* Boston: Little, Brown, 1976, pp 42-43.
130. Federal Trade Commission: *An Analysis of the Funeral Rule Using Consumer Survey Data on the Purchase of Funeral Goods and Services.* Washington, DC: FTC, February 1989, p 6.
131. Basevi, *Burial of the Dead,* p 176.
132. Bendann, *Death Customs,* p 203.
133. Catts EP, Goff ML: Forensic entomology in criminal investigations. *Annual Review of Entomology.* 1992;37:253-72.
134. Mayer RG: *Embalming—History, Theory, and Practice.* Norwalk, CT: Appleton & Lange, 1990, p 23-57.
135. Spitz WU, Fisher RS: *Medicolegal Investigation of Death.* Springfield, IL: Charles C Thomas, 1973, p 16.
136. van den Oever R: A review of the literature as to the present possibilities and limitations in estimating the time of death. *Med Sci Law.* 1976;16:269-76.
137. Polson, Brittain, Marshall, *Disposal of the Dead,* p 283.
138. Eckert, *Medico-Legal Insights,* 1991.
139. van den Oever, *Med Sci Law,* 1976.
140. Ludwig, *Current Methods of Autopsy Practice,* p 17.
141. van der Oever, *Med Sci Law,* 1976.
142. Soren D: Interview. Tucson, AZ: June 6, 1993.
143. Spitz, Fisher, *Medicolegal Investigation of Death,* p 19-20.
144. Selzer, *Mortal Lessons,* p 136-37.
145. Richardson R: *Death Dissection and the Destitute.* London: Routledge & Kegan Paul, 1987, p 15.
146. Kass, *Hastings Center Report,* 1985.
147. Carlson L: *Caring for Your Own Dead.* Hinesburg, VT: Upper Access Pub, 1987, p 59.
148. How to prepare death notices. *American Funeral Director.* 1969; 92(1):33-36+.
149. Ibid.
150. Smyth WH: *Catal. Coins.* Dk. Northumberland: 1856, p 244; As quoted under "Necrological," In: *Compact Edition of the Oxford English Dictionary.* vol 1. New York: Oxford Univ Press, 1971, p 1907.
151. Roger Bacon, From his Will. 1626.
152. Premature report from South Africa. *Prodigy News Service,* May 31, 1993.
153. Two lives to live. *Entertainment Weekly.* October 8, 1993, p 8.
154. Aussie media errs on queen report. *UPI.* November 12, 1993.

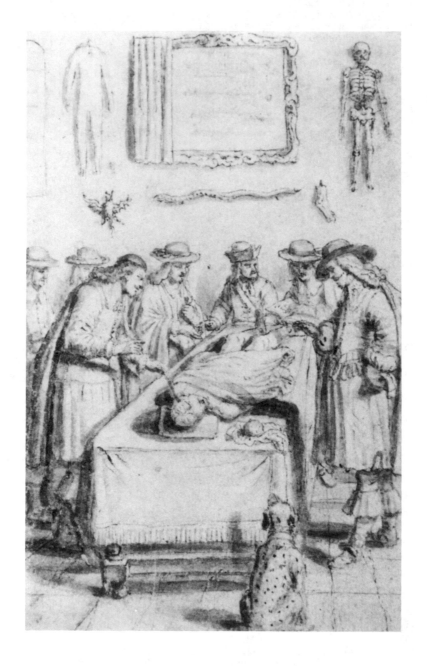

*A lesson in anatomy.* Seventeenth-century anatomical dissection. Originally published in Amsterdam, 1665. (Reproduced with permission. National Library of Medicine.)

# 3: HELP FOR THE LIVING: ORGAN, TISSUE AND WHOLE BODY DONATION

A. What is organ and tissue donation and transplantation?
B. Why donate organs and tissues?
C. Who donates cadaver organs and tissues in the United States?
D. Who donates cadaver organs and tissues elsewhere in the world?
E. Who actually becomes an organ and tissue donor?
F. How do I become an organ and tissue donor?
G. What do religions, law and cultures say about postmortem organ and tissue donation or transplantation?
H. Can I donate blood after death?
I. What are the steps in postmortem organ and tissue donations?
J. How are organs and tissues procured?
K. How are donor organs and tissues distributed?
L. Do donor families know where the organs go? Do recipients know where the organs came from?
M. What happens to the body after donation?
N. What does it cost to donate organs?
O. Can I donate my whole body to a medical school?
P. By what other means have bodies become dissection cadavers?
Q. How else have bodies been obtained for dissection?
R. Have "dead" criminals been used for anatomical dissection?
S. How are bodies prepared as dissection cadavers?
T. Why dissect cadavers?
U. How do medical students dissect cadavers?
V. In what other ways do doctors and researchers use dead bodies?
W. References

*How can the dead aid the living with the gift of life? What need exists for transplantable organs and tissues, how are these organs taken from the cadaver, and can donor bodies still have normal funerals and viewings? How do medical schools use entire bodies for anatomical dissection and research?*

## A. WHAT IS ORGAN AND TISSUE DONATION AND TRANSPLANTATION?

Organ and tissue *donation* refers to the practice of giving part of a person's body, usually after death, for transplant into another person. In *organ transplantation,* surgeons transfer an organ or tissue from one person, called the *donor,* to a second person, called the *recipient.* The transplant recipient usually suffers from an illness or injury requiring new tissue or a new organ, such as skin, bone, bone marrow, or a cornea, kidney, liver, heart, pancreas, or lung. Most donors are cadavers, although kidneys, bone marrow, and portions of livers or lungs may be transplanted from one living patient to another.

The process of organ and tissue transplantation includes three major activities: selection and preparation of a recipient; selection and preparation of a donor; and the surgical transfer of the tissue and organ from donor to recipient. This chapter primarily discusses the organ or tissue donor.

Although we consider organ and tissue transplantation part of modern medical practice, some transplants have been performed for a long time. Pre-Christian writings in Egypt, India and Syria described grafting skin from one area of a person's body to another, and the first successful cornea transplants were done over 100 years ago. These procedures succeeded because they did not require tissue matching and the anti-rejection medications necessary for other transplants.

In 1954, Dr. Joseph E. Murray performed the world's first successful kidney transplant at Boston's Peter Bent Brigham Hospital. The first successful human pancreas transplants occurred in 1966,[1] the first liver and first heart transplants in 1967, and the first single lung and heart-lung transplants took place in 1981. Kidney, heart, liver, cornea, pancreas, skin, bone, cartilage and most other transplants are now routine procedures at major U.S. medical centers. They are recognized and approved therapy, *not experiments.* More than ninety-nine percent of all transplants are done strictly to benefit individual patient needs.

Between July 1988 and January 1990, nearly 93% of kidney transplant patients were alive one year after their operation, as were 89% of patients with pancreas transplants, 82% with new hearts, 74% with new livers, 54% with new lungs, and 53% with a new heart and lungs.[2] Survival rates have increased as experiments have improved transplantation techniques, and new drugs to suppress recipients' immune systems widened the scope of available donors and recipients. The most experienced transplant centers generally have the highest patient-survival rates.[3]

## B. WHY DONATE ORGANS AND TISSUES?

Transplanted hearts, lungs, kidneys and livers save the lives of people with these failing organs. For those whose kidneys have failed, transplants help them avoid years of chronic dialysis. A relatively new, and still experimental, procedure allows children who lack enough intestines to digest food to receive small and large intestine transplants along with a new liver, stomach, and pancreas. (Since these organs have multiple attachments and an inter-connected blood supply, surgeons have more success transplanting them as a unit.)

As Cecil Helman writes of transplant recipients:

The recipient is now a walking collage of the living and the dead. Within him there are kidneys from close kin, and heart and corneas, liver and lungs, cartilage, skin, hair, bone, nerves, lymph nodes, pancreas and parathyroid—all from the bodies of dead strangers. Bottles of blood, plasma and bone marrow donated by other strangers, drip-drip into his veins.[4]

As with organs, donated human tissue is often the key to medical miracles. The difference between *tissue* and *organs* is somewhat arbitrary: the blood supply for tissues comes from millions of capillaries and tiny arterioles, whereas that for organs comes from arteries large enough to have names. Tissue transplants include skin to help seriously burned patients cover and protect their wounds from infection and fluid loss; corneas (eyes) to allow those whose eyes are clouded or deformed to see again; bone and cartilage transplants to provide patients with a foundation on which their own bone may grow or to replace damaged joint tissue; temporal bones including inner ear structures to restore hearing to some who are deaf; heart valves to allow some patients' own hearts to function correctly; and veins to permit others to have coronary artery bypass surgery.

Other tissue grafts are used to repair congenital, surgical, or cosmetic defects caused by illness or injury. Arteries and veins from the legs are used for grafts; cartilage is used to reconstruct noses, other facial structures, and knees—thus avoiding total knee replacements; pliable thigh tissue (fascia lata) helps surgeons reconstruct the covering over brains; discs between the vertebrae are helpful in reconstructing damaged discs; and the spinal bones (vertebrae) themselves are sources of bone marrow for transplantation.

Approximately twenty-five different organs and types of tissue can be used for transplant—and the list is growing.

Yet Americans are not donating.

Fewer than one percent of all those who die in the United States each year have donated their organs for use. Of the approximately 23,000 Americans who are declared dead by brain criteria (and thus are suitable as organ, as well as tissue donors) only about 4,000 (17%) have donated their organs, though two-thirds of those who did donate, donated multiple organs.[5] In 1992, for example, the 4,549 cadaver organ donors in the entire United States provided organs for 14,062 transplants. This was a donation rate of only 19.2 donors per million people in the United States. This represents only a 1% increase over 1991.[6] The breakdown of donations by organ is shown in Table 3.1.

The donation of eyes is an exception, though, because at least fourteen states have *presumed consent* laws that automatically allow authorities to remove cadaver eyes for cornea transplants and other therapeutic and research purposes if there are no objections from the family or no written objections left by the deceased.[7]

As of mid-1992, in the United States there were 27,120 people waiting for organ transplants. A new person goes on the transplant waiting list every 20 minutes. Nearly 60% of these individuals were younger than 45-years old when they were placed on the transplant waiting list; more than 5% were younger than 18-years old. Some individuals on the list were newborns or still in the womb![8] In 1993, there were 32,652 people in the United States on the waiting list for organs (table 3.2).[9]

## TABLE 3.1: Organs Donated in 1992

| Organ | Number Donated |
|---|---|
| Kidney | 8,444 |
| Heart | 2,198 |
| Liver | 3,290 |
| Pancreas | 619 |
| Heart/ Lung | 49 |
| Lung | 616 |
| Total | 5,216 |

Note: Many donors gave more than one organ.

Adapted from: Uninformed next-of-kin thwarts donor process. *The Bank Account.* 1993;14(2):4.

## TABLE 3.2: U.S. Transplant Waiting Lists (1993) and Number of Transplant Operations (1991)

| ORGAN | WAITING LIST(1993) | OPERATIONS (1991) |
|---|---|---|
| Kidney | 24,481 | 9,949 |
| Heart | 2,830 | 2,125 |
| Liver | 2,814 | 2,954 |
| Lungs | 1,214 | 401 |
| Pancreas | 170 | 532 |
| Kidney-Pancreas | 901 | NONE |
| Heart and Lungs | 199 | 51 |
| Intestines | 43 | NONE |
| Totals | 32,652 | 16,012 |

Adapted from: UNOS, *Protocols,* November 1993 & June 1991.

The scarcity of organs is a real concern. Comparison of the numbers of organs donated (15,216 in 1992) and number of organs needed (30,906 in 1993) makes this clear. However, even these figures don't accurately reflect the problem. [Surgeons sometimes speak of "harvesting" organs. While the word "harvesting" makes some queasy, it accurately represents the process. Just as with harvested plants that die, but give life to others, so too with harvested organs.]

The widely known scarcity of transplantable organs dissuades many people from ever going on the waiting list. Ultimately, only one of every nine people who could potentially benefit from a heart transplant actually receives one,[10] and very few of the multitude of Americans with failing lungs are allowed on transplant waiting lists. In spite of the tens-of-thousands of patients waiting for transplants, in 1991 the 266 U.S. organ transplant programs only performed 9,949 kidney transplants (7,722 were from cadaver donors); 2,954 liver transplants; 2,125 heart transplants; 532 pancreas transplants; 401 lung transplants; and 51 heart-lung transplants.[11]

The problem is intensifying. The number of Americans dying while waiting for organ transplants is increasing by twenty percent each year. About 2,500 potential organ transplant recipients die annually in the United States while awaiting transplantation.[12] Of those currently on organ

55

transplant waiting lists in the United States, more than one-third will die without receiving a transplant.[13] In 1990 the United Network for Organ Sharing (UNOS) estimated that 83,028 Americans either died of potentially transplantable conditions or lived with sub-optimal medical treatment because they could not get transplants. While organ donation levels remain stable, the number of potential recipients is climbing dramatically; the waiting list almost doubled in size between 1987 and 1991.[14]

Sociologists Renee Fox and Judith Swazey said of kidney donors, families of donors and recipients:

> The donor who offers a part of his body for transplantation is making an inestimably precious gift. The acutely ill patient who receives the organ accepts a priceless gift. The giving and receiving of a gift of enormous value, we believe, is the most significant meaning of human organ transplantation. This extraordinary gift exchange, moreover, is not a private transaction between the donor and the recipient. Rather, it takes place within a complex network of personal relationships that extends to the families, the physicians, and all the members of the medical team who are involved in the operation. Within the network of these relations, a complex exchange occurs through which considerably more than the organ itself is transferred.[15]

## C. WHO DONATES CADAVER ORGANS AND TISSUES IN THE UNITED STATES?

Who wants to donate their organs or tissues after death and who actually does donate them are different questions. Whether a person donates is affected by rules transplant teams work under, the medical team's behavior, and familial and cultural attitudes.

In the United States, transplant teams will not take organs or tissues unless a deceased person's relatives agree (except where the law allows automatic cornea donation). Asking the deceased's family for permission is not legally required, but it is the standard of practice in the United States. Most states' organ donation laws do not have provisions for next-of-kin involvement.[16,17] Yet in most cases an organ procurement team will remove organs from a cadaver only if the next-of-kin or person responsible for disposition of the cadaver agrees, no matter what the deceased's wishes were. Three reasons for this have been cited: fear of being sued by the next-of-kin, fear of a public outcry which might decrease organ donations, and a wish to give the next-of-kin solace by allowing them to make a gift of the deceased's organs to benefit others. So far these teams have not heeded legal scholars who suggest that where the deceased has left organ donation instructions, transplant teams trample on his rights when they also require

56

family consent. This puts many hospitals, organ donation organizations and physicians at legal risk.[18]

According to two Gallup polls, seventy percent of American adults would be willing to donate a family member's organs, if asked.[19,20] The problem is that in many cases, no one is asking. Because medical teams appeared hesitant to ask the next-of-kin for their consent, the federal "required request" (also called "routine inquiry") law was implemented to encourage more organ and tissue donations. This law mandates that when someone dies in any U.S. hospital, the next-of-kin be asked whether they wish to donate organs or tissues. By itself, however, the routine inquiry law does not appear to be very successful, perhaps because only Kentucky has a penalty for non-compliance.[21] When organs have been donated, physicians initiated the discussion only about 45 percent of the time and families about 30 to 40 percent.[22,23]

In emergency departments where young, healthy, potential donors often die, the situation is even worse.[24] Medical staff, who usually lack training in how to ask relatives about organ donation,[25] dislike adding to relatives' distress when they are already confronted with an unexpected death. Physicians have a limited role, however, since once the subject of donation has been broached, an organ transplant coordinator often takes over to provide the necessary specifics to the family.[26]

Even laws supposedly protecting the transplant team do not necessarily help. Since 1991, Texas law has allowed physicians to recover organs from a body without permission if the next-of-kin cannot be located within four hours of death. Because of the perceived (and probably not real) liability, however, in the twelve months after the law went into effect, it was only used twice.[27]

Family attitudes play a major role in whether an individual donates organs or tissues. Families who have actually donated a loved one's organs often feel that the process helped them make sense out of a tragedy. They believe that their loved one can live through someone else (table 3.3). Most interestingly, eighty-nine percent would donate again, even though more than one-fourth of them ran into problems with the timing of the process (it took too long, they were asked to donate before learning of the death, or they did not know when to schedule the funeral), communication problems (no immediate feedback about the organs' use, or the donation option was presented in a cold and technical manner), or problems with hospital administration (they were incorrectly billed for organ-donation activities).[28]

Cecil Helman describes an attitude that moves some people to donate organs:

> Transplants create an original kind of kinship between recipient
> and donor, both living and dead. In a secular world, this produces
> a type of partial immortality. For when a man dies, his kidney can

57

live on. Heart, liver, cornea and blood become the names of his descendants. Billions of his cells will continue to live, planted like seeds in another man's body.[29]

A 1993 Gallup poll, commissioned by Harvard School of Public Health and the Partnership for Organ Donation, showed that 93% of all Americans would be willing to donate a family member's organs if he or she had expressed the wish before death. If no such wish had been expressed, only 50% would be willing to do so. Yet 89% of would-be donors had *not* discussed their intent with their family or next-of-kin. They could give no reason for not discussing it.[30]

The poll also found that the most common misconceptions about organ donation were:

> 59% of Americans believe that organs are bought and sold in the United States on the black market—they aren't.

> 42% believed that the donor's family incurred a cost to donate—they don't.

> 37% did not know that a "brain dead" person will never recover—they won't.[31]

---

## TABLE 3.3: Differences between Organ Donor Families and the General Public

|  | Donor Families | General Public |
|---|---|---|
| Organ donation makes something positive come out of death. | 86% | 60% |
| Functioning organs should not be wasted. | 75% | 66% |
| Deceased could live on in someone else through donation. | 68% | 41% |
| The government should provide cash incentives for families of brain dead donors. | 16% | 31% |

Adapted from: Batten HL, Prottas JM: Kind strangers: the families of organ donors. *Health Affairs.* Summer 1987, pp 35-47.

---

Minorities in the United States are generally not willing to donate organs after death, although they make up a sizable proportion of those awaiting transplants.[32] In mid-1992, the race and number of individuals waiting for kidney transplants were: white 10,964 (52.9%); black 6,622 (31.9%); Hispanic 1,978 (9.5%); Asian 1,012 (4.9%); and other 165 (0.8%).[33] Although blacks are significantly represented on transplant waiting lists (perhaps because they frequently get diabetes and hypertension and suffer from resulting organ damage) they comprise less than 10% of all organ donors.[34] Kidneys, the most common organs transplanted, are matched by tissue typing. Black recipients have a much higher chance of being a close tissue match with a black donor than with any other donor so the lack of black donors is particularly unfortunate, and causes them to wait twice as long as whites for kidney transplants.[35]

Recent polls show that blacks and Hispanics were less willing to donate than white respondents. Only 69% of blacks and 75% of Hispanics approved of organ donation, compared with 87% of whites. Only 52% of blacks and 57% of Hispanics were willing to donate their own organs, as compared with 72% of whites polled. Yet about one-third of the current 31,000+ patients on the organ transplant lists awaiting organs are minorities.[36]

According to prominent black surgeons, the most common reasons blacks refuse to donate organs are: lack of knowledge about organ transplants and the need for organs by other blacks, religious beliefs, fear that as organ donors they will be declared dead prematurely, distrust of the medical establishment, and wanting the donated organs to preferentially go to black recipients (no one can assure them of this).[37]

Due to the shortage of available organs for transplant, serious consideration is now being given for the first time in the United States to financially compensating the relatives of organ donors, but this practice is not without potential problems.[38] In a recent poll of American adults, however, seventy-eight percent said that financial incentives would not affect their decision to donate a loved one's organs. Nevertheless, in 1993, the American Medical Association's (AMA) Council on Ethical and Judicial Affairs recommended a limited trial of compensating individuals for donating their organs after death. Their proposal was analogous to life insurance, where the person voluntarily enrolled during life, and heirs received money if the person was found appropriate for donation at the time of death. The AMA found the concept unworkable.[39]

## D. WHO DONATES CADAVER ORGANS AND TISSUES ELSEWHERE IN THE WORLD?

Most countries, as in the United States, allow individuals to "opt in" to the system of organ donation if they wish. More than thirteen countries however, mostly in Europe, use an "opting out" or "presumed consent" law

59

that assumes people will donate their organs after death unless they (or in some cases surviving relatives) register an objection to donation.[40,41]

The European Community has considered a presumed consent law covering all member nations, given the success of such a law in Belgium, which increased donated cadaver kidneys by 119% within three years, bringing their donations to 40 per million population.[42,43] Austria has done even better with the system, recovering 53 kidneys per million population, although England's Northern Region achieved the same level of donation with the "opting in" system, by educating the public and medical profession.[44] Some people have suggested that the United States require the removal of all cadaver organs and tissues as needed for medical purposes.[45] Such a law would undoubtedly increase the number of transplantable organs and tissues available. It is doubtful, however, that it could withstand court challenges based on religious freedom and legal due process.[46]

Another option for organ donation, harder to implement but emotionally more acceptable to many, is *mandated choice.* Under a system of mandated choice, all competent adults *would be required* to decide for themselves in advance whether or not they wanted to be organ or tissue donors when they died.[47,48] The decision would be placed on their drivers' license or other identification. Nearly two-thirds of U.S. adults and 90% of college students support a mandated choice system.[49,50] Nearly three-fourths of U.S. adults support the most important part of the system, physicians would have to abide by the deceased's expressed wishes regarding donation without asking permission from the family.[51]

Outside of the United States (and occasionally in the United States), the organs of executed criminals are sometimes taken for transplant.

In Egypt, for example, condemned criminals can agree to donate their organs after death. Both the government and the senior Muslim cleric have approved this procedure. In the first such case under this Egyptian law, the liver and kidneys were removed after the criminal was hanged.[52]

In mainland China, recovering the kidneys of executed criminals is big business and no consent is required. Hong Kong physicians refer patients who pay hard currency to mainland China's Canton University for these transplants. China's *People's Daily* reported that 2,900 of these transplants had been done by 1991. One physician said he welcomed the increased disregard for law-and-order in China since it would lead to even more executions and more opportunity for transplants.[53]

Although it rarely occurs, people are sometimes killed for their organs. The *British Medical Journal* reported in late 1992 that some patients at the state-run Montes de Oca Mental Health Institute, just outside of Buenos Aires, Argentina, had been killed for their corneas, other organs, and their blood. Between 1976 and 1991, more than 1,400 patients "disappeared" from the hospital. When their corpses were found and exhumed, many were missing their eyes and other organs. The physician-director and other hospital staff were arrested in April 1992.[54]

Kidnappers are also reported to be terrorizing Argentinean and Honduran slums to find and kill young donors for their kidneys. They then sell the organs on the black market to Argentine, Brazilian and North American patients in need of transplants, for up to $45,000 each. The Argentinean health minister has vowed to halt the process.[55,56]

## E. WHO ACTUALLY BECOMES AN ORGAN AND TISSUE DONOR?

The most common U.S. organ or tissue donor is a white male between five and fifty-five years of age who dies in the intensive care unit of a large acute care hospital within three days of admission for a brain injury, spontaneous bleeding into the brain, or a primary (not metastatic) brain tumor.[57] This is the usual pattern for donation in most of the world. In one unusual case, however, a Swiss heart-transplant *recipient* became a donor after he suddenly died from bleeding into his brain.[58]

In some countries, infants born without an upper brain (anencephalics) are dead by legal definition and their organs can immediately be taken for transplant if the parents approve. These donations provide tiny livers, hearts and other small organs for transplant into otherwise healthy infants dying of congenital defects. This is not the case in the United States, Canada or Great Britain, however, where attempts to use the organs (within existing laws) of these inevitably and quickly dead (by heart criteria) neonates have been unsuccessful. In most cases, by the time breathing stops (required for "death by whole-brain criteria" criteria, used in organ transplants), anencephalics' organs have been so badly damaged that they are unusable.

There are, of course, specific medical conditions that must be met at the time of death to qualify as an organ or tissue donor. These differ slightly based on the organ or tissue to be donated, as can be seen in Table 3.4.

## F. HOW DO I BECOME AN ORGAN AND TISSUE DONOR?

There are only two steps necessary to become an organ donor after death: signing a donor card (or specifying organ donation in an advance directive) and notifying relatives.

First, a donor signs an organ/tissue donor card (Table 3.5) or the back of a driver's license in any of the 46 states that have organ donation cards on them, and carries it at all times. Unfortunately only about 20% of Americans have even taken this first step.[59] Donor cards can be obtained from local or regional organ or tissue banks, the United Network for Organ Sharing, at 1-800-24-DONOR; The Living Bank, (800) 528-2971; or the American Association of Tissue Banks (703) 827-9582.

## TABLE 3.4 : Criteria for Organ and Tissue Donors

All Tissue and Organ Donors.

Death by brain or heart criteria. *(Many centers only accept organ donation from those dead by brain criteria.)*

No malignancy other than a primary brain tumor without a shunt.
No body-wide infection or injury to tissue
No known neurologic disease or AIDS risk factors.

Tissue Specific

HEART VALVES

Age 3-months to 55-years old with no prior heart surgery.
No disease of heart valves.
No injections into the heart.

BONE

Age 15- to 65-years old.
No steroid or insulin use.
No collagen-vascular disease (e.g., lupus, rheumatoid arthritis).
No neurologic disease.

CORNEAS

Age older than 20 years with no eye disease.
No leukemia or retinoblastoma (eye tumor).

Organ Specific:

KIDNEY

No kidney malfunction or infection.

HEART

Generally younger than 55-years old.
No enlargement of the heart.

LIVER

No liver malfunction or cirrhosis.

LUNG

10- to 50-years old.
No lung disease.
No fluid or infection in the lungs.

PANCREAS

Younger than 60-years old.
No pancreas malfunction.

Adapted from: Information from Arizona Organ and Tissue Bank. Tucson, AZ: May 20, 1993; and United Network for Organ Sharing, November 1993.

As the Uniform Donor Card makes clear, a person may specify which organs or tissues are to be donated. Medical personnel will comply with these wishes if they are aware of them, if it is feasible, and if the family also agrees. Medic Alert[R] or similar identification jewelry help medical personnel identify a person as a potential organ donor, as will a wallet card—if it is carried. If at some point a person changes his or her mind about donation, he can destroy the donor card or mark out the entire section on the back of the drivers license in red ink.[60] There is no national registry that one either has to sign up with or withdraw from if he decides not to donate later on.

Persons under 18-years of age need the consent of a parent or guardian to sign a donor card. Unless the deceased person specified not to donate, or there is opposition from someone at the same level in the family hierarchy (such as a disagreement between two siblings), the senior next-of-kin may donate all or part of a relative's body. Parents can donate for a child.

The second step a potential donor takes is equally, if not more important, than the first. That is to notify one's relatives of this desire since surgical teams require their permission before they will take organs. It is estimated that 25% of adult Americans carry a signed organ donor card.[61] But, as one writer said:

> You could die with an organ-donor card in every pocket, and another one pasted on your forehead, and still no one would touch you if your current or separated but not divorced spouse, son or daughter twenty-one years of age or older, parent, brother or sister twenty-one years of age or older, or guardian, in that order, said no...If you want to be an organ donor, carrying a card is much less important than making sure your relatives know your wishes.[62]

Each year in the United States, relatives refuse donation of and bury at least 5,000 human organs that are medically suitable for transplantation.[63]

Families feel more comfortable about donating a relative's organs if the deceased discussed this with them in advance. Family members must also notify the appropriate agencies (for tissue donation only) if the death occurs at home. If a family refuses permission for organ donation from a patient who has been declared dead by brain criteria, the hospital will immediately remove "life supports" in this now-dead patient and release the body to the medical examiner or family, as appropriate.[64]

There are no age or medical restrictions for donating organs or tissues for biomedical research. An individual family can even specify what research they would like to support with an organ or tissue donation and the surgical recovery team will take the appropriate material.[65] In situations that preclude organ, but not generally tissue, donation for transplantation, the

**TABLE 3.5: Uniform Donor Card**

---

# Uniform Donor Card

_____

**Print or type name of donor**

In the hope that I may help others, I _____
hereby make this anatomical gift, if medically acceptable, to take
effect upon my death. The words and marks below indicate my
desires. **I give**:

(a) ☐ any needed organs or parts
(b) ☐ only the following organs or parts _____

_____
**Specify the organ(s) or part(s)**

(c) ☐ my body for anatomical study if needed.
Limitations or special wishes, if any:

_____

---

Signed by the donor and the following two witnesses in the
presence of each other.


_____
**Signature of Donor**                **Date of Birth of Donor**


_____
**Date Signed**                       **City and State**


_____
**Witness**                           **Witness**

---

This is a legal document under the Uniform Anatomical Gift Act
or similar laws.

organs may still be useful for research. Examples of such situations are those in which a person dies a cardiorespiratory death (the heart and lungs stop and the organs are no longer getting oxygen) or if a medical examiner feels that a medicolegal autopsy is mandatory because of the nature of the death. In some cases, a medicolegal autopsy may be performed after organ donation, especially when the cause of death is obviously from an isolated injury, such as a gunshot wound to the head. Generally, however, if a death falls under the medical examiner's jurisdiction, organs and tissues may be retrieved only if the body is released without an autopsy. When medical examiners grant permission for organ or tissue retreival, they often ask the surgeons to give them detailed notes of their findings or tissue samples from the donor.

Organ donation after death is governed by state statutes, most of which are quite similar. With slight variations, every state in the United States, Washington, D.C., and Puerto Rico have adopted the Uniform Anatomical Gift Act (Appendix E). This Act has *six* key elements:

1. Persons 18 years or older who are of sound mind may give all or part of their bodies upon death for specific purposes.
2. Surviving relatives may donate an entire body or any parts of the body if the deceased left no instructions (the suggested order of decision making is surviving spouse, adult child, parent, adult sibling, and guardian).
3. Medical specialists may determine whether the anatomical gift is suitable for the intended purpose and may refuse to accept any or all parts.
4. Only specified parties may be recipients of anatomical gifts (any hospital, surgeon or physician, accredited medical or dental school, or tissue or organ bank) and the gifts may only be used for education, research, advancement of science, or therapy including transplantation.
5. The donor has the right to revoke or amend a donor card at any time, simply by destroying the card.
6. The state continues to have the right to require an autopsy as stipulated in medical examiner or similar statutes.

Under the Act, hospitals, physicians, teaching institutions, storage banks, and a limited number of others can act as recipients of anatomical gifts. Any donation can be revoked in writing, by changing a donor card, by an oral statement witnessed by two people, or by an attending physician during a terminal illness. Hospital personnel acting in "good faith" under the Act cannot be subject to civil or criminal liability.[66]

The Act specifically does not answer the question of when a person is dead. This is left to state statute or physician discretion. (For how death is determined, see Chapter 2, *I'm Dead—Now What?*)

In Canada, the provinces of Alberta, British Columbia, Newfoundland, Nova Scotia and Quebec have adopted a similar measure, the Human Tissue Gift Act (Appendix F). Similar guidelines for organ and tissue donation are available in most British Commonwealth and European countries.

Individuals can also donate some organs during life. Kidneys, bone marrow, parts of livers and parts of lungs (segmental lung transplant is still experimental) are sometimes donated by living relatives of the recipient.

Even before organ transplants were generally possible, the American writer, H.L. Mencken, believed it was his duty to donate parts of his body to science, yet with an acerbic twist: "When I die my kidneys go to the Municipal Museum of Altoona, Pa., and my liver to Oberlin College, but it would take much eloquence to make me leave even my thyroid gland to Milwaukee."[67]

## G. WHAT DO RELIGIONS, LAW AND CULTURES SAY ABOUT POSTMORTEM ORGAN AND TISSUE DONATION OR TRANSPLANTATION?

Most major religions endorse organ and tissue donation and transplantation.[68] Muslims, Rastafarians, Shintos and Zoroastrians are the major religious groups that oppose donation, although their bans are not observed by all members or in all countries. The laws of most nations also approve of organ or whole body donation, the only exceptions being in some countries where Islam or Shintoism is the state religion. Cultural responses to donation vary greatly, sometimes bordering on the bizarre.

There is no religious objection to organ transplantation by the Sikhs, Hindus, Baha'is, Buddhists, Catholics, most mainstream Protestant denominations, and Jews (although some Orthodox Jews may question the concept of death by brain criteria).[69-71]

Jewish acceptance of organ donation comes from biblical sources. The words "and he shall heal" in *Exodus (21:19)* enjoins men to practice medicine. *Leviticus (19:17)* extends this to a common duty with the verse "You are forbidden to stand idly by when your friend is in danger." They also generally accept death by brain criteria, since the absence of spontaneous respiration that is also absent in these "living cadavers" was the Talmudic definition of death.[72]

Pope Pius XII approved Catholic body donation for anatomical dissection, also implying an acceptance of organ donation, saying:

> ...medical science and the training of physicians demand a detailed knowledge of the human body, and that cadavers are needed for study. What we have just said [about the dignity of the human body] does not forbid this. A person can pursue this legitimate

66

objective while fully accepting what we have just said. It also follows from this that a person may will to dispose of his body and to destine it to ends that are useful, morally irreproachable and even noble (among them the desire to aid the sick and suffering).[73]

Buddhists believe that donating the whole body or parts of the body is an act of generosity, *alobha,* that will be rewarded. "The transplantation of any part of the body—eye, heart, etc. only being Derivatives and as such secondary parts of our body—is merely an act of technology, much like replacing a carburetor in a car, and not of religiosity."[74]

Most Protestant denominations put a high premium on donating to their fellow man, including donating organs and tissues. In general, there is full acceptance of organ and tissue donation, but the wide diversity among Protestant denominations makes blanket statements about all sects difficult.[75]

Strict Muslims will not agree to organ donation, nor will Rastafarians, Shintos or Zoroastrians.[76-78] In some places, such as Singapore, where individuals from groups who donate organs are given priority for the receipt of a transplanted organ, Muslims are reconsidering their position on donation.[79,80] In 1982 the Senior "Ulama" Commission, the highest religious authority in Saudi Arabia and throughout the Islamic world declared that organ donation was *hallal* (permissible). Even so, most Muslims still refuse to donate organs.[81]

Shinto, Japan's state religion, teaches that injuring the *shitai* (corpse) adversely affects the *itai* (soul of the dead). Shintos believe that injuring the *itai* may bring misfortune to the bereaved. Therefore, consent for organ, tissue, or whole body donation is rarely granted by relatives in Japan, even if the deceased made a request to donate before death.[82]

The cultural response to organ and tissue donation usually reflects individual altruism and a concern for personal well-being. Americans, for example, are generally altruistic and concerned about their health. They are, therefore, more concerned about their death than about what will happen to their body afterward, and are, in general, willing to donate organs and tissues.[83] Yet people still do not donate, perhaps because up to one-third of the British and American populace believe (incorrectly) that individuals could be declared dead prematurely so their organs can be removed.[84]

One macabre incident points out American society's struggle between the values of retrieving organs for donation and of inflicting capital punishment.

In the early 1980s, North Carolina executed a Mrs. Barfield by lethal injection. Since she had given permission to retrieve her organs for transplantation after death, a kidney-recovery team stood by until she was pronounced dead when her heart stopped. The well-meaning transplant team attempted to restart her heart, to preserve the kidneys while removing them. Would Mrs. Barfield (presumably not brain dead) have been killed a second time if they had restarted her heart but taken her kidneys? (They didn't start her heart.) One medical writer has even suggested that prisoners be executed by removing their organs under anesthesia.[85]

Some individuals have not donated because of fear—a fear that only the recipient, not the donor, should have. One frightening aspect of being an organ recipient is the risk, albeit small, of contracting a life-threatening infectious disease.

In 1985, for example, a man was shot and killed in Petersburg, Virginia. Although he was tested for the AIDS virus, his disease was at an early stage that could not be detected by tests available at that time. His body parts were transplanted into 58 people. Many tissues (not organs) for transplant are normally freeze-dried or irradiated, killing all viruses, before being sent to a recipient. Because of urgent need in this case, however, four grafts were sent out before either of these procedures could be performed. Seven people became infected with the AIDS virus, four from organs and three from tissues. None of the other recipients had a problem with the disease. While tests for AIDS have markedly improved since 1985, this episode not only caused physicians to reduce their use of transplanted tissue, but also caused the public to reduce their donations![86] This is very similar to the unreasoning scare over AIDS that has slowed blood donations in the United States.

Another, less well-known risk is that of contracting Creutzfeldt-Jacob Disease, a progressive form of dementia. Although it is very rare, this virus may lie dormant in the body for 20 years or more after it is acquired. Some transplant recipients in Britain and Australia have gotten the disease after being treated with pituitary gland extracts for fertility or dwarfism, or after having a tissue transplant (meninges) during brain surgery. All of these transplants or injections have ceased, but no one knows how many people have been affected.[87]

## H. CAN I DONATE BLOOD AFTER DEATH?

Not in the United States.

As everyone knows, there is a chronic shortage of blood for transfusion that has intensified in recent years. The AIDS epidemic has panicked many prospective donors, even though people do not get infected from donating blood. Then what about donating after death?

Since 1930, cadaver blood has been routinely used for transfusions at the famed Sklifosovsky Scientific Research Institute of Emergency Medical Assistance in Moscow. The first patient to receive cadaver blood was a young engineer who was bleeding to death after an attempted suicide. Physicians saved his life by giving him blood from a man who had died in an accident six hours earlier.

Each year the Institute drains about 600 cadavers to obtain their blood. From 1930 to 1960, they transfused more than 50,000 units of cadaver blood. The Russians find that the best cadaver donors are patients who died suddenly, from such causes as heart attack, stroke, accidents, strangling or hanging, acute ethanol (alcohol) poisoning, or electrocution. The blood from these cadavers clots quickly, but liquifies again within 60 to 90 minutes as its clotting chemicals are exhausted. If they drain the cadaver within six hours of death, the remaining mixture of blood cells and serum can be used for transfusion.

To drain the cadaver's blood, technicians tie the body to a table and place two large needles in the neck's largest (jugular) vein, with one needle pointed toward the head and the other toward the feet. They "stand the body on its head," tilting the table so the head is near the floor and the feet are in the air. When blood stops draining through these needles, they place another needle in the large neck artery (internal carotid) and flush the body with an anticoagulant to push out the remaining blood. The average adult cadaver yields approximately three liters (about three quarts) of blood. They then store the blood until all screening tests are run. If the patient has an infectious disease, a low hemoglobin (red-blood-cell count), or indications of liver disease, the blood is not used. About thirty percent of cadaver blood is rejected for these reasons.

U.S. physicians have also investigated the use of cadaver blood in Pontiac, Michigan and Chicago, and it has been used to a limited extent in Kiev, Ukraine. Hopefully, the medical community will give more thought in the future to using cadaver blood, since it may solve the chronic problem of insufficient safe blood for transfusion, and since both the blood and the donor (through autopsy) can be thoroughly inspected before the blood is released for transfusion.[88-91]

## I. WHAT ARE THE STEPS IN POSTMORTEM ORGAN AND TISSUE DONATIONS?

Postmortem organ and tissue donation involves three steps: determining that death has occurred, requesting the donation from relatives, and removing the organs and tissue.

Organs and tissues can only be removed after a person is declared dead by either brain (the entire brain no longer functions) criteria or cardiorespiratory (the heart stops) criteria. To avoid a conflict of interest, the physician treating a patient who is a potential donor is never involved in the transplant process. He or she can then concentrate on saving the patient's life. Likewise, the physician who determines death is neither involved in removing the organs or tissues, nor in transplanting them. Many people do not know this and believe that the medical care necessary for their survival might be curtailed if they were a potential organ donor. Not true! Only when the treating medical team declares a patient dead does the organ transplant team become involved.

Once a person has been declared dead by brain criteria and relatives have agreed to donate organs, the medical team must preserve the organs' functions until they are removed from the body. They keep the body on a respirator (ventilator) to oxygenate the lungs and give medications to keep the body functioning. Some of these procedures are listed in Table 3.6.

If the person is dead by cardiorespiratory (heart) criteria, most U.S. transplant centers will only remove tissues. After 1975, believing that kidney transplants had better success if removed from a donor while blood was still going through the organ, U.S. physicians began to avoid transplanting kidneys from patients whose heart had stopped, using only those from patients declared dead by brain criteria.[92] In some centers, surgeons have reverted to using cadaver kidneys because of the scarcity of donated organs.[93]

Organ donors can be difficult "patients" for the nursing staff, both clinically and emotionally. Since their brains no longer function, they often lack the ability to regulate their body's water content, blood pressure, or temperature, and the clinical staff must often quickly intervene to keep the body functioning. One benefit of today's more rapid organ procurement is the much shorter intensive-care-unit stay for cadaver organ donors.

Surgical teams, usually from the institution where the organ will be transplanted, often fly to the cadaver donor's hospital to remove the organs. Most often this occurs in communities where no transplant team is normally available. The donor's hospital gives the team permission to perform this procedure and the team then leaves with the organ(s).

The organ-procurement team follows a rigid protocol determined by national standards that protects the donor, donor family, institutions at both ends of the procedure, and the recipient. The team verifies that death has been pronounced, ascertains that there is no medical reason why the organs should not be used, and runs additional laboratory tests to evaluate the organ's function before it is removed (Table 3.7). The time taken to do these tests varies, since in some cases many of the necessary test results may already be available.

If a donor has tested positive for the AIDS virus but has not yet shown symptoms of AIDS, recipients in life-threatening situations (if they will die within days without the transplant) or their surrogate decision-makers will be asked whether they wish to take the risk of having the organ transplanted anyway.[94]

## TABLE 3.6: Procedures to Maintain a Brain-Dead Cadaver for Organ Donation

1. Administer medications to keep the blood pressure high enough to send blood to the vital organs.
2. Monitor and record the blood pressure, pulse, respiratory rate (controlled on respirator), and temperature.
3. Give other fluids as required.
4. Keep track of the input and output of fluids.
5. Give antibiotics as required.

Adapted from: United Network for Organ Sharing: *Protocols for Organ Donation,* June 1991.

### J. HOW ARE ORGANS AND TISSUES PROCURED?

Organ procurement looks like any other surgical operation on a critically ill or injured person. In this case, though, the "patient" is a "heart-beating cadaver," and is already dead by brain criteria.

All of the normal surgical procedures are still followed, however, since it is vital to maintain sterility and to keep blood and oxygen flowing to the various organs until they are removed and preservation procedures begun. To accomplish this, an anesthesiologist monitors the heart rhythm, blood pressure, and other body systems; a ventilator pushes oxygen into the lungs; and intravenous fluids drip into the veins. (But, of course, no anesthesia is given, since the dead do not feel pain.) The surgical team scrubs, gowns and prepares the corpse as in any other operation. Complete sterility is preserved, and normal instruments and procedures are used. Scrub nurses pass the instruments and a circulating nurse oversees the scene. The operating theater looks and functions nearly identically to the adjacent operating rooms where recipients may be awaiting some of the organs.

When a cadaver will supply multiple organs, various surgical teams take turns removing the organs. There is some scientific disagreement on the order in which organs should be removed for their optimal survival, although the "life-preserving" organs, i.e., heart, lungs, liver, and in a few centers, small intestines, are usually removed first.

Only when all of the organs are removed does the situation change dramatically. Once the heart is removed, the anesthesiologist simply disconnects the ventilator, since the cadaver can no longer be artificially oxygenated. The surgical teams, once finished with their procedures, sew up the cadaver and leave the room; the body now is in the mortician's realm.[95]

## TABLE 3.7: Procedure for Organ Recovery Team

DONOR IDENTIFICATION
1. Verify death has been pronounced in accordance with state law.
2. Determine that none of the following medical conditions are present:
   a. Malignant tumor (except primary brain tumor without a shunt in place).
   b. Blood-borne infection (sepsis).
   c. Repeated positive immunodeficiency virus (AIDS) tests.

DONOR EVALUATION
1. History and review of all organ systems.
2. Chart review.
3. Physical examination.
4. Vital signs.
5. Laboratory tests:
   a. Complete blood count (CBC).
   b. Electrolytes (sodium, potassium, chloride, bicarbonate).
   c. Blood typing.
   d. Hepatitis screen.
   e. Syphilis screen.
   f. AIDS screen.
   g. Other viral screens.
   h. Blood and urine cultures if hospitalized more than 24 hours.
   i. Other tests are also required for donation of the kidneys, liver, heart and pancreas to assess their function.

Adapted from: United Network for Organ Sharing: *Protocols for Organ Donation.* June 1991.

Unlike organs that must be retrieved while the heart is still pumping oxygen-rich blood through them, tissues are generally removed after a person's heart stops. They survive quite well without oxygen for 12 to 24 hours.

*Eyes* are the most commonly donated tissue, because in fourteen states specific permission is not required, under so-called presumed consent laws. Approximately 43,000 corneal transplants were performed in the United States in 1991, with over ninety percent of those resulting in restored vision.[96] Technicians, who in some areas are also morticians, normally remove the eyes within four hours of death. These technicians are trained in the removal, handling, and preservation of the donated eyes through a short course given by the local ophthalmologists, eye hospital, or organ donor banks. Some morticians remove the eyes without charge, as a community service—whether or not they are involved with any of the burial or funeral arrangements.

To remove the eyes, the technician makes an incision beneath the eyelid, exposing the muscles that control eye movement. He severs the six muscles, then cuts the optic nerve, the eye's connection to the brain. He then removes the eye and places it in neosporin (an antibiotic) and ice. To improve the corpse's appearance, he then places a plastic ball in the eye socket so that as long as the eyelids are closed, no one can tell the eyes have been removed. Although only the cornea, the clear part in the front of the eye, can be transplanted, ophthalmologists use other eye tissue (sclera) to attach muscles to false eyeballs in people who have lost their eyes, and often use the entire eye for research into eye disorders.

*Skin* is also procured to help burn victims. If a cadaver has been refrigerated, skin can be recovered for up to 24 hours after death. In a sterile environment, often the operating room, technicians cleanse the donor area and remove any body hair. They then cleanse the area again, place surgical drapes around the site, and spread sterile mineral oil on the donor area. They then remove a very thin layer of skin with a special instrument, a dermatome, that surgeons also use to take skin grafts from the living. The layer of skin removed is between .005 and .018 inches thick, about the same as the skin that peels after a sunburn. Most of the thirty United States tissue centers routinely remove donor skin from the lower chest, abdomen, back, and the front and back of the legs—all areas covered by clothes to allow an open-casket funeral. The donor must be at least 5-feet tall and weigh 100 pounds to assure that the donated sheets of skin are large enough to be used. While only about 5 square feet of skin can be taken from each donor, about 15 square feet is needed to cover a large child's burns one time—and each burn patient undergoes many such skin grafts. The size of the skin grafts can, however, be increased by converting them from a solid piece to a "fishnet" configuration that looks like a screen with large holes.[97]

Physicians use *bone* grafts to replace bone lost because of tumor, injury or degenerative disease. They also use the minute bones of the ear (within the temporal bone) to restore hearing in people with specific types of deafness. Bone donations are routinely taken from above the hip (iliac crest), the large leg bones (femur, tibia and fibula), and the knee cap (patella). In some cases, and with permission of the family, portions of the ribs, upper arm bone (humerus), jaw bone (mandible), and the bone containing the ear structures (temporal bone) will also be removed. Technicians who remove bones carefully replace them with plastic bracing so that there is no apparent disfigurement of the cadaver. Bone donors must have been 15 to 65 years of age and must not have been bed- or wheelchair-bound for extended periods of time before death. If a cadaver has been refrigerated within 4 hours after death, bone can be removed anytime in the subsequent 24 hours. After removal, the bone is cleaned, cut, air dried, packaged, and sterilized using freeze-drying or gamma radiation. It can then sit on a shelf for many years before use.[98]

If a cadaver has been refrigerated within 4 hours of death, leg (saphenous) *veins* can also be taken in the subsequent 10 hours, and *heart valves* in the subsequent 24 hours.[99,100]

## K. HOW ARE DONOR ORGANS AND TISSUES DISTRIBUTED?

Organs for transplant are sent to compatible recipients who are identified through the United Network for Organ Sharing (UNOS) national computer system. When an organ becomes available for transplant, UNOS ranks the pool of potential recipients by strict medical criteria and by the urgency of their need. A potential recipient's ranking may be affected by how well the tissues match, his blood type, his length of time on the waiting list and his immune status. For hearts, livers, and lungs, matching the size of the organ with that of the recipient is often an important consideration. In all cases, the distance between the recipient and donor is an important factor since organs cannot be preserved for long time periods. Except when a "perfect" tissue match for kidneys warrants sending the organ to the "perfect" recipient, organs are first offered locally, then regionally or nationally.[101] (Whether the geographic area within which UNOS initially distributes some organs should be extended to a range of 2,000 miles or more from the donor's hospital is now a hot topic of debate.)

UNOS offers donated organs through the transplant coordinators at centers with potential recipients. The coordinator determines whether the recipient is available, healthy enough to undergo major surgery, willing to be transplanted immediately, and does not have incompatible antibodies to the donor's organ.

Tissues do not have to be transplanted as quickly as organs and do not usually require elaborate compatibility tests. They can often be set on a shelf in sterile containers and used when necessary on any patient. In 1990, approximately 350,000 bone and tissue grafts were done in the United States alone.[102]

As technology advances, organs and tissues can be maintained for longer periods of time outside of the body before being successfully transplanted. Table 3.8 lists the length of time that organs or tissues can be preserved (in 1993) if properly handled after their speedy removal from the donor corpse. The preservation limit starts at the time that the blood supply to the organ stops and depends on the preservation fluid used.

While the storage time of some tissues, such as frozen and freeze-dried bone, was indefinite in the past, the American Association of Tissue Banks

74

has adopted the pharmaceutical guidelines for the expiration date of medications, at least until the Food and Drug Administration finishes its evaluation and sets guidelines.

Organs must be packaged if they are sent to another institution. The standards for packaging (naturally a bit more stringent than for holiday presents sent through the mail) are: (1) the organ must be protected by a triple-layered sterile barrier and a rigid container; (2) the organ, in a cooled preservative, must be carried in a polystyrene-insulated container 1½-inches thick; and (3) all of this must be placed in an outer container made of double-strength, wax-impregnated fiber or the equivalent. These packages must be labeled inside and out with all identifying information.[103]

## L. DO DONOR FAMILIES KNOW WHERE THE ORGANS GO? DO RECIPIENTS KNOW WHERE THE ORGANS CAME FROM?

No. Although the transplant team may share some basic information with the donor family or recipient, such as the donor's or recipient's age and whether he or she had children, confidentiality is maintained at both ends. This practice is, in part, an attempt to avoid directed donations of organs and tissues, such as to a well-publicized person in need.[104] These donations would nearly always be fruitless anyway, since there is only a minute possibility that any non-related donor is compatible with any recipient. (Overcoming this problem is one benefit of the UNOS system that matches potential donors with the large pool of potential recipients included on all of the U.S. transplant centers' waiting lists.)

Anonymity also forestalls the emotional excesses that have been seen from both the donor family and the recipient, and the rare incidents where donor families have requested money from the recipient.[105] On occasion, it also is necessary to protect a donor family or recipient from the press, as when the donor family for a heart-liver transplant to Pennsylvania's governor was harassed for days after the procedure.

In the early days of organ transplantation, donor families and recipients were told about each other. This frequently led to donor families and recipients trying to become more involved in each others' lives—an extra gift that was often not appreciated. As one transplant surgeon related:

> We've had instances where the donor family has gotten in touch with the recipient family; sometimes that's good and sometimes that's bad. Mostly we think its bad. Donor families think that when they donate something, certainly the heart—the loved one lives on in some way. But a donation is a gift. When you give somebody a gift, you don't ask them, "How's my chess set that I gave you? How's the basketball I gave you?" The same is true with organs...Some people feel that just because you have their

## TABLE 3.8: Length of Time Organs and Tissues for Transplant can be Preserved Outside of the Body

| ORGAN | PRESERVATION TIME |
|---|---|
| Heart | 6-8 hours |
| Heart-Lung | 4-5 hours |
| Lung | Up to 12 hours |
| Liver | 12-24 hours |
| Pancreas | 12-24 hours |
| Kidney | 48-72 hours |

| TISSUE | PRESERVATION TIME |
|---|---|
| Bone | |
|   Fresh (in antibiotics) | 7 days |
|   Fresh frozen | 3 years, then reprocessed |
|   Freeze dried | 3 years |
|   Fixed (inner ear bone) | Indefinitely |
|   Cryopreserved | 5 years |
| Skin | Generally same as bone |
| Tendons | Generally same as bone |
| Heart valves | 5 years |
| Knee cartilage | 5 years |
| Veins | 5 years |
| Bone marrow | Up to 3 years |
| Corneas | 10-14 days |
|   (once put in preservative) | |

Adapted from: Material prepared by UNOS, 1991,1993; and Personal communications with Arizona Organ and Tissue Bank. Tucson, AZ: May 20, 1993.

brother's heart in you, they have some influence over your life. And we don't like to foster that feeling at all. We like to keep them very removed from each other.[106]

Yet this is not a universal sentiment. One organ recipient wrote despondently after discovering that there could be no contact between him and the (dead) donor's family:

I felt somehow deprived because I wanted the family to hear directly from me how much I appreciated their kindness and generosity. It would have been a great deal easier for them to have said "no" than "yes." When I finally came to realize how difficult it would be for parents to know the person whose body contained the kidney of their dead son, it became very clear to me why contact with the donor's family would not be allowed.[107]

## M. WHAT HAPPENS TO THE BODY AFTER DONATION?

After a donation, the surviving kin or those charged with disposal of the body get custody of the remains.

The family is responsible for funeral arrangements and the funeral industry will try to maximize this "sale." Relatives can still arrange for embalming and an open-casket funeral if they wish and if the illness or injury that killed the person does not preclude it. According to the funeral industry, removing organs and tissues *does not* interfere with customary burial arrangements, "regardless of the type or extent of the donation."[108]

The industry has found that embalming donor bodies is good business and it is constantly developing new techniques to restore the appearance of donors when viewing is desired (see Chapter 5, *Beauty in Death*).[109] Jessica Mitford, in her unflattering portrayal of the 1960s funeral industry, quoted a funeral industry publication, *The Funeral Director and His Role as Counselor*:

> Even if the deceased has made ironclad legal arrangements to bequeath his body to a medical school, all is not yet quite lost, because "after the anatomical study is completed, the entire residue of the body may be claimed in a sealed container for a service of committal and burial." In this case, the counselor "should opt for as much funeralization as possible either before the donation or after or both."[110]

What can be done with a donor body that is neither buried in a cemetery nor cremated? One science-fiction writer's suggestion to bury the remains as "human compost" or to send them to the moon to develop soil on "earth's satellite" is definitely a futuristic view.[111]

The tissues and solid organs removed from donors are transplanted whenever possible. If they are found to be unacceptable for transplant, they will often be used in transplantation research. Any residual parts are cremated.

## N. WHAT DOES IT COST TO DONATE ORGANS?

There are no costs to the donor's family to donate organs.

This question arises most often with patients declared dead by brain criteria, since once they have been designated as organ donors, these cadavers must be kept on "life-support" machines to keep blood and oxygen going to the organs until they are removed. Once a person has been declared dead and has been designated an organ donor, the organ-procurement organization covers all hospital and physician costs associated with maintaining the body and recovering the organs and tissues.[112] Hospitals bill these charges to the organ recipient. Hospital costs before the person was declared dead are, of course, still the family's responsibility.

Some philosophers have suggested that the "cost" of being an organ *recipient*, should include being willing to donate organs (before the recipient knows he may need a transplant). Advocates suggest that "buying" this very inexpensive insurance would "avoid 'free loaders' who want the benefits of this costly technology without taking their share of responsibility for the cost."[113] They suggest that this would also increase the number of organs donated. Opponents say it is coercive and "runs counter to the 'pure charity' approach favored in the United States."[114] In the only example of this practice so far, the Republic of Singapore passed a law in 1986 linking priority for receiving an organ transplant to a stated willingness to donate after death. So far, it has proven very successful.[115,116]

Not only does organ and tissue donation cost the family nothing, it is also possible that in the future United States donor families may *receive* some type of payment for their donations. Several transplant experts believe that giving organ donor families $2,000 for funeral expenses would help increase donations, especially from minorities.[117,118] If the plan actually increases the flow of organs, they suggest that the health care system will actually save millions of dollars that are now spent on the treatment of those awaiting transplants. This, of course, would be offset by the money spent on increased transplant surgeries and the necessary follow-up treatment. Currently in the United States, the National Transplant Act of 1984 prohibits the buying or selling of human organs.[119] In other countries this is not always the case. Even in the United States, however, money flows along with tissues and organs. A "processing fee" is charged by those procuring organs, including organs used by biological supply houses for research and teaching. A few unscrupulous operators have made hundreds-of-thousands of dollars in this business.[120]

## O. CAN I DONATE MY WHOLE BODY TO A MEDICAL SCHOOL?

Yes, but arrangements with a medical school must be made well in advance of death. The Uniform Anatomical Gift Act (Appendix E), adopted in one form or another in all fifty states, allows individuals to bequeath their bodies to medical schools or hospitals without permission of the next-of-kin. Most states consider donation of a body to a medical school for dissection its final legal disposition.

As with organ donation, however, the schools themselves normally require relatives' permission. More than ninety percent of the cadavers used by U.S. medical schools have been donated. "These are not street people or people without families," says Cheryl Blumenthal of Pennsylvania's Human Gifts Registry. "Every economic group is represented."[121] Some families have a tradition of leaving their bodies to science, and some individuals leave their bodies to their alma mater or to a school they always dreamed of attending. Typical is the letter received by the coordinator of anatomical gifts at Harvard saying, "I couldn't make it to Harvard as a youngster, but I'm coming now."[122]

The most common reasons people give for donating their bodies to science are to aid medical science and teaching, and to show gratitude to the medical profession. Very few donate because they either lack relatives or cannot afford funeral expenses.[123] Even Oliver Wendell Holmes commented on his experiences as a medical student, "I have been going to Massachusetts General Hospital and slicing and slivering the carcasses of better men and women than I ever was myself or am likely to be."[124]

The Uniform Anatomical Gift Act is remarkably similar to Britain's Anatomy Act which effectively ended body-snatching in England and Scotland. Passed in August 1832, the Anatomy Act allowed those with lawful custody of bodies, except persons entrusted with the body specifically for burial such as undertakers, to permit anatomical examination unless the deceased had previously forbidden it. Once dissected, the remains had to be buried in consecrated ground or in some public burial ground in use for people of the appropriate religious persuasion. Nowadays the remains are usually cremated, as are most bodies in England.

As soon as Britain's Anatomy Act was passed, the Duke of Sussex, sixth son of King George III, said that he wanted a London hospital to dissect his corpse after his death. When he died in 1843, however, the royal family would not stand for this and refused. His body was autopsied, though, with the promise that if he had died of anything "interesting" the findings would be published. He didn't; they weren't.[125]

Anyone wanting to donate his body to a U.S. medical school should contact that school's anatomy department in advance to find out its specific needs and protocol. Each school has written material it can send to potential donors which often includes a wallet card to notify authorities of its claim at the time of death. Table 3.9 is an example of one such card. Note that an autopsy will be performed on the body if legally required or needed by the family or physicians. The body however, will not then be acceptable for anatomical dissection.

Some schools require that bodies come to them immediately; others allow a short delay for funeral services. Most schools do not pay transportation costs for an "out-of-town" body and some require that a mortician deliver the body to them. Others allow the body to be transported by an ambulance, relatives or the school's own vehicle. No school buys bodies, although some desperate schools pay exorbitant shipping costs to receive bodies from out-of-state schools that have excess cadavers. Schools vary widely in the number of donated bodies they receive. The state of Maryland, for example, acquires 700 to 800 bodies each year for its two medical schools. Pennsylvania gets 500 to 600, and the University of California at San Francisco alone receives 300 each year. At the other end of the spectrum is the University of Utah which gets only 49 bodies per year for use by their medical and graduate students, other health-science students, residents, and faculty.[126] Osteopathic and podiatry schools rarely have an adequate number of bodies.

State laws enacted under the Uniform Anatomical Gift Act also allow medical schools or other potential recipients to reject the gift of a body. For example, Grace Metalious, author of the steamy (for its time) novel, *Peyton Place*, willed her body to not one, but two medical schools. Neither wanted it.[127] A school may reject a body because the donor was too young or too old; or because the condition of the body is unacceptable for anatomical study—if it was subjected to an autopsy or amputation, has extensive burns, suffered a violent death, or had extensive surgery. It may also be too obese, emaciated, too tall, or have had a dangerous infectious disease. Schools may also refuse bodies of patients that died in distant places, or because they already have too many bodies and have inadequate storage for more (unique to some regions of the United States). Some of these bodies, however, can still be used by schools of dentistry or podiatry or for special anatomical studies.

Most schools, however, will not allow people to donate a body for a specific purpose (e.g., dissection by orthopedic surgeons) since how a body is used will depend on its condition at the time of death. Though some schools will dispose of any body they receive which they cannot use, others may return it to the family. Virtually all bodies accepted by medical schools are used for anatomical teaching, generally within two years of donation.[128]

If death occurs in another state, complying with the legal requirements necessary to transport the body back to the medical school where the donation has been arranged may take so much time that the body is no longer in a condition suitable for anatomical use. An alternative in such cases is for a relative to locate another medical school in the vicinity of death that would be interested in accepting the body.

Law prohibits the international shipping of bodies as anatomical specimens. But if someone should die in a foreign country, it is frequently possible to donate a body to a foreign medical school for dissection. Many of these schools, due to legal, cultural or religious restraints desperately need anatomical specimens. Up to 200 medical students in Argentina, for example, share one cadaver and Italian medical students have had to travel

## TABLE 3.9: Wallet Card Indicating Whole Body Donation.

NOTICE

I made provision on the _____ day of _____, 19__ in the form required by the laws of Arizona, for the donation of my body to The University of Arizona, Tucson, Arizona, for medical teaching.

No autopsy is to be performed, and the body is to be handled and transported according to instructions from the University. In the event of my death, please notify the College of Medicine, The University of Arizona. (602) 694-0111 Mortician

_____

Signature

to Israel to study anatomy.[129] Unlike some other subjects, anatomy is the same around the world and all physicians need to have this knowledge.

Assuming that one is ready to donate his or her body for medical use, which takes priority, donating organs or using the body for anatomical dissection? The most practical solution is to arrange for both donations, with the removal of needed organs taking precedence, as these donations will often be immediately life-saving. Since many fewer bodies are acceptable as organ donors than as anatomical cadavers (because of the mechanism of death or the diseases at the time of death), it is probable that anatomical dissection will be the result. The best solution, however, is to leave the decision up to the physicians at the time of death.

Even if a body has been accepted for anatomical study, a funeral with the body present can often be arranged. Many medical schools will later return the remains or ashes to the family for interment or disposal if a request is made in advance. Otherwise, the schools generally cremate and dispose of the remains themselves.[130] A stone marker at the gravesite maintained by the University of Cincinnati for the cremated remains of their anatomical cadavers reads, "Through their thoughtfulness knowledge grows."[131] A few schools, such as Harvard, bury rather than cremate the remains.

Forest Lawn Cemetery in Richmond, Virginia, donated a twelve-by-six-foot mound to the state as a memorial garden for the cremains of anatomical cadavers. A tall granite stone describes the garden's purpose: "In memorial to those who gave their bodies to medical science." Since 1986, the Medical College of Virginia has buried the cremated remains of some of their anatomical cadavers there (others are returned to families). They hold an annual service to commemorate the men and women who donated their bodies for use in gross anatomy laboratories. The prayer that begins the service says:

> O God of grace and glory, those who in the silence of death shared of themselves, that we might learn the mysteries of the human body, those who graciously consented that we might discover, those who by circumstances were assigned to offer this last gift to us. We remember our initial fears, our curiosity, our anxious humor, our fascination, our moments of discovery, our hard quest for knowledge, our need to know for excellence in our chosen field.[132]

One woman, whose mother's ashes had just been interred in the mound and whose father had donated his body to science fifteen years earlier said of the process, "I think it is a wonderful way to celebrate a life."[133]

Other medical schools holding such services include Tulane University, the University of Massachusetts at Worcester, West Virginia University, the Mayo Clinic, and the University of Arizona.[134]

Only four institutions will dispose of *all enrolled* donors, whether or not they use the body: University of South Alabama, State Anatomy Board of Maryland, University of South Dakota, and Southwestern Medical School, Dallas, Texas.

The University of Padua, Italy, disposes of some body parts in a unique way. Medical students take their final oral examinations in the majestic fourteenth-century hall of the Faculty of Medicine and Surgery. Looking on, so to speak, are the skulls of past professors who donated their bodies for dissection.[135]

Most religions approve of donating bodies for dissection. Even Orthodox Judaism sanctioned the practice in the early twentieth century. The Right Reverend James A. Pike, Bishop of the Episcopal Diocese of California said:

> A positive, constructive use of the body for medical research is by no means irreverent. It is in fact a noble and fine thing for a person to make such a provision...We believe in the resurrection and the continuous personal life of the individual spirit, not of the earthly remains.[136]

Even so, many individual ministers disapprove of the practice. The religions that disapprove of gifts of this nature are generally identical to those disallowing organ and tissue donation.

## P.  BY WHAT OTHER MEANS HAVE BODIES BECOME DISSECTION CADAVERS?

Throughout history, bodies of executed criminals, unclaimed bodies, bodies robbed from graves, and occasionally murder victims have become dissection cadavers (see also Chapter 8, *Wayward Bodies*). Currently, most dissection cadavers are donated for that purpose, although unclaimed bodies are also still used. The number of unclaimed bodies (some with relatives who just cannot afford burial costs) varies in each state. Though some schools and locales will not accept these bodies as anatomical cadavers, they constitute, for example, ten percent of Maryland's cadavers.[137]

The bodies of executed criminals have long been used as anatomical subjects. During the Roman occupation of Palestine, Talmudic scholars dissected the body of a woman executed by Roman authorities to determine its anatomical structure. In an early attempt to require continuing medical education, the thirteenth-century Holy Roman Emperor Frederick II ordered that the bodies of two executed criminals be delivered every two years to the medical schools for an *Anatomica Publica,* which every physician was obliged to attend. In 1505 the Council of Edinburgh agreed that one executed criminal's body each year should be given to the anatomists for dissection. Agents representing early eighteenth-century surgeons often invited condemned prisoners not already under sentence of dissection to barter their own corpses for money. Occasionally, prisoners agreed so they could pay prison expenses, enjoy a last meal in style, provide for their families or "to purchase the customary decent apparel for their launch into eternity."[138]

Riots beneath the gallows, however, sometimes still robbed the surgeons of the bodies. In 1749, to prevent rioting by family and friends, the Sheriff of London took the bodies of criminals hanged at Tyburn into his own custody. Yet as late as the 1820s, two surgeons in Carlisle, England, after dissecting the body of a hanged man, were set upon by vengeful friends of the deceased. One surgeon was killed and the other was shot in the face.[139] Clearly, the criminal's family was not always enthusiastic about the idea of anatomists dissecting their loved one. After the execution of Charlie Graham, a Gypsy from Fife, his wife, to foil anatomists who planned to exhume his body for dissection, quickly buried him in hot lime and sat, inebriated, on his grave until enough time had passed that she was sure they would not want the corpse.

In 1673, a French royal declaration permitted dissection and anatomical demonstrations with "complete freedom" at the Jardin du Roi, Paris, with "subjects suitable for this purpose" to be provided. One source of the subjects was the public executioner, another the Hôtel Dieu (hospital).[140] As French physicians once said, "My friend was ill: I attended him. He died: I dissected him."[141]

French anatomists, however, with an allotment of only one or two cadavers from the hospital each winter and "a few arms and legs during the summer," still had too few cadavers. Instructors supplemented this supply with cadavers illegally purchased from the keeper of the hospital cemeteries.[142] Eventually grave robbing became the primary source of anatomical specimens. Since body snatching was illegal, some French anatomy students, to hide the remnants of their dissected cadavers, burned the bones and heated "their garrets with the fat of the dead."[143]

In 1752, King George II required the dissection or hanging in chains (or in gibbets) of the bodies of all executed murderers so that "some further terror and peculiar mark of Infamy might be added to the Punishment of Death."[144] "Public anatomies" were held by the Company of Barber-Surgeons in their hall, with compulsory attendance by the Company's members (another early attempt at continuing medical education). Three bodies were dissected at each of these quarterly demonstrations. One body was used to demonstrate the internal organs, one to show the muscles, and one to show the bones.[145]

Between 1805 and 1820, there was an average of eighty executions annually in England and Wales which were supposed to supply dissection cadavers for approximately one thousand anatomy students each year.[146] To assist the anatomists in the 1820s, the British Home Secretary, without legal authority, also gave them the bodies of the dead from prisons and military hospitals for dissection.[147]

America generally followed England's lead with regard to allowing anatomical dissections.

In the United States, Massachusetts donated the bodies not only of criminals but also, occasionally, of those involved in lethal duels, to the anatomists. The coroner was instructed that the dueler's body "be immediately secured and buried without a coffin, with a stake drove through the body, at or near the usual place of execution, or shall deliver the body to any surgeon or surgeons, to be dissected and anatomized." The law demanded that the murderer's body (in a duel) was always to be sent to the surgeons. The law was passed less to aid the study of anatomy than to stop duelling.[148]

After England's Anatomy Act was enacted in 1832, a bureaucratic nightmare ensued, with the poor claiming that they were disproportionately being used as dissection cadavers, which was true. In fact, in 1832, 74% of 607 bodies sent for anatomical dissection came from the workhouse (poorhouse), 22% from the hospital, 2% from the prison, and 1% each from the hulks (prison ships) and asylums (for the mentally ill). By 1914, of 278 bodies sent for dissection, 54% came from the workhouse, 3% from the hospital, and 43% from the asylums.[149] Ruth Richardson comments that, similar to a £10-property qualification that excluded the working classes from the vote (passed the same year as the Anatomy Act), "the Anatomy Act drew a similar line in a similar place, demarcating and isolating the propertyless as its victims."[150] It wasn't until after World War II that there was a major increase in donated bodies. Interestingly, it paralleled a similar increase in the use of cremation.[151]

The shortage of bodies, though, is still with us. The ratio of bodies for anatomical study per student in Britain dropped from about 1.2 per student in 1826 to 0.2 per student in 1970.[152] The United States' supply of cadavers for anatomical dissection currently meets the need, at about 0.25 bodies per student. The distribution of these bodies, however, is quite skewed, with the well-known schools getting more than enough bodies while other schools go begging.

Currently, in the United States, unclaimed-body statutes in many states specify that if a body is not claimed within a certain period of time it can be turned over to a medical school for its use.[153] The number of bodies that go unclaimed varies with the nation's economy; people forego altruistic burials in times of hardship.

## Q. HOW ELSE HAVE BODIES BEEN OBTAINED FOR DISSECTION?

After it became more difficult to steal bodies in Scotland, alternatives were sought to procure them for anatomical study. One suggestion, made by the *Edinburgh Courant* in 1825, was to import bodies. In fact, a brisk trade did develop in bodies from the parts of Europe where corpses were plentiful and inexpensive. Dublin, Ireland became the hub of the illegal body-export trade, with LeHavre, France close behind.

Bodies were usually shipped in innocent-looking containers labeled "books," "pianos," or even "glue." Sometimes, however, things went badly awry. One shipment of bodies destined for anatomical study was encased in cotton bales. The recipient, a secret wholesaler of bodies, unfortunately was unaware of this novel shipment method. Not expecting a shipment of cotton, he refused to accept the bales and they were left on the dock. Only when an appalling odor swept over the area did officials investigate the shipment. They were shocked to discover dozens of bodies of men, women, and children wrapped in the cotton—all in an advanced state of decomposition.[154]

Another method of obtaining bodies was to bribe those in charge of a body to divert it to the dissecting room before it was buried. A coffin suitably weighted with sand by a corrupt church sexton or undertaker was buried in its stead. As one body snatcher said, "the venal undertaker, who having interred sand, inwardly chuckles at the solemn words, 'dust to dust.' "[155] In one London graveyard, body snatching was remarkably easy—the cemetery owner was himself an anatomist, who charged the family for the burial, and then charged the medical students for their fresh cadavers.[156] Many bodies left "unwaked" (unwatched) disappeared in this manner, since bodies suitable for anatomical study could be sold for sizable sums. Children's bodies were often sold by length, with the first foot costing six shillings, and nine pence for each additional inch in 1790s England.[157] Jewish bodies were especially prized and expensive because they were quite fresh, since religious custom dictated quick burial. Obtaining fresh bodies was an important consideration before preservation techniques became common.[158]

In 1830, Dr. John Collins Warren, through a massive lobbying effort, induced the Massachusetts legislature to pass the Anatomy Act legalizing limited anatomical dissection. Two generations later, a Warren descendant, Dr. Thomas Dwight, got the state to liberalize the law so that donating bodies for anatomical dissection became legal.

## R. HAVE "DEAD" CRIMINALS BEEN USED FOR ANATOMICAL DISSECTION?

Criminals condemned to death feared, perhaps more than the hangman's rope, the possibility of waking up on the anatomist's table after a botched execution. Judicial hangings kill by partially decapitating the individual, normally separating the spinal cord at the third and fourth cervical vertebrae. But non-judicial hangings and non-successful judicial hangings do not break the spinal column or usually injure the spinal cord, and may not result in death.[159]

One person who narrowly missed this experience was "Half-Hangit" Maggie Dickson of Musselburgh, Scotland. After being hanged, she was revived only after her family won a struggle with medical students under the gallows for her body. Maggie led a full, although somewhat demented life and went on to bear a large number of children.[160] (Criminals not successfully hanged were generally said to have been spared by God's intervention and were not hanged again.) On at least on one occasion, the victim was not as lucky. As recorded in *Stow's Annals:*

> The 20 of Februarie [1587], a strange thing happened to a man hanged for felonie at Saint Thomas Waterines, being begged by the Chirurgeons of London, to have made of him an anatomie, after he was dead to all men's thinking, cut downe, throwne into a carre, and so brought from the place of execution through the Borough of Southwarke over the bridge, and through the Citie of London to the Chirurgeons Hall nere unto Cripelgate: The chest being opened there, and the weather extreme cold hee was found to be alive, and lived till the three and twentie of Februarie, and then died.[161]

One of the most famous premature "burials" is that of Anne Greene who, after being hanged for a felony, was sent to the anatomy hall to be used for dissection. There she awoke. She lived on for many years afterwards. Her experience was originally published in a pamphlet whose title tells the tale: "News from the Dead, or a true and exact relation of the miraculous deliverance of Anne Greene, who having been executed December 14th, 1650, afterwards revived and by the care of a certain physician, is now perfectly recovered."[162]

Patrick Redmond had a comparable experience in 1773. A condemned robber, he was hanged by Irish officials for twenty-nine minutes. Yet after his friends spirited his body away, they applied tobacco enemas and held lighted pipes to his body, continuously rubbing his limbs. Not long after, his neck wound began to bleed. He was said to have completely recovered and despite the sheriff's attempt to retrieve him, he led a full life in another county.[163]

William Duell had an even closer call. This rapist-murderer was hanged at Tyburn in November 1740, and taken to the barber-surgeons' hall, where he was stripped and washed in preparation for dissection. The assistant, however, noted that he was breathing and had a faint pulse. Two hours later he was sitting in a chair and drinking wine, but was in great pain. He was sent back to prison and later exiled for life.[164]

About this same time, Professor Junkur of Halle University received a sack with the body of a hanged criminal to be used for dissection. The body was dumped in his house after dark when the professor had already gone to bed. During the night, the professor was awakened by the figure of a naked and shivering man—holding an empty sack. The professor decided to help the man escape further punishment and some years later encountered him on the street, a wealthy merchant with a wife and two children.[165]

An eighteenth-century German criminal was not allowed a similar fate. As the surgeon was about to begin dissecting, he felt life in the body. According to the *Newgate Calendar,* he then said: "I am pretty certain, gentlemen, from the warmth of the subject and the flexibility of the limbs, that by a proper degree of attention and care the vital heat would return, and life in consequence take place. But when it is considered what a rascal we should again have among us, that he was hanged for so cruel a murder, and that, should we restore him to life, he would probably kill somebody else. I say, gentlemen, all these things considered, it is my opinion that we had better proceed in the dissection."[166]

As late as 1893, a French physician, Jean-Antoine Chaptal received a 5-hour-dead cadaver which he was preparing to dissect: "...at the first thrust of the scalpel into the cartilage that connects the ribs to the sternum, the cadaver lifted his right hand to his heart and feebly moved his head. The scalpel dropped from my hands, and I fled in terror."[167]

## S. HOW ARE BODIES PREPARED AS DISSECTION CADAVERS?

Adequately preserving bodies for dissection or parts of dissected bodies for demonstration to students has long been a problem.

Anatomists have used many methods to preserve specimens. When the anatomical museum of the British Royal College of Surgeons was founded, its original specimens were preserved in saltpeter, pitch or resin. Others used beeswax, tallow, resin, and turpentine, with coloring added to preserve a natural look. A slight modification, recalling ancient methods, was to use tar, salt, camphor and cinnamon. Two poisons, arsenious oxide and mercuric chloride were also tried. Dr. John Collins Warren, perhaps the first American to embalm anatomy specimens, used a mixture of rum, arsenic and corrosive sublimate. Some of his bodies remained well-preserved for up to eight years.[168] Once alcohol was introduced as a preservative, however, it became the standard for many years.

Formaldehyde, the current standard, was introduced in the nineteenth century, and today is usually used as formalin, a 40-percent solution. Formaldehyde preserves tissues by weakening tissue structures (precipitating proteins) and by destroying chemicals (enzymes) in the body's tissues.

Richard Selzer described bodies that had been prepared for and were awaiting anatomical dissection:

> Forty feet long, four wide, and seven deep is THE TANK. It is set into the ground at the very bottom of the medical school. If Anatomy be the firstborn of Medicine, then the tank is its sunken womb...It is lidded, covered by domed metal, handle at apex, like a casserole of chow mein.
>
> Let me remove this lid. Behold! How beautiful they are, the bodies. With what grace and pomp each waits his turn...forty soldiers standing in the bath, snug as pharaohs, only heads showing, all facing, obediently, the same way...
>
> We review these warriors who, by their bearing, salute us.[169]

The storage method described by Dr. Selzer is no longer common practice at most medical schools where bodies are usually embalmed and stored separately. Bodies for dissection are still, however, much more thoroughly embalmed than are those for funerals. Anatomical embalming uses stronger chemicals in a longer and more complex procedure that often takes from one to three days to complete. The anatomical embalming process may be done up to three times, with the first injection of embalming fluid similar to that in funeral homes, only using much more fluid. A second and usually a third injection of very potent embalming fluid follows. Since preservation of all tissues, rather than a good cosmetic result is the goal, the embalmer injects fluid until the body bloats from the excess liquid. Special injections assure that all parts of the body, such as the brain and lower legs are thoroughly preserved. At some medical schools embalmers also inject dyed latex into the blood vessels so students can more easily identify them during dissection.

According to Grant Dahmer, a chemist devoted to improving the preservation of anatomical teaching specimens, anatomists "don't have to cook the specimens or themselves with harsh chemicals" to provide students with a suitable cadaver. He has used a technique with only an extremely small amount of formaldehyde to successfully preserve anatomical cadavers at the Universities of Arizona, Oklahoma, and Texas. Not only were these specimens less toxic (about one-third of the formaldehyde level in the surrounding air as with the normal technique) but the tissues retained a more realistic color and were more supple.[170]

## T. WHY DISSECT CADAVERS?

Students dissect human cadavers primarily to learn human anatomy, but in the process they are also initiated into the mystique of medicine and many begin to see death as an abstract concept. Many different medical professionals dissect complete or partial cadavers or review dissected or prepared specimens as part of their education. Not only physicians and dentists dissect cadavers, but so do podiatrists, physical therapists, optometrists, medical illustrators and others.

For centuries, the anatomy taught by Galen in second-century A.D. Rome was used as gospel by medical practitioners, whom the Church banned from performing their own dissections. Unfortunately, Galen's writings were highly inaccurate and based on animal, rather than human, dissections. Susutra, the noted surgeon of sixth-century A.D. India, advocated that surgeons learn their craft through dissection of cadavers. His society frowned on this practice, however, and the Indian subcontinent saw little early anatomical study.[171]

Religious contemporaries of Galen did no better with their anatomical studies. In his *Glossa magna in Pentateuchum* (A.D. 210), Rabbi Oshaia said that humans had a bone called *Luz* that never died, just below their eighteenth vertebra. (The name of the bone was derived from *lus,* an old Aramaic word meaning "almond," but early German anatomists called this mystical bone *Judenknöchlein.*) This mystical "bone" could not be destroyed by fire, water, or any other element, nor could it be broken or bruised by any force. God was to use this bone as the nucleus for a new body during resurrection. Other bones would coalesce with it to form the new body. The body would rise from the dead once breathed upon by the divine spirit.[172] Modern anatomists have never been able to locate this structure.

The first semi-accurate anatomy text was Mondino de Luzzi's (aka, Mundinus), *Anathomia*, first published around 1316. It was later reprinted numerous times and became a European medical standard.[173] Subsequently, Antonio Pollaiuolo (ca. 1431-1498) and then other painters, dissected bodies to better represent anatomy in their works.[174] It was not, however, until Galen-basher Andreas Vesalius provided an accurate depiction of human anatomy in his *De Humani Corporis Fabrica* published in 1543, that many people abandoned their belief that a male had one less rib than a female, as described in *Genesis*.[175] His pioneering work, based on dissecting human bodies, made Italy the center of Western anatomical study in the sixteenth and seventeenth centuries. The currently better-known anatomical drawings of Leonardo da Vinci, whose work derived from dissecting at least thirty corpses, did not advance the study of anatomy, since they were hidden from public view until the late eighteenth century.[176]

Continental European medical schools began formal courses in anatomy with human dissection as early as 1340 (Montpellier) and the practice gradually spread: Lerida, 1391; Bologna, 1405; Padua, 1429; Vienna, 1435; and Tübingen, 1485.[177] It was only in the English-speaking countries of England, Scotland, Ireland and North America that anatomical dissection languished. Oxford and Cambridge did not officially recognize anatomical study until the sixteenth century—Caius College, Cambridge intermittently from 1557 until a Chair of Anatomy was established in 1707,[178] and Oxford in 1624. In 1506 the Edinburgh Guild of Surgeons and Barbers received permission to take one executed felon each year for anatomical study (along with their exclusive right to make and sell whiskey). Only in 1531 did David Edwardes write the first English anatomical text, briefly describing a dissection he had performed. By 1800, however, British authors had published more than 500 books on anatomy.[179]

Eventually, the study of anatomy became so fashionable among eighteenth- and nineteenth-century European nobility's pseudo-scientists, that many set up their own dissecting rooms at home. The Marquis de Sade even wrote about it in one of his lesser-known novels, *La Marquise de Gange* (1813). They obtained the bodies they anatomized, of course, from grave robbers.[180]

In the American Colonies, Drs. John Bard and Peter Middleton performed the first well-known dissection to instruct medical students in anatomy in 1750. They "anatomized" the body of Hermannus Carroll, executed for murder in Philadelphia, after injecting his blood vessels with colored dyes so they could be more easily studied.[181] Prior to that, however, at least four other "public anatomies" had occurred in the Colonies. The first was that of Julian, a Native American convicted of murder in the Boston area, in March 1733.[182]

In 1762, the European-educated Philadelphia physician, William Shippen, Jr. began the first series of regular anatomy classes in the colonies, using both models and ongoing dissections. The dissections, though, caused a minor riot since the city's populace believed that all dissections were associated with grave robbing, a practice he vehemently denied.[183] His was an independent school and his income depended on his students' fees. An advertisement for his classes read:

> Dr. Shippen's Anatomy Lectures will begin tomorrow evening at six o'clock, in his father's house, in Fourth Street. Tickets for the Course may be had of the Doctor at five Pistoles [gold coins] each and any gentlemen who incline to see the subject prepared for the lecture and learn the art of Dissecting, Injections, etc. are to pay five Pistoles more.[184]

The fascination with anatomy sometimes has been extreme, as was the case with William T. Morton, one of the first dentists to use ether as an anesthetic. He carried a skeleton with him on his honeymoon. His bride was startled when she awoke to find her groom studying the anatomy of the third-party, rather than hers, in their bed.[185]

In a recent high-tech twist in teaching anatomy, bodies are being computerized for study. Adam Software, Marietta, Georgia, was the first to make the representation of an entire body, available in a computer program, with parts that could be individually manipulated. Their CD-ROM-based program, ADAM[R] (Animated Dissection of Anatomy for Medicine) has been used to instruct both medical students and patients. EVE[R] is the title of the female version.[186] The U. S. National Library of Medicine, in a similar, but more elaborate endeavor, took the body of one man and one woman and sliced each into 1,000 pieces. Each slice is being recorded using computerized tomography (CT scan), magnetic resonance imaging (MRI), and standard photography.[187] This project will provide the first comprehensive digital record of the human body. Once this record is completed, medical students will be able to repeatedly study, rotate, or manipulate the images representing different body sections. This computerized record will take 50 gigabytes of storage. The cost for the project is $700,000.[188] What a way to be immortalized!

Since accurate anatomical texts and computer programs now exist, why do medical students continue to dissect cadavers? Of course they use dissection to learn anatomy and some very basic surgical techniques. But perhaps equally as important is that dissection teaches them to be clinically detached and to overcome the normal societal taboos and revulsion associated with mutilating people (dead, in this instance). As William Hunter, the famous eighteenth-century British anatomist said in his introductory lecture to medical students, "Anatomy is the Basis of Surgery, it informs the Head, guides the hand, and familiarizes the heart to a kind of necessary Inhumanity."[189]

A modern physician, Cecil Helman, points out:

In the dissecting room we come to realize the true paradox of anatomy. For the real agenda of dissection is the taming of Death, or rather the fear of Death. Because of this, we are asked to perform impossible alchemies. We must turn the cadaver into a three-dimensional textbook, a limited edition of tissues and organs...We must give to the body a posthumous life, through the rebirth of its parts.[190]

The anatomy lab also introduces medical students into medicine's guild. Dissecting a human body is a rite-of-passage that the rest of the world knows of, wonders at, and fears. As one medical student said, "When you talk to other people about it they are taken aback. They can't understand how you can do it. Having done it, it sets you apart. It's one of the biggest symbols of medical school...Anatomy is the one thing that medical students do that other people don't."[191]

The late comedian, Gilda Radner, wryly commented on the use of cadavers in physician education:

Doctors are whippersnappers in ironed white coats
Who spy up your rectums and look down your throats,
And press you and poke you with sterilized tools
And stab at solutions that pacify fools.
I used to revere them and do what they said
Till I learned what they learned on was already dead.[192]

Even countries whose religious laws frown on dissection realize the importance of physicians learning anatomy from first-hand experience. Students in Saudi Arabia, for example, study anatomy on corpses imported from non-Islamic countries.[193]

Anatomical dissection, however, is not an autopsy. A determination of the cause of death is not made by the dissectors, who are usually medical students too early in their careers to recognize most diseased tissues.

## U.  HOW DO MEDICAL STUDENTS DISSECT CADAVERS?

At one time, medical students dissected cadavers while fearing for their own lives. Early U. S. medical schools were often besieged by police and angry mobs incensed that cadavers were being "anatomized." The medical schools, however, had their own defense mechanisms.

The University of Maryland School of Medicine in Baltimore, for example, took elaborate precautions to protect their anatomists after angry citizens burned down Dr. John Beale Davidge's first Anatomy Hall in 1807.[194] In the succeeding anatomy building, they built secret passageways hidden behind the lecture halls where students could perform anatomical dissections. Large pictures disguised doorways to this area and massive iron doors, held closed by a giant latch-bar, guarded the building's main entrance. Other secret passageways exited onto nearby streets so students could make fast get-aways. Anatomy was taught in this elaborate amphitheater (the building is now a National Historic Landmark) from the early 1800s until the 1970s. (Medical students visiting the building today are warned to beware of ghosts. They are shown partially dissected sugar-cured anatomical specimens in the old passageways during their tour of this building.)

Other early anatomy schools were also destroyed by rioters. Mobs destroyed the Worthington Medical College in Ohio in 1839, McDowell Medical College in St. Louis in 1844, and forced the Willoughby Medical College in Ohio to relocate to Columbus in 1847.[195]

John Hunter, an early English anatomist, surgeon, and consort of body snatchers, equipped his home-school-anatomy lab with heavy shutters that bolted from the inside. He used these to protect him and his family from the often-angry mobs that gathered "with rope and torches, to scream for his blood."[196]

Until the mid-eighteenth century, experienced surgeons taught anatomy in the United States and Britain by dissecting bodies and showing models and diagrams. William Hunter, who ran a private anatomy school in London, introduced the "Parisian Method" of teaching. This method, now used in most Western medical schools, allowed each student to dissect portions of his own cadaver.

Early anatomy rooms were themselves not very pleasant. John Flint South described St. Thomas' dissecting room:

> The dissecting-room in 1813 was a squeamish room lighted by two windows eastward and a square lantern in the ceiling. The west end of the room was fitted from top to bottom with glass cases for preparations. A large fireplace and a copper vessel used to prepare the subjects for dissection, was on the south side; and a large leaden sink under the windows was indiscriminately used for washing hands and washing subjects and discharging all the filth. In this room were standing usually a dozen tables with their corresponding burdens, and six to eight pupils at each, so that on an average the room was crammed with 70 to 80 people, clad in filthy linen dissecting gowns, so that there was literally scarce possibility of moving.[197]

Today, a trip to a much cleaner, brighter, and roomier anatomy laboratory is part of the first day of medical school. The cadavers are laid out on individual metal tables which the medical students approach, usually very hesitantly, in groups of four—two on each side. Each pair is assigned to dissect one side of the cadaver. The students first cover the head, hands and feet with formaldehyde-soaked cloths and plastic bags to better preserve them for later dissection. This also serves the purpose of partially depersonalizing the corpse, since the body is now (temporarily) faceless. Since many of these students have never even seen a corpse outside of a funeral home, this can be a traumatic experience.

With this procedure behind them, the students turn their cadavers face-down and begin the dissection of the back muscles. Beginning the dissection here serves two purposes. The back is one of the least personal parts of the body and so is the least psychologically threatening to the students. And since these budding physicians have rarely, if ever, held a scalpel (correctly) to cut on human flesh, they can do the least amount of damage to important anatomical structures on the broad expanse of the back.

As one student reads instructions and information from the dissection guide, the other cuts. Under the watchful eyes of the instructors and following the intricate (and sometimes unfathomable) instructions in their dissection guide, the students proceed through the various body areas over a semester or more: back, external chest, arms and shoulders, legs, internal chest, abdomen, pelvis, feet, hands, and finally, the neck, face and head.

Cecil Helman describes his experience in the anatomy lab:

> The human remains lie on symmetrical rows of high stone slabs, while clusters of white-coated students sit on stools around them. Tutors move among the slabs, pointing, advising, cutting. There is the clink of scalpel on skull and bared bone. The greasy pages of someone's *Ellis's Anatomy* lie opened on a nose, a chest, a forehead. There is a shrill laugh somewhere in the formaldehyded air. On all sides you can hear the low Latin murmur, the catechisms of dissection—"latissimus dorsi, flexor pollicis longus, serratus anterior, the inferior vena cava."[198]

Students may have difficulty identifying anatomical structures, either because they inadvertently cut through them or, just as often, because of the wide variations in human anatomy. Some cadavers will not have structures the same size, in the same location, or identical to the pictures in the anatomical atlas. For example, there are numerous variations in the anatomy of some commonly diseased tissues, such as the gallbladder and its associated ducts. Few students can learn all of the thousands of potentially identifiable anatomical structures. However, by the time they complete their residencies seven to twelve years later, they will know the structures that are important in their area of medical practice. The study of anatomy gives them the basis for this practical knowledge.

As students get into the rhythm of identifying the name, location, and relation of each nerve, vessel, tendon, bone, and organ, they lose sight both of the cadaver as a former person and of their natural repugnance to dissection.[199] Late in the dissection process when the face is finally uncovered, however, the cadaver regains for a short interval a human identity with which the student must contend. This recognition quickly passes as they shave all of the hair and dissect away all facial structures.

The unneeded pieces of the cadaver that students remove are discarded into metal pails hanging on each table, to be cremated later. At the end of each anatomy session, the students either wet down the corpse with formaldehyde and cover the body or simply lower the body into its own tank of preservative. The dissection tables have lids that close over the cadavers; between classes the lab appears filled merely with stainless-steel cannisters. The formaldehyde smell, however, lingers on medical students throughout their entire dissection experience, often causing relatives, non-medical-student friends, and the other patrons in stores and movie theaters to move as far away from them as possible.

Practical examinations in anatomy traditionally use all of the cadavers in the anatomy lab. Each student holds a clipboard with an answer sheet containing perhaps 50 or 100 blanks. Standing singly or in pairs at each cadaver, they attempt to identify the anatomical parts their instructors have previously tagged. When a bell rings after one or two minutes, the students move on to the next cadaver, often with moans of frustration at not being able to identify the last item. Anatomical structures can be difficult to identify in cadavers that have become dry and stiff due to prolonged exposure, especially at the end of a school term. Some anatomists now improve a cadaver's condition before exams by spraying or soaking it in commercial fabric conditioner.[200]

Many students find anatomical dissection repulsive, although they understand its necessity, and often view anatomy as their most important first-year medical school course. They frequently feel that they are engaging in a fundamentally disrespectful activity, violating a corpse. They recognize that although the body is "no longer a human presence, it still reminds [them] of the presence which once was utterly inseparable from it."[201] Many medical students find that eating meat is distasteful while they are taking anatomy. A few even become vegetarians from that point on.

Medical students usually dissect a body respectfully, but some feel that the act of dissection itself removes the possibility of respecting a person's remains.[202] This, of course, is false since many if not most cadavers at U.S. medical schools are now donated specifically to teach new physicians their craft. Medical students use tales of macabre humor or horror to help them face the unusual task of dissecting a human body. This is typified by their common practice of naming cadavers and telling apocryphal tales.

Students often give their cadavers names to depersonalize them, although they also constantly discuss where the cadaver may have come from or what may have happened to it during life. Typical names include Abber Cadaver, Kay Daver, Ernest (so you can be "working in Ernest"), Stumpy (one-legged cadaver), and Anne Nomoly (anomaly). These names are often selected by dissection teams before they ever see their cadaver—truly a psychological defense measure.[203]

Medical students have also passed down five types of stories (which might be considered urban legends) about cadavers through at least most of this century. They include stories of students: (1) using anatomical parts to shock "civilians," such as to giving money to a bus driver using a cadaver's hand; (2) manipulating a cadaver's sexual organs to shock other medical students; (3) using part of the cadaver as food—again to terrify others; (4) dressing a cadaver to make it look like he is resurrected; and (5) having a student accidentally find that the cadaver is their recently dead relative or friend.[204] Nearly every physician has heard these stories as a medical student, but as with other urban legends, no one can point to an actual occurrence—except perhaps in literature, such as Edgar Allan Poe's tales. The stories serve as an emotional release for students who see their own vulnerabilities in their cadaver's humanity.[205]

Ernest Morgan, among others, has suggested that the *donor* can aid the development of medical students into physicians by reminding them that the cadaver was once a person. Unsigned and brief notes may be delivered to the students dissecting a body. One particularly good example of such a note is:

> I cannot know who you will be. As I write this you may be a young person in college or a child. You may not even be born. You will never know my name, but this does not matter. I am grateful in the knowledge that my body, when I shall no longer need it will, through your dedication and skill, once more serve mankind.[206]

The power of this type of personalization was brought home to me as a medical student when one dissection group was told that their cadaver had been a physician and another group was told that the young body (our age) they were dissecting was that of a leukemia victim who had been a premedical student before becoming ill. We then really understood that each of these bodies had a human history. Rev. William DeLong, former chaplain at the University of Arizona College of Medicine, held memorial services at the end of the anatomy course for the anonymous people whose bodies were the anatomical cadavers. His purpose was to "encourage us to recall our Anatomy experiences when treating future patients, because it will serve as a reminder of the humanity inherent in all people."[207]

## V. IN WHAT OTHER WAYS DO DOCTORS AND RESEARCHERS USE DEAD BODIES?

In addition to their use in transplants and dissections, cadavers or body parts are used to instruct medical personnel, to supply some rare substances, and for research.

Medical professionals have long used skeletons to help teach anatomy. Students in the health professions generally supplement book-learning with human skeletons prepared for anatomical study. These skeletons were once prepared (by companies that specialized in this) by first removing most of the flesh by boiling or other means and then using special scavenger beetles, *Dermestidae maculatus,* to remove any remaining flesh from the smallest crevices. These beetles, about ten millimeters long (about the size of a grain of rice), are still used to prepare animal skeletons, but the quicker process of prolonged boiling is used for most human specimens. Most bodies used as anatomical skeletons once came from India because they were inexpensive and readily available. (How these bodies were obtained was uncertain and was not questioned). In August 1985, however, the Indian government stopped the practice because they feared that graves were being robbed to obtain these bodies; plastic skeletons are now becoming more common. A real skeleton that sold in 1985 for $400 now costs more than $2,000. An anatomically correct plastic model sells for about $300.[208]

Physicians often practice new surgical procedures, such as laser surgery, on cadavers before they perform them on live patients—a much safer procedure than practicing on the living. This enables the surgeon and the entire surgical team to become familiar with the complexities of a new operation. It provides a dry run, so to speak. Surgical residents may also review specific areas of anatomy on cadavers before performing operations they have never done before (although they will have previously assisted on similar operations and normally have a senior surgeon present in the operating room).

Researchers also first test new medical devices in cadavers. Most of the catheters (tubes) physicians use to look at and to treat the heart, brain and intestines had their first non-animal insertions in cadavers. Most artificial joints, bone nails and other orthopedic appliances had similar tests in cadavers before being used in the living.

Physicians, paramedics and other health professionals involved in emergency and critical care often use fresh cadavers to practice and teach lifesaving skills, such as how to insert a breathing tube in the airway (intubate) or how to insert a catheter into a large vein in the neck or upper chest area. This training normally occurs immediately after death without notifying the deceased's relatives. The clinicians feel that this practice and instruction is essential to help save the lives of patients who need emergency care, that it does not disfigure the body, that the person whose body is being used owes this debt to future patients, and that having to ask permission for this training from grieving relatives whom they have never met would markedly decrease the frequency of this training.[209,210] Maryland's minimum requirement for certifying paramedics and cardiac rescue technicians, for example, is successfully intubating (putting a breathing tube into the airway) of either (1) recently dead cadavers, (2) computer-controlled manikins (*very* expensive), or (3) live patients, twice. One county (St. Marys) requires students to complete five recently dead cadaver intubations to be certified.[211]

The American Heart Association has endorsed the practice of using the newly deceased, especially small infants, to develop and to maintain a high level of skill in intubation.[212] Others advocate using cadavers, rather than live animals to practice and teach procedures.[213] Using cadavers to teach is also much safer than using live patients—as has been done when they are asleep in the operating room (a common practice in teaching hospitals, also usually done without informing the patient). Interestingly, when physicians have established a relationship with relatives of the deceased, they are often granted permission to practice non-invasive procedures, even in the case of deceased infants.[214]

Defending the ethics of practice and teaching on the newly dead, Callahan wrote, "...the reason that all arguments for harm and wrong to the dead must fail is that there simply is no subject to suffer the harm or wrong. Thus, there cannot be a good philosophical reason for holding that the dead can genuinely be harmed or wronged."[215]

Besides being used for instructional purposes, cadavers have also been the source of human hormones that could not be obtained in any other way. For many years pathologists routinely removed the pituitary gland, a pea-sized organ at the base of the brain, during autopsies. This gland provided human growth hormone for some children who otherwise would have been dwarfs and a fertility drug for some women. (Many years after receiving these preparations, some recipients in the U.S., Britain, France, Switzerland, New Zealand and Australia contracted Creutzfeldt-Jacob Disease, a deadly disease that creates holes in the brain and for which there is no cure.)[216] While today these hormones are synthesized, safe, and readily available, research scientists continue to use organs or tissues to extract other naturally occurring substances in an attempt to identify them and to synthesize them for therapeutic use.

Entire corpses are also used in several types of research. Throughout the ages, experiments on dead bodies as well as anatomical dissection have been the basis for medical advances. One of the first well-documented instances of this was William Harvey's treatise, *De moto cordis et sanguinis,* published in 1628, that proved that blood circulates. Part of his work came from autopsies he performed on his father and sister. Later, surgeons such as William Cheselden (bladder stone removal) and the Hunter brothers (aneurysms) developed early life-saving surgeries after experimenting on cadavers. Between 1789 and 1792 (when it was first publicly used) Dr.

Joseph-Ignace Guillotin tested his remarkable new beheading invention, the guillotine, on cadavers (a machine "which makes a Frenchman shrug his shoulders with good reason").[217,218]

Researchers still use cadavers in an unusual array of scientific experiments. At least since the 1970s and continuing to the present, various researchers have used cadavers of both adults and children as dummies to test the effects of car crashes and safety restraints on the human body. In some cases only the head or spine are used for the tests; in most, however, the entire body is involved. These studies have been conducted under the auspices of, among others, private research groups, universities, the U.S. Army, and the Department of Transportation. The Wayne State (Michigan) University's Bioengineering Center, The Medical College of Wisconsin, and the University of Virginia's automobile Safety Laboratory still perform such tests.[219] After the tests, each cadaver normally undergoes a complete autopsy including X-rays. While some researchers have stated that the cadavers were donated for medical purposes, this is not always explicit.[220-226] These studies have helped develop safer cars and safety devices, including seat belts, head restraints, air bags, and helmets. When the German news media revealed in late 1993 that Heidelberg University had used 200 cadavers (eight of them childrens' bodies) for these tests, however, the populace became enraged. Germany's largest automobile club denounced the tests, although Daimler-Benz, the company manufacturing Mercedes-Benz automobiles, defended these studies as being "unavoidable."[227]

Rather than using cadavers, though, most current crash tests use sophisticated, computerized body simulators. Recent studies have suggested, however, that the magnesium headform standardized by the American Society for Testing and Materials (ASTM) and used to test the efficacy of protective helmets, automobile safety devices, and other protective gear, fails to closely simulate the impact acceleration of the human head.[228] Researchers may have to go back to using human cadavers for some tests.

Cadavers have also been used to test weapons. As early as 1892 the U. S. Army tested the effect of bullets on different parts of cadavers' anatomies. Dr. Louis LaGarde, a pioneer in ballistics, performed early experiments on cadavers at Bellevue Hospital.[229] Later, he continued his tests at Philadelphia's Frankford Arsenal thus laying the groundwork for ballistic theories and the "improved" weapons used in modern battles. He initially found it difficult to shoot the exact area he wanted to examine, but found it easier once he suspended cadavers from their necks or heads using a block and tackle so that the area he wanted to shoot was in proper position.[230,231] The French Army had been firing into corpses to teach the effects of gunshot wounds to their medical personnel since about 1800.[232]

Between the Korean and Vietnam Wars, the U.S. Army obtained

## TABLE 3.10: Proposed Guidelines for Using "Brain Dead" Cadavers for Research

1. The dignity and humanity of the body should never be violated, even in the pursuit of the most valuable scientific knowledge.
2. The research must address an important clinical problem.
3. Subjects should be excluded if they are candidates for organ donation.
4. Subjects should be excluded if an autopsy to determine the cause of death is required.
5. The investigators should be prohibited from participating in deciding whether the patient meets the criteria for death and in terminating support systems.
6. Informed consent must be obtained from the next-of-kin; if the next-of-kin is not available, the research should not be conducted.
7. The death certificate must be signed before the experiment begins.
8. The materials to be injected must meet the same purity and production standards as would be required for an investigational new drug for human use under the Food and Drug Administration guidelines.
9. All procedures must be done in a manner identical to those that would be carried out on a living human.
10. Experiments should be designed to minimize the amount of time required for their completion.
11. This research should be reviewed by an Institutional Review Board (federally mandated group to review experiments involving human subjects) to ensure independent assessment by a disinterested and expert group, even though such a review is not legally required.
12. Any charges for the time or resources spent on "life-support" systems after the declaration of death should be paid for by the investigators, not by the patient or the patient's family or their insurance carrier.

Adapted from: Coller BS: The newly dead as research subjects. *Clinical Research.* 1989;37:487-94; and La Puma J: Discovery and disquiet: research on the brain-dead. *Ann Intern Med.* 1988;109:606-608.

cadaver legs and heads from the Baltimore medical examiner's office for field tests. Army experimenters used the legs, clad in routine-issue pants, socks and boots, to test the effect of land mines. The heads were put into newly designed helmets to see if they protected a real head as well as a dummy—they didn't, and many lives were probably saved because of these tests.[233] Tests on the effect of land mines continued through the Vietnam era.

Researchers now occasionally use some very fresh corpses to test new drugs. How fresh are these cadavers? These are cadavers that are dead by brain criteria but not usable as organ or tissue donors. They are still connected to ventilators that "breathe" for them and may have multiple medications being instilled to keep their blood pressure up and their other systems going. Some have suggested that these "living cadavers" be called *"neomorts"* (newly dead) to better designate their status.[234] As first conceived, neomorts "would have the legal status of the dead with none of the qualities one now associates with death. They would be warm, respiring, pulsating, evacuating, and excreting bodies requiring nursing, dietary, and general grooming attention—and could probably be maintained so for a period of years."[235] The term is now used for cadavers declared dead by brain criteria, but whose heart and lungs still function, usually with the aid of mechanical devices.

A number of pregnant women around the world have been kept on "life-support" after being declared dead by brain criteria.[236] Only those near term at the time of death have delivered a viable fetus. One may question, therefore, whether keeping brain-dead women with an early pregnancy on machines to keep their body functioning is not merely another form of research on neomorts, or perhaps, a political statement.

Using neomorts for research is still rare.[237-240] Their use, however, will certainly become more prevalent in the future, since there are many good reasons to test potentially dangerous drugs on the dead rather than on the living. In that case a set of guidelines, perhaps federally mandated, may need to be formulated. Some guidelines have been proposed for this use of the neomort for research. Table 3.10 lists a reasonable, although somewhat idealistic set of rules that could be used for this type of research. At present, they are the best available.

## W. REFERENCES

1. Kelly WD, Lillehei RC, Merkel FK, et al: Allotransplantation of the pancreas and duodenum along with the kidney in diabetic nephropathy. *Surgery.* 1967;61:827-37.
2. Stout H: Organ-transplant rates of survival are high in U.S. *Wall Street J.* September 16, 1992, p B-6.
3. Fox RC, Swazey JP: *Spare Parts: Organ Replacement in American Society.* New York: Oxford Univ Press, 1992, p 9.

4. Helman C: *The Body of Frankenstein's Monster: Essays in Myth and Medicine.* New York: W W Norton, 1991, pp 24-25.
5. The Living Bank. Houston, TX: 1992.
6. Uninformed next-of-kin thwarts donor process. *The Bank Account.* 1993;14(2):4.
7. Mathieu D: *Organ Substitution Technology.* Boulder, CO: Westview, 1988, p 37.
8. United Network for Organ Sharing (UNOS): *Protocols for Organ Donation.* June, 1991.
9. UNOS: *Protocols for Organ Donation.* March 1993.
10. Center for Biomedical Ethics: *Organ Transplantation.* Minneapolis, MN: Univ of Minnesota, 1992, pp 1-8.
11. UNOS, *Protocols,* June 1991.
12. Bond, W. Quoted in: Orndorff B: Wait for organs is fatal to many. *Richmond (VA) Times-Dispatch.* April 20, 1992.
13. Randall T: Too few human organs for transplantation: too many in need...and the gap widens. *JAMA.* 1990;265:1223-27.
14. UNOS, *Protocols,* June 1991.
15. Fox RC, Swazey JP: *The Courage to Fail: A Social View of Organ Transplants and Dialysis.* Chicago: Univ of Chicago Press, 1974, p 5.
16. Peters DA: Protecting autonomy in organ procurement procedures: some overlooked issues. *The Milbank Quarterly.* 1986;64:241-70.
17. Jardine DG: Liability issues arising out of hospitals' and organ procurement organizations' rejection of valid anatomical gifts: the truth and consequences. *Wisconsin Law Review.* Nov/Dec 1990, pp 1655-94.
18. Ibid.
19. Tolle SW, Bennett WM, Hickam DH, Benson JA: Responsibility of primary physicians in organ donation. *Ann Intern Med.* 1987;106:740-44.
20. Koop CE: Increasing the supply of solid organs for transplantation. *Public Health Rep.* 1983;98:566-72.
21. Anderson KS, Fox DM: The impact of routine inquiry laws on organ donation. *Health Affairs.* Winter 1988, p 65-78.
22. Slapak M: New ideas and techniques for vital organ procurement and exchange. *Transplantation Proc.* 1985;17:88-96.
23. Batten HL, Prottas JM: Kind strangers: the families of organ donors. *Health Affairs.* Summer 1987, p 35-47.
24. Riker RR, White BW: Organ and tissue donation from the emergency department. *J Emerg Med.* 1991;9:405-10.
25. Wakeford RE: Obstacles to organ donation. *Br J Surg.* 1989;74:436-39.
26. Batten, Prottas, *Health Affairs,* 1987.
27. Khanna PM: Scarcity of organs for transplant sparks a move to legalize financial incentives. *Wall Street J.* September 8, 1992, p B1.
28. Batten, Prottas, *Health Affairs,* 1987.
29. Helman, *Frankenstein's Monster,* p 25.
30. Painter K: Family key to organ donations. *USA Today.* March 31, 1993, p B1.
31. Ibid.
32. Testimony before the National Kidney Foundation. Atlanta, GA: February 1992.
33. UNOS, *Protocols,* March 1993.
34. Callender CO, Hall LE, Yeager CL, et al: Organ donation and blacks: a critical frontier. *N Engl J Med.* 1991;325:442-44.
35. Blacks: more kidney failure, fewer transplants. *Reuters News Service.* September 15, 1993.
36. *Bank Account.* 1993;14(2):4.
37. Callender et al, *N Engl J Med,* 1991.
38. Khanna, *Wall Street J,* September 8, 1992.
39. American Medical Association (AMA), Council on Ethical and Judicial Affairs: *Financial Incentives for Organ Procurement—Ethical Aspects of Future Contracts in Cadaveric Organs.* Presented at the AMA annual meeting. Chicago, IL: June 1993.
40. Iyer TKK: Kidneys for transplant—"opting out" law in Singapore. *Forensic Science International.* 1987;35:131-40.
41. Stuart FP, Veith FJ, Cranford RE: Death by brain criteria laws and patterns of consent to remove organs for transplantation from cadavers in the United States and 28 other

countries. *Transplantation.* 1981;31:238-44.
42. Roels L, Vanrenterghem Y, Waer M, et al: Three years experience with a 'presumed consent' legislation in Belgium: its impact on multi-organ donation in comparison with other European countries. *Transplantation Proc.* 1991;23:903-904.
43. Taylor RMR: Opting in or out of organ donation: the donor card is not dead, but it could benefit from some intensive care. *Br Med J.* 1992;305:1380.
44. Ibid.
45. Compulsory removal of cadaver organs. *Columbia Law Review.* 1969;69:693-705.
46. Sadler AM, Sadler BL: A community of givers, not takers. *Hastings Center Report.* 1984;14:6-9.
47. Katz BJ: Increasing the supply of human organs for transplantation: a proposal for a system of mandated choice. *Beverly Hills Bar Journal.* Summer 1984, p 152-67.
48. Iserson KV: Volutary organ donation: autonomy...tragedy. *JAMA.* 1993;270(16):1930.
49. Spital A: Mandated choice: the preferred solution to the organ shortage? *Arch Intern Med.* 1992;152:2421-24.
50. Spital A: Consent for organ donation: Time for a change. *Clin Transplantation.* 1993;7:525-528.
51. Ibid.
52. Egyptian condemned criminals can donate organs. *American Medical News.* August 17, 1992, p 34.
53. Sells RA: Traffic in organs. *Br Med J.* 1992;305:63.
54. Journal: Patients at Argentine hospital were killed for organs. *American Medical News.* May 18, 1992, p 11.
55. *World Press Review.* February 1992, p 4.
56. Film charges black market in human body parts. *Reuters News Service.* November 11, 1993.
57. Fruehling JA: *Sourcebook on Death and Dying.* Chicago: Marquis Prof Pub, 1982, p 243.
53. Pasic M, Gallino A, Carrel T, et al: 8euse of a transplanted heart. *N Engl J Med.* 1993;328;319-20.
59. Annas GJ: *The Rights of Patients.* 2nd ed. Carbondale, IL: Southern Illinois Univ Press, 1989, p 230.
60. UNOS, *Protocols,* June 1991.
61. Evans RW, Orians CE, Ascher NL: The potential supply of organ donors: an assessment of the efficiency of organ procurement efforts in the United States. *JAMA.* 1992;267:239-46.
62. Owen D: Rest in pieces. *Harper's.* June 1983, p 74.
63. Evans, Orians, Ascher, *JAMA,* 1992.
64. Annas, *Rights of Patients,* p 232.
65. Arizona Organ and Tissue Bank. Personal communication. May 1993.
66. Bernard HY: *The Law of Death and Disposal of the Dead.* 2nd ed. Dobbs Ferry, NY: Oceana, 1979, pp 57-58.
67. Mencken HL: Letter to Theodore Dreiser, October 30, 1922. Quoted in: Strauss MB, ed: *Familiar Medical Quotations.* Boston: Little Brown, 1968, p 24.
68. UNOS, *Protocols,* June 1991.
69. Green F: Death with dignity: Sikhism. *Nursing Times.* 1989;85(9):56-57.
70. Green F: Death with dignity: Judaism. *Nursing Times.* 1989;85(8):64-65.
71. Green F: Death with dignity: Baha'i Faith. *Nursing Times.* 1989;85(10):50-51.
72. Tendler M: A Jewish approach to ethical issues in death by brain criteria and organ transplantation. In: Kaufman HH: *Pediatric Death by Brain Criteria and Organ/Tissue Retrieval.* New York: Plenum, 1989, pp 31-34.
73. Pope Pius XII. As quoted in: Editors of Consumer Reports: *Funerals—Consumers' Last Rights.* New York: WW Norton, 1977, p 193.
74. Sugunasiri SHJ: The Buddhist view concerning the dead body. *Transplantation Proc.* 1990;22:947-49.
75. Childress JF: Protestant perspectives on organ donation. In: Kaufman, *Pediatric Death by Brain Criteria,* pp 45-53.
76. Green F: Death with dignity: Islam. *Nursing Times.* 1989;85(5):56-57.
77. Green F: Death with dignity: Zoroastrianism. *Nursing Times.* 1992;88(7):44-45.

78. Green F: Death with dignity: Rastafarianism. *Nursing Times.* 1989;85(9):40-41.
79. Iyer, *Forensic Science International,* 1987.
80. Peters DA: Organ Transplantation: issues and recommendations. *J Law Health.* 1988;3:28+.
81. Pallis CA: Death. In: *The New Encyclopaedia Britannica.* vol 16. 1987, p 1040.
82. Namihira E: Shinto concept concerning the dead human body. *Transplantation Proc.* 1990;22:940-41.
83. Kalish RA, Reynolds DK: *Death and Ethnicity.* Los Angeles: Ethel Percy Andrus Gerontology Center, Univ of Southern CA, 1976, p 42.
84. Wakeford, *Br J Surg,* 1989.
85. Spudis EV: Ms. Barfield: a neurologist's view (letter). *Neurology.* 1985;35:941.
86. Transplants down for LifeNet since AIDS scare. *Prodigy News Service.* April 30, 1992.
87. Drug may produce deadly brain disorder. *Prodigy News Service.* September 2, 1993. (from Reuters).
88. Tarasov MM: Cadaveric blood transfusion. *Ann NY Acad Sci.* 1960;87:512-21.
89. Pennell RB: Blood substitutes in the Soviet Union. *Transfusion.* 1969;9:167-68.
90. Vaughn J: Blood tranfusion in the U.S.S.R.: notes on a short visit. *Transfusion.* 1967:7:212-29.
91. Moore CL, Pruitt JC, Meredith JH: Present status of cadaver blood as transfusion medium. *Arch Surg.* 1962;85:364-70.
92. Death by brain criteria. *Br Med J.* 1975;1(15 February):356.
93. Youngner SJ, Arnold RM, and the Working Group on Ethical, Psychosocial, and Public Policy Implications of Procuring Organs From Non-Heart Beating Cadaver Donors: Ethical, psychosocial, and public policy implications of procuring organs from non-heart-beating cadaver donors. *JAMA* 1993;269:2769-74.
94. UNOS, *Protocols,* June 1991.
95. Iserson KV: Organ Procurement in the Acute Setting. In: Mathieu, *Organ Substitution Technology,* p 52-58.
96. UNOS, *Protocols,* March 1993.
97. Skolnick AA: Tissue bank expands facilities, efforts. *JAMA.* 1991;266:1329-32.
98. Ibid.
99. Ibid.
100. Crescenzo D, et al; Human cryopreserved valve conduits: a quantitative analysis of injury associated with variable warm ischemic time, antibiotic disinfection, and cryopreservation using transmission electron microscopy. 28th Annual Meeting, Soc Thoracic Surg. Orlando, FL: February 3-5, 1992.
101. UNOS, *Protocols,* June 1991.
102. Ibid.
103. Ibid.
104. Stiller CR: Ethics of transplantation. *Transplantation Proc.* 1985;17 (suppl):131-38.
105. Carlson L: *Caring For Your Own Dead.* Hinesburg, VT: Upper Access, 1987, p 45.
106. Yalof I: *Life and Death: The Story of a Hospital.* New York: Ballantine, 1990, pp 55-56.
107. Ann Landers Column. In: *Tucson (AZ) Citizen.* June 1, 1993, p B2.
108. National Selected Morticians (NSM) Resources: *A Helpful Guide to Funeral Planning.* (pamphlet). Evanston, IL: NSM, 1987, p 10.
109. Mayer R: *Embalming Techniques—Transplants and Trauma.* (lecture). National Funeral Directors Association (NFDA) Convention. Baltimore: 1989. (audiotape)
110. Raether HC: *The Funeral Director and his Role as Counselor.* (pamphlet). NFDA. Quoted in: Mitford J: *American Way of Death.* NY: Simon & Schuster, 1978, p 298.
111. Arvio RP: *The Cost of Dying and What You Can Do About It.* New York: Harper & Row, 1974, p 1-4.
112. UNOS, *Protocols,* June 1991.
113. Muyskens J: Should receiving depend upon willingness to give? *Transplantation Proc.* 1992;24:2181-84.
114. Ibid.
115. Peters DA, *J Law Health,* 1988.
116. Iyer, *Forensic Science International,* 1987.
117. National Kidney Foundation, Testimony, February 1992.

118. Barnett AH, Blair, Kaserman DL: Improving organ donation: compensation versus markets. *Inquiry.* 1992;29:372-78.
119. UNOS, *Protocols,* June 1991.
120. Englade K: *A Family Business.* New York: St. Martin's, 1992, pp 57-66, 117.
121. Asta LM: The body in question. *The New Physician.* September 1991, pp 13-17.
122. Ibid.
123. Fennel S, Jones DG: The bequest of human bodies for dissection: a case study in the Otago Medical School. *New Zealand Med J.* 1992;105:472-74.
124. Holmes, OW: Quoted in: Lassek AM: *Human Dissection: Its Drama and Struggle.* Springfield: Charles C Thomas, 1958, p 206.
125. Bland O: *The Royal Way of Death.* London: Constable, 1986, pp 153-54.
126. Asta, *The New Physician,* 1991.
127. *Holland v. Metalious* 198 A2d 654 (S Ct NH 1964).
128. Carlson, *Caring for Your Own Dead,* p 48.
129. Ibid., p 50.
130. Grollman EA, ed: *Concerning Death: A Practical Guide for the Living.* Boston: Beacon, 1974, pp 202-203.
131. Asta, *The New Physician,* 1991.
132. MacPherson P: Remembering the donation: memorial service honors those who gave their bodies to science. *American Medical News.* February 9, 1990, p 9.
133. Ibid.
134. Ibid.
135. Hill RB, Anderson RE: *The Autopsy—Medical Practice and Public Policy.* Boston: Butterworths, 1988, p 58.
136. Pike, JA. Quoted in: Mitford, *American Way Of Death,* p 246,
137. Asta, *The New Physician,* 1991.
138. Richardson R: *Death, Dissection and the Destitute.* London: Routledge & Kegan Paul, 1987, p 52.
139. Ibid., p 75-76.
140. Gelfand T: The "Paris manner" of dissection: student anatomical dissection in early eighteenth-century Paris. *Bull Hist Med.* 1972;46:99-130.
141. French Medical Saying. Quoted in: Strauss MB, ed: *Familiar Medical Quotations.* Boston: Little Brown, 1968, p 25.
142. Gelfand, *Bull Hist Med,* 1972.
143. Ariès P: *The Hour of Our Death.* New York: Oxford Univ Press, 1981, p 369.
144. Guttmacher AF: Bootlegging bodies—a history of body-snatching. *Bull Soc Med Hist Chicago.* 1935;4(4):353-402.
145. Ibid.
146. Ibid.
147. Richardson, *Death, Dissection and the Destitute,* p 106.
148. Schultz SM: *Body Snatching: The Robbing of Graves for the Education of Physicians.* Jefferson, NC: McFarland, 1992, p 8.
149. Richardson, *Death, Dissection and the Destitute,* p 369.
150. Ibid., p 262.
151. Ibid., p 259.
152. Ibid., p 290.
153. Sadler, Sadler, *Hastings Center Report,* 1984.
154. Adams N: *Dead and Buried?* Aberdeen, Scotland: Impulse Books, 1972, pp 79-80.
155. Richardson, *Death, Dissection and the Destitute,* p 62.
156. Ibid., p 80-81.
157. Ibid., p 57.
158. Ibid., p 62.
159. Iserson KV: Strangulation—a review of ligature, manual, and postural neck compression injuries. *Ann Emerg Med.* 1984;13(3):179-85.
160. Schultz, *Body Snatching,* p 96.
161. *Stowe's Annals,* 1587. Quoted in Adams, *Dead and Buried?,* p 22.
162. Puckle, BS: *Funeral Customs—their Origin and Development.* London: T Werner Laurie, 1926, p 25.

KENNETH V. ISERSON

163. Gordon R: *Great Medical Disasters.* New York: Dorset Press, 1983, p 208.
164. Adams, *Dead and Buried?,* p 23.
165. Haestier R: *Dead Men Tell Tales: A Survey of Exhumations, From Earliest Antiquity to the Present Day.* London: John Long, 1934, p 130.
166. Adams, *Dead and Buried?,* p 25.
167. Chaptal JA. Quoted in: Ariès, *Hour of Our Death,* pp 362-63.
168. Schultz, *Body Snatching,* p 19.
169. Selzer R: *Mortal Lessons: Notes on the Art of Surgery.* New York: Simon & Schuster, 1987, p 134.
170. Dahmer G: Personal Communication. Tucson, AZ: November 5, 1993.
171. Spiro RK: A backward glance at the study of postmortem anatomy. *International Surgery.* 1971;56(1):27-40.
172. Pallis, Death, p 1037.
173. Spiro RK, *International Surgery,* 1971.
174. Schultz, *Body Snatching,* pp 1-2.
175. Clendening L: *Source Book of Medical History.* Mineola, NY: Dover, 1960, p 122.
176. Richardson, *Death, Dissection and the Destitute,* p 32.
177. Russell KF: Anatomy and the barber-surgeons. *Medical J Australia.* 1973;1:1109-15.
178. Ibid.
179. Ibid.
180. Ariès, *Hour of Our Death,* pp 366-68.
181. Hosack D: Sketch of the origin and progress of the medical schools of New York and Philadelphia. *American Medical & Philosophical Register.* 1812;4 (July):307-11.
182. Schultz, *Body Snatching,* p 13.
183. Gillett MC: *The Army Medical Department; 1775-1818.* Washington, DC: Center of Military History, U.S. Army (GPO), 1981, p 19.
184. Advertisement in *The PA Gazette.* November 16, 1762. As quoted in: Coffin MM: *Death in Early America: The History and Folklore of Customs and Superstitions of Early Medicine, Funerals, Burials, and Mourning.* Nashville: Thomas Nelson, 1976, p 33.
185. Ibid., p 189.
186. Greengard S: Taking a computerized tour through the human body. *American Medical News.* 1993;36(18):27-28.
187. Finding Adam and Eve. *Prodigy News Service.* December 16, 1992.
188. Wanted: 2 perfectly normal bodies. *Prodigy News Service,* January 11, 1993. (reporting on a *Scientific American* article.)
189. Hunter, W. Quoted in: Richardson, *Death, Dissection and the Destitute,* p 30-31.
190. Helman, *Frankenstein's Monster,* p 117.
191. Hafferty FW: *Into the Valley: Death and Socialization of Medical Students.* New Haven, CT: Yale Univ Press, 1991, p 53.
192. Radner G: Unititled poem. *SHHV Student Bulletin.* Knoxville, TN: Society for Health and Human Values, 1991;2:2.
193. Pallis, Death, p 1040.
194. Schultz, *Body Snatching,* p 46.
195. Ibid., p 47-48.
196. Franklin J, Sutherland J: *Guinea Pig Doctors.* New York: Wm Morrow, 1984, p 30.
197. Felton CT: *Memorials of John Flint South.* London: T Murray, 1884. Quoted in: Guttmacher, *Bull Soc Med Hist Chicago,* 1935.
198. Helman, *Frankenstein's Monster,* p 115.
199. Kass LR: Thinking about the body. *Hastings Center Report.* 1985;15:20-30.
200. Blaney SPA, Johnson B: Technique for reconstituting fixed cadaveric tissue. *Anatomical Record.* 1989;224:550-51.
201. Hill, Anderson, *The Autopsy,* p 8.
202. Kass, *Hastings Center Report,* 1985.
203. Hafferty, *Into the Valley,* pp 55-58.
204. Ibid.
205. Ibid., pp 58-65.
206. Morgan E: *A Manual of Simple Burial.* Burnsville, NC: Celo Press, 1966, p 54.
207. DeLong, Rev. William: Personal Communication. January 1993.

106

208. Noonan P: Oh, dem bones. *OMNI.* May 1991, p 28.
209. Iserson KV: Requiring consent to practice and teach using the recently dead. *J Emerg Med.* 1991;9(6):509-10.
210. Iserson KV: Postmortem procedures in the emergency department: using the dead to practise and teach. *J Medical Ethics.* 1993;19(2):92-98.
211. State of Maryland EMS Division. Personal Communication. June 4, 1993.
212. American Heart Association Emergency Cardiac Care Committee and Subcommittees: Guidelines for cardiopulmonary resuscitation and emergency cardiac care. Part 8: Ethical Considerations. *JAMA.* 1992;268(16):2282-88.
213. Ellis RE: Use cadavers, not dogs for training (letter). *American Medical News.* May 3, 1993, p 21.
214. Benfield DG, Flaksman RJ, Lin TH, et al: Teaching intubation skills using newly deceased infants. *JAMA.* 1991;265:2360-63.
215. Callahan JC: On harming the dead. *Ethics.* 1987;97:341-52.
216. Study cites people injected with hormones from corpses. *Reuters News Service.* October 1, 1993.
217. Bierce A: *Devil's Dictionary.* New York: Dover Publications, 1958, p 50.
218. Gordon, *Great Medical Disasters,* p 149.
219. Clements M: Corpses used in automobile crash tests. *USA Today.* November 26, 1993, p B1.
220. Pritz HB: Comparison of the dynamic responses of anthropomorphic test devices and human anatomic specimens in experimental pedestrian impacts. *Proc 22nd Stapp Car Crash Conf.* Soc Automotive Engineers, 1978, pp 341-57.
221. Kallieris D, Barz J, Schmidt G, et al: Comparison between child cadavers and child dummy by using child restraint systems in simulated collisions. *Proc 20th Stapp Car Crash Conf.* Soc Automotive Engineers, 1976, pp 513-42.
222. Hu AA, Bean SP, Zimmerman RM: Response of belted dummy and cadaver to rear impact. *Proc 21st Stapp Car Crash Conf.* Soc Automotive Engineers, 1977, pp 587-635.
223. Jones AM, Bean SP, Sweeney ES: Injuries to cadavers resulting from experimental rear impact. *J Forensic Sciences.* 1978;23:730-44.
224. Kallieris D, Mattern R, Härdle W: Belastbarkeitsgrenzen und Verletzungsmechanik der angegurteten Fahrzeuginassen beim Seitaufprall. *FAT-Schriftenreihe.* 1986;2:60.
225. Allsop DL, Perl TR, Warner CY: Force/deflection and fracture characteristics of the tempero-parietal region of the human head. *Proc 35th Stapp Car Crash Conf.* Soc Automotive Engineers, 1991, pp 269-78.
226. Yoganandan N, Skrade D, Pintar FA, et al: Thoracic deformation contours in a frontal impact. *Proc 35th Stapp Car Crash Conf.* Soc Automotive Engineers, 1991, pp 47-63.
227. Crash tests used cadavers. *Associated Press.* November 23, 1993.
228. Lewis LM, Naunheim R, Pittman T, et al: A comparison between magnesium headforms and instrumented human cadaver heads in measuring peak accelerations of impact (abst). *Ann Emerg Med.* 1993;22:900.
229. Douglas Lindsey, MD, DrPH (Col, U.S. Army Medical Corps., ret.). Interview. Tucson, AZ: May 1992.
230. LaGarde LA: *Gunshot Injuries: How They are Inflicted, Their Complications and Treatment.* New York: William Wood, 1914, pp 41-43, 68.
231. LaGarde LA: *Preliminary Report of a Board of Officers.* Convened October 16, 1903, Springfield Armory, Springfield, MA.
232. LaGarde, *Gunshot Injuries,* p 42.
233. Douglas Lindsey, Interview, June 1, 1993.
234. Gaylin W: Harvesting the dead—the potential for recycling human bodies. *Harpers Magazine.* 1974:9:28.
235. Ibid.
236. Seibert S, Waldrop T, Marshall R: A matter of death and life. *Newsweek.* November 16, 1992, p 55.
237. Fost N: Research on the brain dead. *J Pediatrics.* 1980;96;54-56.
238. Coller BS: The newly dead as research subjects. *Clin Research.* 1989;37:487-94.
239. Robertson JA: Research on the brain-dead. *IRB: Rev Human Sub Res.* 1980;2:4-6.
240. Martyn SR: Using the brain dead for medical research. *Utah Law Review.* 1986, pp 1-28.

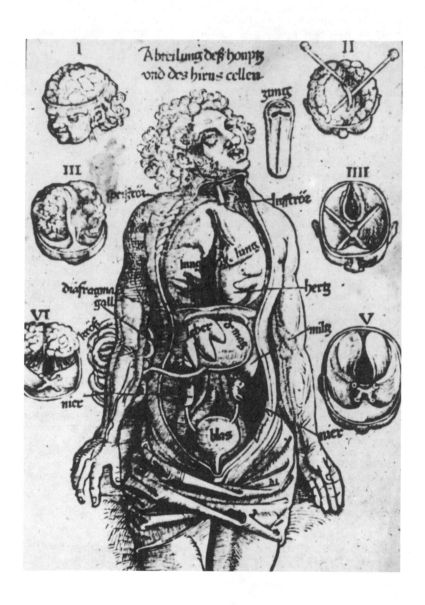

An anatomical drawing. Originally published by Lorenz Fries: *Speigl der Artzny,* Straszburg: Getruckt von Johanni Grieninger, 1519. (Reproduced with permission. National Library of Medicine.)

# 4: MY BODY AND THE PATHOLOGIST: THE AUTOPSY

A. What is a morgue and how long will my body be there?
B. How do nurses prepare bodies for the morgue?
C. What if I die at home?
D. What is an autopsy and who performs it?
E. Why do an autopsy?
F. Will I have an autopsy?
G. Who gives permission for an autopsy?
H. After an autopsy, can I still be embalmed?
I. Why doesn't everyone get autopsied?
J. How is an autopsy done?
K. How do autopsy techniques vary?
L. Are autopsies harmful to pathologists?
M. What is a medical examiner/coroner?
N. How long have physicians been doing medicolegal autopsies?
O. What is special about a medicolegal autopsy?
P. Why is an autopsy done on a decomposing or dismembered body?
Q. How can a person be identified from partial or decomposed remains?
R. What happens if they cannot identify my body?
S. How is the time of death determined?
T. What happens to the organs and tissues examined at autopsy?
U. What is an exhumation?
V. What happens to miscarried fetuses and stillborn infants?
W. What are common religious views about autopsies?
X. How do I get the autopsy report?
Y. What does an autopsy cost?
Z. References

*This chapter sheds a little light into the morgue. How and on whom are autopsies performed? What special techniques do pathologists and medical examiners use? How do pathologists perform routine hospital autopsies? How do these differ from the investigations and autopsies performed by the medical examiner (e.g. Quincy)? Can the pathologist really determine an accurate time of death? What do pathologists really do at the scene of major disasters? How do individuals get copies of autopsy reports?*

## A. WHAT IS A MORGUE AND HOW LONG WILL MY BODY BE THERE?

The *Morgue*, first called the *Châtelet*, was originally the name of a vacant butcher shop in Paris where authorities often displayed bodies to the public for identification. (Street murders in eighteenth-century Paris were very common.)[1]

Today, morgues are places where bodies are stored temporarily until their final dispositions are decided. For convenience, hospitals usually locate their morgues in the basement, adjacent to the autopsy room. The modern morgue is a large room with tile floors, tile covering at least halfway up the walls, stainless-steel tables, operating room sinks, and refrigerators. While the original morgue-type corpse cooler (see illustration, p. 444), patented by Charles Kimball in 1868, was a large refrigerator with one compartment for the body, the other for ice, modern morgue refrigerators are built into the wall with stainless steel doors and trays.[2] The trays slide out so bodies can be easily loaded, unloaded, and exhibited for identification. Morgue refrigerators are kept at 2°C to 8°C (35.6°F to 46.4°F). Corpses do not visibly deteriorate for four days or longer if they are adequately refrigerated. Due to limited space, hospitals try to limit the time that bodies are in their morgues, encouraging morticians to quickly remove bodies after death, autopsy, or organ donation. Medical examiners also try to quickly empty their morgues, since more bodies continually arrive.

When funeral home workers "remove" a corpse from a hospital morgue in the United States, the morgue attendant opens the morgue and identifies the correct body. Before the days of individual pagers, attendants were often audibly paged as *Mr. Post* (as in *post*mortem). A gratuity often speeds the process.

Disasters causing multiple deaths often require temporary morgues, which may take many forms. During the 1977 Beverly Hills Supper Club fire in northern Kentucky, rescue workers laid 150 bodies dressed in their evening finery in a temporary morgue on the grass of the outdoor wedding chapel. They laid there until the still-raging fire threatened to engulf them. After airplane crashes, disaster workers commonly use airplane hangers as morgues, often with adjacent refrigerated trucks (sometimes from food

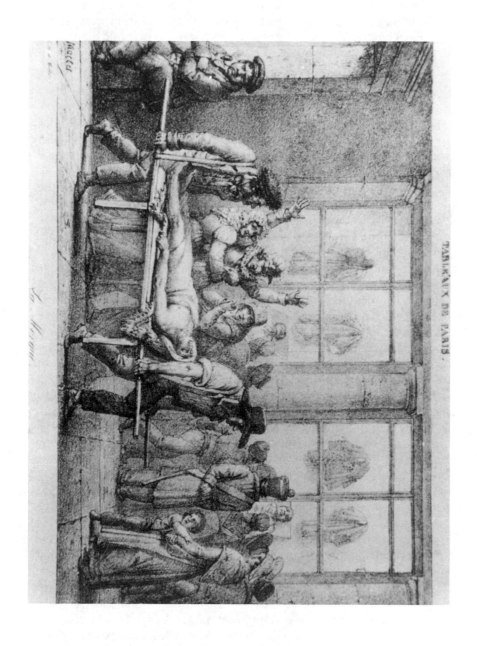

*Le Morgue.* Originally published by Jean Henri Marlet: *Tableaux de Paris,* 1840. (Reproduced with permission. National Library of Medicine.)

111

wholesalers) to preserve the bodies while they are processed.[3] Hangers provide the forensic teams with the large areas they need to process bodies and pieces of bodies. They use the morgue to X-ray the parts, do dental and fingerprint examinations for identification, autopsy bodies, and embalm them when possible.

## B.  HOW DO NURSES PREPARE BODIES FOR THE MORGUE?

Between 1930 and 1950 the usual place of death in the United States shifted from home to the hospital, nursing home, and hospice. In these institutions, doctors and other high-status health care workers rarely touch a body once they terminate a resuscitation attempt or declare a person dead. Other health care workers sometimes avoid both the work and the unpleasantness of dealing with death and dead bodies by letting the next shift "discover" a death.[4]

In the United States, nurses traditionally prepare the corpse for transport to the hospital morgue.[5] The nurse first cleans the body of any excreta and sometimes bathes the entire corpse. Then, using a tongue depressor, she packs the rectum and often the vagina with cotton batting. If the patient had dentures, she inserts them into the mouth and closes the corpse's mouth and eyes. Although nurses still tie the jaw closed and the hands together before they transfer a body to the morgue, medical examiners dislike this practice since it leaves marks that may distort their autopsy findings. Embalmers also dislike these ties, facetiously suggesting an award for the nurse who can most distort the face or hands by tying them tightly.[6] The nurse then covers the body with a sheet or a paper drape. The drape, sometimes contained in a "mortuary pack," fits over the head, extends the length of the body, and ties around the legs. They attach an identifying tag to the great toe, often with a "twisty." Recently, many hospitals have diminished the nurse's role in what the British call "last offices," cleaning or shrouding the corpse. While some nurses feel that these actions are rightfully the mortician's responsibility, others argue that performing them actually helps the nurse, who then has a chance to grieve for her patient.[7]

Attendants then place the corpse in a vinyl, zippered body-bag. This complicates embalmers' work since the plastic retains the body's heat and makes the corpse "sweat." In some hospitals nurses then transport the bodies to the morgue, although in large facilities this is now done by in-house morticians or morgue attendants. They transport the cadaver on a stretcher with a false top or a covering that makes it appear to be simply a large, rectangular wheeled container. Sometimes called a "cadaver carrier," this disguise prevents patients, relatives and staff from being disturbed by the sight of a corpse being pushed through the halls.

Emergency department nurses do much less corpse preparation. This is partly due to medical examiners' restrictions that prohibit the removal of disposable equipment from the corpse, excess cleaning of the corpse, or manipulations of the body that might cloud autopsy findings. (The mechanism or timing of death puts most emergency department deaths within the medical examiner's domain.) Emergency department nurses only remove nondisposable medical equipment and cover the body with a sheet. If relatives will view the deceased patient in the emergency department, the nurses also clean the corpse's face and hands.

Operating room nurses rarely deal with cadavers except for the bodies of organ donors. Any death in an operating room immediately comes not only within the medical examiner's jurisdiction, but also under the scrutiny of multiple hospital review committees. Surgeons and anesthesiologists assiduously try to avoid this administrative burden, and the associated paperwork, by attempting to keep patients alive until they at least get out of the operating room. New rules, however, have extended medical examiners' oversight jurisdiction to deaths which occur within 24 hours of surgery.[8]

Hospital personnel must be sensitive to the special corpse handling that some religions require. Hindus, for example, frown on non-Hindus touching the body, so non-Hindu nurses or morticians must wear disposable gloves. The corpse must be wrapped, unwashed and with jewelry or sacred objects intact, in a plain sheet without religious emblems.[9] Muslims want attendants, immediately after death, to tie a corpse's jaw closed and straighten the body after first flexing the large joints of the shoulders, hips, elbows, and knees. Muslims also want the corpse's head turned toward the right shoulder, so the body can face Mecca when buried. Attendants may wash the body, but only after they completely cover it with a white sheet.[10]

## C. WHAT IF I DIE AT HOME?

Home deaths must be reported to the appropriate authorities.

In ideal circumstances, relatives first notify a physician of the death. He or she agrees to sign the death certificate, and then the family contacts a mortuary. The medical examiner takes control of the body if no physician is willing to sign the death certificate or if the circumstances of death make his office legally responsible. (See *What is a medical examiner/coroner?*)

Most bodies are then transported either to the medical examiner's office or directly to the funeral home/crematorium. If the medical examiner is involved, his workers remove the body. A mortician later collects the body from the medical examiner's office.

But if one calls the emergency line (911 in most U.S. jurisdictions) ambulance personnel *must* attempt resuscitation on patients who are not *clearly* dead. Many people have had ambulance personnel attempt unwanted resuscitations on their loved ones after simply trying to notify authorities of a death.[11,12]

For this reason, many members of the Hemlock Society recommend that relatives wait ninety minutes or more after a death to notify authorities. If the home is warm, however, it is prudent to turn off the heat or run an air conditioner so that the body does not quickly begin to decompose. Since most people do not feel comfortable around a corpse, they also suggest that survivors should leave home for that time period. When officials arrive about two hours after death, *livor mortis* (pooling of blood in the vessels in the lowest parts of the body) will be evident, indicating that they should not attempt resuscitation.

Some states, such as Arizona, Connecticut, Colorado, Montana and New York have statewide protocols whereby individuals can prevent unwanted resuscitation through "prehospital advance directives." They are a type of living will which is recognized by ambulance personnel.

When removing a body from the home, funeral directors carefully stage the event so that they appear to show respect for the corpse. They refer to the deceased by name and gently manipulate the body, treating it reverently. After placing the corpse's hands carefully at its sides, they cover the body with a nice sheet and quietly snap and cinch the straps holding the body on the stretcher. They then quietly close the stretcher cover and gently move the stretcher out of the home. This contrasts markedly with the way they handle a body when no onlookers are present. They then swing the body onto the stretcher, yank the straps tightly, and cavalierly propel the stretcher toward the hearse.

Once a funeral home takes possession of a body, it very rarely transfers it to another local funeral home. For this reason, the United States Federal Trade Commission (FTC) says that the choice of the funeral home to be used for body "removal" is "the most critical decision which a bereaved consumer must make, and the decision with the tightest time strictures...in many instances a consumer may be called upon to select a funeral home on extremely short notice, wholly unexpectedly. The consumer has no time to plan or to arrange finances, or to put the purchase off until a better time. If the home selected does not offer the particular goods or services desired by the consumer, essentially all options have been foreclosed."[13]

Since the Funeral Rule (Appendix I) went into effect in April 1984, however, funeral homes must promptly relinquish or transfer bodies at a family's request.

In many parts of the world, bodies can be prepared and viewed at home. In the Netherlands, for example, the only legal requirement is for an official to seal the casket. Rather than embalming, they use cooling tables or "koeltafels" to preserve bodies for home viewing. If a Dutch body goes to the morgue and no family members are present, an individual who nursed the person at home accompanies the body to the morgue to ensure a chain-of-custody.[14]

114

## D. WHAT IS AN AUTOPSY AND WHO PERFORMS IT?

In an autopsy, also known as necropsy or postmortem examination, the physician dissects a corpse to determine, if possible, a cause of death and, sometimes, to add to medical knowledge. "Autopsy" comes from the Greek, *autopsia*, which means seeing with one's own eyes. Autopsies are performed by pathologists, physicians who specialize in the anatomy of the human body.

In the modern autopsy, pathologists not only remove and inspect the major organs, but also use all of the sophisticated tools of modern medicine to analyze body fluids, tissues and cellular components.

There are three levels of autopsy: (1) *Complete*—in which all body cavities, including the head, are exposed for examination; (2) *Limited*—which generally excludes the head; and (3) *Selective*—in which the physician examines only one or more organs of special interest.

The autopsy only gradually developed into its present form as an important medical tool. Greek physicians performed autopsies as early as the fifth century B.C., although Hippocratic writings described the procedure as "an unpleasant, if not cruel, task." The famous Egyptian physicians Herophilus and Erasistratus used autopsies to teach anatomy and pathology between 350 and 200 B.C. in Alexandria. They supposedly obtained criminals "for dissection alive, and contemplated, even while they breathed, those parts which Nature had before concealed."[15] Galen, the famous second-century A.D. Greek physician, first correlated findings in life with those after death through autopsy. Unfortunately, most of his autopsies were performed on animals. Doctors who followed the Roman legions, however, autopsied dead barbarians after battles.

Christian Europe generally frowned on autopsies throughout the Middle Ages. The Council of Tours (1163) stated that "the church abhors blood," suggesting that physicians, most of whom were clergy, should abstain from both autopsies and surgeries. When Pope Alexander V died suddenly in 1410, however, physicians performed an autopsy to determine whether his successor had poisoned him; they did not find any evidence for that. Subsequently, Pope Sixtus IV (1471-1484) permitted medical students at Bologna and Padua to open plague-ridden bodies to search for the cause of this fearful disease.

The first reported autopsy in the New World was performed on July 19, 1533 in Santo Domingo, on the island of Hispaniola. Its purpose was ostensibly religious—to determine whether a set of Siamese twins had one soul or two, so the priest would know how many postmortem baptisms to perform. Johan Camacho, the surgeon-dissector found evidence to support two souls and two baptisms were performed. He said "they had everything that is to be found in two human bodies...[except that]...the livers were joined one to the other, with, however, a furrow or line between the two which clearly showed the part that belonged to each."[16] The babies' father refused to pay for both, though, saying "as far as he was concerned, a single soul was enough."[17]

The next reported autopsies in the Americas were performed at the insistence of the French explorer, Samuel de Champlain. While exploring the St. Croix River (which now divides Maine and Canada) in 1605, his party developed scurvey. He ordered his surgeons to repeatedly dissect the dead to determine the cause of this deadly disease.[18] While they accurately recorded their findings, their autopsy could not reveal that the deaths were due to a vitamin C deficiency.

An early autopsy in the American Colonies was ordered by the General Court in Hartford, Connecticut in 1662. Consistent with the times, the autopsy was performed at the graveside of an 8-year-old girl to determine whether she had died of witchcraft. (We can now tell from the autopsy record that her death was due to upper airway obstruction, probably caused by diphtheria or epiglottitis. The dissector, Dr. Rossiter, wrote "The gullet or swallow was contracted like a hard fish bone that hardly a large pease could be forced through."[19]) The suspected witch, Goody Ayers, fled the colony.[20]

In 1769, the Italian physician, Giovanni Batista Morgagni (1682-1771) published *De Sedibus et Causis Morborum per Anatomen Indagatis (The Seats and Causes of Diseases Investigated by Anatomy)*. This was the first comprehensive pathology text, correlating autopsy findings with clinical disease, thereby giving rise to the specialty of anatomic pathology (which trains physicians who perform autopsies).

The first English pathology texts were Matthew Baillie's *Morbid Anatomy* (1793) and John Hunter's (he of body-snatching fame) *A Treatise on the Blood, Inflammation, and Gun-Shot Wounds* (1794).[21] Rudolf Virchow (1821-1902), advanced the science of pathology with his *Cellular Pathology* (1858), which added descriptions of the microscopic appearance of diseased tissues and cells to gross visual observations.

Into the early twentieth century, many physicians performed autopsies on their own patients, often at the deceased's residence. Both William Osler, the most renowned of modern physicians, who died in 1919, and Beethoven, who died in 1827, were autopsied in their own homes.[22]

Eventually, the medical specialty of anatomical pathology (and later forensic pathology) arose. One role of these specially trained physicians is to perform autopsies, and few other U.S. physicians now do the procedure. A traditional medical maxim describes the physician's view of the pathologist:

> The psychiatrist knows everything and does nothing.
> The surgeon knows nothing and does everything.
> The dermatologist knows nothing and does nothing.
> The *pathologist* knows everything but is always a day too late.

This suggests that, due to the nature of their work, pathologists are sometimes set apart from other physicians. Richard Selzer described the modern image of an anatomical pathologist:

> The best place to see a pathologist is in the basement of a medical school. ...Among these dews and damps, he nethers, shouldering from tank to slab and back again, his eyes hooded, and always in hand a bottle or tray the contents of which are best left unspecified. Where he passes, a chill gathers; you catch the rank whiff of formaldehyde.[23]

Yet pathology has become the most exacting of medical specialties, using breakthroughs in all scientific areas to advance its understanding of disease processes.

## E. WHY DO AN AUTOPSY?

The primary reason for an autopsy is to determine the cause of death.

Autopsies also ensure quality control in medical practice, help confirm the presence of new diseases or the recurrence of old and unsuspected diseases, educate new physicians, and enhance the investigation of criminal activity (Table 4.1). A survey of Kansas hospitals found that autopsy results are actually used for multiple purposes. More than 68% of the hospitals used autopsy results to assess their physicians' quality-of-care. They also found that 47% of the autopsies at these hospitals were used in clinical conferences, 38% in departmental reviews, 17% in organ procurement, 15% in other teaching, 9% in research, and 23% for other reasons including family or physician curiosity and medicolegal uses.[24]

As Angrist said, "The autopsy is the moment of truth for all medical care and the time of reckoning to improve the care of the patient...It becomes a stimulus and incentive for better care and increases both empathy and science in medicine...It crystallizes errors, exposes abuses and points out fads and fancies."[25]

Pathologists mainly use the autopsy to determine the cause of death. This also acts as a quality control, identifying physicians who repeatedly diagnose or treat the wrong diseases. John Stone extracted the essence of the autopsy in his poem, *Autopsy in the Form of an Elegy:*

> In the chest
> in the heart
> was the vessel
>
> was the pulse
> was the art
> was the love

117

was the clot
small and slow
and the scar
that could not know

the rest of you
was very nearly perfect.[26]

Modern techniques of clinical medicine have not, as some believe, assured that a correct diagnosis will always be made. One extensive 1967 study found that the actual cause of death as found at autopsy correlated only about *half* of the time with the cause of death listed by the patient's physician. This was a study of all in-hospital deaths over a six-month period.[27] Advanced medical techniques and impressive medical technology have not helped much. Today, more than one-third of patients autopsied still have discrepancies between their clinical and autopsy diagnoses that may have adversely affected their survival.[28] In some cases, over-reliance on new technologies has actually led to missed diagnoses. Because doctors rely on these technologies, such as lung scans, to be definitive, other back-up diagnosis techniques are seldom used to confirm negative results. As a result of this phenomenon, only about half of the blood clots to the lung are diagnosed before death (the correct diagnosis drops dramatically after age 40),[29] as are only about half of all heart attacks, half of all abdominal infections (peritonitis), and about two-thirds of all intestinal hemorrhages, lung abscesses and metastatic cancers.[30-32] Even coronary artery arteriography (dye injected into the heart vessels) often fails to show how extensively the affected vessels have narrowed.[33]

In British hospitals, pathologists found that surgeons missed the diagnosis on two-thirds of the patients who were autopsied, and that a quarter of those might have lived if the correct diagnosis had been made.[34] As might be expected, these discrepancies are more common in community hospitals.[35] Diagnosis is least accurate in both infants and elderly patients.[36] People over 60-years old who die are the least likely to have an autopsy, perhaps because the aged are expected to die of "old age."[37] As Hill and Anderson said, "invaluable knowledge is being interred daily with the unautopsied bodies."[38]

Determining the cause of death can help a family's grief process or can assuage guilt. Autopsy results can sometimes reassure the family that nothing else really could have been done to save the deceased, that they were not the cause of their loved one's death, that there was no disease known to be familial, or that tissues removed or findings discovered at autopsy will help other people. This use for autopsies has long been known.

## TABLE 4.1: The Uses of Autopsies

BENEFITS TO MEDICAL PRACTICE AND SCIENCE
> Discover or elucidate new diseases
> Explain unknown or unanticipated medical complications
> Assist development/quality assurance of new technology, procedures and therapy
> Educate medical students
> Continue physician education

BENEFITS TO THE JUDICIAL SYSTEM
> Classify and explain sudden, unexpected and/or unnatural deaths

BENEFITS TO PUBLIC WELFARE
> Identify infectious and contagious diseases
> Identify and monitor occupational and environmental health hazards
> Quality control and risk assessment in hospital practices
> Provide a source of organs and tissues for medical and scientific purposes
> Provide materials and hypotheses for research
> Improve accuracy, and therefore usefulness, of vital statistics

BENEFITS TO THE DECEASED'S FAMILY
> Assist grief process
> Provide a vehicle for contribution
> Discover contagious diseases within family
> Assist in genetic counseling and identification of family health risks
> Provide information for insurance/death benefits

Adapted from: Svendsen E, Hill RB: Autopsy legislation and practice in various countries. *Arch Pathol Lab Med.* 1987;111:846-850.

After a high official in fifteenth-century Florence, Italy lost a son, the physician said in his autopsy report, "To lose one's offspring is hard, harder to lose a son, and hardest [to lose him] by a disease not yet fully understood by doctors. But for the sake of the other children, I think that to have seen his organs will be of the greatest utility."[39]

To aid his son, Napoleon demanded that his corpse be autopsied. He believed (correctly) that he was dying of the same disease, cancer of the stomach, that killed his own father. In transmitting the report to his son, the surgeon was to "Indicate to him what remedies or mode of life he can

119

pursue which will prevent his suffering from a similar disease."[40] This turned out to be for naught. The boy died at age 21 from tuberculosis.

Society also benefits from autopsies. Through autopsies, physicians have repeatedly discovered how the body works, recognized new diseases, and found alternative treatment methods. Hermann Boerhaave, an early anatomist, recognized this, telling his fellow physicians, "A disease which is new and obscure to you, Doctor, will be known only after death; and even then not without an autopsy will you examine it with exacting pains."[41]

One famous case, thwarted by the family, would have provided just such information. Alexis St. Martin was the most famous patient in the history of gastroenterology. The hapless trapper was accidentally shot in the stomach in 1822 while in upper Michigan. The wound to the stomach never healed and was used by physicians to determine how the stomach digests food. When St. Martin died, Sir William Osler, one of the greatest modern physicians, tried hard to get permission to do the autopsy. St. Martin's family was determined to prevent an autopsy and therefore "kept the body at home much longer than usual and during a hot spell of weather, so as to allow decomposition to set in and baffle the doctors."[42] The family was successful. By the time the funeral took place the body was so foul it had to be left outside of the church.

While successfully obtaining specific information from an individual's autopsy is common, the following famous incidents from the past century demonstrate the autopsy's importance to the development of modern medicine. This includes recognizing both the cause and the potential treatment for disorders we now consider commonplace. In 1886, for example, Reginald Fitz recognized during autopsies that appendicitis caused many people to die with pus in their belly, and that early surgery might prevent this.[43] Appendectomies then became a routine procedure, and countless lives have been saved as a result. In the early twentieth century, autopsies defined the causes of heart attacks and angina pectoris, thus leading the way to the medical and surgical treatments we now use for these diseases.[44] Autopsies also helped differentiate AIDS as a new disease and continue to provide fresh information about this epidemic.

Over the past two decades autopsies have been instrumental in identifying the causative organisms in Legionnaire's disease, toxic shock syndrome (an acute and severe disease that mainly strikes women in their childbearing years), and the new strain of Hantavirus initially killing people in the American southwest. Hill and Anderson compiled a list of 87 diseases or groups of diseases that were discovered or clarified through the use of autopsies between 1950 and 1983.[45] Table 4.2 contains an abbreviated and updated list.

Autopsies also help clinicians develop safe and effective methods of treating acutely injured patients.

## TABLE 4.2: Some Diseases Discovered or Explained by Autopsy Since 1950

Acquired immunodeficiency syndrome (AIDS)

Acute tubular necrosis (shutdown of kidney after shock)

Asbestosis (injury from asbestos in the lungs)

Cardiomyopathies (the reason for most heart transplants)

Child abuse syndrome

Complications of diabetes mellitus in various organs

Course and spread of various cancers

Fetal alcohol syndrome

Legionnaire's disease

Lung cancer from passive smoke

Medication injuries (e.g., halothane, a common anesthetic and methotrexate, a common cancer and antirheumatoid drug)

Mitral valve prolapse (mitral click syndrome)

Occupational and environmental diseases

Oxygen toxicity

Radiation fibrosis (injury to organs from radiation treatment)

Respiratory distress syndrome in infants

Retrolental fibroplasia (oxygen-induced infant blindness)

Steroid therapy complications

Sudden infant death syndrome (SIDS)

Toxic shock syndrome

Tumors from oral contraceptives

Viral hepatitis

---

The standard methods now used to insert chest tubes in traumatized patients were perfected due to autopsy findings. (Chest tubes are large polyvinyl tubes put into the chest to drain out air, blood and other substances surrounding a lung so the patient can breathe easier.) In the early 1970s, modern protocols for treating acutely injured patients were first being developed because of the Vietnam experience and the medical community's recognition of civilian trauma as a serious disease. Pathologists doing autopsies found an inordinate number of chest tubes were going into livers and spleens (in the abdomen) instead of into the chest. They discovered that the problem was two-fold: first, that many of these patients' diaphragms were high enough to allow the tube to enter the abdomen even though it first passed through the ribs, and second, that the common insertion technique did not allow physicians to recognize incorrect placement before damage was done. The pathologists passed on this autopsy-derived information, the technique was modified, and the complication now rarely occurs.

Autopsies have long been a vital educational tool in Western medicine. As a classic medical maxim states, *Mortui vivos docent* – the dead teach the living.

At the beginning of the twentieth century, Dr. Richard Cabot amazingly found diagnostic inaccuracies in 3,000 patients he had autopsied at Massachusetts General Hospital.[46] This precipitated a landmark report that led to marked changes in U.S. medical education – eliminating scores of medical schools, providing a uniform curriculum, and paving the way for advanced specialty training.[47]

For medical students, as sociologist Renee Fox said, exposure to autopsies is a 'landmark,' or 'milestone' event along the road to becoming a doctor. Participating in autopsies is "an emotionally important experience...[that] significantly challenges their ability to act and feel like doctors." [48] Unfortunately, fewer than half of all medical schools currently require students to attend even one autopsy; few students ever see more than one autopsy.[49,50]

The most dramatic autopsies (or at least their outcomes) are the medicolegal or *forensic* autopsies which often discover evidence of unnatural deaths that were initially thought to be unremarkable. Over one five-year period in London, more than five percent of all unnatural deaths had been unsuspected before the autopsy. These included cases of poisoning, head injuries, child abuse and suffocation.[51] (See the sections on medicolegal autopsies further along in this chapter.)

Before reading the sections on how autopsies are done (necessarily somewhat morbid), remember that the substantial benefits that this procedure provides cannot be obtained in any other way. The autopsy helps improve medical practice, assists society by providing public health and legal information, and benefits the deceased's family by discovering family health risks.

## F. WILL I HAVE AN AUTOPSY?

Whether or not your body is autopsied depends mainly on the circumstances surrounding your death, where you die, and the sentiments of your next-of-kin. In some circumstances it may also hinge upon your wishes as expressed in an advance directive or upon the insurance policy you have. Relatively few non-medicolegal autopsies are now done in the United States, although they are more frequent elsewhere.

Autopsies were once routine medical procedures in the United States. In the 1940s, 50% of in-hospital deaths had postmortem examinations and by the late 1950s some teaching hospitals autopsied 80% to 90% of all deaths.[52] The number of autopsies performed in the United States, however, has drastically declined over the past twenty-five years. This decline has been variously ascribed to medicolegal concerns, lessened emphasis on getting autopsy permission from families, the elimination of a minimum autopsy requirement by hospital accrediting bodies, the negative attitude of funeral directors and embalmers, and an assumption that modern medical technology can provide most necessary diagnostic information.[53,54] Today pathologists conduct autopsies on less than 12% of non-medicolegal deaths.[55-57] In the United States, less than half the number of adults who died in hospitals with fewer than 250 beds were autopsied as compared with those who died in larger hospitals. Those dying in the smaller hospitals with only part-time pathologists on staff were autopsied one-fourth as often. For non-homicide-related deaths, the frequency of autopsy ranges from 6% in Connecticut and 10% in Oklahoma, to 95% in Hawaii.[58,59]

Most U.S. jurisdictions have "medical examiner laws" that require a pathologist or coroner to determine whether or not an autopsy will be performed in cases of sudden, unexpected, mysterious, unusual, unnatural, unexplained or violent deaths, or those that might pose public health hazards. In some states this jurisdiction also includes sudden infant deaths, executed prisoners, deaths from malnutrition, or deaths associated with child or sexual abuse. In some areas a local health officer, judge, district or county attorney, or director of a state mental hospital may also order autopsies.[60]

Medical examiner cases require no consent for an autopsy. Specifically, many of these laws state that any death from violence (including motor vehicle deaths), deaths within 24 hours of general anesthesia, deaths in which the patient has not been seen by a physician in the past 24 hours (eliminates expected in-hospital deaths), deaths in prison or jail, and any other suspicious deaths come under the purview of the medical examiner. Even if death from violence is delayed many years, such as an when an individual finally succumbs to infection after being paralyzed by a gunshot wound, it falls within the medical examiner's domain.

Medical examiners may also order an autopsy in cases where a body will become permanently unavailable due to cremation (Connecticut, Delaware, District of Columbia, Florida, Kentucky, Minnesota, Oklahoma, and Tennessee) or burial at sea (Connecticut, District of Columbia, Florida and Minnesota).

Medical examiner laws have been quite effective. Autopsies on victims of blunt and penetrating trauma increased more than 14% in the United States during the 1980s, and pathologists now autopsy 59% of all such deaths. Among trauma deaths, the rate of autopsy varies by state, but homicide victims and trauma deaths in metropolitan areas are autopsied most often. The rate of homicide-victim autopsies ranges from less than 80% in Mississippi to 100% in six other states.[61]

Some states may honor religious objections to medicolegal autopsies, although officials will always conduct an autopsy if they feel it is in the public interest. In some states, an otherwise-mandated autopsy may be waived if the deceased was being treated by prayer or spiritual means alone in accordance with the tenets and practices of a "well-recognized" church or religion. These exemptions, however, are quickly disappearing as states prosecute parents who deny their children medical care for painful or lethal conditions.

In some European countries, including Hungary, Austria, France, Spain, and England medical examiners or their equivalent must grant permission for burial or cremation and may order an autopsy if they think it appropriate.[62] In 1992 an Australian government commission began reviewing the entire process of "coronial" (medicolegal) autopsies, emphasizing increased next-of-kin involvement in the process and in the disposition of body parts.[63]

## G. WHO GIVES PERMISSION FOR AN AUTOPSY?

Survivors must usually give their permission before pathologists perform a non-medicolegal autopsy. State statutes clearly specify who has legal custody of the corpse and the right to authorize an autopsy. In most states this is the next-of-kin, but in a few states the individual who assumes custody of the corpse for burial may give autopsy permission.[64-68]

The order in which next-of-kin may authorize an autopsy is usually: surviving spouse, adult children, adult grandchildren, parents, siblings and others per statute.[69] Sometimes even a minor may authorize the autopsy.[70]

Permission can normally be given in writing, by a witnessed (and usually recorded) telephone call, telegram, or by other telephonic means, such as a FAX. More than two-thirds of the states in the United States require only one person to give consent for the autopsy, even if more than one person has taken custody of the body.[71]

If an autopsy is done without legal approval or proper consent, or the pathologist conducts a more extensive examination than is authorized, survivors may sue for damages based on their mental anguish. This practice derives from an English common law holding that "the person with the right and duty to dispose of the body is entitled to possession and receipt of the body without delay, in the same condition as it was at the time of death."[72] An unauthorized autopsy interferes with this quasi-property right.[73,74]

In general, however, monetary awards for violations have been relatively small, with one California court awarding the plaintiff only 6 cents.[75,76] Some states provide immunity to those who, in good faith, perform or order autopsies.

Where death occurs also plays a factor in whether a body will be autopsied. Consent is not required for autopsy in some foreign countries (Table 4.3) such as Austria, Bulgaria, Hungary, Italy, and Poland. In Austria, autopsies have been required on the bodies of those who have died in public hospitals since the mid-eighteenth century when Empress Maria Theresa made it law. Czechoslovakia, even with a requirement for permission, and Austria both have close to a 100% autopsy rate. In Denmark, France, Iceland, and Norway no consent is required, but families may object to non-forensic autopsies. According to the *British Medical Journal,* in Great Britain "many coroners' necropsies are done not only without the permission of the relatives but also in the face of their active antagonism."[77]

## TABLE 4.3: International Legal Requirements for Autopsies

| | HOSPITAL AUTOPSIES | | FORENSIC CASES |
|---|---|---|---|
| | Consent Required? | Rate | Rate |
| Austria | Not in public hospitals | High | 100% |
| Belgium | Yes | Low | 10% |
| Czechoslovakia | Yes | High | 100% |
| Denmark | No;family may object | High | 25% |
| Finland | Yes | High | High |
| France | No;family may object | Low | Variable |
| Germany | Yes | Low | Variable |
| Greece | No hospital autopsies | Zero | 100% |
| Iceland | No;family may object | High | High |
| Irish Republic | Yes | ? | 50% |
| Israel | Yes | Low | ? |
| Italy | No | Low | ? |
| Netherlands | Yes | Low | 5% |
| Norway | No;family may object | High | 100% |
| South Africa | Yes | Low | ? |
| Spain | Yes | Low | 50% |
| Sweden | Yes | High | 100% |
| Switzerland | Yes, in most cantons | Variable | 30% |
| United Kingdom | Yes | Low | 70%-90% |
| United States | Yes | Low | Variable |

Adapted from: Svendsen E, Hill RB: Autopsy legislation and practice in various countries. *Arch Pathol Lab Med.* 1987;111:846-50; and Hill RB, Anderson RE: *The Autopsy—Medical Practice and Policy.* Boston: Butterworths, 1988, p 169.

United States military authorities determine whether to autopsy active duty military personnel. A base commander may order an autopsy to determine the true cause of death, to complete military records, to protect the welfare of the military community, or for an aircrew member. Even on military bases, however, next-of-kin permission is required to autopsy non-military personnel.

Some insurance policies with special accidental death clauses may give an insurance company the right to demand an autopsy.[78] For some individuals who die in foreign countries, even if they are autopsied there, a second autopsy may be requested or required upon the bodies' return to their home country to clarify insurance claims or to investigate criminal activity.[79] If the next-of-kin refuses an autopsy in these cases and there is no reason for the medical examiner to "post" the body, a private pathologist will probably also be unwilling to do the autopsy, since some courts have held them to be liable for damages in such cases.[80-83]

Similarly, authorities sometimes financially pressure survivors to authorize an autopsy. In Vermont for example, if survivors refuse the state's request for a Worker's Compensation-related autopsy, they may be excluded from receiving death benefits.[84] Similarly, if relatives refuse autopsy permission for a patient who has died in a Veteran's hospital from a potentially service-related cause, they may not receive VA death benefits.[85]

Some advance directives (living wills, health care durable powers of attorney, etc.) include provisions through which people can advise survivors whether they desire an autopsy. New advance directive laws, such as the one in Arizona, give people this right, as does an 1881 New York statute which states "A person has the right to direct the manner in which his body shall be disposed of after death."[86,87] (New York did not give the living the same right to direct their health care until 1914.)[88] California, Illinois, Nebraska, Nevada, Pennsylvania and Utah also allow a person to authorize an autopsy on his corpse. In Pennsylvania, however, a surviving spouse must also give written permission.[89]

## H.  AFTER AN AUTOPSY, CAN I STILL BE EMBALMED?

Yes, although it is sometimes more difficult to embalm a body after an autopsy. These difficulties have caused an historical antagonism between pathologists, who frequently did not understand the embalmer's needs, and embalmers, who often gave scant heed to the importance of the pathologist's work. When both worked in concert, however, each could do his work successfully.

Dr. Jesse Carr, former Chief of Pathology at San Francisco General Hospital gives the pathologist's classic view of embalmers, saying, "It's generally the badly trained or avaricious undertaker who is resistant to the autopsy procedure...[they] are obstructive, unskilled and can be nasty to the point of viciousness. They lie to the family, citing all sorts of horrible things that can happen to the deceased."[90] Some individuals in the funeral industry also feel this way. One funeral director quoted by Jessica Mitford said, "Most funeral directors are still 'horse and buggy undertakers' in their thinking and it shows up glaringly in their moronic attitude towards autopsies."[91]

Embalmers, however, cite the horrible condition of some bodies after autopsies, delays in getting bodies prepared for viewing, and major problems in preparing some bodies after autopsy. "Not too many years ago," said one funeral industry notable, "mention of the word 'autopsy' to someone in funeral service was like the use of one of the more vulgar profanities...There are several extremely objectionable practices which some pathologists still engage in."[92] While eighty percent of funeral directors and embalmers believe there is a benefit to autopsies, nearly half counsel families not to permit them. And almost one-third of families take their advice.[93]

Common embalmers' complaints include receiving bodies that have not been properly cleaned after postmortem examination, tying the wrists with string or gauze which leave disfiguring marks and may obstruct the entry of embalming fluid into the hands, not using a head rest during the autopsy causing the face to become stained with pooled blood, and tying the sheet or shroud so tightly that the nose is flattened.[94] Others describe pathologists "butchering" bodies when they cut arteries too short to be injected, or cut into areas of the body that would be exposed in a viewing, such as the face and hands.[95] Funeral directors particularly dislike bearing the brunt of the family's wrath over the condition of the body, how long it takes to embalm the body, or for delays in the viewing—all problems they believe are due to the pathologist's lack of cooperation.[96,97] Some embalmers suggest that they should keep pictures of autopsied bodies they embalm, both before and after restoration, and a complete autopsy record on any difficult-to-embalm body. They can then show these to the family if there is a dispute, and they can also be used to defend against litigation. This very negative attitude toward autopsies, however, markedly contrasts with the industry's acceptance of, and even promotion of, organ donation.[98]

Because they need not be concerned about embalming or viewings, autopsies performed outside of the United States and Canada often are very disfiguring, with incisions running up to the chin. In London, autopsied bodies take at least three days to be released to the morticians, often requiring them to schedule funerals a week after the death.[99]

The embalming process for autopsied bodies is different than the usual procedure (see Chapter 5, *Beauty in Death*). Embalmers use the ends of abdominal arteries that are cut during the autopsy as injection sites. They then dry the abdominal cavity and dust it with embalming powder. The organs are placed in a thick plastic bag and embalming fluid is poured over them. They are then removed from the bag, put into the abdomen and also covered with embalming powder.[100] In the past, embalmers occasionally filled the empty abdomen with sawdust-containing material, but when wet, it emitted a sour odor. They now use other fillers.[101] The embalmer finally resews the abdominal autopsy incision and coats it with a liquid sealant.[102]

One simple solution to the difficulties may seem to be embalming the body *before* the autopsy. Pathologists, however, never voluntarily permit this, since embalming interferes with the examination. Embalming changes the color and consistency of the tissues, eliminates much of the body's bacteria, and confuses or obliterates signs of intoxication or poisoning. The alcohols used in embalming fluids, for example, render useless one of the most commonly positive findings, the presence of alcohol. Similarly, cyanide can no longer be identified after it reacts with formaldehyde.[103]

## I. WHY DOESN'T EVERYONE GET AUTOPSIED?

Bodies are not autopsied because physicians do not ask and relatives refuse permission when they are asked.

Most modern U.S. physicians don't ask for autopsies on their patients who die. Physicians tend to request autopsies mostly on young patients, when they are unsure of their diagnoses, and when relatives appear favorably disposed to granting permission.[104] These situations have not generated a sufficient number of autopsies for teaching and to check on the quality of medical care. Therefore, as the rate of autopsies decreased at major teaching hospitals in the 1960s and 1970s, faculty physicians pressured their trainees (residents) to obtain autopsy permission from families. Sometimes amoral techniques were used to get the permits. In a 1982 *Esquire* article, Dr. Hellerstein related the instructions he received as an intern:

> "Number one," said Jerry, "when you ask the family for the post (autopsy), don't reason with them. It's a waste of time...Number two: Tell them 'I'll be there, not some pathologist down in the morgue, but *me*, the guy who took care of Mom or Dad.' Am I always there? Not always...Number three:...don't go into detail. They don't want to hear about...the liver cut into little pieces." The overriding principle, it appeared, was to tell them whatever they wanted to hear.[105]

They also offered prizes to those who were most successful and publicly blamed those who failed to obtain permissions. In the infamous book, *The House of God*, Samuel Shem's characters discuss the "Black Crow Award":

> The [Chief of Medicine] said that the terns (interns) were not getting enough postmortem permissions, and since he knew "how

hard it is to approach the family for permission in their hour of need," he thought of "a way to raise the incentive: an award. The award will go to the intern with the most postmortem permissions for the year. The prize will be a free trip for two to Atlantic City to the AMA in June."[106]

Milder techniques to encourage physicians to ask for autopsies, such as informative lectures, have been unsuccessful; the number of autopsies is still decreasing.[107] One group found that they could achieve a forty to fifty percent autopsy rate for in-hospital deaths if they: (1) required the physician certifying death to sign the forms in the morgue, so they would frequently come in contact with the pathologists and staff who encourage autopsies; (2) discussed death and autopsies with relatives in a special room removed from the patient areas; (3) designated morticians to act as "bereavement officers" who are in contact with every physician pronouncing death; and (4) held frequent conferences between clinicians and pathologists so the former could see the benefits derived from autopsies.[108] These techniques have yet to be widely adopted.

Even when physicians do ask for autopsies, relatives often balk at giving their permission. While most people would permit an autopsy on themselves, their next-of-kin or surrogate often refuses permission. (Writing out or stating directions in advance both allays relatives' unease and guides survivors in their decision making.) Helen Brown discovered seven common beliefs that cause survivors to refuse autopsy permission:

1. Medical diagnosis is excellent and diagnostic machines almost infallible; an autopsy is unnecessary.
2. If the physician could not save the patient, he or she has no business seeking clues after that failure.
3. The patient has suffered enough.
4. Body mutilation occurs.
5. An autopsy takes a long time and delays final arrangements.
6. Autopsy results are not well communicated.
7. An autopsy will result in an incomplete body, and so life in the hereafter cannot take place.[109]

Each of the first six points have just enough truth to make them almost believable. Whether they warrant declining autopsy permission for a loved one, however, is a personal decision.

Individuals from several religious traditions may worry about body integrity and resurrection. The only relevant question here, especially for Christians, is the one Lord Shaftesbury asked. If a whole body is required for an afterlife, "What would in such a case become of the Blessed Martyrs?"[110] (See also Chapter 6, *What do religions say about cremation?*) Questions of faith, however, do not normally succumb to rational analysis.

In general, college-educated young adults are most likely to approve autopsies on their relatives.[111] Reluctance to permit autopsies has led some to suggest that the government ensure a sufficient number of autopsies to meet society's needs for education, research and health statistics.[112] English physicians have fewer problems obtaining autopsy permission from relatives than their colleagues in the United States do, since most English bodies are cremated without a viewing.[113]

Some cultures, however, resist autopsies, even when they may quickly prevent deaths in a community. When the unknown epidemic (eventually identified as a Hantavirus) began killing mainly Navajos in New Mexico and Arizona in mid-1993, Dr. Beulah Allen, a Navajo internist working in the Indian Health Service, explained the continuing resistance to autopsying the dead: "They do not understand why a body needs to be cut up and explored after a person has died. It's dishonoring to the person who has died."[114]

Clinicians' perceived disinterest in autopsies is another reason that few relatives permit autopsies. Several major teaching centers have, therefore, trained specific individuals to sensitively request autopsies, inquire about organ and tissue donations, assist families with the paperwork surrounding a death, and coordinate their work with funeral homes. This generally leads to an increase in the incidence of non-medicolegal autopsies.[115]

## J. HOW IS AN AUTOPSY DONE?

The complete autopsy can be divided into four sequential steps: (1) inspecting the body's exterior; (2) examining the internal organs' position and appearance; (3) dissecting and examinating the internal organs; and (4) the laboratory analysis of tissue, fluids and other specimens. At each step of the autopsy, the pathologist may photograph unusual findings.

The *first step* is examining the corpse's exterior. In most autopsies this is perfunctory, since it does not add much to the findings. In medico-legal (forensic) autopsies, however, this step is crucial and meticulously documented with notes, diagrams and photographs. In John F. Kennedy's autopsy, for example, it is the record of the external examination that has caused the most controversy. Radiographs (X-rays), commonly taken at this stage, may reveal unsuspected injuries to the bones, the presence of bullets and other foreign bodies, old fractures or bone infections, congenital abnormalities, or unusual collections of gas, any of which can explain the cause of death.[116] In one case, for example, where a man supposedly "dropped dead" and his body had been extensively eaten by hogs, X-rays revealed that he had been shot three times from three different distances with a shotgun.[117]

The pathologist then moves to the *second step* of the autopsy by opening the thoraco-abdominal (chest-belly) cavity. The incision, generally Y-shaped, begins at each shoulder or armpit area and runs beneath the breasts to the bottom of the breastbone. The incisions then join and proceed down the middle of the abdomen to the pubis, just above the genitals. The front part of the ribs and breastbone are then removed in one piece. This procedure exposes most of the organs and their containers (the pleura and ribs on the inner side of the chest; the peritoneum on the inside of the belly) for examination. The pathologist then examines the relationship of the organs to each other and sees if any abnormality in one organ affects an adjacent organ.

At this stage, the pathologist also examines the brain, unless it is clear that no useful information will be obtained or if relatives do not permit it. To expose the brain, the hair is parted and an incision is made behind the ears and across the base of the scalp. The front part of the scalp is then pulled over the face and the back part over the nape of the neck, exposing the skull. The pathologist opens the skull using a special high-speed oscillating saw, identical to that used by a neurosurgeon when doing brain surgery and similar to that used for removing plaster casts. Some pathologists form a notch in the skull so that the "skull cap" does not move when replaced. Morticians appreciate this. After the skull cap is separated from the rest of the skull with a chisel, the pathologist examines the covering of the brain (meninges) and the inside of the skull for signs of infection, swelling, injury or deterioration.

For cosmetic reasons, pathologists normally do not disturb the skin of the face, arms, hands, or the area above the nipples unless it is required in a forensic autopsy or they have obtained special permission.[118] Also, in U.S. autopsies, they rarely remove the large neck vessels (carotid arteries and jugular veins), even when there is known disease in that area. If they do remove the neck vessels, pathologists often insert rubber tubes so embalmers can later infuse the head with preservatives. In some instances, embalmers infuse bodies in the autopsy room before the neck vessels are removed.[119]

If a patient has a pacemaker, that is also removed at this stage. In many institutions, the pacemaker is sent to the local pacemaker technician to check it for defects. It is then returned to the family or discarded.

In the autopsy's *third step,* pathologists remove the body's organs for further examination and dissection. In a few cases where relatives have religious objections to a legally required autopsy, the organs are not removed, but examined and dissected *in situ,* although less extensively than in Rokitansky's method. (See *How do autopsy techniques vary?*)

Normally, however, pathologists either remove organs from the chest and belly sequentially or *en bloc.* If the organs are removed *en bloc,* the following procedure is common: major vessels at the base of the neck are tied and the esophagus and trachea are severed just above the thyroid cartilage (Adam's apple). They pinch off the aorta above the diaphragm and cut it along with the inferior vena cava, allowing the heart and lungs to be removed together, but leaving the esophagus in place. The spleen is then separately removed from the abdomen, as are the small and large intestines. The liver, pancreas, stomach and esophagus are removed as a unit, followed by the kidneys, ureters, bladder and abdominal aorta. Finally, the testes are removed. The pathologist then takes small samples of muscle, nerve and fibrous tissue from various organs for microscopic examination. The spinal cord itself is rarely removed. However, if it is to be examined, the backbone is cut with a special saw and the cord is lifted out.[120]

Richard Selzer provides a graphic description of the autopsy's third step:

> Above each of the slabs, there is a hanging scale such as is used in delicatessen stores. Now and then, a kidney will flop up on the scale, then bounce itself to stillness. "Right kidney ... 200 grams," a voice calls out. Somewhere this is recorded. The kidney is retrieved from the scale; cubes and slices of it are taken and arranged on trays. From these pieces, microscopic slides will be made.[121]

After the pathologist examines and weighs the organs to determine deviation from age and sex norms (for example, lungs in people dying from congestive heart failure, i.e., water on the lungs, are heavier than normal), they are opened to check for internal pathology. Pathologists open the heart, for example, to visualize the valves and internal walls. They make small incisions along the coronary arteries that run on the outside of the heart to check for blockages, and routinely open and clean the entire intestine to check for growths, bleeding or other abnormalities. They remove minute tissue fragments from each organ in any area where they see abnormalities, as well as representative sections from at least the left ventricle of the heart, the lungs, kidneys, and liver. These, as well as representative body fluids, are examined in step four.

To remove the brain from the skull with its connection to the spinal cord (the brainstem), the pathologist cuts the nerves to the eyes, the major blood vessels to the brain, the fibrous attachment to the skull, the spinal cord, and several other nerves and connections. After gently lifting the brain out of the skull and checking it again for external abnormalities, he usually suspends it by a thread in a two-gallon pail filled with ten percent formalin. This "fixes" it, firming the tissue so that it can be properly examined ten to fourteen days later. If the brain must be examined immediately, he infuses formalin solution under pressure through the carotid arteries before he opens it. This method, however, results in some tissue distortion. The pathologist then slices the brain into one-half- to one-inch sections and spreads the pieces like a deck of cards for examination of its internal structures.[122]

Pathologists rarely remove large portions of bone at autopsy unless there is specific pathology, such as an infection or degenerative disease of the area. If they do remove bone, they usually insert wooden, metal, plastic or plaster prostheses (at the end of the autopsy) to replace the missing segment.[123]

At the end of step three, they sew closed any large incisions.

In a somewhat unusual twist on autopsy procedure, research pathologists at the Shock-Trauma Center at the University of Maryland in Baltimore, at one time went to the bedside of dying patients and removed small samples of tissues for examination as soon as clinicians declared a patient dead. This provided some early information about cellular and subcellular changes in patients (who had recently been) in shock. They also rapidly preserved the brains by injecting them with chemicals, subsequently taking samples for research.[124]

*Step four* consists of examining minute tissue and fluid specimens under the microscope and by chemical analysis in the laboratory. This is the most time-consuming part of the autopsy and often causes delays in releasing autopsy results. The pathologist's laboratory arsenal includes culturing specimens for bacteria and viruses, using immuno-flourescence to identify abnormal proteins, and searching for abnormal tissue patterns with an electron microscope (on samples only 1/20,000th of an inch thick magnified 10,000 times). Recently, pathologists have also begun using the new polymerase-chain-reaction (PCR) technique to multiply and then identify minute amounts of DNA-containing material. In forensic autopsies, it is routine to test fluid from the eye, gallbladder, urine, and blood for alcohol, drugs and other chemical agents.

Miscarried fetuses and stillborns, and infants with congenital defects are commonly tested for chromosome abnormalities. In an autopsy on a fetus or infant, the pathologist must look carefully for malformations that suggest congenital abnormalities due to genetic defects or maternal disease of which the parents should be informed. These include a cleft palate, closed nasal passages (choanal atresia), a closed anus or vagina, or abnormalities of the face, ears, hands, kidneys, heart, intestines and other organs. Most pathologists will also routinely check for collapsed lungs, which are common in infants. When available, the placenta and umbilical cord are also studied to detect abnormalities. Pathologists have special techniques for opening the skull of a small child or fetus because of its soft bone and small size.[125]

After completing the autopsy, the pathologist synthesizes the information and determines, when possible, both a "cause of death" and the factors contributing to the death. They try to describe the findings so that future pathologists will be able to interpret them whether or not they still use the same syndrome names or other medical-shorthand terms. Autopsy results from early eighteenth-century England, for example, are written so clearly that modern pathologists can often make diagnoses (that the original authors could not) from their findings.

The final autopsy report may not be available for many weeks, depending on the time needed to prepare tissues (such as the brain) in chemicals before examining them, and the number and type of laboratory tests performed. The College of American Pathology (professional organization of anatomic pathologists) requires all pathology laboratories that they accredit to complete their autopsy reports within thirty days .

## K.  HOW DO AUTOPSY TECHNIQUES VARY?

Although most modern pathologists use the autopsy technique described in the prior section, autopsy techniques and limitations change over time and with the extent of survivor's permission for the procedure.

Modern autopsy techniques began with Rudolph Virchow (1821-1902) who standardized the method of removing and examining each organ in order. Few pathologists still use his method routinely, although some use it on patients who have died of communicable diseases. Later, Rokitansky developed the now-discarded technique of dissecting the organs *in situ* (in place) combined with removing some of them *en bloc* (together).

Modern pathologists use methods developed by Ghon and Letulle for removing groups of organs *en bloc*, determining their relationships, and then examining them separately. Using the Letulle method, they remove all organs from the neck to the perineum (all of the "insides" from the throat to the groin) in one large group and later dissect them. With this procedure, the body can be delivered to the mortician within 30 minutes or less after beginning the autopsy; the organs can be stored in the refrigerator and examined at a later time.[126] Otherwise, the entire surgical part of an autopsy in which the organs are removed and then examined with the naked eye normally takes between one and three hours.[127]

The conventional (complete) autopsy involves all major organs in the chest and abdomen, as well as the brain and brainstem. The patient's disease, complaints, or external marks may also lead to investigation of other parts of the body. When autopsy permission is limited, the examination may be restricted to the abdominal or chest cavities, to examination through recent surgical incisions, to not removing the organs, or in other ways that may limit the value of the pathologist's findings.[128] Commonly, autopsy permission forms include options for "complete postmortem examination," "complete postmortem examination—return all organs" (this does not include microscopic slides, fluid samples or paraffin blocks pathologists are required to keep), "omit head," "heart and lungs only," "chest and abdomen only," "chest only," "abdomen only," or "head only."

In some cases, relatives will only give permission for limited autopsies. At the extreme, organs may only be sampled through needle biopsies, without opening the body. This technique has decreasing success when used on the liver, heart, lung and kidney.[129,130] In other cases, permission to autopsy may be limited to a single body cavity (such as the abdomen). Although difficult, an autopsy limited to an abdominal incision still allows all organs from the neck down to be removed if relatives give their permission. Prior to and during the Middle Ages, physicians even performed autopsies through the anus or vagina because of religious and cultural taboos on mutilating the body.[131] While traditionalists frown on limitations, some community-based pathologists have recommended limited autopsies as a way to reduce autopsy costs and the time spent doing the (poorly reimbursed) procedure.[132]

## L. ARE AUTOPSIES HARMFUL TO PATHOLOGISTS?

Autopsies can be deleterious to a pathologist's health. Many famous (and not so famous) pathologists over the past two centuries have died or become seriously ill from diseases they acquired while doing autopsies.

Before the introduction of antibiotics, autopsies were sometimes lethal to the pathologist. The most dangerous autopsies for pathologists to perform were those on women who died from childbirth infections (puerperal peritonitis). The death in 1847 of Dr. Ignaz Semmelweis' colleague, Dr. Jacobus Kolletschka, from a cut finger received during an autopsy on a woman who died from puerperal peritonitis led Semmelweis to discover how to prevent this dread disease.[133] Many pathologists have been infected through tiny cuts in their hands during an autopsy. Rubber gloves were not used routinely for autopsies until after World War II.[134]

Even with antibiotics and gloves, pathologists still worry about deadly viruses. They worry most about hepatitis B, HIV virus (AIDS), and Creutzfeldt-Jakob virus (which causes a rare but relentlessly progressive dementia). In modern times pathologists have acquired both pulmonary (lung) and skin tuberculosis (affectionately called "prosector's warts"), smallpox (although this virus now only exists in two research laboratories), and hepatitis B from doing autopsies. Pathologists have not acquired other infectious diseases, including HIV, by performing autopsies, although they are concerned about their risk.[135] To avoid disease, modern pathologists prepare for an autopsy by changing into surgical "scrubs," and donning surgical masks, caps, shoe covers, goggles, waterproof aprons and usually three pairs of gloves: latex, steel or kevlar mesh, and surgical gloves in that order. If they suspect the presence of an infectious agent, pathologists will often use the "Virchow" technique, removing organs separately for examination. In these cases, they use special procedures to limit the possibility of aerosolizing body fluids. They usually open the skull, for example, while the head is covered by a special container. Unfortunately, many people die with unsuspected infectious diseases, so most pathologists take these precautions in all cases. Pathologists also face other dangers. When autopsying a body containing radioactive materials (usually inserted for treatment of a tumor), a radiation safety officer is normally present to ascertain whether it is safe to perform the procedure.[136]

However, Dr. Jesse Carr, while Chief of Pathology at San Francisco General Hospital in the 1950s, moved the morgue from the basement to near his third-floor office to demonstrate that "we have so little apprehension of disease being spread by dead bodies that we have them up here right among us...Ten to twenty students attend each autopsy. No danger here!"[137]

After the autopsy, specimens not used for study or returned to the body are usually incinerated in special bags labeled as contaminated and hazardous waste.

One of the most dangerous sets of autopsies ever performed was done by Joe Kahn, at one time professor of pathology at Case Western Reserve University. During World War II, Dr. Kahn went ashore with the first wave of soldiers onto the South Pacific beaches of New Guinea and New Britain to autopsy natives who had died in the crossfire. In a hail of bullets, he sought evidence of biologic-warfare diseases with which the Japanese had been experimenting.[138]

## M.  WHAT IS A MEDICAL EXAMINER/CORONER?

Medical examiners and coroners investigate violent, suspicious or unexpected deaths, and deaths that were unattended by physicians. In the United States, state laws specify the types of death that are investigated, the official(s) who are responsible for investigations, and those officials' qualifications. The 1954 *Model Post-Mortem Examination Act* recommends forensic examination of all deaths that: (1) are violent; (2) are sudden and unexpected; (3) occur under suspicious circumstances; (4) are employment-related; (5) occur in persons whose bodies will be cremated, dissected, buried at sea or otherwise unavailable for later examination; (6) occur in prison or to psychiatric inmates; or (7) constitute a threat to public health.[139] Many states have adopted this law.

Not all deaths in the United States that come under the medical examiner's jurisdiction are investigated or autopsied. But police, physicians and morticians must notify the medical examiner's office of cases that fall within its domain. A record of this notification usually appears on the death certificate. Since medical examiners work within a tight budget, they often decline to examine bodies in which the cause of death appears clear. Approximately 20% of all deaths fall under the medical examiner/coroner's purview, but the percentage of deaths undergoing medicolegal autopsy varies greatly by location.[140]

Medical examiners use many types of scientific analysis in their investigations. These include techniques from pathology, hematology, odontology (teeth), anthropology, criminology, ballistics (bullets), and most recently, genetics. When warranted, they examine suspected crime scenes to determine as accurately and scientifically as possible, the specific cause of death and how the person died (natural causes, accident, homicide or suicide). They must also determine the person's identity when the body is badly mutilated or only fragments remain.[141]

Scene investigation, however, can be both dangerous and tedious. While examining a corpse in a badly burned house, one Iowa medical examiner narrowly missed being hit on the head when a bathtub fell from the floor above. On another occasion, he traipsed along more than a mile of busy train track gathering body parts from a pedestrian killed by a train.[142]

Formal training in forensic pathology began at the Harvard Medical School in 1937. Current training and certification in forensic pathology generally requires four years of medical school, four more years of basic pathology training (residency) and an additional one to two years of special training in forensic pathology. These last years include training in medicolegal autopsies, criminal investigation, judicial testimony, toxicology and other forensic sciences.

The position of coroner, unlike that of the medical examiner, predates the *Magna Carta*. England's *Charts of Privileges* first granted the office to St. John of Beverly in 925,[143] and before the 1194 publication of the *Articles of Eyre*, the office of coroner had become an official position throughout the country. These individuals were called "keepers of the pleas of the crown," a phrase later shortened to "crowner" and then "coroner." The position was initially that of a formidable and prestigious judicial officer, collecting monies due the king, trying felony cases and controlling treasure-troves, shipwrecks and salvage matters, but the job gradually narrowed to the investigation of unusual, untimely or suspicious deaths. By the thirteenth century, coroners had to examine all bodies before burial, appraising all wounds, bruises and other signs of possible foul play.[144] In Shakespeare's *Hamlet*, for example, it is the coroner who rules, questionably, that Ophelia did not kill herself and so is entitled to a Christian burial.[145]

A recent case illustrates the use of medical examiners, rather than coroners: In Wyoming, a man was convicted of his wife's murder because she had a small wound in her back and a large wound in front. A coroner (who qualified for that position by being a funeral director with a four-wheel-drive vehicle to collect bodies from remote areas) testified that it was clearly a murder. After the widower had served two years in prison, a forensic pathologist was called in and showed that the evidence clearly demonstrated that the woman had committed suicide. He was released from prison.[146]

The first American coroner was Thomas Baldridge of St. Mary's, Maryland Colony, who, appointed on January 29, 1637, held his first death inquest two days later. (He ruled the cause of death to be accidental.)[147] It wasn't until 1890 that Baltimore appointed two physicians as the United States' first medical examiners.

In 1915 New York City followed suit, eliminating its coroner system and replacing it with medical examiners[148] who were authorized to investigate deaths "resulting from criminal violence, casualties, suicide, or suddenly while in apparent health, or when not attended by a physician or imprisoned or in any suspicious or unusual manner." The mayor-appointed medical examiner could make the decision to autopsy any case. Most U.S. medical examiner systems still follow this pattern. In 1939 Maryland initiated the nation's first statewide medical examiner system.

Currently in the United States, nineteen states and the District of Columbia have chief medical examiners responsible for investigating deaths for the entire state (Table 4.4). This individual is usually appointed and must be a licensed physician with training in pathology, usually specializing in forensic pathology, as did television's medical examiner, *Quincy*. Deputy or county medical examiners assist this individual. Eleven states have county or district coroners who are likewise responsible for investigating deaths within their jurisdiction. This elected position has no educational requirements. Seventeen states have death investigation systems mixing coroners and medical examiners. With the complexities of modern forensic science, however, pathologists almost always direct at least the autopsy investigation, and in some instances the field investigations in cases of unusual deaths.

Some places still use coroner's juries or inquests, a less formal group than a court or grand jury, to conduct the preliminary inquiry into suspicious deaths. They decide whether the cause of death was accidental, natural or criminal. In the United States, coroner's inquest findings are not binding on anyone—although they often help the prosecuting attorney's case. In England, the findings act as an indictment of an accused person, just as a grand jury does in the United States.[149]

## N. HOW LONG HAVE PHYSICIANS BEEN DOING MEDICOLEGAL AUTOPSIES?

Physicians have performed medicolegal autopsies for at least 2,000 years.

The Roman physician Antistius performed one of the earliest recorded forensic examinations so he could determine the exact cause of Julius Caesar's violent death in 44 B.C. He opined that of the twenty-three wounds Caesar received, only the blow to the chest was fatal. A Chinese handbook on autopsies published about A.D. 1247, *Hsi Yuan Chi Lu* (*The Washing*

*Away of Unjust Wrongs*), includes descriptions of various kinds of wounds and comments on how to determine whether persons found drowned or burned died before or after entering the water or fire.[150] (Fire victims have soot in their lungs; drowning victims may still be difficult to differentiate from those who died before entering the water.)

## TABLE 4.4: State Death-Investigation Systems.

### MEDICAL EXAMINER SYSTEMS

#### State Chief Medical Examiner

| | | |
|---|---|---|
| Connecticut | Mississippi | Rhode Island |
| Delaware | New Hampshire | Tennessee |
| Dist of Columbia | New Jersey | Utah |
| Iowa | New Mexico | Vermont |
| Maine | North Carolina | Virginia |
| Maryland | Oklahoma | West Virginia |
| Massachusetts | Oregon | |

#### District/County Medical Examiners

| | | |
|---|---|---|
| Arizona | Florida | Michigan |

### CORONER SYSTEMS

| | | |
|---|---|---|
| Colorado | Nebraska | Pennsylvania |
| Idaho | Nevada | South Dakota |
| Kansas | North Dakota | Wyoming |
| Louisiana | Ohio | |

### MIXED MEDICAL EXAMINER/CORONER SYSTEMS

| | | |
|---|---|---|
| Alabama | Illinois | New York |
| Alaska | Indiana | South Carolina |
| Arkansas | Kentucky | Texas |
| California | Minnesota | Washington |
| Georgia | Missouri | Wisconsin |
| Hawaii | Montana | |

Adapted from: Combs DL, Parrish RG, Ing R: *Death Investigation in the United States and Canada, 1992.* Atlanta, GA: U.S. Dept of Health & Human Services, 1992, p 9.

Thirteenth- and fourteenth-century European physicians also performed medicolegal autopsies. In the fourteenth century, Emperor Charles V of France decreed that medical testimony be offered at trials where the court was considering death by infanticide, homicide, abortion, or poisoning. In the latter half of that century, Ambrose Paré performed official medicolegal autopsies, later reporting his findings about smothered children and sexual assault victims to the medical community.[151]

Medicolegal autopsies rarely occurred in the American Colonies, but when they did, it was to investigate possible murders. The autopsy of a Massachusetts apprentice who died of a skull fracture in 1639 led to the arraignment of his master. When John Dandy of Maryland killed an Indian boy in 1643, the body was autopsied to determine the exact cause of death. During the late 1600s, other medicolegal autopsies occurred in Massachusetts and Maryland to determine the causes of suspicious deaths. The most famous early medicolegal autopsy, however, was that of New York Governor Slaughter, who died under mysterious circumstances on June 23, 1691. While some thought the governor had been poisoned, the examining physicians found that he died of a blood clot in the lung (pulmonary embolus).[152]

After 1778 there was a steady increase in the number of British homicide trials that included autopsy findings. This may have reflected the presence of textbooks in, noted teachers of, and a recognition of the importance to the courts of pathology.[153] In 1829 John Gordon Smith complained in a self-serving manner that; "I do not believe there is a medical man educated in England who can open a dead body, certainly not one who could name the instruments required to perform this operation—for judiciary purposes unless he may be found among my own pupils, or those of my friend Professor Christison of Edinburgh."[154]

In 1831, a surgeon-pathologist testified about the results of his extensive autopsy on a 14-year-old boy, supposedly killed for sale to the anatomists by Bishop, May and Williams (see Chapter 8, *When were "grave-robbed" bodies not dead?*):

> There was a wound on the temple, which did not injure the bone—that was the only appearance of external injury; on the scull beneath the scalp or bone there was some blood effused; on opening the body the whole contents of the abdomen and chest were found to be in a healthy condition...[the brain] was perfectly healthy, as well as the spinal part...some coagulated blood was found laying in the [spinal] cavity opposite the blood found in the muscles of the neck...I think these internal marks of violence were sufficient to produce death...I think a blow from a stick on the back of the neck would have caused those appearances.[155]

This report to the court is so complete that it would still be acceptable today.

## O. WHAT IS SPECIAL ABOUT A MEDICOLEGAL AUTOPSY?

A medicolegal autopsy differs from a regular autopsy in several ways. It usually includes an extensive investigation of the death scene, extra documentation of the autopsy itself, an increased emphasis on determining the time and manner of death, and frequently, identification of the body under examination. Most people know some of these steps from watching *Quincy* and other TV shows, or from reading crime novels. Much of that information is incorrect, as was pointed out in Petty's "Devil's Dozen: popular misconceptions about medicolegal autopsies" (Table 4.5).

The *first step* in a medicolegal (forensic) autopsy takes place at the death scene where, as Ludwig said, "masterly inactivity is the keynote."[156] Major medical examiner offices often have teams of investigators trained in criminal detection to assist them at a death scene. Investigators glean many clues from the position and state of the body, physical evidence, and the body's surroundings. They also photograph the body, the evidence, and the scene for possible use, if necessary, in court. Any evidence collected must be connected to the scene or body by a "chain-of-custody" that is documented in the police and autopsy records. When not in use, the evidence must be secured and labeled for positive identification.

In the *second step*, the body is brought to the morgue, where the pathologist carefully examines clothing on the still-dressed body for any clues to the mechanism of death, including the effects of penetrating objects and the presence of blood or body-fluid stains. The pathologist often dictates the autopsy while performing it so that no details are forgotten or omitted. Forensic pathologists know that courts and other investigatory agencies will use their autopsy reports, so they must be done in exacting detail. They use specific measurements instead of words such as "extreme" or "large." These measurements must be recorded two ways—scientifically in metric (centimeters, grams) for the autopsy records and in English foot-pounds-inches for any related legal documents.[157]

The body is disrobed and carefully examined for identifying marks and characteristics as well as for any sign of injury or violence. The feet and hands are of great importance to forensic pathologists. Scrapings from under the corpse's nails can often help identify a killer, and gunpowder on a hand may indicate a suicide. Paint, glass fragments or tire tracks on a hit-and-run victim's body or clothes may later be matched with a suspect vehicle. X-rays are frequently taken, if not of the whole body, at least of areas that might have been injured.

## TABLE 4.5: Popular Misconceptions about Medicolegal Autopsies.

1. The time of death can be precisely determined.
2. The autopsy always yields the cause of death.
3. An autopsy can be properly done without a history of the events surrounding death.
4. The autopsy is over when the body leaves the morgue.
5. Embalming will not obscure autopsy findings.
6. Only homicide victims (or suspected victims) need be autopsied.
7. The only finding from the medicolegal autopsy is the cause of death.
8. Any pathologist can properly do a medicolegal autopsy.
9. The autopsy must be done immediately.
10. Poisons are always detected at autopsy.
11. All physicians are good "death investigators."
12. Medicolegal autopsies are slanted toward the prosecution.

Adapted from: Petty CS: The devil's dozen: Popular medicolegal misconceptions. *Southern Medical J.* 1971;64(8):919-923.

This is also when the pathologist first tries to determine the number of gunshot wounds and to differentiate where a bullet entered the body (entry) from where it came out (exit). This is not always an easy process. (Treating physicians misinterpret the number of entry/exit wounds more than half the time in single wounds going through the body, and more than three-quarters of the time with multiple wounds.)[158]

The *third step*, the internal examination, generally follows standard autopsy procedures, except when specific injuries are known or suspected. In strangulation deaths, for example, the pathologist carefully dissects the larynx (trachea, hyoid bone, cricoid and thyroid cartilages, and surrounding tissues). When a rape-murder is suspected, the reproductive organs may be removed, examined for any tissue injury, tested for sperm and DNA samples, and sent for chemical analysis. The medical examiner has the authority to keep any organs or tissues that may be needed for evidence in a criminal or civil legal case. The forensic pathologist may be required to actually bring parts of the autopsied body to court, although photographs now normally suffice.[159] Bringing the body parts to court can disconcert participants, as with one woman whose father's heart was presented at a workman's compensation hearing long after he had been buried.[160]

Medical examiners normally test for drugs and poisons (toxicology screens) in all medicolegal autopsies. Tests may be done on the spinal fluid,

142

eye fluid (vitreous humor), blood, bile, stomach contents, hair, skin and urine. According to these tests, alcohol, cocaine, tobacco and marijuana are the most commonly found toxins at death in many parts of the United States.

## P. WHY IS AN AUTOPSY DONE ON A DECOMPOSING OR DISMEMBERED BODY?

Forensic pathologists perform autopsies on decomposing bodies or partial remains primarily to identify the deceased. Corpse identification may be difficult with victims of war or major disasters, remains that have been purposely hidden, bodies found in historical burial places, and some individuals buried prior to obtaining forensic evidence for criminal prosecution. Not only must the forensic specialist attempt to identify the remains, but he also must determine the cause and time of death in cases of homicide victims and non-homicidal deaths discovered after the corpse was hidden or abandoned.[161] In some instances, they must first determine whether remains are, in fact, human and whether they represent a "new" discovery or simply the disinterment of previously known remains. This becomes particularly difficult when the corpse has been severely mutilated or intentionally given a wrong identity.[162]

Forensic pathologists autopsy all victims of major disasters, the most common of which are commercial airline crashes, train accidents, and large fires. A forensic team must identify not only the victims, but the pattern and mechanism of injury, the cause and mechanism of death, the presence of intoxicants in the victims, any evidence of explosives or other intentional trauma, any pre-existing disease, the time of death, and the last survivor in deaths of spouses (for insurance and inheritance distribution).[163] This is not always a simple task, as can be seen from Tom Wolfe's description of a burned airman:

> "burned beyond recognition," which anyone who had been around an air base for very long ... realized was quite an artful euphemism to describe a human body that now looked like an enormous fowl that has burned up in a stove, burned a blackish brown all over, greasy and blistered, fried, in a word, with not only the entire face and all the hair and the ears burned off, not to mention all the clothing, but also the *hands* and *feet*, with what remains of the arms and legs bent at the knees and elbows and burned into absolutely rigid angles, burned a greasy blackish brown like the bursting body itself, so that this husband, father, officer, gentleman, this *ornamentum* of some mother's eye, His Majesty the Baby of just twenty-odd-years back, has been reduced to a charred hulk with wings and shanks sticking out of it.[164]

143

Where multiple bodies or parts of bodies scatter over a relatively confined area, as in most airline crashes, wooden stakes or indelible paint (on concrete) mark where every body part, article of clothing, or other possibly identifying item is located, to help later identify and piece together victims. Investigators note each marker on a grid map and the remains themselves are photographed and tagged. Body parts may then be brought to the morgue or covered for later removal. While workers commonly retrieve only parts of bodies, the forensic team must identify as many victims from the airplane (and sometimes victims on the ground) as possible. They often get amazing results. In the December 1988 explosion and crash of Pan American Flight #301 over Lockerbie, Scotland, for example, all but six of the 259 people on the plane were eventually identified, even though the investigation site and evidence were scattered over an 845-square-mile area. No bodies or parts of the remaining airline victims or any of the eleven ground victims were ever recovered.[165]

The forensic team also tries to determine a cause of death for each victim. While an aircraft accident may appear to make the cause of death obvious, the pathologist can often determine whether a victim died from a premortem event (such as a heart attack), an explosion in the air, hitting the ground, a subsequent fire, gas inhalation, or drowning after falling into water.[166] One problem the forensic team faces in such cases is that no standard set of identifying information, such as dental records, DNA patterns, or X-rays will be available on such a diverse group of people—and identifiable parts may not be available for each victim.

On rare occasions, such as during the bombing of England during World War II, non-pathologists may be asked to assist in piecing together a large number of bodies. One such volunteer who had some anatomy training described her work:

> The bodies—or rather the pieces—were in temporary mortuaries. It was a grim task...but someone had to do it...We had somehow to form a body for burial so that the relatives could [without seeing it] imagine that their loved one was more or less intact for that purpose. But it was a very difficult task—there were so many pieces missing and, as one of the mortuary attendants said, "Proper jigsaw puzzle, ain't it, miss?"...It became a grim and ghastly satisfaction when a body was fairly constructed—but if one was too lavish in making one body almost whole then another one would have sad gaps. There were always odd members which did not seem to fit and there were too many legs.[167]

If there is any question of the victims' identities or of foul play after major disasters, authorities prevent cremation or embalming since they may later need to do further investigations. They also bury unidentified parts or bodies in separate graves so they can be retrieved if further information becomes available.[168] Losing information about a body or body part in a disaster morgue is a major concern, so any identifying data are stored with the body or part.[169] Death certificates are issued and the remains released only after they have been identified as well as possible. This reduces the possibility of error in a chaotic situation.[170]

Forensic entomologists also investigate the cause of death when there is a decomposing corpse. They can often determine the deceased's drug use, even when only a skeleton remains. Entolomological investigators now test maggots, rather than the body's putrefied remains, for drugs. This is because the chemicals from a body are more concentrated, and therefore easier to detect, in the maggots.[171] The drugs that have been found include phenobarbital, triazolam, oxazepam, alimemazine, chloripriamine, organophosphates, cocaine and heroin. Cocaine and heroin stimulated maggot growth.[172] Even insect carcasses in or around skeletonized remains can also aid investigators.[173] FBI experts also predict that investigators will soon be able to tie a suspect to a corpse by matching the blood sucked by mosquitos in the area. In one case, a grasshopper's leg in a murderer's pants cuff was matched with the rest of the grasshopper at the site of death.[174]

Forensic specialists sometimes perform or repeat autopsies centuries after death. For example, the bodies of Edward V and Richard, Duke of York, the boy princes murdered in the Tower of London, have been examined twice—once when they were found buried in a chest in 1674, and again during a more scientific inquiry in 1932. Pathologists and anatomists examined and X-rayed the remains during this later examination and confirmed the previously questioned identity of the remains.

Authorities call forensic specialists when bodies or parts of bodies appear unexpectedly. In modern societies, corpses are frequently disinterred for a variety of reasons, such as vandalism, natural events such as floods, during construction, or through criminal activity. Forensic specialists must determine if these parts are: (1) really human (animal parts may look similar; twenty-five percent of the bones the forensic anthropologists at the Smithsonian Institution get are from animals);[175] (2) the result of accidental disinterment of legal burials (recent or ancient); or (3) evidence of criminal activity.

Clues that a body or body parts were originally buried in a cemetery come from the embalming process. If the body was embalmed, medical examiners often find that the corpse's head and face tightly retain its hair, the skin is cracked and flaky like old paint, the trunk and face are better preserved than the rest of the body, the face has impressions from fabric on the coffin lid, and fungus grows on the face and hands. If the fungal growth is white, it indicates that embalmer's cosmetics were used to prepare the body for viewing; the cosmetics used frequently contain fungal spores. If the brain was embalmed, there may be a fracture of the bone where the nose meets the skull (cribiform plate) through which the embalmer injected chemicals. Other evidence of the mortician's trade that may be found include eye caps, mouth formers, injector needles, trocar buttons, waxed sutures, cotton packing, molding wax, specific types of funerary clothing, and ornamental devices associated with coffins.[176] High levels of alcohol in the tissue may also indicate a modern embalming, although the body's natural fermentation will also produce alcohol in smaller quantities. Older embalming leaves traces of metals such as aluminum, zinc, copper, arsenic, and mercury.[177] Evidence of a prior autopsy also means the person was accidentally disinterred.

Utilitarian items found with a body that may suggest it is not from a cemetery include money, keys, lighters and other accoutrements of the living rather than the dead.[178]

## Q. HOW CAN A PERSON BE IDENTIFIED FROM PARTIAL OR DECOMPOSED REMAINS?

Forensic teams use multiple techniques to discover the identity of decomposing or dismembered remains. These include examining identifying skin marks, tattoos, fingerprints, the condition and prior repair work on the teeth, metal medical implants, and the condition of the bones.

The first famous British forensic pathologist, Sir Bernard H. Spilsbury, used these techniques in the case that brought him to public attention. In July 1910, a woman's torso was found, missing the head, limbs, and genitals. (Spilsbury was well acquainted with dismembered bodies since, before World War II, many British murderers hacked apart their victims and stuffed the pieces in trunks.) He was able to identify the remains as a Cora Crippen, and found that she had been poisoned with hyoscine. Her medically trained American husband was convicted of her murder after authorities apprehended him through an international telegraph message as he arrived back in the United States with his lover.[179]

The military has become expert at identifying even the bits and pieces of corpses that remain after death.

Authorities identified only 10% of the U.S. dead in the Mexican War (1846 to 1847) and 58% of American Civil War dead. Some Union and Confederate soldiers were so fearful that their corpses might go unidentified that they pinned their names to their backs before they went into battle at Gettysburg, Sharpsburg, Cold Harbor, and elsewhere. Authorities, however, gradually improved their record of identifying American war dead, identifying 86.4% in the Spanish-American War, 96.5% in World War I, 96.9% in World War II, 97.1% in Korea, and nearly all victims in

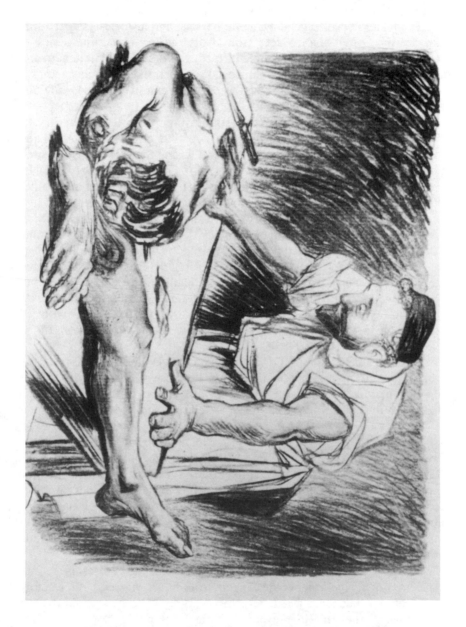

*Le Médecin légiste.* A physician attempts to identify a corpse from the few remaining body parts. Originally published 1902 by Jules Abel Faivre. (Reproduced with permission. National Library of Medicine.)

Vietnam.[180] The military accomplished this by using the services of physical anthropologists, medical examiners, forensic dentists, military mortuary officers and, more recently, specialists in genetics or tissue typing.

The team first collects all available physical and historical information. They are then often able to determine, from the few remaining bones or pieces, the individual's age, sex, height, race, and the approximate date and time of death. Identification had improved so much that when an unknown soldier was selected to memorialize the Vietnam conflict in 1984, only one body met the criteria.[181]

In future conflicts, nearly all U.S. soldiers' remains will be identifiable, even if only a scrap is left. New U.S. Army recruits give blood samples and mouth scrapings to act as "genetic dog tags." Using these specimens, stored at the Armed Forces Institute of Pathology's new Armed Forces DNA Identification Laboratory, the Army claims that "there will never be another body buried in the tomb of the unknown soldier." The blood is stored in a vacuum-packed plastic bag at -20°C for forty years, while the mouth scraping is stored at room temperature. To decrease costs of the program, the records will only be tested if a soldier is missing in action or killed.[182]

Operation Desert Storm, however, occurred before DNA records were established. Because of this, pathologists attempting to identify one Gulf War pilot had to match the DNA from hair found in his electric razor with the DNA in his remains.[183] The first military units deployed with all members having DNA "dog tags" on record were the U.S. forces sent to Somalia in December 1992.[184]

Scientists used similar DNA testing to check the remains recently found in Yekaterinberg, Russia, thought to be those of Czar Nicholas II, his wife and children, executed in 1918. Prince Philip of England, Queen Elizabeth's husband, and other (distant) relatives supplied blood samples for these tests.[185]

Tattoos, used as body decoration for at least 20,000 years, sometimes play an important role in identifying battlefield dead and wounded. In 1066, after the Battle of Hastings, for example, Edith the Swan Neck identified the body of King Harold from his tattoos. The irony is that few modern military personnel know that the intricate tattoos they proudly display have long been used to identify dead soldiers. In Africa, women once identified their stolen children and their dead through unique filed and chipped teeth, sometimes called slave or tribal marks.

The FBI's Disaster Squad often lifts fingerprints from disaster victims. Sometimes they must remove the fingers from badly charred bodies before they clean and ink them for fingerprinting. Where the surface skin is too badly burned, they cut it away and obtain fingerprints from underlying tissue.[186] Occasionally palm or sole prints can also be used, but relatively few people have usable prints on record. (Those taken at birth are usually poorly done and are often later discarded.)[187] Civilian bomb squad members, however, often have their footprints taken when they begin their dangerous job. Often, when they are working on a bomb that explodes, feet inside of their boots are the only identifiable pieces left.[188]

Forensic dentistry also plays an important role in identifying decomposed or dismembered corpses. Teeth are particularly useful as identifiers, since aside from the unique characteristics of restorations, crowns, and missing teeth, each tooth has 5 surfaces (usually 160 in a complete set) available for comparison with a suspected victim's dental records.[189] They also help narrow the age range of subjects under twenty-five-years old.[190] In many countries survivors can FAX the dental (and medical) records and X-rays of possible decedents to forensic teams who then can match identifying details for postmortem identification. When bodies are badly charred or decomposed, dentists sometimes remove the bones containing the teeth (mandible and maxilla) from the body before they attempt dental identification.[191] New computer systems now speed the dental identification process.[192]

Forensic dentistry existed as early as the American Revolutionary War when Paul Revere, a dentist as well as a silversmith, identified the remains of Dr. Joseph Warren, a patriot killed at Bunker Hill, from his teeth. Dental evidence has also helped to identify criminals' bodies, such as those of John Wilkes Booth and Adolph Hitler, and victims such as Dr. Parkman (a Harvard Medical School faculty member killed and cremated in 1849 by someone he considered his friend). Scientists have used similar techniques to identify the charred remains of David Koresh and his followers at the Branch Davidian cult compound in Waco, Texas. Even using the teeth was tricky, because according to Dr. Nazim Peerwani, the Tarrant County Medical Examiner, the remains were so fragile, some of the faces turned to powder.[193] In other cases, such as that of Eva Braun, Adolph Hitler's mistress, forensic dentists could convincingly identify her remains only decades after her death when her dental records became available.[194]

Identification through dental records works nearly as well for those without teeth.[195] In some cases forensic dentists have identified victims from jaw abnormalities or the placement of tooth sockets, even though their teeth were pulled after death by medically sophisticated killers.

Joint prostheses can also help identify some remains, as can other nondestructible internal devices, such as pacemakers, metal bone nails or screws, or metal skull plates.[196] Healed or partially healed fractures also provide identifying information.[197]

Occasionally, forensic scientists must laboriously rearticulate (piece together) the remaining and sometimes scattered bones of the deceased so that new X-rays can be taken and compared to those taken while the person was alive.[198] Modern techniques, however, are now replacing the more time-consuming methods. In addition to direct visualization of the person's remains, modern-day forensic sleuths can use scanning electron microscopes, new genetic technologies, and ground-penetrating radar to peer into unopened graves.

### R. WHAT HAPPENS IF THEY CANNOT IDENTIFY MY BODY?

That depends on many factors. Unidentified bodies will be stored, then cremated or buried. How long they will be stored depends on the amount of available storage space, whether there is a suspicion of foul play, and the investigator's tenacity.

Approximately 1,500 bodies that cannot initially be identified are found in the United States each year. Many of these badly decomposed corpses are thought to be those of transients, teenage runaways, prostitutes or kidnap victims. While some may have died by exposure, accident or suicide, more than two-thirds of them may be victims of foul play. Many, usually corpses of illegal immigrants, carry false identification papers.

California still has nearly 2,000 unidentified bodies (or parts of bodies) in morgues and Texas has 600. To assist in identifying these bodies, law enforcement officials may submit information on unknown corpses to the FBI's National Crime Information Center. There, specialists compare the corpse's physical make-up, fingerprints, dental work and distinguishing marks with over 70,000 missing-person reports on file. Unfortunately, not all jurisdictions submit information to this system.[199]

Facial features of unidentified corpses can now be reconstructed using the skull and other available information. Authorities use this method to identify crime victims in selective cases. The techniques involve video superimposition of faces on skulls, computer modeling, and the use of modeling clay and other materials to reconstruct the face directly on the skull. When authorities think they know whose skull they have, they rely on the more rapid video superimposition or computer modeling methods.[200] This was done with the skeletons of Czar Nicholas and Czarina Alexandra Romanov unearthed in a pit in Yekaterinburg, Russia, more than seventy years after their July 17, 1918 execution by the Bolsheviks. Investigators matched the skulls with old photographs of the couple.[201] The newest computer-assisted methods of facial reconstruction can produce a recognizable face from a skull in only two hours, and in the future should completely replace the need for sculptors to reconstruct faces.[202]

Eventually, authorities bury or cremate the unidentified remains. Disposal of unidentified remains, however, may present problems when multiple unidentified victims were known to be of incompatible religions or sects.[203] After World War II, for example, bodies interred as unknown soldiers had combined Protestant, Catholic and Jewish religious ceremonies—just to cover all bases.[204]

## S. HOW IS THE TIME OF DEATH DETERMINED?

Although their ability to pinpoint the moment of death serves as the main plot element in countless movies and novels, and has been the most popular research topic in forensic medicine over the past 150 years, forensic pathologists can still only give an approximate time of death.[205,206] (Forensic entomologists sometimes can be more exact.) Several parameters can suggest an approximate length of time since death, with varying degrees of accuracy. These include the body's temperature, amount of food in the stomach, pressure in the eyeball, reaction of the pupil to medications, and changes in chemicals in the spinal fluid, blood, or eye fluid (vitreous humor).[207-208] For example, using the body's postmortem temperature (*algor mortis*) to determine the time of death, can be complicated by the size of the body, cause of death, ambient temperature, air movement, amount of clothing on the body or site at which the measurement is taken.[210]

Although the timing of death plays an important role in criminal cases, it is more often used to settle questions about who died first when two or more people appear to have died simultaneously. This is especially true in circumstances in which a married couple both died at approximately the same time or were found dead together—legally termed *commorientes*. Time of death estimates help determine the pattern of inheritance or insurance payments, as in the case of a couple who were dancing under the skywalk of the Hyatt Regency in Kansas City when it collapsed. The medical examiner determined that the man had been instantly crushed, while the woman had lived a short time after her injury, surviving her spouse. In another case a couple's car was hit head-on while on a country road; both people died. The medical examiner determined that the husband's injury, a ruptured heart, had been immediately lethal, while his wife had bled after her injury. Since she bled, she was alive after her injury; she was the "survivor."[211]

Forensic entomologists often can determine the time of death from the types of insects present on a body more accurately than the pathologist. They can also ascertain if a body has been moved, since most fly subspecies stay within a mile or so of where they hatched; and whether the victim died during the day or night, since certain flies rest at night and do not feed, slowing the corpse's decomposition. Insect evidence has also been successfully used to determine the time of burial, place of death, cause of death, the social status of the victim and, in at least one case, to establish that a specific automobile was used to transport a corpse.[212-214] One method formerly used to determine the time of death was to identify the largest of the approximately 150,000 maggots found on an exposed corpse. Forensic entomologists could then calculate when the first egg was laid and establish the time of death. A newer method involves estimating the fly-larval stage that is present in the greatest number.[215] A common problem facing forensic entomologists is that maggot specimens collected from corpses are themselves usually dead and poorly preserved. This complicates identification.[216]

## T. WHAT HAPPENS TO THE ORGANS AND TISSUES EXAMINED AT AUTOPSY?

After an autopsy, the major organs are usually put in plastic bags and stored in body cavities unless pathologists have written permission to keep them.[217] When permitted to do so, many teaching hospitals will keep most of the organs for later study and teaching.[218] The pathologist routinely keeps small pieces of organs (about the size of a crouton) that show or might show evidence of disease or injury, for subsequent microscopic and chemical analysis. They may also keep and analyze fluid from the eye, heart, gallbladder, stomach, urinary bladder, spinal canal, vagina, and other sources. National standards require that "wet tissue" from autopsies be held for six months after issuing a final autopsy report, tissue in paraffin blocks (from which microscope slides are made) must be kept five years, and the slides themselves along with the autopsy reports must be retained for twenty years.[219]

At one time pathologists commonly removed tissues from a body during autopsy for research, teaching or therapy. Beginning in 1963, pathologists started removing pituitary glands, (small grape-size pieces of brain) during autopsies in Great Britain and the United States to obtain human growth hormone. The U.S. program, under the auspices of the National Institutes of Health, treated children who lacked this hormone and would otherwise have been dwarfs. Approximately 200 pituitary glands were needed to maintain normal growth in one child for one year and up to 7 million glands were needed annually. The practice slowed when it became public knowledge in the mid-1960s. From then on pituitary glands were only taken with the family's permission.[220,221] (Human growth hormone is now synthesized and readily available.)

At one time kidney and lung tissue from the autopsies of some premature infants were used as growth media for the study of viruses. Other tissues were frequently removed at autopsies for use as grafts, such as heart valves, arteries, bone, cartilage, skin and dura mater (the covering of the brain).[222] In the past, these tissues were generally removed without permission.

Into the 1970s, permanently removing most of the organs and storing them for later study was not unusual, especially when cases were unique or useful for teaching purposes. While this practice still sometimes occurs without asking, it is increasingly likely that permission will be requested. If organs are kept by the pathologist, they can simply be stored in formaldehyde or can be prepared for display in an anatomical or pathology museum, such as the National Medical Museum at Walter Reed Medical

Center, Washington, D.C. An old method of displaying organs was in thick glass jars. In the last sixty years, plastic has replaced glass. The specimens are first mounted on glass, dissected to display specific pathology, then injected with dyes to demonstrate the vessels or "cleared" to demonstrate the bones or injected blood vessels. The specimens can also be mounted in a gel or clear plastic, mummified, or infiltrated with wax or resins.[223] Plastination or biopolymerization is the newest method of preserving these specimens for future study. It allows the specimen to remain flexible, odorless, and indefinitely preserved.[224]

One argument against asking a family for permission to remove organs is "the distress caused by the adding of gruesome details to the discussion with the bereaved relatives."[225] Physicians have used this same excuse for not telling patients and families the truth for at least two millennia. It is called paternalism and is neither ethical nor legal.

United States courts have held that autopsy permission does not grant the right to permanently remove tissue other than small samples, unless specifically stated.[226] Under English law, however, it is doubtful that someone could be prosecuted for unauthorized use of corpses for medical education or research. The most that could happen would be to charge them with the "common law offence of unlawful interference with a corpse."[227]

Tissue stored from old autopsies can be helpful not only for teaching, but also for research. Blood from old autopsies has helped researchers trace the early patterns of AIDS and the U.S. Hantavirus. In another study, researchers at Washington State University used old autopsy tissue to study the effects of radiation on people working with radioactive substances. Starting with their substantial tissue archive, called the U.S. Transuranium and Uranium Registries, the Department of Energy has added the remains of 20,000 human tissue samples collected over many years from people who had worked with radioactive substances. From studying the tissues and correlating the findings with each person's medical and work history, the researchers hope to better understand the effect of radiation on the human body.[228]

## U. WHAT IS AN EXHUMATION?

Exhumation or disinterment is the removal of a corpse from a grave or other burial site. Pathologists rarely undertake this procedure; it is more commonly done by archaeologists, paleontologists, and construction workers (usually by accident), or caused by natural events, such as floods. Pathologists usually exhume bodies only for criminal or civil investigations. Their exhumations are to: (1) investigate the cause or manner of death; (2) collect evidence (such as bullets or hair fragments); (3) determine the cause of an accident or the presence of disease; (4) gather evidence to assess malpractice; (5) compare the body with another person thought to be

153

deceased; (6) identify war and accident victims who were hastily buried without identification; (7) settle accidental death or liability claims; or (8) search for lost (often valuable) objects.[229,230] The British claim to have less cause for exhumations than in the United States, since they say that "it is very unusual for a victim of death from violence to escape a coroner's necropsy before burial."[231] The most sensational disinterments have been done to investigate homicides—suspected homicides disguised as suicides, suspected homicidal poisonings, and deaths as a result of other criminal activity (in the past, criminal abortions).[232] When bodies are accidentally exhumed, forensic pathologists and anthropologists must determine whether the body was a routine burial accidentally uncovered or evidence of criminal activity.[233] (see *Why is an autopsy done on a decomposing or dismembered body?*)

Criminal cases may warrant disinterment if new evidence appears after a victim has been buried without recognition of foul play. In one instance a 9-year-old girl died in a fire, and only a decade after her burial did a repeat autopsy find that she had actually died from a stab wound to the neck.[234] (Attempting to hide a murder with a fire, however, is relatively common, and forensic pathologists rarely miss this.) In another case, an initial autopsy ruled that a man had died as a result of being run over by a car. A second autopsy after exhumation, however, revealed three bullets in his brain, the actual cause of his demise.[235]

Pathologists have also used exhumation to delineate the extent of therapeutic catastrophes. In 1964 and 1965 up to twenty-four Belgians with prostatic cancer were inadvertently given pills containing large doses of digitoxin, a long-acting heart medication and potential poison, instead of estradiol, a hormone. They died and were buried before anyone suspected there was a problem. A forensic team disinterred the bodies 17 to 40 months after death and determined the true cause of their deaths—accidental poisoning.[236]

Exhumation has also been used to investigate massacres and to reconstruct historical events. Exhumations of remains and forensic techniques were used to investigate the Russian massacre of Polish soldiers in the Katyn Forest in World War II, the German massacre of Italian civilians in Rome's Ardentine caves, the deaths of prisoners in the German concentration camps, and in the 1990s, the fate of thousands of civilians who "disappeared" under the former Argentine dictatorship.[237] Disinterment techniques also aided in identifying the body of the American naval hero, John Paul Jones, and in reconstructing the events at General Custer's last battle at Little Bighorn.[238,239]

Perhaps the ultimate example of an autopsy after embalming was the examination of a 2,100-year-old woman, the so-called "Chinese Princess," whose embalmed corpse was found in the Hunan Province of China in 1972.

When Chinese pathologists examined her body, they found she had suffered from heart and gallbladder disease, been afflicted with three types of intestinal parasites and tuberculosis, as well as having a poorly healed arm fracture and arthritis of her spine. Pathologists were also able to determine that she had borne children.[240]

Normally a court order is required before a body can be exhumed. In Britain, if the body is to be reinterred in the same churchyard gravesite from which it is exhumed, a church license (Bishop's Faculty) is required.[241] Objections to exhumations often come from family members, others who for political reasons do not want further investigation of a case, or law enforcement officials who may be embarrassed by the results.[242]

Exhumed bodies are not pretty. According to Dr. Jesse Carr, former Chief of Pathology at San Francisco General Hospital, "An exhumed embalmed body is a repugnant, moldy, foul-looking object. It's not the image of one who has been loved. You might use the quotation 'John Brown's body lies a-moldering in the grave'; that really sums it up. The body itself may be intact, as far as contours and so on; but the silk lining of the casket is all stained with body fluids, the wood is rotting, and the body is covered with mold."[243] To counteract the odor, pathologists put benzoin on their masks, spray fragrant aerosols, or freeze the remains before the examination. Before they routinely used gloves during autopsies (in the mid-twentieth century), pathologists often put soap under their fingernails before starting an autopsy on decomposed or exhumed bodies to prevent the smell from lingering on their hands.[244]

While pathologists now autopsy exhumed corpses in the morgue, these autopsies were once routinely conducted at the graveside, on the ground or on overturned coffins. This practice was also used, by necessity, in disinterments carried out during the post-World War II war-crimes investigations.[245] Disinterment may take place behind screens, although not only exhumations, but also the subsequent autopsies have occasionally been done in full view at the graveside—and some have resulted in court-imposed damages to the family.[246] The next-of-kin or their representatives are commonly invited to be present for the disinterment.[247]

In a disinterment for medicolegal reasons, photographs are taken as soon as the casket is opened. After the remains are removed and transferred to a standard autopsy table, the body is weighed, measured and, in many cases, X-rayed. Fingerprints and hair samples are obtained whenever possible. Mold is cleaned off to reveal scars, tattoos, birthmarks or other identifying information. Dental structures and abnormalities are carefully recorded for use in identification. Dental X-rays may be taken. Pathologists perform as much of a forensic autopsy as possible, including tests for toxins, on what remains of the body.[248] After the examination, which may include a full autopsy, the body is reburied.

When a pathologist examines the bones from a body that has been buried long enough that very little else remains, he often boils the bones to macerate them and to assist in a diagnosis. According to Ludwig, "maceration of bone yields instructive specimens which are esthetically satisfying and of unlimited durability."[249]

Occasionally, bodies have been exhumed for very unusual reasons. In 1960, an English man disinterred his mother, who had been buried earlier that morning. He took the body to an empty house where he attempted to revive her by feeding her a mixture of plasma, sugar, lime juice and milk. He then used electric shocks, connecting her foot to the house current until it short-circuited.[250] Perhaps this was life imitating art; Alfred Hitchcock's *Psycho* came out the same year.

## V.  WHAT HAPPENS TO MISCARRIED FETUSES AND STILLBORN INFANTS?

Nearly all U.S. hospitals routinely cremate fetal remains with other tissue specimens. If requested, they will usually return fetal remains to the parents for burial.

Miscarried fetuses (spontaneous abortions) are usually smaller than the end of an adult's little finger and occasionally as long as an index finger. Most other tissue passed in a miscarriage is placenta and blood clots. The fetus is normally sent to the pathologist for examination for any congenital defects of which the parents should be aware. In many places the parents may see the aborted fetus before it goes to the pathologist; most do not avail themselves of this privilege.

In the United States, all but two states require a death certificate for fetal deaths. However, the majority of these only require a certificate if the fetus was older than 20-weeks gestation.[251] In Britain, a developing fetus that dies before 28-weeks gestation is considered an *abortus*, but if it has developed 28-weeks or more, it is a *stillborn* and a death certificate must be completed. In Britain, until recently, fetal tissue was discarded by laboratory personnel in waste disposal units. A new British organization, Stillbirth and Neonatal Death Society published a report in 1991 urging their hospitals to follow a more humane standard.[252] Sweden has recently done an about-face in its treatment of aborted fetuses. Until July 1990, aborted fetal tissue had merely been considered a waste-disposal problem, and treated accordingly. At that point, the Swedish National Board of Health and Welfare issued guidelines governing the treatment of aborted fetal tissue.[253] Now, Pathology Departments hold aborted fetal tissue (anonymously with a coded identification number) for two to four weeks, allowing the parents enough time to decide if they want to inter the remains, place cremated remains in a separate grave, or anonymously scatter the ashes in a cemetery with other fetal ashes.[254]

Both pathologists and parents treat stillborn infants as they would any infant death. Pathologists, however, must take special care when handling a stillborn. Too much or too rough handling easily peels off the skin and distorts the head.[255]

Since the establishment of fetal tissue banks, some women who abort spontaneously may be asked or ask to donate this tissue. Unfortunately, the tissue will often be at too early a stage or be too deformed to be used.

## W. WHAT ARE COMMON RELIGIOUS VIEWS ABOUT AUTOPSIES?

Religious views about autopsies generally parallel attitudes about organ or tissue donation. They vary not only among religions, but also sometimes within religious sects and among co-religionists in different countries.

Jewish religious custom forbade autopsy until the eighteenth century, when it was permitted only to save another life, such as that of an accused murderer (by proving him innocent). They based their objection on the belief that the autopsy is a disgrace to the human body and a dishonor to the dead. Opposing this was the stronger traditional duty to save and maintain life, so autopsies are now permitted in select cases. Throughout the 1970s, the Chief Rabbinate of Israel permitted Hadassah University Hospital in Jerusalem to do autopsies if the cause of death was uncertain, information was needed to save a life, foul play was suspected, or genetic counseling information would result.[256]

Even in these cases the body had to be buried as a "whole," requiring that the organs be examined while still in the body, and disallowing the common practice of removing the organs for examination. The pathologist could remove only small blood, fluid and tissue specimens for later analysis. The body was first placed on a sheet so that any fluids that spilled during the procedure could be buried with the body; the paper towels used to clean the instruments were also placed in the body.[257] In 1981, the Israeli parliament, under pressure, tightened the criteria under which an autopsy could be performed with the Anatomy and Pathology Law. For a full autopsy, the permission of three physicians and approval of all next-of-kin are required, thus making autopsy permission extremely difficult to obtain. Postmortem biopsies are common, however.[258] Modern Reform Responsa suggest that not only is there no biblical or Talmudic prohibition on autopsies, but that the Talmud also states that students of anatomy had dissected an executed woman, and their teachers had previously dissected other men and women.[259]

Islam forbids autopsies, except those required by law, based on the Prophet Muhammad's ruling that "The breaking of the bone of a dead person is like the breaking of the bone of a live person." Yet in about the twelfth century A.D., the Islamic legal maxim, "Necessity permits the forbidden" was used to permit autopsies to investigate crimes. In some Islamic countries, permission for an autopsy for a man, when not given by the court, may be given by next-of-kin in this order: father, son, mother, siblings, and only then his wife. In the past, if an autopsy could not be performed in the country where the death occurred, it was not uncommon for the body to be sent to England for the examination.[260,261]

Rastafarians and Hindus find an autopsy extremely distasteful.[262,263] Shintos, the Greek Orthodox Church and Zoroastrians forbid autopsies except those required by law.[264-266]

The Baha'i faith, most non-fundamentalist Protestants, Catholics, Buddhists, and Sikhs permit autopsies.[267-268] The Catholic Church had Pope Alexander autopsied in 1410, and the Vatican allowed and approved of da Vinci's, Vesalius' and Morgagni 's study of anatomy by dissection.[270]

Although modern Catholics generally accept the need for autopsies, Mexican-Americans frequently believe that autopsies are useless, hasten death, destroy the necessary "wholeness" of the body, and that the soul remains near the body and feels pain from the autopsy.[271] This may stem from the rarity of the autopsy in Mexico, where physicians have only used it for 50 years, and then only in the major government-run hospitals.[272] Nevertheless, they give permission for autopsies at the same rate as do Anglo-Americans, who tend not to hold these beliefs.[273]

Some medical examiners' offices now have procedures to accommodate religious objections to autopsies as best as they can. Some Florida medical examiners currently try to stress values of "respect, compassion, kindness and courtesy beyond the minimum required by any policy or guideline" as recommended by a state ethical advisory committee. Their investigators are taught that in some cases an autopsy will not be needed if they: (1) perform an in-depth investigation to exclude a suspicion of a criminal act; (2) do an external examination of the body; (3) get necessary X-rays; (4) test blood, urine and stomach contents for poisons; and (5) perform other procedures without opening the body. They work with religious leaders to accommodate special needs, and even allow them to be present during required autopsies.[274]

## X. HOW DO I GET THE AUTOPSY REPORT?

If the autopsy was done at the family's request or with the family's permission at a hospital, the person who signed the authorization needs only to request a copy of the report. It is probably best to request the report in writing at the time that the authorization for the autopsy is given. Getting these results is worthwhile, since family members often learn unexpected and valuable information from these reports that can help them or their children. A physician may be needed, however, to interpret the report.

If a medical examiner performs the autopsy, the nature of the case will determine how a copy of the results is obtained. In routine cases of sudden or accidental death where no foul play is suspected, the next-of-kin can usually obtain a copy by requesting it in writing from the medical examiner's (or coroner's) office. In cases where the autopsy results will be introduced into court as evidence, a lawyer involved in the case may need to formally request the report.

Postmortem results may not be completed for a month or more after the examination of the body. Some tests and examinations take considerable time; some tissues, such as the brain, require prolonged periods in preservatives before they can be adequately examined. In unusual cases, small tissue or fluid specimens may be sent to outside laboratories or to consultants for their review before a final report can be generated. Ultimately, the autopsy report goes into the patient's medical record. Normally the patient's physician also receives a copy.

Since the onset of the AIDS epidemic, morticians have requested all information about communicable diseases in the deceased. Some pathologists will not release this information unless they have explicit permission from the next-of-kin who authorized the autopsy.[275] New York is the only state that requires that every medical examiner's case include a test for HIV. This information is kept confidential except for notifying other people who had an identifiable risk of contracting AIDS from the deceased.[276] Some states, such as Kansas, also allow the pathologist to release this information to morticians.[277]

## Y. WHAT DOES AN AUTOPSY COST?

A modern autopsy for medical, rather than medicolegal, purposes cost more than $1,000 in the mid-1980s and is higher now.[278] This fee is "eaten" by the hospital, since the charge is reimbursed neither by Medicare nor insurance companies. Nor is there a charge to either the family or the deceased's estate for an autopsy, whether performed by a hospital pathologist or the medical examiner.

## Z. REFERENCES

1. Gelfand T: The "Paris manner" of dissection: student anatomical dissection in early eighteenth-century Paris. *Bull Hist Med.* 1972;46:99-130.
2. Habenstein RW, Lamers WM: *The History of American Funeral Directing.* 2nd ed. Milwaukee, WI: National Funeral Directors Association (NFDA), 1981, p 201.
3. McCarty VO, Sohn AP, Ritzlin RS, Gautnier JH: Scene investigation, identification, and victim examination following the accident of Galaxy 203: disaster preplanning does work. *J Forensic Sciences.* 1987;32:983-87.
4. Sudnow D: *Passing On.* Englewood Cliffs, NJ: Prentice-Hall, 1967, pp 42-51.
5. Interview with Jean Lindsey, R.N. and Kathy Schaffer, R.N. Tucson, AZ: 1992.
6. Sawyer DW: *Embalming Techniques—Restoration after Organ Donation.* (lecture). National Funeral Directors Association Annual Convention. Louisville, KY: 1990. (audiotape)
7. Speck P: Care after death. *Nursing Times.* 1992;88(6):20.
8. *Arizona Revised Statues 11-593:* Reporting of certain deaths; failure to report; classification.
9. Green F: Death with dignity: Hinduism. *Nursing Times.* 1989;85(6):50-51.
10. Green F: Death with dignity: Islam. *Nursing Times.* 1989;85(5):56-57.
11. Iserson KV: Prehospital DNR orders. *Hastings Center Report.* 1989;19(6):17-19.
12. Iserson KV: Foregoing prehospital care: should ambulance staff always resuscitate? *J Medical Ethics.* 1991;17:19-24.
13. *Federal Register.* 1982;47:42265-66.
14. van der Woude J: De Wet op de lijkbezorging en de verpleegkundige. *TVZ.* 1991:12:402-404.
15. Guttmacher AF: Bootlegging bodies—a history of body-snatching. *Bull Soc Med Hist Chicago.* 1935;4(4):353-402.
16. Hektoen L: Early postmortem examinations by Europeans in America. *JAMA.* 1926;86(8):576-77.
17. Chavarría AP, Shipley PG: The siamese twins of Espanola: the first known post-mortem examination in the New World. *Ann Med Hist.* 1924;6:297-302.
18. Hektoen, *JAMA,* 1926.
19. The first postmortem recorded in the country. *JAMA* 1893;21:661-2. Reprinted as: Flanagin A: JAMA 100 years ago. *JAMA.* 1993;270(16):1891
20. Cone TE: The earliest recorded autopsy in America performed in 1662 on the 8-year-old Elizabeth Kelly. *Pediatrics.* 1978;61:572.
21. Forbes TR: *Surgeons at the Bailey: English Forensic Medicine to 1878.* New Haven, CT: Yale Univ Press, 1985, p 33.
22. Hill RB, Anderson RE: *The Autopsy—Medical Practice and Public Policy.* Boston: Butterworths, 1988, pp 19, 32.
23. Selzer R: *Confessions of a Knife.* New York: Quill, 1979, p 180-81.
24. Travers H: Mortui vivos docent: the dead teach the living. *Kansas Medicine.* December 1986, pp 329-33+.
25. Angrist A: Plea for realistic support of the autopsy. *Bull NY Acad Med.* 1971;47:758-65.
26. Stone J: Autopsy in the Form of an Elegy. In: *The Smell of Matches.* New Brunswick, NJ: Rutgers Univ Press, 1972, p 76.
27. Prutting J: Lack of correlation between antemortem and postmortem diagnoses. *NY State J Med.* 1967;67:2081-84.
28. Battle RM, Pathak D, Humble CG, et al: Factors influencing discrepancies between pre- and post-mortem diagnosis. *JAMA.* 1987;258:339-44.

29. Goldhaber SZ, Hennekens CH, Evans DA, et al: Factors associated with correct antemortem diagnosis of major pulmonary embolism. *Am J Med.* 1982;73:822-26.
30. Battle et al, *JAMA,* 1987.
31. Zarling EJ, Sexton H, Milnor P: Failure to diagnose acute myocardial infarction: the clinicopathologic experience at a large community hospital. *JAMA.* 1983;250:1177-81.
32. Ludwig J: *Current Methods of Autopsy Practice.* Philadelphia, PA: WB Saunders, 1972, p 308.
33. Dietz WA, Tobis JM, Isner JM: Failure of angiography to accurately depict the extent of coronary artery narrowing in three fatal cases of percutaneous transluminal coronary angioplasty. *J Am Coll Cardiology.* 1992;19:1261-70.
34. Mosquera DA, Goldman MD: Surgical audit without autopsy: tales of the unexpected. *Annals of the Royal College of Surgeons of England.* 1993;75:1115-17.
35. Battle et al, *JAMA,* 1987.
36. Polson CJ, Brittain RP, Marshall TK: *The Disposal of the Dead.* 2nd ed. Springfield, IL: Charles C Thomas, 1962, p 56.
37. Ahronheim JC, Bernholc AS, Clark WD: Age trends in autopsy rates: striking decline in late life. *JAMA.* 1983;250:1182-86.
38. Hill, Anderson, *Autopsy,* p 42.
39. Thorndike L: A fifteenth-century autopsy by Bernard Tornius. *Ann Med Hist.* 1928;10:270-77.
40. Hill, Anderson, *Autopsy,* p 133.
41. Boerhaave Hermann: Atrocis, nec Descripti Prius. *Morbi Historia.* Translated in: *Bull Medical Library Assoc.* 1955;43:217.
42. Osler W. As quoted in: Selzer, *Confessions of a Knife,* p 130.
43. Fitz RH: Perforating inflammation of the vermiform appendix, with special reference to its early diagnosis and treatment. *Boston Med Surg J.* 1886;115:13-14.
44. Hill, Anderson, *Autopsy,* pp 44-48.
45. Ibid., pp 51-52.
46. Cabot RC: Diagnostic pitfalls identified during a study of three thousand autopsies. *JAMA.* 1912;59:2295-98.
47. Flexner A: *Medical Education in the United States and Canada.* New York: Carnegie Foundation for the Advancement of Teaching, 1910.
48. Fox RC: *Essays in Medical Sociology.* New York: John Wiley & Sons, 1979, p52.
49. Hill, Anderson, *Autopsy,* p 58.
50. *Liaison Committee on Medical Education (LCME) Annual Survey.* LCME. 1991 & 1992.
51. Johnson HRM: The incidence of unnatural deaths which have been presumed to be natural in coroners' autopsies. *Med Sci Law.* 1969;9:102-106.
52. Hill, Anderson, *Autopsy,* p 41.
53. Heckerling PS, Williams MJ: Attitudes of funeral directors and embalmers toward autopsy. *Arch Pathol Lab Med.* 1992;116:1147-51.
54. Anderson RE, Hill RB: The current status of the autopsy in academic medical centers in the United States. *Amer J Clin Pathol.* 1989;92(suppl 1):S31-S37.
55. Hill RB, Anderson RE: The autopsy crisis reexamined: the case for a national autopsy policy. *Milbank Quarterly.* 1991;69:51-78.
56. Pollack DA, O'Neil JM, Parrish G, Combs DL, Annest JL: Temporal and geographic trends in the autopsy frequency of blunt and penetrating trauma deaths in the United States. *JAMA.* 1993;269:1525-31.
57. Travers, *Kansas Medicine,* 1986.
58. Kircher T, Nelson J, Burdo H: Descriptive epidemiology of the autopsy in Connecticut, 1979-1980. *Arch Pathol Lab Med.* 1985;109:904-909.
59. Pollock et al, *JAMA,* 1993.
60. Schmidt S: Consent for autopsies. *JAMA.* 1983;250:1161-64.
61. Pollock et al, *JAMA,* 1993.
62. Habenstein RW, Lamers WM: *Funeral Customs the World Over.* Milwaukee: Bulfin Printers, 1963, multiple pages.
63. Coronial autopsies inquiry. *Applied Ethics: Newsletter of the Kingswood Centre for Applied Ethics.* Perth, Australia: 1992;7:4.

161

64. *Hawaii Rev Stat* §453-165.
65. *Md Ann Code art 5,* §501.
66. *Mich Stat Ann* §14.45(2855).
67. *Miss Code Ann* §41-37-25.
68. *Ariz Rev Stat Ann* §36-382.
69. Ludwig, *Current Methods of Autopsy Practice,* p 299.
70. Schmidt, *JAMA,* 1983.
71. Ibid.
72. Ibid.
73. *Jackson v. Rupp,* 228 So 2d 916, Fla 1969.
74. *Larson v. Chase,* 50 NW 238, Minn 1891.
75. Waltz JR: Legal liability for unauthorized autopsies and related procedures. *J Forensic Sciences.* 1971;16:1-14.
76. *Gray v. Southern Pac. Co.,* 68 P2d 1011 (Cal App 1937).
77. Postmortum tissue problem. *Br Med J.* August 5, 1978, p 382.
78. Ludwig, *Current Methods of Autopsy Practice,* p 301.
79. Cordner SM: The second post-mortem and deaths overseas: a case report. *Med Sci Law.* 1984;24:261-64.
80. *Louisville and Nashville Ry Co v. Blackmon,* 59 SE 341, Ga 1907.
81. *Streipe v. Liberty Mutual Insurance Co,* 47 SW 2d 1004, Ky 1932.
82. *Aetna Insurance Co v. Burton,* 12 NE 2d 360, Indiana 1938.
83. Holder AR: Unauthorized autopsies. *JAMA.* 1970;214:967-68.
84. *Vt Stat Ann title 21,* §1018.
85. *38 CFR* §3.312.
86. *Arizona Revised Statute: Living Wills and Health Care Directives Act.* Title 36, Chapter 32 (1992).
87. *New York Public Health Law,* § 4201 (Supp. 1967).
88. *Schloendorff v. Society of New York Hospital,* 211 NY 125, 129, 105 NE 92 (1914).
89. Schmidt, *JAMA,* 1983.
90. Carr J. As quoted in: Mitford J: *The American Way of Death.* New York: Simon & Schuster, 1963, p 85-86.
91. Mitford J: *The American Way of Death.* New York: Simon & Schuster, 1963, p 86.
92. Sawyer D: Autopsies. *The Dodge Magazine.* 1982;74:1.
93. Heckerling, Williams, *Arch Pathol Lab Med,* 1992.
94. Sawyer, Autopsies, *The Dodge Magazine,* 1982.
95. Heckerling, Williams, *Arch Pathol Lab Med,* 1992.
96. Ibid.
97. Williams MJ: *The Funeral Director's and Embalmer's Role in Medical Technology.* (lecture). National Funeral Directors Association Annual Convention. Louisville, KY: 1990. (audiotape)
98. Sawyer, *Restoration after Organ Donation,* 1990. (audiotape)
99. Mayer R: *Embalming Techniques—Transplants and Trauma.* (lecture). National Funeral Directors Association Annual Convention. Baltimore, MD: 1989. (audiotape)
100. Kalfofen RW: After a child dies: a funeral director's perspective. *Comprehensive Pediatric Nursing.* 1989;12:285-97.
101. Sawyer, Autopsies, *The Dodge Magazine,* 1982.
102. Kalfofer, *Comprehensive Pediatric Nursing,* 1989.
103. Ludwig, *Current Methods of Autopsy Practice,* p 18.
104. Start RD, Hector-Taylor MJ, Cotton DWK, et al: Factors which influence necropsy requests: a psychological approach. *J Clin Pathol.* 1992;45:254-57.
105. Hellerstein D: The battle for the dead. *Esquire.* February 1982, p 83-90.
106. Shem S: *The House of God.* New York: Doubleday Dell, 1978, p 152.
107. Sidorov J: An attempt to motivate internal medicine housestaff to obtain consent for autopsies. *Acad Med.* 1990;65:647-49.
108. Champ C, Tyler X, Andrews PS, Coghill SB: Improve your hospital autopsy rate to 40-50 percent, a tale of two towns. *J Pathol.* 1992;166:405-407
109. Brown HG: Lay perceptions of autopsy. *Arch Pathol Lab Med.* 1984;108:446-48.

110. Mitford, *The American Way of Death,* p 163.
111. Wilke A, French F: Attitudes toward autopsy refusal by young adults. *Psychol Rep.* 1990;67:81-91.
112. Hill, Anderson, *Milbank Quarterly,* 1991.
113. Mitford, *The American Way of Death,* p 211.
114. Navajo seeks answers for illness. *Prodigy News Service.* June 3, 1993.
115. Haque AK, Cowan WT, Smith JH: The decedent affairs office: a unique centralized service. *JAMA.* 1991;266:1397-99.
113. Ludwig, *Current Methods of Autopsy Practice,* p 224-26.
117. Fatteh A, Mann GT: The role of radiology in forensic pathology. *Med Sci Law.* 1969;9:27-30.
118. Ludwig, *Current Methods of Autopsy Practice,* p 6.
119. Ibid., p 190.
120. Univ of Arizona Dept of Pathology: *Post Mortem Examination.* Tucson, AZ: August 1990.
121. Selzer, *Confessions of a Knife,* p 179.
122. Ludwig, *Current Methods of Autopsy Practice,* p 157-88.
123. Ibid., p 199.
124. Ibid., pp 5-6.
125. Ibid. pp 160-62.
126. Ibid., p 2.
127. Hill, Anderson, *Autopsy,* p 5.
128. Ludwig, *Current Methods of Autopsy Practice,* p 301.
129. West M, Chomet B: An evaluation of needle necropsies. *Am J Med Sci.* 1957;234:554-60.
130. Wellmann KF: The needle autopsy: a retrospective evaluation of 394 consecutive cases. *Am J Clin Pathol.* 1969;52:441-44.
131. Ludwig, *Current Methods of Autopsy Practice,* p 5.
132. Dorsey DB: Limited autopsies: defined benefits, limited costs. *Arch Pathol Lab Med.* 1984;108:469-72.
133. Gordon R: *Great Medical Disasters.* New York: Dorset Press, 1983, p 68.
134. Foster WD: *A Short History of Clinical Pathology.* Edinburgh: E & S Livingstone, 1961, pp 9-10.
135. Univ of Arizona Dept of Pathology: *Autopsy Procedures—How to do an autopsy: the twenty steps.* Tucson, AZ: 1992.
163. Univ of Arizona, *Post Mortem Examination,* August 1990.
137. Mitford, *The American Way of Death,* p 83.
138. Hill, Anderson, *Autopsy,* p 141.
139. Uniform Law Commissioners: *Model Post-Mortem Examinations Act, 1954.* As cited in: Combs DL, Parrish RG, Ing R: *Death Investigation in the United States and Canada, 1992.* Atlanta, GA: U.S. Dept of Health & Human Services, 1992, pp 323-31.
140. Carlson L: *Caring for Your Own Dead.* Hinesburg, VT: Upper Access, 1987, p 53.
141. Grollman EA, ed: *Concerning Death: A Practical Guide for the Living.* Boston: Beacon Press, 1974, p 183.
142. Wooters RC: A medical examiner recalls an array of experiences. *American Medical News.* June 2, 1992, p 27.
143. Wilson EF, Fisher RS: The medical examiner system in Maryland. *Maryland State Medical J.* 1968;17(Dec):51
144. Hill IR: The coroner—12th and 13th century development of the office. *Med Sci Law.* 1990;30:133-37.
145. Shakespeare W: *Hamlet.* Act 5, scene 1.
146. Randall T: Clinicians' forensic interpretations of fatal gunshot wounds often miss the mark. *JAMA.* 1993;269(16):2058-61.
147. Browne WH, ed: *Archives of Maryland.* Baltimore Historical Society. vol4. 1887. Cited in: Spitz WU, Fisher RS: *Medicolegal Investigation of Death.* Springfield, IL: Charles C Thomas, 1973, p 6.
148. American Forensic Sciences 1776-1976. *Inform Letter.* 1976;8(3):5.
149. Bernard HY: *The Law of Death and Disposal of the Dead.* 2nd ed. Dobbs Ferry, NY: Oceana Pub, 1979, pp 65-67.

150. Spitz WU, Fisher RS: *Medicolegal Investigation of Death*. Springfield, IL: Charles C Thomas, 1973, p 3.
151. Ibid., p 3-4.
152. Schultz SM: *Body Snatching: The Robbing of Graves for the Education of Physicians*. Jefferson, NC: McFarland, 1992, pp 9-10.
153. Forbes, *Surgeons at the Bailey*, p 35.
154. Ibid., p 34.
155. Ibid., p 73.
156. Ludwig, *Current Methods of Autopsy Practice*, p 12.
157. Ibid., p 14.
158. Randall, *JAMA*, 1993.
159. Grabuschnigg VP, Rous F: Konservierung menschlicher Leichen im Wandel der Zeit—ein Beitrag zur Entwicklung und Methodik. *Beitrage zur Gerichtlichen Medizin.* 1990;48:455-58.
160. Carlson, *Caring for Your Own Dead*, p 53.
161. Hawley DA, Doedens DJ, McClain JL, Pless JE: Concealment of the body in drug deaths. *J Forensic Sciences.* 1989;34:495-99.
162. Mant AK: The identification of mutilated and decomposed bodies (with special reference to air crash victims). *Med Sci Law.* 1962;2:134-42.
163. Eckert WG: The Lockerbie disaster. *The Inform Letter.* 1989;21.
648. Wolfe T: *The Right Stuff.* New York: Farrar, Strauss and Giroux, 1979, p 5.
165. Eckert, *The Inform Letter*, 1989.
166. Busuttil A, Jones JSP: The certification and disposal of the dead in major disasters. *Med Sci Law.* 1992;32:9-13.
167. Faviell F: *A Chelsea Concerto*. London: Cassell, 1959.
168. Hooft PJ, Noji EK, van de Voorde HP: Fatality management in mass casualty incidents. *Forensic Science International.* 1989;40:3-14.
169. Randall B: Body retrieval and morgue operation at the crash of United flight 232. *J Forensic Sciences.* 1991;36:403-409.
170. Busuttil, Jones, *Med Sci Law*, 1992.
171. Kintz P, Godelar B, Tracqui A, et al: Fly larvae: a new toxicological method of investigation in forensic medicine. *J Forensic Sciences.* 1990;35;204-207.
172. Catts EP, Goff ML: Forensic entomology in criminal investigations. *Ann Rev Entomol.* 1992;37:253-72.
173. Rodriguez WC, Bass WM: Insect activity and its relationship to decay rates of human cadavers in east Tennessee. *J Forensic Sciences.* 1983;28;423-32.
174. Richards B: The maggot test: bugs on dead bodies have tales to tell. *Wall Street J.* April 27, 1992, p A1.
175. Goodman S: Advances in forensics help in solving more crimes. *Tucson (AZ) Citizen,* May 4, 1993, p 4NE.
176. Berryman HE, Bass WM, Symes SA, Smith OC: Recognition of cemetery remains in the forensic setting. *J Forensic Sciences.* 1991;36:230-37.
177. Ibid.
178. Ibid.
179. Browne DG, Tullett EV: *Bernard Spilsbury—His Life and Cases.* London: George G Harrap, 1951, pp 38-54.
180. Wood WR, Stanley LA: Recovery and identification of World War II dead: American graves registration activities in Europe. *J Forensic Sciences.* 1989;34:1365-73.
181. Raether HC: *Funeral Service: A Historical Perspective.* Evanston, IL: National Funeral Directors Assoc., 1990, p 90.
182. Cauchon D: Another GI wait: in line for DNA sampling. *USA Today.* December 7, 1992, p 6A.
183. GIs now getting genetic dog tags. *Tucson (AZ) Citizen.* June 11, 1992, p 4A.
184. Cauchon, *USA Today*, December 7, 1992.
185. Russia's royal mystery finds clue in Prince Phillip's blood. *Prodigy News Service.* December 15, 1992.

186. McCarty et al, *J Forensic Sciences,* 1987.
187. Mant, *Med Sci Law,* 1962.
188. Interview with a member of the Tucson Police Department Identification Unit. Tucson, AZ: March 1993.
189. Spitz, Fisher, *Medicolegal Investigation of Death,* p 66-67.
190. Ibid., p 75-77.
191. McCarty et al, *J Forensic Sciences,* 1987.
192. Lorton L, Langley WH: Decision-making concepts in postmortem identification. *J Forensic Sciences.* 1986;31:190-96.
193. Medical examiner to begin cult autopsies. *Prodigy News Service.* April 23, 1993.
194. Keiser-Nielsen S, Strom F: The odontological identification of Eva Braun Hitler. *Forensic Science International.* 1983;21:59-64.
195. Lorton, Langley, *J Forensic Sciences,* 1986.
196. Busutti, Jones, *Med Sci Law,* 1992.
197. Mant, *Med Sci Law,* 1962.
198. Vanezis P, Sims BG, Grant JH: Medical and scientific investigation of an exhumation in unhallowed ground. *Med Sci Law.* 1978;18:209-21.
199. Castaneda C: Nameless bodies burden, baffle law enforcers. *USA Today.* April 24, 1992, p 10A.
200. Iten PX: Identification of skulls by video superimposition. *J Forensic Sciences.* 1987;32:173-88.
201. Skeleton confirmed as Czar's. *Chicago Tibune.* June 23, 1992, Section 1, p 15.
202. Ubelaker DH, O'Donnell G: Computer-assisted facial reproduction. *J Forensic Sciences.* 1992;37(1):155-62.
203. Busuttil, Jones, *Med Sci Law,* 1992.
204. Wood, Stanley, *J Forensic Sciences,* 1989.
205. Knight B: The evolution of methods for estimating the time of death from body temperature. *Forensic Science International.* 1988;36:47-55.
206. van den Oever R: A review of the literature as to the present possibilities and limitations in estimating the time of death. *Med Sci Law.* 1976;16:269-76.
207. Ibid.
208. Ludwig, *Current Methods of Autopsy Practice,* p 16-17.
209. Eckert WG: Timing of death and injuries. *Medico-Legal Insights.* Cited in: *Inform Letter.* Fall 1991.
210. van de Oeuver, *Med Sci Law,* 1976.
211. Eckert, *Medico-Legal Insights.* Cited in: *Inform Letter,* Fall 1991.
212. Catts, Goff, *Ann Rev Entomol,* 1992.
213. Keh B: Scope and application of forensic entomology. *Ann Rev Entomol.* 1985;30:137-54.
214. Erzinclioglu YZ: Entomology, zoology and forensic science: the need for expansion. *Forensic Science International.* 1989;43:209-13.
215. Erzincliogul YZ: On the interpretation of maggot evidence in forensic cases. *Med Sci Law.* 1990;30:65-66
216. Catts, Goff, *Ann Rev Entomol,* 1992.
217. Univ of Arizona, *Post Mortem Examination,* 1990.
218. Univ of Arizona, *Autopsy Procedures,* 1992.
219. *CAP Today.* August 1988, p 25. (From the rules of the National Laboratory Accreditation Program.)
220. Postmortem tissue problem. *Br Med J.* August 5, 1978, p 382.
221. Sadler AM, Sadler BL: A community of givers, not takers. *Hastings Center Report.* 1984;14:6-9.
222. Ludwig, *Current Methods of Autopsy Practice,* p 310.
223. Ibid., pp 253-61.
224. Dahmer G: Personal communication, November 5, 1993.
225. Postmortem tissue problem, *Br Med J,* 1978.
226. *Hendrikson v. Roosevelt Hospital,* 297 F Supp 1142, DC NY, 1969.

227. Skegg PDG: Criminal liability for the unauthorized use of corpses for medical education and research. *Med Sci Law.* 1992;32:51-54.
228. A glowing gift of human tissue. *Prodigy News Service.* March 27, 1993.
229. Eckert WG, Katchis GS: Disinterments—their value and associated problems. *Am J Forensic Med & Path.* 1990;11:9-16.
230. Ludwig, *Current Methods of Autopsy Practice,* p 305.
231. Necropsy after exhumation. *Br Med J.* October 4, 1969, p 6.
232. Ludwig, *Current Methods of Autopsy Practice,* p 305.
233. Berryman, *J Forensic Sciences,* 1991.
234. Eckert, Katchis, *Am J Forensic Med & Path,* 1990.
235. Ibid.
236. Thomas F, La Barre J, Renaux J, Draux E: A therapeutic catastrophe, entailing 16 exhumations, following the administration of digitoxin instead of oestradiol benzoate to prostatic cancer patients: identification of the poison. *Med Sci Law.* 1979;19:8-18.
237. Eckert, Katchis, *Am J Forensic Med & Path,* 1990.
238. Ibid.
239. Eckert WG: Identification of John Paul Jones. *Am J Forensic Med & Pathol.* 1982;3:143-52.
240. Wei O: Internal organs of a 2100-year-old female corpse. *Lancet.* Nov 24, 1973, p 1198.
241. Balfour AJC: His honour'd bones. *Aviation, Space & Environmental Med.* 1989:60(10, Suppl.):B24-B26.
242. Eckert, Katchis, *Am J Forensic Med & Path,* 1990.
243. Carr J. As quoted in: Mitford, *American Way of Death,* p 84.
244. Mant AK: Changes in the practice of forensic pathology, 1950-1985. *Med Sci Law.* 1986;26:149-57.
245. Mant, *Med Sci Law.* 1986.
246. *Hill v. Traveler's Insurance Co,* 294 SW 1097, Tenn 1927.
247. Ludwig, *Current Methods of Autopsy Practice,* p 306.
248. Eckert, Katchis, *Am J Forensic Med & Path,* 1990.
249. Ludwig, *Current Methods of Autopsy Practice,* p 201-206.
250. Polson, Brittain, Marshall, *The Disposal of the Dead,* p 253.
251. Carlson, *Caring for Your Own Dead,* p 52.
252. Dignified in death. *Nursing Times.* 1991;87(29):16-17.
253. Swedish National Board of Health and Welfare: *Guidelines SOSFS 1990:8,* 1990.
254. Kallenberg K: The disposal of the aborted fetus—new guidelines: ethical considerations in the debate in Sweden. *J Medical Ethics.* 1993;19:32-36.
255. Kalfofen, *Comprehensive Pediatric Nursing,* 1989.
256. Mittleman RE, Davis JH, Kasztl W, Graves WM: Practical approach to investigative ethics and religious objections to the autopsy. *J Forensic Sciences.* 1992;37(3):824-29.
257. Ibid.
258. Meyers N: Medicine confronts Jewish law. *Nature.* 1985;318(Nov):97.
259. *Talmud: B. Bechorot 45a.*
260. Green, Islam, *Nursing Times,* 1989.
261. Ghanem I: Permission for performing an autopsy: The pitfalls under Islamic law. *Med Sci Law.* 1988;28(3):241-42.
262. Green, Hinduism, *Nursing Times,* 1989.
263. Green F: Death with dignity: Rastafarianism. *Nursing Times.* 1992;88(9):56-57.
264. Namihira E: Shinto concept concerning the dead human body. *Transplantation Proc.* 1990;22(3):940-41.
265. Green F: Death with dignity: Zoroastrianism. *Nursing Times.* 1992;88(7):44-45.
266. Mittleman et al, *J Forensic Sciences,* 1992.
267. Green F: Death with dignity: Baha'i Faith. *Nursing Times.* 1989;85(10):50-51.
268. Green, Rastafarianism, *Nursing Times.* 1992.
269. Green F: Death with dignity: Sikhism. *Nursing Times.* 1989;85(9):56-57.
270. Hill, Anderson, *Autopsy,* p 167.
271. Perkins HS, Supik JD, Hazuda HP: Autopsy decisions: the possibility of conflicting cultural attitudes. *J Clinical Ethics.* 1993;4(2):145-54.

272. González-Villalpando C: The influence of culture in the authorization of an autopsy. *J Clinical Ethics*. 1993;4(2):192-97.

273. Perkins, Supik, Hazuda, *J Clinical Ethics*, 1993.

274. Mittleman et al, *J Forensic Sciences*, 1992.

275. Memo from the Chief Mortician. University Medical Center. Tucson, AZ: September 25, 1990.

276. American Medical Association Council on Ethical and Judicial Affairs: *Confidentiality of HIV Status on Autopsy Reports*. Presented to the AMA House of Delegates. Chicago, IL: June 1992.

277. *Kansas State Ann.* §65-2438.

278. Hill, Anderson, *Autopsy*, p 15.

# ΝΕΚΡΟΚΗΔΕΙΑ:

## OR, THE

# Art of Embalming;

### Wherein is fhewn

# The Right of Burial,

## THE

# FUNERAL CEREMONIES,

### And the feveral Ways of

# Preferving Dead Bodies

## IN

# Moft Nations of the WORLD.

### With an Account of

The particular Opinions, Experiments and Inventions
of modern Phyficians, Surgeons, Chymifts and Anatomifts.

## ALSO

Some new Matter propos'd concerning a better Method of *Embalming* than hath hitherto been difcover'd.

## AND

A *Pharmacopœia Galeno-Chymica, Anatomia
ficca five incruenta,* &c.

### In Three PARTS.

*The whole Work adorn'd with variety of Sculptures.*

*By* THOMAS GREENHILL, *Surgeon.*

LONDON: Printed for the Author.

# 5: BEAUTY IN DEATH

A. What do undertakers do?
B. What does a funeral director do?
C. Who composes the funeral industry?
D. What training do embalmers have?
E. What are funeral industry buzzwords?
F. How do funeral homes differ?
G. What are some traditional preparation rites for bodies?
H. What is embalming?
I. Why embalm a body?
J. How has embalming occurred in the past?
K. How is a body prepared for embalming?
L. What is restoration?
M. How are cosmetics used on the corpse?
N. What restoration techniques are used for organ and tissue donors?
O. How is a body embalmed today?
P. Are embalming and restoration always successful?
Q. How is a body prepared for viewing?
R. How does a mummy differ from an embalmed body?
S. Can all bodies be embalmed?
T. Must all bodies be embalmed?
U. What are religious & legal attitudes toward embalming?
V. How much does embalming cost?
W. References

*To most of the world's amazement, if not disgust, embalming is a common and accepted custom in the United States. What happens within the secretive world of the embalmer? Who comprises the funeral industry? What special restoration techniques do embalmers use? What legal requirements exist for embalming? What are religious attitudes toward the process and how much does it cost?*

## A. WHAT DO UNDERTAKERS DO?

*Undertaker*, a term in use by 1698, originally meant one who "undertook" to make funeral arrangements and to keep a body safe.[1] However, the duties of an undertaker have evolved from ancient times, and continue to do so. *Undertaker* is a traditional term deplored by members of the industry. The term "funeral director" was coined by 1885, and it has taken a long time and much effort on the part of the industry for it to catch on. Into the 1960s, the *New York Times* continued to use the term "undertaker" to describe this vocation.[2] In the early twentieth century, the term *mortician* was devised, but it has never been popular. In spite of the industry's dislike, however, the term "undertaker" persists and is used interchangeably with mortician, embalmer, and funeral director by the general public. In this section, the term "undertaker" refers to early practitioners of the funerary trade.

The undertaker's job began when that of the physician ended.[3] Undertakers saw that the corpse, in one sociologist's words, "conformed to the expectations of its audience, particularly the bereaved family. In this he functioned to save responsible members of the family and their friends from performing the menial and unpleasant tasks necessary to prepare a body for burial. He did the physical work of taking the ritually unclean, usually diseased, corpse with its unpleasant appearance and transforming it from a lifeless object to the sculptured image of a living human being who is resting in sleep."[4]

In ancient Rome *libitinarii* managed the temple of Venus Libitina where funeral supplies were sold, and from which slaves called *pollinctores* operated. These slaves bathed corpses, while their assistants, the *designators*, collected money, kept records of the dead, sold funeral supplies, assigned places in funeral processions, and managed other aspects of the funerals.[5,6] Ancient Scythian undertakers suffered for their trade when attending dead kings. They had to cut off one of their own ears, shave their heads, and wound themselves in the arms, forehead, nose, and left hand with arrows.[7]

In Britain, William Boyce opened his undertaking business in "ye Grate Ould Bayley, near Newgeat" in 1675.[8] Within a decade, undertaking had begun to broaden its scope when, to increase profits, individuals in the "Dismal Trade" gradually began to procure and sell coffins; furnish materials for mourning; preserve bodies using ice, embalming and other

170

methods; and rent hearses or similar transportation to the cemetery.[9] British undertakers announced their duties by posting a person at the front doorstep, usually in top hat and frock coat, to symbolize the family's mourning; many British undertakers still wear this garb.[10]

British royalty first used a professional undertaker in 1751, when the unpopular Frederick, Prince of Wales, died. A Mr. Harcourt sent the royal family a bill for laying out the corpse and providing the coffin and winding sheet. (A winding sheet is a cloth wrapped or wound around the corpse until burial, normally leaving the face exposed. It is tied or sewn above the head and below the feet to resemble a double-ended sack.) He also supplied "two wooden urns covered with lead and lined with silk for ye Bowells," and "six men to move the Body under the canopy."[11] The royal family refused to pay the bill, believing that the undertaker had charged for some services he did not provide.[12]

Early undertakers usually combined their funeral business with other trades. Many tradesmen, desperate to get any type of work, combined undertaking with child care, dentistry, picture-framing, messenger services, church sexton, coroner, and city lamplighting.[13] Many were furniture makers who began making coffins as a sideline, and only gradually branched out into supplying the other materials and personal services needed for funerals and burials. In the American colonies the earliest record of an undertaker was Blanch White, who set up a New York business in 1768 that combined upholstering and undertaking. Her advertisements promised to supply "all kinds of Field Equipage, Drums, Etc. Funerals furnish'd with all things necessary and proper Attendance as in England."[14] Mrs. Benjamin Birch set up a similar combined business in Montreal, Canada, in 1820. She added cabinet-making to her trade, a combination that spread through North America.[15]

Undertakers continued to stress the "furniture" part of undertaking—the coffin—which remained their major income producer. Businesses combining furniture sales and funeral directing were common in the American Midwest through the mid-twentieth century. In the post-Civil War era, however, undertakers began to rely on specialized coffin manufacturers and lost control of coffin and casket prices. The coffin manufacturers formed the National Burial Case Association and set industry-wide prices—with a forty percent price increase in 1881. This spurred undertakers to organize their trade, so they could control funeral prices and collectively bargain with manufacturers for funeral merchandise.[16]

In nineteenth-century United States cities, retired carpenters, gravediggers, and owners of horse carts began making their livings as undertakers. By the 1820s, some enterprising owners of livery stables found themselves doing increasing amounts of business renting coaches and horses for funerals, so they attempted to eliminate the middleman by becoming undertakers.[17] Eventually, new transportation methods allowed enough corpses to be brought to them so that they could support themselves by undertaking alone.[18] The personal services associated with funerals, however, were rarely performed by undertakers. By the early 1800s, most U.S. cities had women identified as "layers out of the dead," who survived by preparing corpses for funerals and burials.[19]

Undertakers gradually incorporated embalming into their work, taking the job over from the surgeons, the earliest embalmers in Western society. This added status to the trade since, as Renouard wrote in 1883, "the public had once believed that any fool could become an undertaker. Embalming, however, made people marvel at the 'mysterious' and 'incomprehensible' process of preservation, and made them respect the practitioner."[20]

The U.S. Army was forced to establish the first licensing rules for embalmers and undertakers during the Civil War. There was such severe competition among embalmers that on at least one occasion, one burned down another's embalming tent.[21] After the 1863 battle, "a whole slew of them descended on Gettysburg in the high spirit of profit. Setting up their places of business within a macabre distance of the field hospitals, they did not wait long for a flourishing trade. A plank across a couple of barrels made a handy establishment...The embalmers pumped the bereaved for all the cash they could get and then pumped in their preservative."[22]

The trade first organized in the United States as the Undertakers' Mutual Protection Association of Philadelphia in January 1864. By 1881 they had also organized in eight other states as "undertakers."[23] By the end of the nineteenth century, embalming had become a career in the United States, with licensing required in some jurisdictions. Yet, in 1920, when the organization had nearly 10,000 members, National Funeral Directors Association (NFDA) President John F. Martin told their convention that funeral directors had not yet become professionals.[24]

Social stigma has always surrounded undertakers. Diodorus Siculus said of ancient embalmers, "All there present pursue him with execration and pelt him with stones, as if he were guilty of some horrid offense, for they look upon him as an hateful person, who wounds and offers violence to the body in that kind, or does it any prejudice whatsoever."[25] This position was well illustrated by W. Lloyd Warner when he said, "The deep hostilities and fears men have for death, unless very carefully controlled and phrased, can turn the undertaker into a scapegoat, the ritual uncleanliness of his task being identified with his role and person."[26]

"In performing these ritually unclean tasks," said one sociologist, "the undertaker reduces the horror the living feel when in contact with the cold and 'unnatural' remains of a loved person, particularly during the uncertain in-between stage of the funeral rites of passage, when anxieties are greatest."[27] At the first meeting of the NFDA in 1882, the mayor of Rochester, New York, astutely observed that "the varied improvements in your art enable you to conceal much that is forbidding in your calling."[28]

In China, especially in Cantonese rural society, the equivalent of undertakers are the funeral specialists (*ng jong lo*) who constantly come in contact with dead bodies. Because of this contact, they become social pariahs and many people believe them to be living ghosts. Traditionally, when these men enter a village, all doors and windows quickly close, parents remove children from their paths, no one speaks to them, and heads turn to avoid their glance. The shops selling coffins hire these men, many of whom have been illiterate opium addicts, to wash, dress and arrange the corpses, dig graves and carry coffins.

These men have been shunned for two reasons: they profited from death and they touched dead bodies. The villagers feel that these men thrive on others' sorrow and misfortune, buying their food with money tainted by anguish. This behavior contradicts their society's norms. In addition, Chinese lore says that, "After a man touches seven corpses, he can no longer be made clean again." (Women are not considered affected in the same way.) To avoid this stigma, the more skilled, higher orders in the Chinese funerary trade neither touch nor look at the corpse and are treated with more respect.[29]

As Charles Berg admitted in *The Confessions of an Undertaker*, "The question has yet to be decided, whether the undertaker made the modern funeral or the demand for the modern funeral made the undertaker."[30] Nevertheless, by the beginning of the twentieth century, undertaking was becoming a vocation. By the 1950s, at least in the United States, it had been transformed into the "profession" of funeral directing, represented by practitioners who referred to themselves as "doctors of grief." (Many still question whether it is, or can ever be, a profession).[31-33] Some U.S. federal and state authorities have questioned whether embalmers or funeral directors even need to be licensed.[34]

## B. WHAT DOES A FUNERAL DIRECTOR DO?

According to the National Funeral Directors Association (NFDA), a funeral director is one who serves the public in all aspects of funeral service.[35] Funeral directors coordinate and sometimes conduct funeral services, and often supervise embalmers. They also instruct and assist the pallbearers, arrange transportation to the funeral for the family, orchestrate transportation for both the family and the corpse to the cemetery or crematorium, assist the clergy who run the services, help lodge members run separate services, seat mourners, provide music, and maintain guest registers. The funeral director may also place death notices in newspapers. About seventy-five percent of persons licensed in funeral service hold both a funeral director's and an embalmer's license.[36]

As Charles Berg pointed out, however, "It is one thing to furnish the casket and other necessary requirements, and quite another to conduct the funeral in a manner pleasing and satisfactory to the parties concerned. Unfortunately, these two requisites are not found coupled together in all undertaking establishments."[37] Most funeral directors, like actors, have both public and private personae. As Pine says, "...in his funeral home, the funeral director is an expert at impression management. There the funeral director conducts himself in such a way as to guide and manage the impressions of himself that he emits to any individual or set of individuals."[38]

Funeral directors are usually very active in community activities. This is in part an attempt to offset the gruesome perception of their profession which, they feel, has been badly and incorrectly portrayed in the popular media, especially the movies.[39] As Raymond Arvio said, however, "the funeral director is not merely a local friendly citizen, serving the needs of neighbors and friends, but part of a hard-hitting, well-organized, well-financed lobby, whose network of trade associations, of legislative lobbyists and lawyers strives to maintain the hold the funeral director has on the market and, of course, on the consumer's personal fortune."[40]

Said a modern sociologist of the funeral profession,

> Despite the fact that the undertaker performs a necessary, useful service and provides necessary goods for an inevitable event, that the skills and services he brings to bear are of a high order, and that he is usually well paid and very often successful as an entrepreneur, there is considerable evidence that neither he nor his customers are content with his present symbols and status within the occupational and social hierarchy... There is an increasing tendency on the part of the undertaker to borrow the ritual and sacred symbols of the minister and other professional men to provide an outward cover for what he is and does.[41]

Although modern society recognizes that funeral directors fulfill a necessary function in society, it is seen as an unfavorable role that many would just as soon ignore. Paralleling society's view, many Protestant ministers hold a negative view of the funeral director's role, as Robert Fulton stated, "In a word, the funeral director, by virtue of his close association with death, and by the 'relative' attitude he takes toward all funerals, is, in a religious sense, 'unclean.' "[42]

In Cantonese China, funerary priests, who learn their trade through years of apprenticeship, fulfill the funeral director's role. These are the priests for "white affairs" (*pai-shih*), associated with funerals. They are usually called *nahm mouh lo*, a pejorative term. Although they attempt to invent more flattering titles, the villagers ignore them. They often live in the village they serve, but are said to be *in* the village, but not *of* the village. As with the public persona of funeral directors, they make every effort to avoid direct contact with corpses or coffins and rarely go to the graveside. They are the only ones who communicate in public with the body-handling specialists, the *ng jong lo*, but do so only in curt and formalized phrases. Interestingly, they describe their function using an ancient quote from the *Li chi* that sounds close to a description of the modern U.S. funeral director:

> During the funeral it is my job to make sure everything keeps going forward and that nothing stops. Everyone has to be told what to do, quickly, or there will be trouble. The worst thing that can happen is for a funeral to start but not be finished properly.[43]

Most funeral directors in the United States are men between the ages of 40 and 49, with an average of 25 years in the funeral industry. Only 2.5% are under 30 and only 19% over 60.[44] Women still have a difficult time entering the funeral industry, but their numbers are increasing, and they now comprise more than one-fourth of current mortuary students. One-third of this group, however, already have family ties to the funeral industry.[45] In Australia, women-run and staffed funeral homes have become very popular. Survivors especially desire the "White Ladies" (dressed in white) services for deceased children, women, gays, and those whom the survivors consider to have been "womanizers" during life.[46]

The majority of funeral directors in the United States have completed four or more years of college. Fewer than 9% have only a high school education supplemented by a mortuary science certificate.[47] (See *What Training Do Embalmers Have?*) In most countries, such as Australia and England, there are no licensing or educational requirements for funeral directors.[48] Colorado does not require licensing; funeral directors simply apply to the board of health for registration.

Paralleling the increased education among funeral directors has been a rise in their professional fees. The item showing the greatest increase among funeral costs in the past decade has been the charge for the funeral director's services. Between 1981 and 1987 the inflation-adjusted charge for these services increased by 70%.[49] Owners and managers of funeral homes in the United States work from forty to sixty hours a week and have an average annual income of $59,574; funeral directors/embalmers average $27,421 per year. According to the NFDA, however, the average starting salary for a funeral director is $17,489 per year.[50]

## C. WHO COMPOSES THE FUNERAL INDUSTRY?

The funeral industry includes the individuals who run funeral homes, cemeteries and crematories, those who work for them, and the industries

175

that supply them with their materials.

Funeral homes form the backbone of the U.S. funeral industry. According to the NFDA, the average U.S. funeral home conducts 160 funerals per year and has been in business for 59 years. Nearly 85% of all funeral homes are family operated, with some having been in existence for more than a century, passing through many generations of the same family.[51] One must wonder how they have remained in operation so long while averaging fewer than one funeral every two days. The low volume of funerals per funeral home may explain why fewer and fewer students are attending U.S. mortuary schools. In 1992, a study of 1700 students who had graduated from these schools found that one-third entered their family-owned business and another one-third left the funeral industry within five years.[52]

Many independent funeral homes are now being acquired by giant conglomerates. By 1992, Houston-based Service Corporation International (SCI), the nation's largest holding company of funeral homes and cemeteries, had acquired 670 funeral homes and 169 cemeteries in the United States.[53] Its chairman, Robert Waltrip, told *Business Week* that he was attempting to turn the company into "the True-Value hardware of the funeral-service industry." Others have described the company's concept less generously as running funeral homes "like K-Marts."[54] SCI targets areas with higher-than-average death rates, such as Texas and Florida. The company buys local funeral homes and cemeteries, but usually keeps the original name on the property and allows the original owners to manage the business, making the public believe that it is still family owned. They organize the funeral homes into "clusters" that share services, such as transportation and embalming, helping to reduce costs. The company also buys materials in bulk, manufactures some of its own merchandise, and at one time expanded into related areas, such as florist shops and insurance companies. The company's 1992 profits (before taxes) were $86.5 million.[55]

A variety of people work for funeral homes, including embalmers, cosmetologists, hairdressers, and hearse/limousine drivers. Some work as full-time employees, but many are employed on an on-call basis, earning only a minimal income. Many embalmers eventually attempt to start their own funeral homes.

Cemeteries are the other large public side of the industry. No love is lost between funeral directors and cemetery operators, who often compete to sell some of the same merchandise and services. Cemetery or memorial park operators may be funeral directors who have taken another route in the industry, or other people with no background whatsoever in funerary services. Land speculators financially back many large cemeteries, having found this end of the funeral industry a lucrative source of income. Both funeral directors and cemetery operators usually operate crematories.

Wholesale suppliers to the funeral industry include the large companies that sell caskets, embalming chemicals, monuments, urns, and columbaria. Caskets alone constitute a multimillion dollar industry. Hillenbrand Industries, a family dominated company, controls over 70% of the U.S. casket business. In either a bit of business irony or shrewd investment, the company recently "backward integrated" from caskets to hospital beds. The *Wall Street Journal* quoted Mr. D. Mark Cunningham (a money manager with Alliance Capital Management L.P.) as saying the company "looks like a jumbo jet taking off."[56]

The two large chemical companies that supply materials to embalmers are the Champion Company and the Dodge Chemical Company. Not only do they supply chemicals and the latest information on embalming techniques to practitioners, they have their own publications that are widely read within the industry. Dodge also runs educational seminars to enhance its image, although they are expensive ($300 to $500 each) by industry standards. Smaller chemical companies compete with a few specialized products.

Other groups that have a vested interest and a great involvement in the funeral industry include the airlines (who make a tidy profit shipping bodies and families to funerals), organ manufacturers, the music business, funeral-clothing manufacturers, hearse manufacturers, professionals who teach embalming and funeral directing, and the manufacturers of embalming, crematory, and funeral equipment. Insurance companies also earn money from insuring the industry against loss, as well as defending them in suits brought by disgruntled families, states, and the federal government.

## D. WHAT TRAINING DO EMBALMERS HAVE?

For centuries, embalming was a mysterious art passed down by surgeons and anatomists to selected students. Only during the past century has there been formal embalming instruction.

While the U.S. Army required licenses for embalmers and undertakers during the Civil War, most embalmers at the time only had certificates from travelling instructors whose courses lasted from a few days to a week. The first textbook devoted to embalming in the United States was *The Undertaker's Manual*, published in 1878.[57] Formal schools for embalmers first appeared in the United States in the 1880s, and gradually increased in number, with many sponsored by the companies that made embalming chemicals.[58]

Many schools now exist to educate embalmers and funeral directors in "mortuary science." As of mid-1990, there were 41 schools approved by the American Board of Funeral Service Education. Many of these schools are housed within community colleges, but a few are in large universities, such as those at the University of Minnesota, Wayne State University in Detroit, and Southern Illinois University. Embalming schools can be accredited either by the American Board of Funeral Service Education or the state's own board of education.[59] The typical curriculum stresses embalming, but also includes anatomy, physiology, pathology, bacteriology, funeral service management and practice, restorative art, cosmetology, chemistry, funeral service law, counselling and psychiatry.[60] The emphasis on education stems, in part, from the NFDA's three main goals for the organization: education, professionalization, and financial security. Yet the amount of science would make the organization's early leaders cringe. As one early NFDA convention speaker said, "If necessary, we will develop a scientific body of knowledge as the basis of the profession."[61]

More than half of all U.S. funeral service professionals now have at least four years of college education and fewer than nine percent have only a high school education.[62] As of 1990, the American Board of Funeral Service Education recommended that an associate's degree be the minimum academic requirement for licensure, and industry educators believe a bachelor's degree should be required.[63]

Licensing requirements forced embalmers to obtain increasing amounts of education. The first state to regulate and license embalmers was Virginia in 1893. By 1900, 25 states required licenses for embalmers, and by 1920, Illinois required embalmers to study embalming for six months at a school, serve a one-year apprenticeship, and pass a licensing examination.[64,65] England still does not require a license for embalmers. In Russia, however, embalmers must take three years of schooling to become licensed as "non-commissioned doctors." They only embalm bodies at hospitals, and then usually only work on foreigners whose bodies will be shipped home.[66]

Requirements for a funeral service license in the United States (funeral director or embalmer) now generally include:

1. at least a high school education;
2. at least one year of college in most states;
3. at least one year of professional education in a college of funeral service education or mortuary science (except in Hawaii which accepts two years of apprenticeship in the state in lieu of schooling);
4. passing the state licensing examination; and
5. a period of apprenticeship, usually one, but occasionally up to three years during which they must have embalmed a specific number of bodies (from twenty in Maryland to one hundred in California).[67,68]

As of late 1993, the profession is currently revising these criteria. They will probably require a Bachelors degree in the future.

Continuing education is available for license renewal for funeral directors and embalmers. The courses cover new techniques to deal with difficult cases, newly available chemical preservatives, and new regulations or issues affecting the industry. As of 1992, 14 states required between five and twelve continuing education hours each year.

## E. WHAT ARE FUNERAL INDUSTRY BUZZWORDS?

As with all professions, the funeral industry uses its own jargon to discuss its work. This avoids both the strain morticians feel in their unusual societal role and any appearance of ghoulishness when they discuss their work. It also helps them sell their services more easily[69] and adjust to any insecurity over their professional status.[70]

Funeral professionals speak of "removing" or "transferring" the corpse from the place of death to the funeral home.[71] After they prepare the body, they "casket" it. They then prepare the "set up," the embalmed and dressed body arranged in the casket, surrounded by flowers. They often refer to the funeral as a "call," as in "how many calls (funerals) does a funeral home handle in a year?" The term derives from the call a funeral director receives from the family after a death. Some embalmers, echoing surgeons (their predecessors) also speak of funerals as "cases." Comparisons of other common words and their funeral industry euphemisms are listed in Table 5.1.

The funeral industry also uses jargon to deepen the mystery surrounding working with the dead. Mystery enhances income (as with the medical profession). When the industry speaks of "serving families" rather than arranging funerals, their thrust is to move the funeral director into the role of counselor, rather than merely embalmer. The role suggested by these terms also connotes an entire line of business services they can provide.

## F. HOW DO FUNERAL HOMES DIFFER?

Traditionally, funeral homes differentiate themselves by religious affiliation, cost, aggressiveness, and location. The services they offer may also vary, although most will now arrange any service survivors desire. Alternatives to traditional funeral homes are available. (See Chapter 12, *What are memorial societies?*)

Currently, there are about 18,000 funeral homes in the United States.[72] When people select a funeral home, they are primarily concerned with four factors: knowing the funeral director, the home's reputation, personal experience with the home, and the home's location.[73]

## TABLE 5.1: Funeral Industry Jargon

| Ordinary Words | Euphemisms |
| --- | --- |
| Ashes | Cremated remains |
| Autopsy | Postmortem; Necropsy |
| Body fluids | Purge |
| Bury | Inter; Inhume; Final rest |
| Coffin | Casket |
| Corpse; Body; Stiff | Remains; Mrs. Z; Loved one |
| Cost (casket) | Investment |
| Crematorium grounds | Garden of remembrance |
| Dead | Expired; Passed away; Deceased |
| Death certificate | Vital statistics form |
| Digging a grave | Opening a vault |
| Embalming | Preservative treatment; Lasting memory picture; Preparation |
| Family | Prospects; Clients |
| Funeral | Service; Ceremony; Rite; Case |
| Grave; Plot | Pre-need memorial estate |
| Graveyard | Memorial park; Cemetery; Remembrance park |
| Hearse | Coach; Casket coach |
| Job | Case; Call; Service |
| Keep; Hold | Maintain preservation |
| Makeup | Cosmetics |
| Morgue | Mortuary; Preparation room |
| Pulverize (Ashes) | Process |
| Oven; Retort | Cremation chamber; Vault; Cremation vault |
| Shroud | Slumber robe; Clothing; Suit; Dress; Garment |
| Showroom | Display room; Selection room |
| Stillborn | Baby; Infant |
| Tombstone | Monument; Memorial tablet |
| Tools | Instruments |
| Undertaker | Funeral director; Mortician; Bereavement Counselor |

Few Americans know a funeral director, although funeral professionals make an effort to actively participate in community and religious groups. Therefore, they must rely more on information about the funeral home itself.

Most U.S. funeral homes today are designed for that purpose. This was not always true. Funeral homes were once part of the embalmer's house, with some rooms set aside for embalming and funeral services. Later they became part of other businesses, such as furniture stores that could provide the caskets, or ambulance companies that transported the dead and nearly dead. As late as the 1960s, one-sixth of all funeral firms were "combination establishments."[74]

Today's funeral home has been designed to accommodate the needs of both the funeral professionals and their clients (living and dead). The building typically has both private and public areas. The private areas contain rooms for embalming, restoration and storage of bodies, administrative offices, and in some cases, crematory ovens. Living or recreation facilities may also be provided for the employees. The public areas include a chapel, adjoining family rooms and often a larger reception area that can be used for visitations with the family. They also, of course, usually include a display room where caskets, vaults, burial garments and cremation urns are shown and sold. The goal, as the industry says, is for "furnishings [to be] always appropriate, creating an atmosphere of comfort, beauty and reverence in keeping with the occasion, while easing the burden of your loss."[75]

No matter how gracious they appear, funeral homes are not always welcomed by their community. For many years the courts have wrangled over the question of whether funeral homes constitute a nuisance in a residential neighborhood. While most have found that they are not a nuisance per se, the presence of the hearse, the morgue, the funeral procession and the service "with all the incidents of grief-stricken relatives forced upon frequent attention of those entitled to the quiet, peace, and happiness of the home, bring depression and discomfort to the normal person."[76]

While funeral homes are generally considered nonsectarian or oriented towards certain religions, no religion bars its members from using any funeral home; the choice is merely custom. Nonsectarian homes hold funerals for those of any or no religious persuasion, while those that cater to specific religious groups in the United States are usually classified as Christian or Jewish. African-American, Chinese-American and other communities also often use only specific funeral homes for their funerary rites. While repeated use of one funeral home by one group or faith allows the funeral home personnel to become familiar with their rituals, funeral costs usually increase due to the lack of competition.

Funeral homes also differ greatly by price. Funerals are one of life's most expensive functions (along with the cost of homes, cars and weddings), so a funeral home should be selected with care. Few people, however, carefully select a funeral home. (See Chapter 11, *What do funerals cost & is comparison shopping possible?*)

The aggressiveness of a funeral home can also distinguish it from others. Since the death rate is relatively constant, funeral homes often ruthlessly compete with each other for business. In the United States, funeral homes (and cemeteries) rely on obnoxious telephone and direct-mail advertising. This is mild, however, compared to Thailand where two "charity" burial organizations, the *Por Teck Tueng* and *Ruamkatany* monitor police radios and use lights and sirens to speed to accident scenes to retrieve bodies, often arriving before the police. Not infrequently, their representatives fight over the right to collect a body. Each group claims that the other does this to extort money from the victims' relatives.[77]

## G. WHAT ARE SOME TRADITIONAL PREPARATION RITES FOR BODIES?

In speaking of traditional ways of dealing with the dead, Leon Kass said, "each people thinks its own customs and mores are the best; moreover, people generally do not believe that their own customs are merely *customary*, but think them inherently—naturally—right or good or best."[78] Persia's King Darius came to understand this after questioning his kingdom's Greek citizens who cremated their dead, and the Calatians (Indians) who ate their dead. Neither would abide the other's customs, each feeling their own was superior.[79]

The rites people use to prepare their dead still vary by social status, nationality, and religion.

In the early nineteenth century, American and British poor often prepared their own dead for burial, in a process called "laying-out," "streeking" or rendering the "last offices." Women normally washed the corpse, plugged its orifices, closed its eyes and mouth, straightened its limbs and dressed or shrouded it.[80] It was ritually important to close the eyes quickly, since they are the first to rigidify in *rigor mortis*, and it was thought that a corpse with open eyes posed a threat to its kin. As has long been the case in many cultures, they used coins to keep the corpse's eyes closed. The practice of using coins still endures, representing a feeling that money, so important in life, may also be important to the dead.

The Ghia Gallery in San Francisco, California, no friend of the traditional funeral industry, says "a traditional funeral means every service they can sell you."[81] Only in the United States are the dead routinely embalmed, viewed and stored in concrete.[82] Americans consider their funerary practices the norm, although the rest of the world looks at them in wonder, if not horror. American death rites are seen as exotic by non-Americans, since they are more elaborate than those in any other industrialized Western country. People outside of the United States think Americans are "barbarians in the way we treat our dead."[83] Interestingly, although many different cultural groups have been added to the U.S. population in the past century, most have adopted American funerary customs.[84]

Outside of the United States, each culture has its unique traditions when preparing a corpse for burial. Only a few of these are described below.

The Swedes customarily bury an unmarried woman with a mirror so she might arrange her hair on Resurrection Day. Married women braid their hair, so do not need the mirror. Russians often place a certificate of good conduct in the corpse's hands, to be used as a pass into heaven.

Scots often put a bell under the head of a corpse to announce its coming, and place a salt shaker representing immortality and bread symbolizing the corruptible body on the chest. Traditionally the Scots' undertaker was also the carpenter who built the coffin. He and his helpers, often with the assistance of relatives, lifted the corpse into the coffin with a "death sheet" (a special white sheet kept for the purpose) or with three towels, three bolster covers, or a plank of wood. Often the Scottish wake was concluded by putting the corpse in the coffin, a rite they called "kisting." (U.S. funeral homes use hoists to transfer the body into the casket—a process called "casketing" for which there is often a separate charge).

In Iran, a person who dies during the day is immediately placed in a coffin. Those who die at night have a copy of the Koran laid on their chest and a lighted candle placed at their head. A person reading the Koran keeps watch over the body through the night. Most bodies are washed three times, first with lotus water, then with camphor water and finally with pure water. They are then wrapped in large seamless cotton cloths that have generally been carried around Mecca or another holy site.[85]

In Jordan, attendants clean, perfume and otherwise prepare the corpse in a traditional way. When they wash the corpse, all body orifices are cleaned, and the nostrils and anus are stuffed with cotton; they also put cotton between the toes and fingers and in the armpits. They then perfume the body. "Perfume is for the good of the dead one, *halal*," said one woman. "Perfume—nowadays *Eau de Cologne*—is sprinkled on the body in the grave. They open the great cloth, the winding sheet, to do it."[86] While the usual Islamic grave preparations are used for most people, "a virgin who dies is considered a bride, and she is decorated as a bride. Her face is painted and gilded, gold is strewn over it. Her eyes are blackened. Henna is dusted over her body, and she is sprinkled with perfume."[87] If a person has been martyred, the blood is not washed off.

The Japanese bathe their dead, shave part of the hair, and dress the body in white, topped with a ceremonial hat or triangular piece of white paper tied to the forehead.[88] Koreans wash the corpse's face with perfume and dress the body in hemp or silk garments tied in seven places to correlate with the seven stars in the lucky Ursa Major constellation.[89]

The Chinese customarily place a coin in the corpse's mouth, so that it is readily available to pay those who might obstruct its ethereal trip. Chinese dead are also traditionally bathed. In southern China, relatives "buy" the water for bathing from the God of a well or stream for a small amount of money. What then happens to the money is uncertain. The bathing ranges from scrubbing the whole body to ritually daubing the forehead.[90] Paid professionals often perform this service, as well as other rituals involving the dead. In northern China, buying the coffin, locating a burial site and readying grave clothes is often done prior to death. When death occurs, the body is immediately dressed in grave clothes, with an unpadded quilt serving as shroud. Pearls, coins or other special objects are placed in the mouth, the face is covered with a piece of cloth or paper, and the feet are tied with colored string. As soon as it is deemed auspicious (by a yin-yang master), the body is placed in the coffin. The eldest son or wife wipes the corpse's eyes with cotton floss and the coffin is closed. After the funeral, the body may be stored for many years, so that a husband and wife can be buried together, or to wait for a favorable burial date.[91]

The traditional method of preparing a corpse among the Ashanti of Ghana is to wash the corpse in hot water with a new sponge and then towel it off. Rum is poured down the throat to preserve the body and gold dust is sometimes sprinkled in the ears. A handkerchief is put between the palms so the spirit can wipe its hands as it ascends the hills to eternity.[92]

Religions also have their own customs for body preparations. Washing, anointing and clothing the corpse in garments suitable to its rank was instituted in ancient times, when it was believed that the departed required such attentions to enable them to appear at their best in a future material state. This custom was later incorporated into Christian rites.

Jewish dead, in a rite called *taharah*, are traditionally cleansed and clothed by two or more Sabbath-observing Jews of the same sex as the deceased, who are specially qualified, and who are not relatives. The body is covered by a sheet during this entire process. After the body is undressed, they rinse the front of the body from head to foot with tepid water. They then turn the corpse on its right side and rinse, then on the left side and rinse again. After they clean the fingernails and toenails, a final three-gallon rinse is poured over the head and allowed to run down the body. They then carefully dry the body with sheets and dress it in at least three garments made of either pure white linen or calico. If the deceased died from a wound, the body is buried in the clothes worn at the time of death and they place the shroud, made with neither a hem nor knots, over the other garments. Persons performing these rituals are forbidden to speak while they are working. Once the body is casketed, the *shomrim*, or sitters, stay with the body until burial.

In Islam, preparation for burial begins when the person assigned to wash the body, either a professional washer or a coreligionist of the same sex as the deceased, turns the body's head toward Mecca. After washing, he clothes the body in three pieces of white, unsewn cloth, nine yards long—one beneath, one above and one wrapped around the midsection. In some countries, white is used for men, colored cloth for women. Burial clothing is a very important part of Islamic tradition. As one Jordanian woman said, "Everyone who dies should be given a shroud. That is a decree...To give someone dying in poverty his death clothes is considered a good deed for which a reward—*ajer*, a reward from Heaven—may be expected."[93]

Members of the Church of Jesus Christ of the Latter-Day Saints (Mormons) are dressed for their funerals by Church members of the same gender who have permission to be admitted into the temple. They dress the deceased in white one- or two-piece undergarments that reach to the knees, which are covered by a robe and a cap, with an apron similar to that worn by Masons. Prior to burial, women's faces are veiled and white caps are placed on men.

## H. WHAT IS EMBALMING?

"Embalming is the art of disinfecting dead bodies and thereby slowing the process of decomposition," according to *The Funeral Director's Practice Management Handbook*.[94] The American Board of Funeral Service Education agrees, saying that it is "a process of chemically treating the dead human body to reduce the presence and growth of microorganisms, to retard organic decomposition, and to restore an acceptable physical appearance."[95]

Chemists describe the process as coagulating the body's proteins (like dropping raw egg white into a hot frying pan), temporarily hardening and preserving them from destruction by the body's enzymes or bacteria. Bacteria, also composed of proteins, suffer the same fate. The unpleasant smell of embalming chemicals also dissuades insects and animals from molesting the body.

Embalming has, over time, meant different things to different cultures. Originally, embalming meant placing balm, essentially natural sap and aromatic substances, on a corpse.[96] Unlike embalming, *embalmment* was the old technique of removing the internal organs, soaking and packing the body cavities with chemicals, and then allowing the body to dehydrate.[97] To disinfect and preserve the tissues, modern embalmers replace a corpse's fluids with chemicals. Most embalmers will rarely talk about this process to outsiders, since it involves very invasive treatment of the cadaver to deliver a suitable "product."[98] They believe that the public would disapprove of the process if they knew what was actually involved.[99]

A remarkable instance of early embalming was seen in the body of Litsang, wife of the Marquis of Tai, the Chancellor of Hunan Province, Central China. She died in 167 B.C. during the early Western Han Dynasty. When her body was discovered at Mawangtui in the early 1970s, more than

2,100 years after burial, scientists found that her body had been immersed in a liquid preservative within an airtight coffin, and then nested within six other boxes. It was then packed in five tons of charcoal and clay and buried under 60 feet of earth. At the time her 76-pound body was unearthed, the flesh remained moist, the hair was firm in her scalp, her joints remained flexible, and all organs except the brain were shrunken, but well preserved.[100]

British sailors used makeshift embalming when Lord Nelson died at Trafalgar. Surviving officers decided to return his body to England rather than bury this famous admiral at sea. Reportedly his body was immersed in the ship's brandy stores, the only preservative available. The sailors, though, not wanting to go without their alcohol, siphoned out portions for drinking through a piece of macaroni, eventually draining the brandy dry. The British navy still uses the term "tapping the Admiral" for getting a drink of rum.[101] Similarly, when Prince Henry of Battenberg died from malaria on a British expeditionary force to West Africa in 1895, his body was transported back to England for a royal burial in an improvised tank made from biscuit tins and filled with navy rum.[102]

This type of preservation was also occasionally used for the less exalted. In 1857, Nancy Martin, a 27-year-old American woman was on a cruise with her father. When she suddenly died at sea, her father had her body placed in a cask of alcohol to preserve it. Upon his return to Wilmington, North Carolina, he buried her body, still in the cask, in the Oakdale Cemetery.[103]

Before 1880, embalming was viewed by most Americans "only as an historical phenomenon, an exotic custom of the ancient Egyptians."[104] Up to that time most American undertakers used ice to cool the body for preservation until burial. Some used patented "preservers" or "corpse coolers" that surrounded the body with ice and cool air and temporarily slowed putrefaction. (See illustration, p 444.) Ice was packed around a metal liner surrounding the upper body. A glass window made the face visible. Openings allowed workers to replenish the ice and a hose drained off the water. They were, however, unwieldy, unsightly, and difficult to maintain. If the undertaker failed to frequently drain off the water and replenish the ice, the body occasionally exploded, and often spoiled,[105-107] as described in a song from *Oklahoma!*:

He looks like he's asleep.
It's a shame that he won't keep,
But it's summer and we're runnin' out of ice...[108]

"Pore Jud is Daid" *Oklahoma!*

Before embalming was a common practice, newly interred coffins occasionally exploded, especially if they were encased in lead coffins that were truly airtight.[109] It was a common practice to "tap" a leaden coffin that was bulging to let out the accumulated gas. This was done by boring a hole in the coffin and igniting the jet of gas that instantly emerged. The flame lasted from ten to thirty minutes, and the workers had to be extremely careful during the procedure.[110]

In the early 1880s, methods were perfected whereby the average undertaker, after minimal instruction, could embalm a body more or less successfully. Ice preservation quickly gave way to embalming. "By 1920, almost all dead bodies were embalmed, not just those intended for transport."[111]

The Russians developed a unique embalming technique to preserve Vladimir Lenin's body after he died in 1924. Every 18 months, scientists from the Institute of Biological Sciences removed Lenin's body from his mausoleum and immersed it in a glass tub of glycerol, potassium acetate and other chemicals. After removing the corpse from the vat and letting some of the liquid drip off, they bound the body with rubber bandages to prevent further leakage, and dressed it. They bathe the corpse's exposed head and hands with embalming fluids and check them for bacteria twice a week.[112] The public mausoleum (now closed to the public) keeps the body at 61°F (16°C), and 70% relative humidity.[113] Lenin's widow, who opposed putting the body on display, would be pleased that the new Russian government will probably bury the corpse. Ilya Zbarsky, whose father helped develop the embalming technique and who himself tended the body from 1934 to 1952, said "I put a lot of energy and time into this in my life, but as a citizen, I say it's time to bury him."[114] Moscow's Institute of Biological Sciences now peddles its expertise in preservation to anyone willing to spend at least $250,000.[115]

According to Ariès, embalming is almost unused in Europe. Yet embalming is now routine in the United States, Canada, and Australia, and is becoming more common in England. The English, however, do not use cosmetics on bodies as is routine in the United States. In other parts of the world, authorities consider embalming so unusual that before it can be done, it is necessary to get a special permit. Embalmers in non-English-speaking countries are often physicians.

## I.  WHY EMBALM A BODY?

Corpses are embalmed for two main reasons: public health and public viewing. Public health reasons are, at best, questionable; public viewing is an American cultural phenomenon.

Advocates suggest that embalming ensures public health by preserving the corpse for transport over long distances and by preventing the spread of infectious disease to mourners or into the ground when the body's fluids disperse after burial.[116] An early reason for embalming a body in the United States was to preserve the body during transport to the site of burial. This solved a practical problem. Embalming a corpse to protect public safety is highly questionable.

The funeral industry claims embalming lessens the chance that disease-causing bacteria will infect mourners, funeral personnel and ultimately the ground in which the corpse is buried. In support of this they cite their *Snell Report*, a study that found that more than 99 percent of these organisms were killed in bodies thoroughly embalmed for anatomical study.[117] The process used in the study to embalm these bodies, however, was much more extensive than that used for a funeral.[118] As one sociologist wrote:

> While preservation was the first reason (and probably the primary motivation) for embalming, disinfection quickly became a strong second rationale for the process...After 1883, funeral directors linked preservation and disinfection as reasons for embalming. One funeral director drew the medical analogy, saying that 'the surgical operation saves but one life. Who can not say how many lives are saved sometimes by proper embalming and disinfecting of a tubercular body and of the home?'...After 1883, funeral directors consistently hitched themselves to the star of sanitary science.[119]

Healthy people carry potentially infectious organisms; not surprisingly, so do corpses. Researchers at Wayne State University found virulent pathogens in the unembalmed bodies of patients who died from non-infectious causes, such as strokes and heart attacks. Another study at Rush-Presbyterian-St. Luke's Medical Center, Chicago, showed that the Human Immunodeficiency Virus (HIV; AIDS virus) survived for nearly 22 hours after the heart stopped in about half the people dying of AIDS.[120] To date, the U.S. Centers for Disease Control and Prevention (CDC) have not yet determined how long HIV (AIDS virus) or similar viruses remain viable in an unembalmed corpse.[121]

Yet in 1969 Dr. Fredrick, a funeral industry leader claimed somewhat hysterically, "... the only *safe assumption* is to regard the unembalmed body as a 'bacterial bomb'—fully capable of exploding with disastrous effect on public health and the well-being of mortuary personnel ... let me remark that *never before in the entire history of embalming has the hazard of personal and public infection from unembalmed human remains been as great as it is today!"*[122] A few months earlier he had written:

> Irresponsible novelists in their self-seeking quest for easy dollars also contribute to public complacency [about the public health need for embalming]. A deluge of controversial books have descended upon the public in a flood of half-truths and blatant untruths ... fostering distorted concepts about the high cost of funerals and picturing the embalming of dead human remains as

'an unnecessary frill.' With artful sophistry, these calculating writers play upon the gullibility of the public—taking advantage of its readiness to adopt any expedient which promises to slow the inflationary trend to save dwindling economic reserves.[123]

Embalmers say they now fear two particular diseases, hepatitis B and AIDS. Yet U.S. embalmers rarely act like they fear infections from their "customers." While the U.S. Occupational Safety and Health Administration (OSHA) requires that workers protect themselves from infectious diseases whenever *any* body is handled, fewer than 1% of funeral directors use the "universal precautions" of gloves, masks, waterproof gowns, and eye coverings. Only one-third have had immunizations against hepatitis B.[124,125]

Nevertheless, "many funeral practitioners refuse to handle or embalm AIDS bodies," says Robert Inman, former president of the Cremation Association of North America. How can they then justify embalming non-AIDS bodies for the public's health? He wonders if the rationale is "just to sell better merchandise" to funeral consumers?[126] Some funeral directors feel that this refusal to handle AIDS victims is a violation of their license, since in some states it reads, "we are caretakers of human remains dying of contagious diseases."[127]

When they do handle bodies suspected of having died from AIDS or other communicable diseases, however, some funeral directors often charge extra fees, although laws will soon outlaw such extra charges.[128] In cities with a high number of AIDS deaths, such as San Francisco, Houston, Washington, DC, and Los Angeles, a single funeral home with a reputation for treating the families decently often handles the vast majority of these cases.[129]

Part of an embalmers training includes how to avoid illness from contact with dead clients. The highest risk comes from sources with the highest bacterial counts: "first drainage" of the corpse, disinfecting instruments and surface areas of the preparation room. Commenting on the industry's normal standards, an industry leader said, "The most dangerous instrument in a preparation room is a dull and dirty trocar. Running cold water through the barrel does not constitute disinfecting procedure."[130]

In reality, public health authorities feel that embalmers have minimal health risks and those could be reduced by using standard protective garments, such as gloves.[131] Embalmers' incidence of hepatitis B, the most common serious blood-borne pathogen, is about the same, or only slightly higher (13%), than that of the general population, even though they are exposed to the virus twice as often.[132,133] Embalmers without risk factors for AIDS are not at risk for the disease.[134]

Dead bodies present considerably fewer risks to the living than do other people, according to Dr. Jesse Carr, former Chief of Pathology at San

189

Francisco General Hospital. " 'There are several advantages to being dead,' he said...'You don't excrete, inhale, exhale, or perspire'."[135] Arizona's Auditor General's office, while reviewing that state's funeral industry also found that the "public health risks associated with disposal of human remains are minimal."[136] As a Canadian health minister said:

> ...embalming serves no useful purpose in preventing the transmission of communicable disease. In those few cases where a person dies of a highly infectious disease, a far better procedure would be to wrap and securely seal the body in heavy plastic sheeting before removing it from the place where death occurred.[137]

One teacher of mortuary science candidly admitted, however, that "Sanitation is probably the farthest thing from the mind of the modern embalmer. We must realize that the motives for embalming at the present time are economic and sentimental, with a slight religious overtone."[138]

Despite the debate regarding the public health benefits of embalming, the reason survivors have corpses embalmed is mainly to perpetuate the American custom of viewing the body over an extended period of time. In the United States, Canada, and some other countries where American culture has influenced the populace, embalming techniques are also used to enhance the corpse's appearance for viewing and to permit a leisurely disposal of the corpse.

Jessica Mitford, in *The American Way of Death*, said that the purpose of embalming "is to make the corpse presentable for viewing in a suitably costly container."[139] Emphasizing this, Frederick and Strub, in *The Principles and Practices of Embalming* say, "A poorly prepared body in a beautiful casket is just as incongruous as a young lady appearing at a party in a costly gown and with her hair in curlers."[140]

When the body will be viewed before or during a funeral, it is normally embalmed. Embalmers, of course, promote viewing of the corpse, saying that it helps mourners realize a person has died and it improves their memory of the person. "The concern with the appearance is made openly by the funeral director and draws attention to his work, his importance, and his practical value."[141] According to the industry, corpse restoration is not meant to make the dead look alive, but rather to provide an acceptable image for recalling the deceased. Yet Frederick and Strub say, "Basically, the embalmer is a creator of illusions—of pleasant illusions which banish the traces of suffering and death and present the deceased in an attitude of normal, restful sleep. In the practice of embalming we call this illusion a 'memory picture.' "[142] Others say that embalming is "the most literal example of saving face."[143]

An even earlier funeral industry writer said, "one idea should always be kept in mind, and that is to lay out the body so that there will be as little suggestion of death as possible."[144] Thomas Greenhill, an early English embalmer, wrote in his 1705 *Art of Embalming*:

> Some have spared no means to render themselves immortal...but finding death inexorable and irresistible, they altered their measures by inventing a thousand ways to perpetuate their memories after their dissolution...It may justly be said of embalming, that [it is] undeniably the most considerable and efficacious means to answer their intention. For the utmost care in erecting monuments etc. yields but an obscure and imperfect idea of the person deceased, whereas by embalming, that very person is known to be preserved...[145]

A contemporary sociologist who observed the funeral industry, says:

> Once the family gets the message that the funeral director's questions are concerned with the appearance of the body, they usually make it clear that they are pleased or that something could be modified. Such modifications are handled in an interesting fashion. In most cases, the family is asked to leave the room while the funeral director makes an effort to correct things. Change at this time often is not easy, and it is common that the funeral director actually does not do much. He might make minor readjustments in the vicinity of the requested change, or, as is more common, he does almost nothing at all. In the vast majority of the cases observed, the family came back and said, 'Oh, that's wonderful. That's just perfect. That makes so much difference.'[146]

This "memory picture" is, of course, sometimes distorted when the family has already seen the body just after death in the emergency department or hospital. These memories, which emphasize to relatives that their loved one is really dead, may actually be the ones that last.

Not everyone approves of embalming corpses for viewing. One nineteenth-century writer, appalled by embalming for any reason other than to preserve anatomical specimens said there is "something revolting in the artificial conservation of what, by the law of nature, should undergo chemical dissolution...a senseless homage to cling to the shattered chrysalis when the winged embryo has soared away."[147] More recently, Rabbis Lamm and Eskreis wrote, "By making a display of the flesh minus the mind we are in fact demonstrating our life-long emphasis on appearance over value."[148]

## J. HOW HAS EMBALMING OCCURRED IN THE PAST?

Corpses have always been naturally preserved, but until the Egyptians developed embalming for religious purposes around 3200 B.C., preservation had been a purely accidental process. The Egyptian period of formal embalming lasted until about A.D. 650, after which embalming became primarily the anatomists' domain until modern arterial embalming appeared in the nineteenth century. The Book of Genesis contains one of the first references to embalming, "So Joseph died, being an hundred and ten years old: and they embalmed him, and he was put in a coffin in Egypt."[149] Although both Jacob and Joseph were "embalmed," the Egyptian method of "embalming" was to anoint the body and wrap it in spices, perhaps with a special shroud, rather than to inject any preservatives. Early Christians rejected embalming as a pagan practice that mutilated the corpse, although some exceptions were made for exalted persons, such as Charlemagne who died and was embalmed in A.D. 814. It was not until the time of the American Civil War that modern embalming, again for religious or at least sentimental purposes, took hold.[150]

Natural embalming occurs in several situations.

A natural process, called "pit-tanning," preserved the "bog people" of Europe when the humic and tannic acids in the bog's soil slowly tanned and preserved the bodies. This process can take millennia as with the so-called "Grauballe man," whose skin was found in 1952 to be only partially tanned after lying in the bog for more than one thousand six hundred and fifty years. It took almost two more years for technicians to complete the tanning process in the laboratory. (Scientists then used some modern embalming methods, such as collodion injection, to restore the shape to parts of the body so that he could be exhibited. He now lies under glass in the Museum of Prehistory at Aarhus, Denmark.) Bog people, while mainly found in Denmark, have also been found in Germany, Holland, Great Britain, Ireland, Norway and Sweden. Most have been ancient, but the preservation process can be rapid, with some bog bodies belonging to German and Russian soldiers and airmen killed in the Masurian lakes region of Europe during World Wars I and II.[151]

Shakespeare humorously suggested in *Hamlet* that natural embalming might start in some people *before* death:

> Hamlet: How long will a man lie i' the earth ere he rot?
>
> 1st Clown: I' faith, if he be not rotten before he die -- as we have many pocky corses [sic] now-a-days, that will scarce hold the lying in — he will last you some eight or nine year. A tanner will last you nine year.
>
> Hamlet: Why he more than another?
>
> 1st Clown: Why, sir, his hide is so tanned with his trade, that he will keep out water a great while; and your water is a sore decayer of your whoreson dead body.[152]

Over the millennia, essential oils, aloe, salt, myrrh, precious spices, honey, plaster, wax and sugar have all been used to preserve bodies. The Egyptians varied their method of embalming not only from dynasty to dynasty but also between clients, based on the amount each could afford. Some of their preparation methods, resulting in what are now generally referred to as *mummies,* are described in Section R (*How does a mummy differ from an embalmed body?*). Egyptian lore held that embalming began on the doomed isle of Atlantis, spread to the Canary Islands, and only then to Egypt. Indeed, the Guaches, the native people of the Canary Islands, did use methods similar to the Egyptians to preserve their dead. So too did the Ethiopians, who also covered their mummies in plaster and painted lifelike pictures on them.[153]

Other ancient cultural groups independently developed methods for preserving their dead. Persians, Syrians and Babylonians immersed some of their dead in honey to preserve them. This method was supposedly used on the body of Alexander the Great during its trek from Babylon to Egypt.[154] The ancient Scythians disemboweled their kings, "cleaned out the inside, fill[ed] the cavity with a preparation of chopped cypress, frankincense, parsley-seed, and anise-seed, after which they sew[ed] up the opening, [and] enclose[d] the body in wax."[155]

Prehistoric Americans also developed corpse preservation methods. The Paraca Indians of Peru preserved their dead with significant embalming skill from at least A.D. 600. Incan rulers are also thought to have been eviscerated, frozen and then painted with a resinous substance. None of these bodies have been found, but many mummies of common people, naturally preserved by the dry climate, do exist. Early accounts of Native Americans suggest that at least some tribes removed the skin from their chiefs, cleaned and reconnected the bones, and reinserted them into the preserved skin. The skin was then filled out with sand. Aleutian islanders also have preserved their dead since at least A.D. 1000 by cleaning out the internal organs, removing the fatty tissue in a running stream and then forcibly bending and tying the body into a fetal position.[156]

Early Mongols also attempted to embalm their greatest leaders. According to tradition, when he died in 1405, Tamerlane's body was embalmed with musk and rose-water. When the sarcophagus was opened in the mid-twentieth century, however, only a skeleton remained.[157] Marco Polo described the Chinese method of preserving bodies with camphor and spices to keep them for up to three years until the signs were propitious for cremation.

European embalming was performed on royal corpses by monks and surgeons as early as the thirteenth century. Embalming royalty became important when the person died far from home, so that relatives could positively identify the body, declare the monarch dead, and crown the new king.[158] Excavations of royal bodies suggests that some of these embalmers were quite successful in preserving the bodies, while others simply hoped that no one would discover their ineptitude.[159] In many instances, and despite the use of fifty or more different substances in the embalming process, intolerable odors necessitated rapid transit of the bodies from the church funeral to an underground grave.[160] By the sixteenth-century, only barber-surgeons performed embalming in England, graphically described as "ripping the corpse."[161] The process involved opening the abdomen and chest, removing the organs and washing the cavity. They then filled the chest and abdomen with cotton moistened in aloe, myrrh, rosemary and other spices, and closed the opening.[162]

In seventeenth-century-Puritan New England, bodies were only embalmed if the corpse had to be transported some distance for burial or when they smelled badly enough to offend the mourners. The most expeditious method of eliminating the smell was to quickly bury the body—which was frequently done. If "embalming" was necessary, they removed the body fluids and disemboweled the corpse.[163]

Two of the early popularizers of embalming were the famous anatomist and surgeon brothers, Drs. John (1728-1793) and William Hunter (1718-1783), who embalmed many bodies that were later put on public display.[164] John injected a mixture of vermilion and the oils of turpentine, lavender, and rosemary into arteries to preserve his cadavers. He then vigorously massaged the body to work the chemicals into the tissues.[165] Other early anatomists tried several methods to preserve their specimens, drying cadavers through exposure and in slow ovens in an attempt at mummification. They also forced warm air through the blood vessels to both dry the body and remove the blood.

Girolamo Segato, a seventeenth-century Italian physician, supposedly converted some bodies to stone by injecting them with potash solutions and then immersing the body in acid. These processes eventually gave way to curing bodies with sugar or molasses, salt solutions, and many proprietary methods that remain unknown. Preserving bodies by coating them with concentrated sugar solutions, such as molasses, was actually an extension of a method early man used to preserve meat. Sugar inhibits the growth of surface bacteria and fungi as well as helping to dehydrate the body.[166]

Well into the twentieth century, some Spaniards preserved bodies by placing them on wood shavings soaked with deodorizing and absorbing substances and then pouring thymol, formalin, alcohol and benzoic acid over them. This method was obviously successful, since these bodies were then often displayed in glass coffins—a practice most modern embalmers would not relish.[167] Even in twentieth-century Missouri, some farmers wrote, "A mixture of soda and cold water is put hourly on corpses to keep the skin from turning dark before the burial. This is done where embalming doesn't take place."[168]

Modern arterial embalming had a precarious start. As early as 1663, Robert Boyle, the famous scientist, published the results of his experiments involving the preservation of animals using vascular injection of "spirits of wine."[169] Early embalmers eventually turned to various arterial injection methods that used turpentines, salt and nitrate solutions, and alcohols. They also used solutions of metals, including arsenic, zinc, aluminum, and mercury. After an 1840s French murder trial in which the presence of arsenic in the embalming fluid thwarted convicting a woman of murdering her husband with the substance, arsenic was banned from use in French embalming solutions. In 1906, New York banned the use of arsenic and various heavy metals for similar reasons.[170]

The first U.S. patent for embalming was granted in 1856. The patented process involved injecting the body with an arsenic-alcohol mixture, electrically charging it, then washing it in chemicals, covering it in oils, and filling the hermetically sealed coffin with alcohol. The body was probably not particularly viewable after this process, but it effectively preserved the corpse for lengthy transport.[171]

U.S. embalmers trace their modern professional lineage to "Dr." Thomas H. Holmes, who, perhaps because of his overt passion for cadavers and dissection, and his cavalier way of leaving corpses in inappropriate places, was expelled from New York University's medical school. (Nevertheless he occasionally practiced medicine and called himself "Doctor" for the rest of his life.) During the Civil War he got a commission in the Army Medical Corps but spent most of his time privately embalming soldiers. He claimed to have personally embalmed 4,028 cadavers in four years—a rate of nearly three bodies per day. Concentrating on embalming officers (whose families could usually pay for the service), he charged $100 each and returned from the war a rich man. Holmes claimed that bodies he embalmed would be preserved "forever, or at least as long as stone." He never revealed his embalming formulae, but they are now thought to have included various combinations of zinc chloride with an arsenic base.[172] Interestingly, he demanded that when he died, his body not be embalmed.[173]

During the American Civil War, embalmers began to come into their own. A major impetus for embalming came from displaying in an open casket at the White House, at New York's City Hall, and again in Albany, New York, the corpse of the military hero, Col. Ellsworth, whose body Dr. Thomas Holmes embalmed in May 1861.[174,175] Military authorities permitted civilian embalmers, like other sutlers, to work within military-controlled areas. Only in the last year of the war did the U.S. Army require embalmers to be examined by a board to prove their qualifications. If successful, they were licensed.[176] Always entrepreneurial, some embalmers even offered to dig up bodies they had embalmed to show how good their work was, advertising that "Bodies embalmed by us never turn black." Given the dissatisfaction of some of the families they dealt with, however, it is clear that they did not exhume too many of these bodies.[177] Estimates are that between 30,000 and 40,000 Civil War dead were embalmed. In 1864 and 1865, all those who died at Armory Square Hospital in Washington, DC were embalmed.[178]

It was not until 1867 that August Wilhelm von Hofman discovered formaldehyde, the chemical basis for all modern embalming fluids. Although its preservative properties were recognized by 1888, it was several years until the chemical became cheap enough to be regularly used for embalming.[179]

During the late nineteenth century, most embalmers only swabbed the corpse with embalming fluid, since both the tools and skills to inject vessels (that we now consider quite common) were usually not available to either embalmers or physicians.

As modern medicine has advanced, embalmers have constantly had to change the chemicals they use. Many medications now used on patients cause abnormalities in the body that no single arterial embalming chemical will overcome. The liver, kidneys and blood vessels are most affected. Drug addicts are difficult to embalm because of the effects of the drugs they have taken as well as their low protein levels and frequent jaundice (abnormally yellow skin and eyes). Embalmers now use computer programs to determine what preservative chemicals to use, based on the medical history of the patient.

Even the site where embalming occurs has changed over time. Around the turn of the century, embalming was often done in private residences, with the embalmer bringing his own "table-cooling board," a device he used to cool the corpse. Some embalmers still did in-home embalming in the United States into the late 1950s, with the body's drainage going into the sink.[180] Today, embalming is considered strictly private work.

Robert Habenstein defends this, saying:

> If the bereaved are to be given the illusion that the dead one is really in a deep and tranquil sleep, then the undertaker must be able to keep the bereaved from the workroom where the corpses are drained, stuffed, and painted in preparation for their final performance.[181]

Although a family may legally request that a representative be present during the embalming process, this is rarely done and vehemently discouraged by the funeral industry. Relatives rarely see the embalmer. When they do, he is usually in an immaculate surgical gown, as if to indicate that embalming is neither messy nor offensive. It is both.

## K. HOW IS A BODY PREPARED FOR EMBALMING?

When a body arrives at a funeral home, it is subjected to a series of steps before the actual process of embalming commences.

First, funeral home personnel lay the body out on a stainless steel or porcelain embalming table, not unlike those used for an autopsy. They then remove all of the corpse's clothes and either clean and return them to the family or destroy them as they do with any bedclothes that accompany the body. Next, funeral home personnel carefully inventory any jewelry on the body, usually taping or tying rings in place, so they do not disappear. Other jewelry and glasses are removed during embalming and then replaced on the body.

The embalmer then cleans the body surface with a disinfectant spray or solution by sponging it onto the body. This kills any insects, mites or maggots on the body and decreases any odor from the corpse. Occasionally they will use commercial preparations or kerosene to kill infestations. The embalmer disinfects the mouth and nose using cotton swabs. If fluid from the lungs or stomach seeps into the mouth (both are called "purge" in the industry) the mortician rolls the body over to drain it out. Nasal suction is also used for this purpose. To avoid further secretions from the mouth or nose, some embalmers cut and tie off the trachea (windpipe) and esophagus when they cut open the neck to expose the arteries for embalming.

Next, the embalmer positions the body. He relieves *rigor mortis* by flexing, bending and massaging the arms and legs. He then moves the limbs to a suitable position, usually with legs extended and arms at the sides or hanging over the sides of the table so that blood can drain into and expand the vessels for better embalming. Once embalming fluid enters the hands, they will be placed in their final position over the chest or abdomen. The fingers are often kept together by using cyanoacrylate (e.g., Superglue[R]). Where arthritis or other illness has deformed the arms or legs or pushed them into unnatural positions, the embalmer may straighten them by attaching them to splints or occasionally cutting tense tissues. In some instances they will be left as they are, and will be hidden from view. The embalmer elevates the head above the chest so that blood in the heart will not gravitate "northward" and discolor the head and neck tissues, a condition termed "embalmer's gray." He then tilts it slightly to the right (facing the viewers in most funeral homes) and lifts the chest above the abdomen. This final position "makes the body appear comfortable and restful in later repose in the casket."[182]

The embalmer then washes the body with warm water, often adding a soapy, germicidal solution containing bleach (sodium hypochlorite) to kill viruses such as those causing AIDS and hepatitis. He then cleans the fingernails, uses solvents to remove any stains on the body, and applies other chemicals to remove scaling on the hands and face. Blood in the hair

197

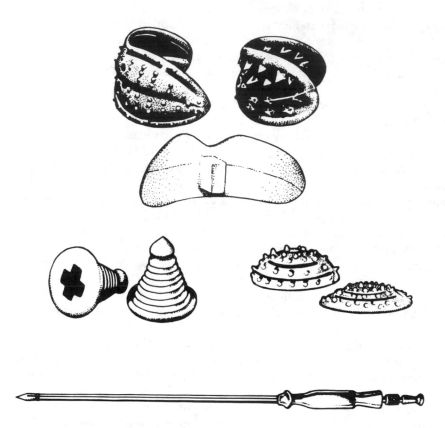

Mouth formers (top), trocar buttons (left), eyecaps (right), trocar (bottom)

is removed with washing or chemicals. The embalmer or a professional hair dresser then washes and styles the hair. Embalmers may do this either before or after embalming; hairdressers normally wait until after embalming has been completed. In his standard text on postmortem body preparation, Mayer states that male embalmers are apathetic about hairdressing, and most "funeral directors have a beautician 'on call' or have a competent wife."[183]

Any hair stubble on the corpse is shaved with an electric razor. Facial hair and any visible nose hair are removed from all bodies, including those of women and children who may have excess facial hair because of medications they received, or because they have downy hair on their upper lips and cheeks. Ear hairs are sometimes burned off with a candle's flame, and other unsightly facial hairs are removed or trimmed. Embalmers must be careful with beards and mustaches, since once accidentally removed, they can be difficult to properly replace. He then removes any fever blisters from the lips or crust from the eyelids with a damp cloth. The nose is straightened with the insertion of little pieces of cotton.

The embalmer then closes the eyes using cotton or an *eyecap*, a plastic disk with knobs on the surface which is inserted under the eyelids to keep the eyelids closed (p. 198). Alternatively, the eyelids are glued closed with Superglue[R] or rubber cement. The embalmer often massages the forehead to relax the muscles that control the eye area, achieving a peaceful look with the upper lids just meeting the lower lids two-thirds to three-fourths of the way down. If the upper and lower lids meet in the middle, the corpse takes on a pained look; if they overlap, it looks as if the face is squinting.

Just before embalming commences, the embalmer packs the throat with gauze, inserts dentures, and replaces missing teeth with cotton or a mouth former. The mouth former is a plastic or metal device which looks like an eye mask, but has surface knobs to help keep the lips closed.

The embalmer then permanently closes the mouth by passing a needle and thread through the upper and lower lips and gums or into the nose (from the inside of the mouth). The thread is then tied, securing the mouth shut. An alternative is to pass a barbed wire into the upper and lower gums, twisting it until it closes the mouth. This device looks like a wire "T" with the end of a fish hook on two ends.

There are several methods of closing the mouth. The prime consideration is to have the lips meet naturally. If the mouth is closed too loosely, the embalmer cannot produce a pleasant look, and if the mouth is closed too tightly, the area under the nose puckers, giving the upper lip a distinctly unnatural expression, sometimes appearing to scowl at the mourners. The embalmer will occasionally widen the lower lip to improve a face's appearance.[184,185] (See illustration p. 198.)

The primary "character lines" of the face run from the corner of the nose to the corner of the mouth, the nasolabial folds. Embalmers can distort these lines if they insert ill-fitting dentures or mouth former, or too much packing to fill out the cheeks. Some embalmers now inject a mastic compound into the mouth to fill out the cheeks and better preserve the nasolabial folds. If the material spills out, however, wiping it up with cotton leaves fuzzy fibers over the face.[186]

The corpse is often a forgiving canvas on which to work, with natural changes assisting the embalmer. While mourners sometimes comment on "how much younger" the person appears, this is as much a result of the natural effect of gravity on facial wrinkles, as it is the artistry of the embalmer.

The embalmer then packs the vagina and anus with cotton soaked in cavity fluid or autopsy gel. He then places the body in tight-fitting plastic clothing to control leakage of embalming fluid and undrained body fluids. These plastic undergarments also control odor if they are dusted with powdered deodorants (sometimes called "safe powder") and preserving chemicals. After the embalmer places a light coating of greasy massage cream over the face, neck and hands, the embalming begins.

An important aspect of preparing stillborns and infants for embalming is that the body's shape must be maintained, since the parents may want to pick the child's body up after it is embalmed. To accomplish this, the embalmer first makes a bed of soft cotton on which to lay the body so that the back, buttocks and legs do not become flattened by laying on a hard surface. Also, an attempt is usually made to smooth and conceal the autopsy incision.[187]

## L. WHAT IS RESTORATION?

Restoration is the attempt to revive the deceased's natural form and color. To do this, the restorer tries to remove the visible effects of injury and disease and to hide postmortem changes. As one funeral industry writer said, "People don't tend to die pretty; they generally die ugly! It's up to the embalmer to restore a peaceful, pleasant appearance."[188] While many embalmers use simple techniques to improve the corpse's appearance, they reserve intensive restorative measures for bodies that are discolored or deformed. The techniques they use often depend on the corpse's condition. (See Appendix G for a method embalmers use to categorize the types of corpses.)

Ancient Egyptians used aromatic ointments and oils to enhance a corpse's appearance and to hide its odor. Today, embalming takes care of the odor and cosmetics are only used to improve the appearance.[189]

Restoration is an art that combines color sense, manual dexterity, and an artist's vision—qualities that not all embalmers have. The ability to restore a body varies with an individual's experience and aptitude for the art.

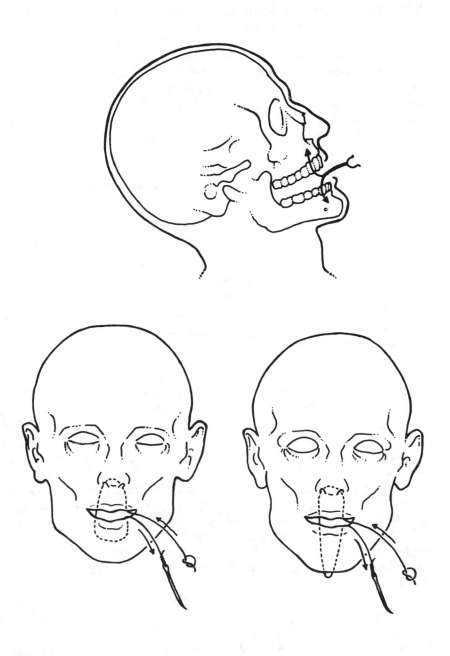

Two mouth-closing techniques: wire barb (top), sutures (bottom)

201

Embalmers without this ability simply embalm a body without altering features. This is known as "what you see is what you get."[190] Embalmers normally work alone. Only in rare cases (usually on very important clients) will an embalmer call in a restorative expert to assist in difficult cases.

Even the best embalmers have limitations, however. The general rule of restoration is that if there is damage to more than one-third of the face, the embalmer should think twice about trying any reconstruction. The basic principle for all restoration, however, is that embalmers should never call attention to their work since this only makes families concentrate on areas that may look less than optimal.[191]

The difference an embalmer can make in the corpse's appearance can be inferred from this 1920 advertisement for a Boston undertaker:[192]

> For composing the features, $1
>
> For giving the features a look of quiet resignation, $2
>
> For giving the features the appearance of Christian hope and contentment, $5

Restoration techniques are applied before, during and after the actual embalming. The restorer first closes any wounds or drainage sites. Superglue[R] (or a similar cyanoacrylate product) is the restorer's best friend in this process. A little dab can close many wounds and intravenous catheter sites effectively. One nationally known embalmer even suggested that he could endorse Superglue[R] on the radio, but he didn't believe listeners would like to hear about his uses for the product while they were eating lunch.[193]

The restorer then disinfects and sews closed any larger wounds. If the body will eventually be cremated, he removes pacemakers during this step. If the body has been autopsied, he will fill the neck, abdomen and pelvis with cotton- or kapoc-soaked preservatives to achieve a natural look. The body cavities and scalp are then sewn closed very tightly and the wounds are sealed.

Swelling in a corpse can result from injury, medications or hospital-administered fluids. The restorer first tries to reduce this swelling by instilling a very strong embalming fluid. If this fails, he may cut away tissue to obtain an acceptable appearance or apply cold packs to reduce the swelling. If tissue has been removed, the restorer tightly sews the area closed and seals the area with mortuary putty or hardening compound to prevent leakage of body or embalming fluid.[194]

If parts of the anatomy are missing, they will usually be replaced with plaster, plastic, clay, wax or wire-mesh substitutes that are covered or, when necessary colored, to match the body. If the body has been decapitated, the restorer trims the skin edges and sews the head back on with dental floss, adding splints to avoid having it sag to one side. The suture line is sealed with a chemical and the stitching is hidden with a high collar, scarf or tie. If

202

an ear is missing, a wooden dowel or wire is placed in the ear canal and a replica, often made of clay or wax, is centered on the dowel. As one professional said, "You can make a thousand mistakes with (restoring) ears—nobody will know the difference."[195] Lips are similarly easy to reconstruct, while restoring the nose or eyelids is much more difficult, since they are easily noticed by mourners. With any restoration, however, families will notice if it falls off, the coloring is incorrect, the hair around it is not appropriate, or body or embalming fluids leak.

If the spine has been removed at autopsy, embalmers place a rigid splint, sometimes even a broom handle, up the spine and into the head to keep the body reasonably stiff. They straighten and splint any badly aligned arm or leg fractures. If the skull is deformed, many embalmers use plaster-of-Paris-soaked cotton under the skin or bone to reform it. If the hands, feet, arms or legs are missing, they are easily replaced with commercially made or plaster substitutes. These substitutes can then be covered with clothing. Mangled hands are sometimes covered by latex gloves to which cosmetics are applied.[196] The cost of reconstruction for lower extremity damage is spared when only the top of the casket is opened for viewing (half-couch casket).

Embalmers remove bruises with bleaching agents, such as "Bruise Bleach," a compound of carbolic acid (phenol). They cover remaining discoloration with an opaque paint or wax. Burned skin is removed before embalming and rough skin can be sandpapered before cosmetics are applied.[197]

At this point the restorer rewashes the hair and body and then thoroughly dries them. He then moves the body to a dressing table in preparation for cosmetic treatment.

## M. HOW ARE COSMETICS USED ON THE CORPSE?

Embalmers normally apply cosmetics (in the United States, but not elsewhere) to the "warm color areas" or "prominent eminences" of the face, such as the chin, lips and nose, forehead, cheeks and ears.

Mayer says there are seven reasons to apply cosmetics to the visible part of a corpse: (1) To replace the coloring lost in death, illness, or embalming; (2) To compensate for the effect of funeral lighting; (3) To present a well-groomed appearance consistent with the best characteristics of the deceased; (4) To create a memory picture of peaceful rest, free from pain; (5) To accent or de-emphasize parts of the face or features; (6) To harmonize the corpse's complexion with color of the clothing and casket interior; and (7) To conceal discolorations.[198]

Different funeral homes vary the order of whether the body is dressed before cosmetics are applied (most funeral homes), or are partially dressed first, cosmetized first, or dressed and placed in a casket before cosmetics are applied.

Whatever the order, the face and hands are initially covered with cosmetic oil or massage cream, a blend of fatty alcohols, waxes, oil, glycerin, and often lanolin. If a denser coating is needed to prepare an area for restoration, petroleum jelly is used. The hair, when necessary, is dyed using standard color rinses. Liquid, cream and powder cosmetics are then applied to the exposed areas of the face, neck and hands. Both mortuary and theatrical cosmetics are used (Table 5.2). Some areas of the face can be emphasized or deemphasized, and discolorations hidden using cosmetics. Cheeks or foreheads can appear narrowed or widened, the forehead or chin height can appear increased or decreased, and the basic head shape can appear to be changed. Even better, the nose can be made to look smaller, dimples can be exaggerated, a double chin can evaporate into the background, and sagging lower eyelids can be firmed up.

Defects in the skin or injuries can be eliminated by applying waxes under the cosmetics. Funeral lighting greatly affects the way cosmetics and other restorative efforts are applied. Emphasis is normally placed on the right side of the body, since this is the "viewing side" in most U.S. funeral homes. If a "kneeler" is used during the viewing, it is placed in line with the shoulders so that the mourners will only see the right side of the face. If it placed further towards the feet, both sides of the face will be seen, and the embalmer will need to do extra work to be certain that both sides look acceptable.

The amount and type of cosmetics applied may depend, in part, on the mechanism of death. If the person was jaundiced when he died, not only will special embalming fluids with colorant be used, but a much larger amount of make-up than normal may be needed to mask the yellow-green skin tinge that is accentuated by normal embalming chemicals. If death was from carbon monoxide, however, the rosy color of the skin aids the embalmer immeasurably, reducing the work that is needed.

There are six types of cosmetics used to give color to the face and hands. Transparent liquids are usually applied by brush or sprayed on the skin and are meant to impart a very natural-looking-diffused color simulating flesh tones. Opaque liquids are used to mask blemishes without obliterating skin pores or altering the natural texture of the skin. Tinted emollient creams are applied by massaging them into the skin to "condition" and color the skin. Opaque creams and soft pastes can cover more resistant surface blemishes. "Pancake makeup" is occasionally used to color the face and hands.[199]

Age also determines the color and distribution of the cosmetics, with more red being used over wider areas on the corpses of younger people. Adult women, because of their cultural use of cosmetics, usually warrant

## TABLE 5.2: Typical Color Names of Pigment Powders

### MORTUARY

| | |
|---|---|
| Caucasian | Black |
| Pink | Light Brown |
| Rachel | Dark Brown |
| Dark Flesh | Chocolate |
| Brunette | Cinnamon |
| Suntan | Peach |
| Flesh | Orchid |
| Natural | |

### THEATRICAL

| | |
|---|---|
| Caucasian | Black |
| Flesh | Light Brown |
| Light Pink | Othello |
| Rachel | Spanish |
| Ruddy | Panchromatic Tans |
| Healthy Old Age | Mongolian |
| Outdoor Natural | Chinese |
| Dark Sunburn | Indian |
| Spanish Olive | Hindu |
| Sallow Old Age | Japanese |
| Dark Brunette | East Indian |
| | Red Brown |

Adapted from:Mayer JS: *Color and Cosmetics: The Consummation of Restorative Art.* New York: Graphic Arts Press, 1973, p 277.

more red when dead, although the coloring added by the restorer is immeasurably aided by a photograph of the person in good health. Placing cosmetics on the forehead, ears and cheeks is especially tricky, since any variation from side to side will be very noticeable.[200] Compounding this difficulty is the fact that the corpse is usually only illuminated from one side for viewing. To compensate for this, some cosmeticians use this same lighting in their preparation areas.

## N. WHAT RESTORATION TECHNIQUES ARE USED FOR ORGAN AND TISSUE DONORS?

Embalmers can usually restore and embalm the bodies of organ donors for open-casket viewings. Donations of internal organs, such as the heart, lungs, pancreas, kidneys or liver pose few problems for embalmers, and may even make their job technically easier. Morticians are already very involved in eye donation, since in many states they harvest eyes for the eye bank, having taken special courses to learn this technique. The key to restoring the eye area is to effectively seal the hole where the optic nerve exits the skull by filling the orbit with mastic, cotton, or similar material. One embalmer reported that a family became rather agitated when they "saw tears" coming from their loved one's eyes. It was really only embalming fluid leaking out of the skull.[201]

Donations of skin, ribs and the spine also result in only minor embalming problems. Since donated skin is usually only a few cells thick, the area is restored by simply painting it with an embalming solution. Normally only every other rib is taken when ribs are donated, so the chest remains rigid. Missing spines are replaced, as they are in many autopsies, with rigid poles.[202]

Other donations pose special embalming difficulties, although the norm is for surgical teams to work with their local embalmers so bodies can be embalmed as easily as possible. Both groups have a vested interest in a good outcome for the family. When transplant surgeons harvest the temporal bones (the bones that make up the sides of the skull and contain the hearing part of the ear) the embalmer must make a special effort to seal the skull and boney sinuses. When they harvest a jawbone (mandible) the organ bank usually sends the body to the funeral home with a prosthesis that the embalmer substitutes for the bone. Many organ banks, however, will not harvest mandibles unless the families want to cremate the bodies.[203]

When an arm, leg or pelvic bone is harvested, embalmers use splinting material to keep the area rigid. They often place the legs in plastic hosiery and fill the leggings with embalming gel.[204] Overall, the embalmer's art is good enough in nearly all cases of organ donation to accommodate a family's wish for an open-casket viewing.

## O. HOW IS A BODY EMBALMED TODAY?

Modern embalming prepares a corpse so it will look acceptable for viewing, remain preserved until buried (and often longer), not smell bad, and not leak body or embalming fluids. These technical goals are often difficult to achieve, and practitioners vary greatly in their grasp of the craft and its artistry. Jessica Mitford succinctly described modern embalming as bodies being "sprayed, sliced, pierced, pickled, trussed, trimmed, creamed, waxed, painted, rouged and neatly dressed—transformed from a common corpse into a Beautiful Memory Picture."[205]

To achieve this memory picture, modern embalmers use four methods: (1) *arterial* embalming, in which they inject chemicals into the blood vessels; (2) *cavity* embalming, in which the abdomen and the chest are injected with chemicals; (3) *hypodermic* embalming, in which they inject chemicals under the skin in certain areas; and (4) *surface* embalming, in which they apply chemicals in liquid or gel form directly to the body surface. Early in the twentieth century animosity existed between advocates of the more technically demanding arterial embalming ("throat cutters") and cavity embalming ("belly punchers").[206] The arterial embalmers finally triumphed, although cavity embalming is still an important part of the process. (See illustration, p. 208.)

In *arterial embalming*, the most commonly used method in the United States, embalmers inject three or four gallons of chemicals into a large artery, while simultaneously removing blood from a large vein. To do this, they position the body on an embalming table that is ringed by a gutter used to collect the blood that comes out by funnelling it into pails or a sewer. Next, the embalmers select large arteries and veins, expose them, and then insert the hollow metal tubes they will use to inject chemicals and aspirate blood and fluids. The arteries they select for injection depend on the state of the body, and whether organ donation, autopsy, or a major injury has occurred or a deformity is present. In an unautopsied body, they commonly use four arteries for injection: the right or left common carotids (neck), right femoral (groin), and right axillary (upper arm). They "raise" the arteries by cutting the skin over the vessel and dissecting it out of the body—actually lifting a portion of each out to identify it, so they can insert metal cannulae. This technique is very similar to the "cutdown" physicians do to place an intravenous (IV) catheter when no other method is available. Embalmers generally inject fluid through both neck vessels and drain it from the right internal jugular (neck) vein in obese bodies. They often use the femoral (groin) vessels in thin bodies.

If the body has undergone an autopsy or extensive organ donation, embalmers inject the head, arms and legs separately, and drain the blood into the chest and abdomen. This type of embalming is called a "six-point injection" (two carotid arteries, two axillary arteries, and two femoral arteries). Occasionally embalmers will have to drain fluid and blood from the body by piercing the heart with a *trocar* (a large hollow tube with a sharpened end, illustrated on p. 198). They pass it through the abdominal wall and up into the heart. In infants and young children, the embalmer often makes a three- to four-inch incision in the abdomen and injects preservatives directly into the aorta ("big red") or the heart (left ventricle). They call this a "heart tap." Heart taps can also be used by inexperienced embalmers when a corpse is grossly obese, has severe atherosclerosis making the vessels rigid, or if congenital anomalies or surgical changes make finding the vessels difficult.[207]

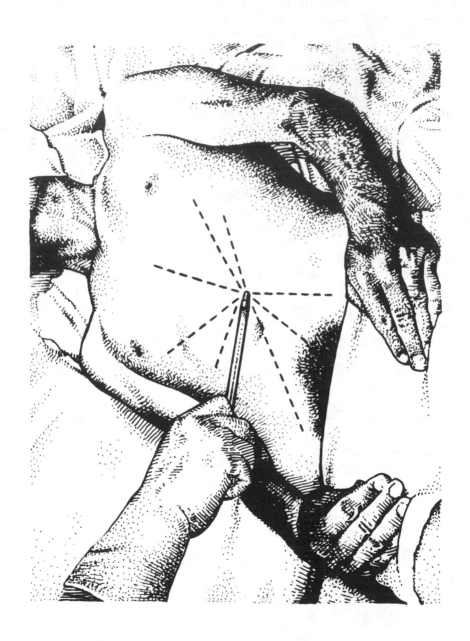

Cavity embalming using a trocar.

There are eight types of chemicals embalmers routinely use: preservatives, germicides, modifying agents (buffers, humectants, water conditioners, and inorganic salts), anticoagulants, surfactants, dyes, perfuming agents, and chemical vehicles. These are combined by commercial manufacturers into a wide variety of products used by embalmers. Embalmers use different types of chemicals, solution strengths, and injection rates depending on the size of the body, its water content, age, amount of decomposition, temperature, the condition of the body's vessels, and medications that the deceased took before death. (Some medications, such as the common hospital antibiotic, gentamycin, inactivate embalming fluid in its normal concentration.)

The main preservative chemicals, formaldehyde and methyl (wood) alcohol, change the nature of the body's cell proteins so that they will not putrefy. They do the same thing to any bacteria still in the body. Embalmers use other chemicals to color the tissues (dyes), help retain moisture in the tissues (humectants), prevent blood clotting (anticoagulants), and purify the water used to dilute the embalming fluid (water conditioners). Additional chemicals allow the fluid to flow through the smallest blood vessels (surfactants), mask the smell of the chemicals being used (perfuming agents), and allow these various chemicals to mix together (vehicles). Some surface disinfectants also contain chemicals to kill bacteria (germicides). They are not needed in arterial injections—the formaldehyde is strong enough. Other materials, such as hardening agents to dry tissues, embalming powder to preserve surface tissues, and sealing agents to help close physician- or embalmer-made wounds, are used in special circumstances.

Embalmers inject these chemicals by using hand-held syringes, gravity drainage (like a medical intravenous fluid drip), or most commonly, a centrifugal pump. The pump pushes embalming fluid into the body with five to ten pounds-per-square-inch of pressure. Simultaneously, embalmers drain blood and fluid from the body using gravity or an electrically or water-powered (hydro) aspirator. As the injection proceeds, embalmers look for evidence that the fluid is moving into the important (visible) areas, such as the face and hands. To aid the process, they massage and reposition the corpse or inject additional chemicals. Any holes they make in the body are sewn shut.

No matter what stage of *rigor mortis* a body is in, once embalming fluid is injected, the muscles begin to firm up or "set." (Without embalming, they would gradually lose their firmness over a period of hours and then be flaccid.) After embalming, the muscles harden gradually over an eight- to twelve-hour period. Once they are set, the body's position cannot be altered by the embalmer.

*Cavity embalming* takes little or no skill, but when used alone rarely preserves the body. It is often used as a supplement to arterial embalming.

The process begins with the embalmer blindly inserting a *trocar* into the belly to remove any gas or liquids remaining in hollow organs such as the stomach, urinary bladder, and large intestines. (Embalmers also usually do this after arterial embalming when that method is used alone.) One industry writer said of the procedure, "Some embalmers almost appear to imagine themselves amateur fencers. Their idea of aspirating is to make very rapid thrusts and lunges with the trocar. In fact, the trocar has to remain long enough in any given position to allow time to build up vacuum to remove gases and liquids in the cavities."[208] The embalmer then infuses about sixteen ounces of a very strong undiluted chemical preservative into the abdomen through a trocar and the same amount into the chest. The embalmer will often direct the trocar into the scrotum and penis of males who have not received adequate arterial embalming fluid.

Trocar holes are then sewn shut or closed with *trocar buttons*, beveled plastic screws that are pushed into the holes. In bodies that have recently had surgery or been organ donors, the embalmer reopens incisions, aspirating organ contents and performing cavity embalming under direct view. He then sews the incision closed. If cavity aspiration and embalming are not done, it is likely that bowel contents will seep up through the mouth and nose. This seepage is known in the industry as "purge." "In many funeral homes where embalmers do not routinely embalm the abdominal organs (cavity embalming), the embalmer places cotton under the pillow in the casket so the attendant can use it to wipe off 'purge' (dark liquid) that comes out of the mouth and nose."[209]

A trocar can also be passed through the nose and into the skull through the thin bone at the top of the nose (cribiform plate). Early users of this method inserted the trocar along side the nose at the corner of the eye ("the eye process").[210] Embalmers remove gas and fluid from the skull and instill cavity fluid. They then pack the nose with cotton to avoid leaks. Cavity embalming can also be used to preserve organs replaced in the chest or abdomen after an autopsy.

*Hypodermic embalming* refers to the injection of preservatives under the skin in specific areas that appear to need additional chemicals. This is often necessary because the arterially injected chemicals did not reach those sites. Hypodermic embalming is routinely used after autopsies by injecting fluid into the buttocks, chest and abdominal walls, shoulders and the back of the neck. It may also be used as the sole method of preserving an infant, fetus, a removed body part, or mutilated portions of a body.[211]

*Surface embalming* is normally used to supplement other forms of embalming. In this process, embalmers apply liquid chemicals in cotton or gauze packs, and apply gels with a brush. They often use surface embalming for eyelids, the inside of the mouth, and to injured areas of the body, especially those that are cut, abraded or mangled. They also apply gel to the

210

inside of the chest, abdomen and scalp if the body has been autopsied. This technique can also be used to preserve an infant or fetus.

The type of embalming, the chemicals, and other techniques the embalmer uses are governed, in part, by the "type" of cadaver with which the embalmer is presented. Corpses are classed into six types, each having embalming techniques that are usually successful, as well as specific problems associated with it (Appendix G). Success for embalmers rests much less with knowing the disease that killed the person, as it does with the condition of the body.

Embalmers obviously use many different types of implements and materials to embalm bodies. The most common are listed in Table 5.3. Embalming is not always the quiet procedure the public imagines, so the embalming or "preparation rooms" are usually well sound-proofed to avoid the sound of machinery or dropped instruments radiating into the public areas.[212]

The chemicals embalmers use on corpses are quite hazardous, and many are now regulated by the Occupational Safety and Health Administration (OSHA). According to industry experts, the most danger to embalmers comes not from the bodies they embalm, but from the chemicals they use.[213] Formaldehyde, acetone, phenol are the most common of these dangerous compounds that require special handling, storage, reporting and employee training. At least 42 other OSHA-regulated dangerous chemicals are also commonly used in embalming and body preparation.[214] Scientists have found that embalmers are at significantly greater risk than the general populace of getting cancers of the skin, brain, colon, sinuses, nose, throat and blood, kidney failure, arteriosclerotic heart disease, chromosomal damage, and cirrhosis of the liver.[215-219] This is presumably a direct result of their exposure to these toxins, particularly formaldehyde. Canadian researchers found embalmers to be more susceptible to chronic bronchitis, dyspnea, skin irritation, and nasal and eye irritation because of their exposure to formaldehyde.[220] As a result, OSHA recently reduced the permissible exposure limit to formaldehyde (0.75 parts per million).[221] Male embalmers have also suffered from breast enlargement, other feminizing characteristics, and a loss of sexual drive—all caused by estrogens in a massage cream they were applying to bodies.[222,223] As Donald W. Sawyer, a noted industry spokesman says about the new federal safety standards, "OSHA is probably a godsend to the funeral service."[224]

**P. ARE EMBALMING AND RESTORATION ALWAYS SUCCESSFUL?**

No. In his standard text on embalming, Mayer states that "embalming is effective when the commercially available embalming chemicals are used in proper concentrations and in adequate total volumes, and are administered under conditions of proper techniques."[225]

## TABLE 5.3: Instruments and Materials used in Embalming

| | |
|---|---|
| Surgical Knives (Scalpels) | Cosmetics |
| Tissue Scissors | Artery Forceps |
| Dissecting Forceps | Artery Tubes |
| Separator | Director (Knife Guide) |
| Aneurysm Needle | Surgical Needles |
| Containers and Pumps | Syringes |
| Trocar | Drainage tubes |
| Embalming Fluids | Massage Cream |

Adapted from: Polson CJ, Brittain RP, Marshall TK: *The Disposal of the Dead.* Springfield, IL: Charles C Thomas, 1962, pp 295-307.

The proper techniques he describes are to: (1) Inject the body in multiple arteries and drain through multiple veins; (2) Use only a moderate rate of flow (10 to 15 minutes per gallon) at a relatively low injection pressure (2 to 10 pounds per square inch); (3) Use venous drainage intermittently; (4) Inject at least 1 gallon of chemical preservatives with no less than a 2% formaldehyde concentration for each 40 pounds the corpse weighs; (5) Use additional chemicals as indicated by the body condition; and (6) Use cavity embalming to supplement arterial embalming.[226]

Each of these steps helps ensure the flow of preservatives to various parts of the body. Yet each of these steps costs the embalmer time, effort and money, and he may skimp at any stage, producing a less-than-optimal result. For example, if he injects preservatives too quickly, they do not flow into the smaller blood vessels, and therefore are not effectively distributed to the surface tissues. They will, rather, take the path of least resistance through the larger vessels leaving sizable areas of the body unpreserved.

Mayer's predecessors, Frederick and Strub, were more candid about embalming failures. They said that embalming failures are numerous and are often due to both errors in judgement and problems with the corpse too difficult to remedy (Table 5.4).

Many embalmers put dyes in the injected fluid to actually see whether embalming fluid is reaching all surface areas of the body. Available dyes are colored (suntan and pink) or are fluorescent that can only be seen with an ultraviolet light. The embalmer can tell which surface areas of the body need additional chemical infusion by using any of these dyes.

The embalming clearly was inadequately done on George IV of Britain. Of his funeral in 1830, one observer wrote,

They were very near having a frightful accident for, when the body was in the leaden coffin, the lead was observed to have bulged very considerably & in fact was in great danger of bursting. They were obliged to puncture the lead to let out the air & then to fresh cover it with lead. Rather an *unpleasant operation*, I should think, but the embalming must have been very ill done.[227]

Embalming can also lead to some embarrassing situations as noted by a description of what happened to Cardinal Donnet in 1872:

> On his death...an outstanding surgeon was dispatched to Bordeaux to perform the embalming...The fluid in this case was allowed to flow in by force of gravity...then it was further dispersed through the arterial tree and body by kneading and massage...By the time this...manipulative process had been applied from stem to stern, one intercurual strategic part had become quite turgid and assumed a grossly erectile character. The organ proved so refractory on further manipulation that it had to be slit altitudinally in order to release the pent-up fluid under pressure.[228]

A similar episode is recorded in a traditional Afro-American "toast" called *'Flicted Arm Pete*. The toast is a recitation, usually performed in celebrations and passed down through oral tradition.

> They took old Pete and buried Pete down in the graveyard,
> Pete was stone dead and Pete's prick was still hard.
> Say they put old Pete about six feet down,
> about four inches of Pete's prick still stood up above the ground.
>
> They had to put old Pete about ten feet down,
> but when they finally got old Pete buried all the undertakers frowned
> because they had to jack Pete off to let the coffin lid down.[229]

Lack of successful embalming is still evident. When Pope John Paul I died after only 33 days in office, his body began to bloat and emit noises while it was kept unburied so the ceremony could be broadcast live during prime-time in the United States.[230] When Pope John XXIII died, his body was inadequately embalmed when it was simply immersed in formaldehyde gas. The inadequacy of the embalming was demonstrated when an attendant had to continually wipe purge from the body's mouth during public ceremonies.[231]

## TABLE 5.4: Seven Common Causes of Embalming Failures

1. Too little time devoted to the preparation of the corpse. This is often evidence of sloppy technique and little interest in the procedure.

2. Using too little embalming solution. Injecting adequate amounts of solution takes time—and the solution can be expensive.

3. Using too strong an embalming solution. This may be done in error, or as a method to hurry the process. The result can be a partially embalmed body because the embalmer must halt the process when the parts of the body exposed to the solution become wrinkled and darkened.

4. Using only the rigidity caused by the embalming fluid as a test for the adequacy of tissue perfusion. *Rigor mortis* can simulate this rigidity and lead to incomplete embalming.

5. Excessive injection speed and pressure. As with the first point, this is done out of sloppiness.

6. Excessive drainage. If too much liquid is drained from the vessels, it normally means that the embalming fluid is being "short-circuited" and the whole body is not receiving an adequate amount of preservative chemicals.

7. Failing to thoroughly preserve the internal organs. This shortcut is taken because the embalmer knows that there is no cosmetic effect in not preserving the organs. Putrefaction of the body, however, will be markedly speeded up if the viscera are not embalmed.

Adapted from: Strub CG, Frederick LG: *The Principles and Practice of Embalming.* 4th ed. Dallas, TX: LG Frederick, 1967, pp 393-397.

---

### Q. HOW IS A BODY PREPARED FOR VIEWING?

Preparation, restoration and the use of cosmetics are not meant to make the dead look alive, but to provide an acceptable image and recollection of the deceased person, a "beautiful memory picture." Mayer says that the goal "is the achievement of a natural, non-cosmetic effect, simulating the appearance of color coming from within the skin."[232] He goes on to say that "the faithful representation of the deceased's best appearance is desirable. Neither glamorization nor slovenliness is desirable."[233]

The final grooming includes removing any excess cosmetics, and "touching up" the hair, eyebrows and eyelashes with an eyebrow pencil, mascara, a hair-crayon, or a hair tint spray.

Embalmers may feel that they can accomplish miracles with restoration, but there *are* limits. In 1989 two men died and were sent to the same Florida funeral home. The bodies were switched when they were sent to different cities for their funerals. The first funeral, with an open casket, went well and nobody appeared to notice the switch, but the same did not happen at the second funeral. The second family said that "Dad did not look right, he didn't have a mustache." The embalmers shaved the mustache. The family then said that his nose was too thin; they stuffed the nose with silicone. Only after they had also cosmetically adjusted the eyebrows and the family said their father still didn't look right did the embalmers realized they had the wrong body.[234]

The body is finally "casketed," placed in the coffin or casket. The standard position for a body in a coffin is to place the right shoulder lower than the left, to decrease the impression of a body flat on its back. The body is also raised high enough in the box so that the perception of being in a casket is reduced, yet it must also be low enough so that the lid does not hit the nose when closed. The hands are positioned according to local custom, either at the sides or crossed over the body. In some cases flowers or a favorite memento, such as a picture, book or stuffed animal (for children) is put in the hands.

## R. HOW DOES A MUMMY DIFFER FROM AN EMBALMED BODY?

Mummies are corpses that have been poorly preserved through complete dehydration.[235] They are "merely a bag of bones," according to Dr. Richard Froede, an experienced forensic pathologist.[236] A mummy's skin, muscles and even some bones (especially the ribs) are often so dry and brittle that any disturbance causes them to collapse into dust. In other cases the skin has become so rigid that it is almost impossible to cut with a scalpel.[237] A mummy could, in fact, be termed a "skeleton," since that word comes from the Greek *skeletos*, meaning dried up or withered.[238] The derivation of the word *mummy* is uncertain. It may alternatively come from the word for a resinous liquid the Greeks used to preserve bodies, called *mumia* or *momie*, the Arabic noun *mum* meaning wax, or the Persian word *múmiyà* meaning bitumen or mineral pitch.

Mummies have developed both through a natural drying process and through the use of chemicals. People have repeatedly attributed magical, religious and healing properties to mummies. Even modern man is now trying to mummify corpses.

Bodies mummify naturally under the right conditions. Natural mummification results in permanent preservation, although there is considerable tissue shrinkage. Any destruction of the body is generally the work of rodents and moths.[239] Exposure to dry, cold air, as in the highlands of Peru or cave areas in the western Andean and sub-Andean provinces of Argentina has naturally mummified bodies. Several natural mummies have also been found in U.S. caves, such as Mammoth Cave, Kentucky. Similarly, burial in hot, dry sand was used to intentionally mummify bodies in coastal Peru and in Egypt prior to the pharaohs.[240] Most ancient Egyptians could not afford the elaborate mummification of their dead. Instead, they buried their dead in a coarse shroud on beds of charcoal to reduce any seepage from the body into the Nile.[241] In Europe, some cemeteries were known for their ability to preserve bodies, as are those in Guanajuato, Mexico. Several natural mummies are well known, and in some cases this "incorruptibility of the flesh" has been given religious significance.

Theresa of Avila is one of the best-known examples of the incorruptibility of the flesh. After dying on October 4, 1582, at Alba, her body was buried without any special preparation. Her corpse was placed in a wooden coffin, and then interred under stone, chalk, and damp soil in a very deep ditch beneath the nuns' choir screen. During the following nine months a very strong smell of lilies, jasmine, and violets rose from the grave, filling the chapel and convent. Intrigued with this unusual event, religious authorities exhumed the body. Although the coffin had broken and filled with soil and water, and the corpse's clothes had disintegrated, the body remained intact. They reinterred the body in a new coffin. In 1585 when religious authorities planned to take the body to Avila, the tomb was reopened; the body was found to be as intact as before. When exhumed again in 1604 and in 1616, the body remained unaltered. Since it was believed that this was miraculous and due to the woman's saintliness, Theresa of Avila's heart was removed and placed in a crystal vase, and later a rib, her right foot, and several pieces of flesh were given away as relics.[242]

On April 18, 1485, workers quarrying marble along the Appian Way in Rome discovered a totally preserved, beautiful girl's body in a 1,500-year-old sarcophagus. John Addington Symonds, in *Renaissance in Italy: the Age of the Despots* recounts that it was "Julia, daughter of Claudius," a 15-year-old girl "preserved by precious unguents from corruption and the injury of time. The bloom of youth was still upon her cheeks and lips; her eyes and mouth were half open; her long hair floated round her shoulders...her beauty was beyond imagination or description; she was far fairer than any woman of the modern age could hope to be."[243] To prevent a cult from developing around the corpse, Pope Innocent VIII ordered that the body be secretly buried somewhere outside of Rome.[244]

The body of Saint Francis Xavier has reportedly remained intact since the sixteenth century, and was once exhibited to the masses each year at the Bom Jesus Cathedral in Goa, an enclave on the Indian subcontinent.

Around 1900, however, a supplicant supposedly bit off one of the cadaver's big toes, suggesting more protection was needed. Now the body is shown, behind glass, only every twelve years. In intervening years, the toe (also behind glass) is paraded through the streets.[245]

In Kampehl, Germany, 100,000 people a year visit the mummified remains of the 17th-century Count Christian Friedrich von Kahlbutz. The body of the Count (1651-1702) was discovered to have naturally mummified when his crypt was opened in 1783. By the 1850s, people began paying to view the mummy, which now weighs only 13 pounds. Since the reunification of Germany, this former East German town has used the income from the mummy's visitors to bolster its economy, and has fended off attempts by a neighboring town to kidnap the mummy for its own use.[246]

Russians traditionally believed that natural mummies, *morchi*, were miraculous. "To convince them of the absurdity of this belief the Soviet government allowed the mummies to crumble no less miraculously into dust under the eyes of the crowd in 1919."[247]

Litten, author of *The English Way of Death*, witnessed the discovery of a natural mummy.

> I was present in 1983 during the clearance of the vaults beneath St. Marylebone parish church when the coffin of a two-year-old boy who had died in 1815 was opened. Once the lids of the outer case and the leaden shell had been removed, the workman prised off the lid of the inner coffin; the slightly yellowed silk sheets were drawn back and there lay the body of the child, looking as if he had gone off to sleep but a few moments before. This child had not been embalmed and his preservation was due to nothing more than the construction of the coffin, for the wood was no less thick—1½ inches—than that of an adult's coffin, and the lead was likewise no different gauge.[248]

Could Norman Bates' mother really have become naturally mummified as Alfred Hitchcock depicted in *Psycho*? Absolutely. Numerous examples exist of bodies that have mummified when left in homes with very low humidity and protected from insect and other carnivore activity. Modern forensic pathologists encounter naturally mummified bodies that have been kept in warm, dry places, such as the corpses of infants kept in drawers, cupboards or boxes near fireplaces or heaters.[249]

Well known for their process of using natural drying and the soils surrounding their monastery, the Capuchin and Franciscan monks of Italy have long put their mummies, preserved with a year-long process of burial and drying, on display. Just off the Piazza Barberini on Rome's Via Veneto stands the unobtrusive Capuchin church of Santa Maria della Concezione. Cowled skeletons and mummified remains of long-dead friars stare out from niches in the crypts. Not only are friars buried here, but because of the great honor of this burial site, so are princes and princesses, mostly relatives of Popes.[250] As Ragon describes it:

> In the eighteenth century, quite ordinary mortals were, after being dried in the air, usually in church towers, placed in a row, standing or sitting and presented to visitors in their everyday clothes. In the Franciscan church in Toulouse these mummies are visited and presented as in a spectacle. In Rome where in a vault of the Capuchin church one can see the standing mummies of the monks and the lay brothers of Saint Francis, there existed a confraternity of gravediggers who organized an annual festival in which purgatory was represented using real corpses.
>
> But the most astonishing use of mummies in a spectacle, and one which in any case can still be visited today, is to be found in the Capuchin monastery at Palermo. From the mid-seventeenth century to 1881 the rich families of Palermo sent their dead to this monastery. There are at present 8,000 in the Capuchin catacombs, standing in rows, labeled, with the date of their death, bearing on their faces expressions that relate not so much to the cause of death, as the hazards of their drying and preservation.[251]

Lucien Augé described the Capuchin catacombs at Palermo in Les Tombeaux in 1879, saying:

> Vaulted galleries spread out and intersect like streets of a city. The dead stand there, lining our route, a sinister company, a hideous mob...They have been cooked, arranged, dressed, some wearing only a shroud, others the clothes of which they were perhaps most proud when alive. Death is turned into a masquerade...Here is a magistrate who still wears on his hollow chest a lace jabot; there is a child, yellowed and shriveled, and a little further on a girl lying in her wedding dress. On her black, desiccated head, she wears a white crown—gloomy irony...Cats and rats haunt these sad places, and, rolling skulls across the floor, stirring the tattered garments into motion, they pursue their mad chases through the galleries.[252]

According to Jean Baudrillard, these tombs "had for a long time been a place for Sunday walks for the nearest and dearest of the deceased, who came to see them, recognize them, show them to their children, in living familiarity, a 'dominicality' of death like that of going to mass or going to the theater."[253]

Various other cultures and sects have periodically used mummification for their dead. In the Hayti Islands, bodies were traditionally smoke-cured or partially burnt, then dressed in their finest apparel and kept in the homes of relatives. Mummified former brothers of the monasteries of Krewzberg in Bonn were dressed in the habit of their order and arranged row by row, in lifelike attitudes.[254]

In Chile 5,000 to 6,000 years ago, some bodies were prepared for an afterlife in a somewhat unusual form of mummification. The bodies were "flayed, skinned, opened, and cleaned, stuffed with vegetable matter and herbs, baked, propped up with sticks, reinserted into their skins, and fitted with wigs and clay masks."[255] Hill and Anderson wryly suggest that this is also the method great French chefs use to prepare game.[256]

The most famous mummies are, of course, Egypt's. Mummification was introduced into Egypt in the III dynasty (2980-2900 B.C.) and initially reserved for the bodies of pharaohs. The process became almost universal in Ptolemaic times (332-30 B.C.).[257] It took 70 days to mummify the body of Pharaoh Tutankhamun, who died in 1343 B.C. All that remains now is skin and bones. The special technicians, known as *paraschistes*, who performed embalming in Egypt were "held in such aversion that they were driven away with curses, pelted with stones, and otherwise roughly handled, if caught."[258] Herodotus, a Greek historian described the Egyptian process of embalming:

> The body is carried away to be embalmed. There are a set of men in Egypt who practice the art of embalming, and make it their proper business. These persons, when a body is brought to them, show the bearers various models of corpses, made in wood, and painted so as to resemble nature. The most perfect is said to be after the manner of him whom I do not think it religious to name in connection with such a matter; the second sort is inferior to the first, and less costly; the third is the cheapest of all. All this the embalmers explain, and then ask in which way it is wished that the corpse should be prepared. The bearers tell them, and having concluded their bargain, take their departure, while the embalmers, left to themselves, proceed to their task. The mode of embalming, according to the most perfect process, is the following: They take first a crooked piece of iron, and with it draw out the brain through the nostrils, thus getting rid of a portion, while the skull is cleared of the rest by rinsing with drugs; next they make a cut along the flank with a sharp Ethiopian stone and take out the whole contents of the abdomen, which they then cleanse, washing it thoroughly with palm wine, and again frequently with an infusion of pounded aromatics. After this they fill the cavity with the purest bruised myrrh, with cassia, and every other sort of spicery except frankincense, and sew up the opening. Then the body is placed in natrum for seventy days, and covered

entirely over. After the expiration of that space of time, which must not be exceeded, the body is washed, and wrapped round, from head to foot, with bandages of fine linen cloth, smeared over with gum, which is used generally by the Egyptians in the place of glue, and in this state it is given back to the relations, who enclose it in a wooden case which they have had made for the purpose, shaped into the figure of a man. Then fastening the case, they place it in a sepulchral chamber, upright against the wall. Such is the most costly way of embalming the dead.

If persons wish to avoid expense, and choose the second process, the following is the method pursued: Syringes are filled with oil made from the cedar-tree, which is then, without any incision or disembowelling [sic], injected into the abdomen. The passage by which it might be likely to return is stopped, and the body laid in natrum the prescribed number of days. At the end of the time the cedar-oil is allowed to make its escape; and such is its power that it brings with it the whole stomach and intestines in a liquid state. The natrum meanwhile has dissolved the flesh, and so nothing is left of the dead body but the skin and the bones. It is returned in this condition to the relatives, without any further trouble being bestowed upon it.

The third method of embalming, which is practised in the case of the poorer classes, is to clear out the intestines with a clyster, and let the body lie in natrum the seventy days, after which it is at once given to those who come to fetch it away.[259]

It has been estimated that the most expensive method of mummification cost ancient Egyptians about $1,200 (in current dollars), that the intermediate method cost about $300, and the least expensive about $75.[260] Part of the cost may have been related to the gold used to sew on some mummy's fingernails.[261]

During mummification, the lungs, intestines, stomach and liver were removed and separately preserved in *canopic jars* (named by early Egyptologists for Canopus, an ancient Egyptian city where a diety of the same name was supposedly buried). The brain was discarded as of no use, and the heart was left in the mummy, as it was thought to be the seat of intellect and would be needed in the next life. Finally, the mummy was placed in a wooden sarcophagus.[262]

The essential process in Egyptian mummification was similar to the preservation of meat with salt. It dehydrated what remained of the body after the internal organs were removed. Natron, also applied to the mummy for this purpose (not used to soak the mummy as is commonly thought), damaged and discolored the skin so badly that it was rarely used on the head and neck.[263,264]

During the mummification process, the ancient Egyptians attempted to restore the body to a beautiful appearance. Facial features were adjusted by packing the mouth with sawdust to pad the cheeks and by stuffing linen pads under the eyelids. Other body contours were altered by forcing padding under the skin in various parts of the body, splinting broken extremities, replacing eyes with stones or small onions, and in at least one case, straightening a crooked spine.

Geochemists have found that the Egyptians also applied hot pitch or bitumen to further protect their mummified dead. They obtained the substance from the Hit-Abu Jir region of Iraq or from the Dead Sea, where asphalt occurs in floating blocks. Its use was related not only to its preservative powers, but also to the fact that the color black was associated with rebirth.[265] Unfortunately, rather than protecting the mummy, the application of these hot substances caused significant damage. The heat from the pitch and bitumen burned underlying skin and hair, and frequently singed through facial features, fingers and toes. The embalmers probably did not know this, however, since they could not see through these dark substances once they were applied.[266]

The bodies of Egyptian mummies have long been a subject of research. Johan Czermack first successfully examined microscopic slides of Egyptian mummy tissue in 1852. Subsequently, mummies have been X-rayed, dissected, and cultured. Yet for studies of the skin, the bodies of peasants buried in Egypt's desert have proven to be the best preserved, since the preservatives used in mummy preparation actually destroyed the skin structures.[267]

Modern man has not always respected Egyptian mummies. Locals reportedly used them for fuel—even possibly to power their railways.[268] Mark Twain parodied this in *Innocents Abroad*, having the train engineer tell the fireman, "These common folk don't burn worth a damn. Send me a King!"[269] They were also reportedly used as fertilizer and to supply linen rags to make paper.[270]

"Mummy medicine" was once prescribed as a magical cure for many ills. Avicenna, the ancient physician, spoke of using powdered mummy to treat abscesses, migraines, epilepsy, fractures, vertigo, concussions, paralysis, heart palpitations, poisoning, and disorders of the stomach, liver, and spleen.[271] English apothecaries sold mummy medicine as late as the eighteenth century and several European medical museums, including the medical and pharmaceutical museums in Budapest, still have samples of mummy powder. This "medicine" fell out of use primarily because it could no longer be obtained.[272]

After Egyptian authorities halted trafficking in mummies in the early twentieth century, Egyptian traders gathered modern corpses and treated them with asphaltum, a cheap preservative, bound them in winding cloths and exposed them to the sun. They then appeared to the uninitiated, to be ancient mummies, and they were frequently sold to naive foreigners.[273]

Some Chinese corpses were also mummified. Shun-chih, the first Manchu emperor of China (1644-1661), had his body mummified and lacquered in gold when he died in 1670. His body still serves as a memorial to him at the monastery of *Tien Tai Ssu,* where he spent the last years of his life.

Corpses are still mummified in Tibet using an ancient technique in which the corpse is put in a large box and packed in salt for about three months.[274] Modern mummies are on exhibit at several places around the world, including the Pantheon of Guanajuato, Mexico. The soil in the Guanajuato region naturally mummifies buried bodies. The locals have disinterred dozens of these mummies and display them as a tourist attraction. The mummies, many of whom still wear their burial clothes, stand shoulder-to-shoulder in long halls. Many of the mummies' descendants, some of whom are locally prominent, have given permission for this unusual display. The exhibition is enhanced by the sale of elaborate candy figures depicting the mummies in Guanajuato and surrounding communities. (See illustration, p 364.)

It is also claimed that contemporary man can be intentionally mummified—and kept in much better condition than Egyptian mummies.

In 1975, Claude Nowell (now called Summum Bonum Amon "Corky" Ra) founded a Salt Lake City-based company, Summum, to mummify the dead. While he has so far only mummified animals, at least one embalmer who has enrolled to be mummified believes the process will preserve bodies for thousands of years. Unlike the water-draining chemicals the Egyptians used, his process uses phenol, a small amount of formaldehyde, DMSO (a solvent), and a secret recipe of salts and other chemicals. The hundreds of people who have already signed up with Nowell, for $40,000 per person, will have their bodies immersed in the chemicals for several months after death. He will then wrap them in gauze, seal them with latex rubber, and cover them with layers of fiberglass and an epoxy-like resin. For an extra $7,000 to $10,000, he will cover the body in a gold-leaf veneer. And for $25,000 extra, the body will be welded into a custom-made quarter-inch-thick cast bronze molded shell, decorated to the subscriber's specifications. Most of those who have signed up for this service are health devotees who do not want their perfectly trim bodies to decompose after death. Says Ra of his clientele, "They're not necessarily vain, but they find the idea of being preserved for all eternity very appealing."[275] However, as one writer said, "in this recycling-conscious age, many may bristle at the idea of hanging around in the environment indefinitely like some glorified lump of Styrofoam."[276]

## S. CAN ALL BODIES BE EMBALMED?

No. But embalmers have many techniques to restore mutilated (but not decomposed) bodies.[277] Their goals are to restore mutilated remains, conceal injury and restore "a recognizable appearance to the features." Embalmers promise, however, only that they will improve the corpse's appearance—perfection is not guaranteed.

Before they begin the embalming process on a difficult case, they often have friends or family members view unrestored bodies to emphasize the challenging task ahead. When working on a mutilated corpse, the embalmer completes as much embalming as he can, and then covers the corpse with clothes. As much as possible, he uses long-sleeved garments, high-necked collars, and veils over the open portion of the casket to filter the features and prevent anyone from touching the restored corpse. One must wonder what type of clothing hid the rather unsightly wound left by the beheading axe when surgeons embalmed the body of Mary, Queen of Scots.

Difficult bodies to embalm include those that have been frozen, have marked *rigor mortis*, are either dried out or markedly swollen, are badly damaged, or are decomposing. Bodies, or portions of bodies, sometimes freeze while being stored in a morgue's refrigerator. Frozen bodies can be embalmed as soon as they thaw, but embalmers must be wary of dehydration and damage caused by ice crystals. Bodies with marked *rigor mortis* can be embalmed by injecting fluid into available arteries, then massaging the extremities to relax the *rigor*.

Embalmers worry about maintaining the body's correct water content. Bodies can dry out from refrigeration, from exposure after death or from dehydration before death. They can also be swollen from extra fluid caused by their disease or injury or from their therapy. Embalmers vary the strength and type of embalming solutions to correct water imbalances.

There are limits to what embalmers can do.

If decomposition is too far advanced, trying to restore the body may be futile. They may only be able to preserve and disinfect what remains, kill any vermin on the body, and eliminate the nauseating odor of the decomposing corpse. In these instances, the embalmer first destroys maggots by applying kerosene, carbon tetrachloride or similar chemicals. He then sprays the body with a disinfectant-deodorant solution. If arterial injection is not possible, the embalmer will inject chemicals through each shoulder, hip, elbow, knee to reach the various parts of the trunk and extremities. Additional injections are made in the hands, feet and parts of the head, and into the abdominal and chest cavities. He preserves all remaining parts of the face with injections through the mouth, nose, and beside the eyes.[278] When the brain has decomposed, it is sucked out through the nose and embalming fluid is instilled into the head. In cases of gunshot or other open head wounds, some embalmers draw the brain through the wound itself and then close the hole with a trocar *button*.[279] They then usually cover bodies for several hours with packs containing embalming fluid.

When a body or a part of a body is so badly mangled, crushed, burned or decomposed that no other method will work one alternative is to "vat" the body. As may be inferred from the term, the part is dunked in a strong solution of embalming chemicals. Knowing the strength of the solution and how long it needs to be kept there is a part of the art of embalming.[280]

In those instances when a badly decomposed body must be taken for a funeral service without embalming, morticians often pack the body in dry ice and then wrap it in a heavy quilt or blanket. Within an hour or so this freezes the outer shell of the body, temporarily reducing or eliminating any smell and fluid leakage. The danger of doing this in a sealed casket, however, is that it could result in an explosion from the buildup of carbon dioxide gas. Another method of quickly reducing the smell is to put the body in a waterproof pouch and cover it with a generous amount of slaked lime. While this is neither as fast nor as effective as using dry ice, it may be more readily available in some situations.[281]

## T.  MUST ALL BODIES BE EMBALMED?

No. Even if a body will be viewed, it need not be embalmed. However, the U.S. Federal Trade Commission (FTC) has repeatedly found that more than 90% of those not opting for cremation purchase embalming services.[282] Even among families who choose cremation, 25% opt for viewing and 14% of all corpses are embalmed.[283] More than half of all Americans believe that the law requires embalming.[284] This is patently untrue, as is shown by New York's Potter's Field that contains many thousands of unembalmed bodies.

Today, funeral directors are more likely to get permission before they "prepare" the body for viewing than they were in earlier, less litigious, times. Before the FTC's Funeral Rule went into effect in 1984 (Appendix I), it was common for funeral homes to embalm bodies (and charge for this service) if they had been asked to "remove" them from homes or medical facilities.[285] The Funeral Rule prohibits funeral providers from embalming a "deceased human body *for a fee* unless: (1) State or local law or regulation requires embalming in the particular circumstances regardless of any funeral choice which the family might make; or (2) Prior approval for embalming (expressly or so described) has been obtained from a family member or other authorized person...".[286]

Embalming is rarely required within the United States for public health reasons. That is because corpses carry little disease risk, and if they did, embalming might not prevent it. As C. J. Polson, a noted British forensic pathologist noted, "the principal value of embalming lies in the prevention or delay of putrefaction. A further advantage is that the body remains free from the odour of putrefaction and is not offensive to those who may have to live in the same house or who wish to pay their last respects where the body lies...Death, in itself, appreciably reduces the danger which results from contact with a body. The mortality rate amongst funeral directors is no greater than the average rate for the community as a whole, and their occupation does not appear to hold special danger of infection."[287] This is also the conclusion drawn by the U.S. Centers for Disease Control and Prevention (CDC) and many other professionals who have independently researched this without financial support from the funeral industry.[288] The CDC rates the risk to funeral industry workers from infectious disease as no greater than that of other medical professionals. In fact, their risk may be lower as their "patients" don't move. Mourners obviously have a much lower risk.

Despite the claims of the funeral industry, normal embalming does not kill all disease-causing organisms in a cadaver. One study showed that many common pathogens, including the bacillus that causes tuberculosis, were present in twenty-two of twenty-three cadavers within 24 to 48 hours after being embalmed.[289] Other infectious organisms are virtually unaffected by normal embalming practices, including those that cause anthrax, tetanus, and gas gangrene.[290] Students in the health professions have little if any risk of contracting infectious diseases from the cadavers used for anatomical dissection, since the corpses undergo much more intense embalming than those in funeral homes. No transmission of disease from anatomical cadavers has ever been documented.

## U. WHAT ARE RELIGIOUS & LEGAL ATTITUDES TOWARD EMBALMING?

Embalming in modern times is primarily a Christian practice. In the Middle Ages Christianity discouraged embalming, although King Henry I of England was reportedly embalmed (or mummified) by Egyptian methods in 1135.[291] All mainstream Christian denominations now allow embalming, although none require it. In some subcultures, however, embalming, if physically possible, is considered mandatory. Other major world religions generally discourage embalming or adamantly oppose it. This group includes Sikhs, Muslims, Jews, Buddhists, and Hindus.

The only legal requirement to embalm a body is normally associated with transit across state or international lines—and even then it may not always be mandatory.

## V. HOW MUCH DOES EMBALMING COST?

According to data from the NFDA's 1991 Survey of Funeral Operations, the average price for embalming listed on funeral homes' FTC-required price lists was $226.23. This, however, did not include other body preparation, such as cosmetology and hair styling, that averaged $90.71. The total is $316.94.[292] (For other funeral costs, see Costing it out: a cost-comparison chart of postmortem activities, Chapter 13.)

## W. REFERENCES

1. *The Compact Edition of the Oxford English Dictionary.* vol 2. New York: Oxford Univ Press, 1971, p 3494.
2. Mitford J: *The American Way of Death.* New York: Simon & Schuster, 1963, p 231.
3. *People v. Ringe,* 197 NY 143, 148, 90 N.E. 451.
4. Warner WL: *The Living and the Dead: A Study of the Symbolic Life of Americans.* New Haven, CT: Yale Univ Press, 1959, p 315.
5. Tegg W: *The Last Act: Being the Funeral Rites of Nations and Individuals.* London: William Tegg & Co, 1876, p 46.
6. Habenstein RW, Lamers WM: *The History of American Funeral Directing.* 2nd ed. Milwaukee, WI: National Funeral Directors Association, 1981, p 26.
7. Herodotus: *History.* Book IV, verse 71.
8. Litten J: *The English Way of Death: The Common Funeral Since 1450.* London: Robert Hale, 1991, p 17.
9. Habenstein, Lamers, *History of American Funeral Directing,* pp 139-40.
10. Koosman S: *Cultural Variations in Funeral Practice.* (lecture.) National Funeral Directors Association Annual Convention. Baltimore, MD: 1989. (audiotape)
11. British Public Record Office: LC 2/26. As quoted in: Bland O: *The Royal Way of Death.* London: Constable, 1986, p 100.
12. Bland O: *The Royal Way of Death.* London: Constable, 1986, p 100.
13. Habenstein, Lamers, *History of American Funeral Directing,* p 146.
14. *The New York Journal of General Advertisers.* January 7, 1768. As quoted in: Habenstein, Lamers, *History of American Funeral Directing,* p 140.
15. Habenstein, Lamers, *History of American Funeral Directing,* p 140.
16. Farrell JJ: *Inventing the American Way of Death, 1830-1920.* Philadelphia, PA: Temple Univ Press, 1980, pp 148-49.
17. Habenstein, Lamers, *History of American Funeral Directing,* p 143.
18. Gittings C: *Death, Burial and the Individual in Early Modern England.* London: Croom & Helm, 1984, p 95.
19. Habenstein, Lamers, *History of American Funeral Directing,* pp 146-48.
20. Renouard A: Merchantable Wares. *The Casket.* 1883;8(Jan):2.
21. Mayer RG: *Embalming: History, Theory, and Practice.* Norwalk, CT: Appleton & Lange, 1990, p 44.
22. McLaughlin J: *Gettysburg—The Long Encampment.* New York: Bonanza Books, 1963, p 183.
23. Kansas State Board of Embalmers: *The Kansas State Board of Embalmining.* Kansas City, KS: Univ of Kansas 1966, pp 11-19.
24. Farrell, *Inventing the American Way of Death,* pp 155-56.
25. *Historical Library.* London: 1700. As quoted in: Jackson PE: *The Law of Cadavers and of Burial and Burial Places.* New York: Prentice-Hall, 1937, p 163.
26. Warner, *Living and the Dead,* p 317.
27. Ibid., p 316.
28. Farrell, *Inventing the American Way of Death,* pp 146-47.
29. Watson JL, Rawski ES, eds: *Death Ritual in Late Imperial and Modern China.* Berkeley, CA: Univ of California Press, 1988, p 109-34.
30. Berg CW: *The Confessions of an Undertaker.* Wichita, KS: McCormick-Armstrong Press,

1920, p 27.
31. Kansas State Board of Embalmers, *Kansas State Board of Embalmining,* pp 11-19.
32. *O'Rielly v. Erlanger,* 108 App. Div. 318, 320, 95 NY Supp. 760.
33. *Building Com'r of Brookline v. McManus,* 263 Manss. 270, 273, 160 N.E. 887.
34. State of Arizona, Office of the Auditor General: *A Performance Audit of the Board of Funeral Directors and Embalmers.* Phoenix, AZ: August 1983. Report 83-13.
35. National Funeral Directors Association: *Funeral Service—Meeting Needs...Serving People.* (pamphlet). Milwaukee, WI: NFDA (no date).
36. Ibid.
37. Berg, *Confessions of an Undertaker,* p 31.
38. Pine VR: *Caretaker of the Dead.* New York: Irvington, 1975, p 41.
39. Sime JH: In review. *The American Funeral Director.* 1992;115(4):16-17.
40. Arvio RP: *The Cost of Dying and What You Can Do About It.* New York: Harper & Row, 1974, p X.
41. Warner, *Living and the Dead,* p 317.
42. Fulton RL: The clergyman and the funeral director: a study in role conflict. *Social Forces.* 1961;39(4):317-23.
43. Watson, Rawski, *Death Ritual,* p 120.
44. NFDA: 1991 Survey—How do you compare? *The Director.* November 1991, pp 42-44.
45. Finch MG: Women still face hurdles in funeral service. *The American Funeral Director.* 1992:115;24-26+.
46. Palmer G, exec. producer: *Death: The Trip of a Lifetime.* Seattle, WA: KCTS-TV Public Broadcasting Station, 1993. (video production)
47. NFDA, 1991 Survey, *The Director,* Nov 1991.
48. Tobin D: Bereaved families and funeral directors. *Australian Family Physician.* 1983;12:263-64.
49. Daniel TP: *An Analysis of the Funeral Rule Using Consumer Survey Data on the Purchase of Funeral Goods and Services.* Washington, DC: Federal Trade Commission, February 1989, p 7.
50. NFDA, 1991 Survey, *The Director,* Nov 1991.
51. Ibid.
52. Isard D: Teaming: the wave of the future. *The Director.* 1992;64(3):26-28.
53. Jacob R: Acquisitions done the right way. *Fortune.* 1992;126(Nov. 16):96.
54. Englade K: *A Family Business.* New York: St. Martin's Press, 1992, p 42-43.
55. *Valueline.* May 14, 1993, p 1390.
56. White JA: When employees own big stake, it's a buy signal for investors. *Wall Street J.* February 13, 1992, p C1+.
57. Habenstein, Lamers, *History of American Funeral Directing,* p 328-29.
58. Mayer, *Embalming,* pp 48-52.
59. Kansas State Board of Embalmers, *Kansas State Board of Embalmining,* pp 11-19.
60. College executives assess ABFSE recommendations. *The American Funeral Director.* 1992;115(4):22-30+.
61. Farrell, *Inventing the American Way of Death,* pp 150-51.
62. NFDA survey of funeral operations, 1991. *The Forum.* March 1992, p 20.
63. College executives assess ABFSE recommendations. *The American Funeral Director.* 1992;115:4:22-30+.
64. Mayer, *Embalming,* p 53.
65. Farrell, *Inventing the American Way of Death,* p 153.
66 Koosman, *Cultural Variations in Funeral Practice,* 1989. (audiotape)
67. Grollman EA, ed: *Concerning Death: A Practical Guide for the Living.* Boston: Beacon Press, 1974, p 191.
68. Chronicle Guidance Publications: *Brief 38.* Washington, IN: The Conference of Funeral Service Examining Boards. (no date)
69. Kubasak MW: *Cremation and the Funeral Director—Successfully Meeting the Challenge.* Malibu, CA: Avalon Press, 1990, p 90.
70. Metcalf P, Huntington R: *Celebrations of Death.* 2nd ed. New York: Cambridge Univ Press, 1991, p 20.
71. Kubasak, *Cremation and the Funeral Director,* p 37.

72. Isard, *The Director*, 1992.
73. Market Facts: *Report on the Survey of Recent Funeral Arrangers*. Washington, DC: Federal Trade Commission, 1988, pp II 5-6.
74. U.S. Senate: Subcommittee on antitrust and monopoly of the Committee on the Judiciary: *Hearings, Antitrust Aspects of the Funeral Industry*. 88th Congress, 2nd Session, 1964, p 90.
75. *Facts about funerals every family should know*. (pamphlet). Forest Park, IL,: Wilbert, 1987, p 8.
76. *White v. Luquire Funeral Home*, 221 Ala. 440, 443, 129 So.
77. *Prodigy News Service*, February 29, 1992.
78. Kass LR: Thinking about the body. *Hastings Center Report*. 1985;15:20-30.
79. Herodotus: *History*. Book 3, verse 38.
80. Richardson R: *Death, Dissection and the Destitute*. London: Routledge & Kegan Paul, 1987, p 17.
81. *Ten Forbidden Funeral Facts & the Rules Funeral Directors Break Most Often*. (pamphlet) San Francisco, CA: Ghia Gallery, no date. (distributed in 1992)
82. Metcalf, Huntington, *Celebrations of Death*, p 22.
83. Alex Ghia: Interview. San Francisco, CA: January 23, 1992.
84. Metcalf, Huntington, *Celebrations of Death*, p 200.
85. Habenstein RW, Lamers WM: *Funeral Customs the World Over*. Milwaukee, WI: National Funeral Directors Association, 1963, p 167-68.
86. Granqvist H: *Muslim Death and Burial—Arab Customs and Traditions Studied in a Village in Jordan*. Helsinke-Helsingfors: Societas Scientiarum Fennica, 1965;34:62-63, 67.
87. Ibid.
88. Habenstein, Lamers, *Funeral Customs the World Over*, p 55.
89. Ibid., p 65.
90. Watson, Rawski, *Death Ritual*, p 12.
91. Ibid., pp 439-42.
92. Habenstein, Lamers, *Funeral Customs the World Over*, p 218.
93. Granqvist, *Muslim Death and Burial*, pp 58-59.
94. Raether HC, ed: *The Funeral Directors Practice Managment Handbook*. Prentice-Hall, 1989. As quoted in: Kubasak, *Cremation and the Funeral Director*, p 88.
95. American Board of Funeral Service Education. As quoted in: Kubasak, *Cremation and the Funeral Director*, p 88.
96. Grabuschnigg VP, Rous F: Konservierung menschlicher Leichen im Wandel der Zeit—ein Beitrag zur Entwicklung und Methodik. *Beitrage zur Gerichtlichen Medizin*. 1990;48:455-58.
97. Oatfield H: *Literature of the Chemical Periphery—Embalming*. Advances in Chemistry Series. vol 16. American Chemistry Society, 1956, pp 112-42.
98. Adams J: The importance of basics. *The Dodge Magazine*. 1992;84(2):6+.
99. Coriolis (pseudonym of a Canadian undertaker): *Death, Here is Thy Sting*. Toronto: McClelland & Stewart, 1967. Cited in: Editors of Consumer Reports: *Funerals—Consumers' Last Rights*. New York: WW Norton, 1977, p 257.
100. The Group for Research on the Han Cadaver of Mawangtui: The state of preservation of the cadaver of the Marquise of Tai found in the Han Tomb No. 1 in Mawangtui near Changsha as revealed by the fine structure of the muscle and other tissues. *Scientia Sinica*. 1976;19:557-72.
101. Haestier RE: *Dead Men Tell Tales: A Survey of Exhumations from Earliest Antiquity to the Present Day*. London: John Long, 1934, p 78.
102. Bland, *Royal Way of Death*, pp 183-84.
103. Coffin MM: *Death in Early America: The History and Folklore of Customs and Superstitions of Early Medicine, Funerals, Burials, and Mourning*. Nashville: Thomas Nelson, 1976, p 138.
104. Farrell, *Inventing the American Way of Death*, p 157.
105. Holman JM: The undertaker's lot in America. *Casket and Sunnyside*. 1972;101(13):14-15.
106. Farrell, *Inventing the American Way of Death*, p 159.
107. Coffin, *Death in Early America*, p 108-109.

228

108. Rogers & Hammerstein: *Oklahoma!*: "Pore Jud is Daid." As quoted in: Barber P: *Vampires, Burial, and Death: Folklore and Reality.* New Haven, CT: Yale Univ Press, 1988, p 166.
109. Curl JS: *The Victorian Celebration of Death.* Detroit: Partridge Press, 1972, p 82.
110. Walker GA: *Gatherings From Grave Yards.* London: Longman, 1839. Reprinted by Arno Press, New York, 1977, p 204.
111. Farrell, *Inventing the American Way of Death,* pp 158-59.
112. Tanner A: Lenin exposed: Preservationist reveals tricks of the trade. *USA Today.* December 1, 1993, p 4A.
113. Taking care of Lenin's body. *The American Funeral Director.* 1992;115(4):13-14.
114. Tanner, *USA Today,* December 1, 1993.
115. Ibid.
116. Mendelsohn S: Embalming from the medieval period to the present time. *Ciba Symposia.* May 1944, pp 1805-12.
117. Burke PA, Sheffner AL: The antimicrobial activity of embalming chemicals and topical disinfectants on the micobial flora of human remains. *Health Laboratory Science.* 1976;13(4):267-70.
118. Inman R: *Cremation Liability.* (lecture). National Funeral Directors Association Annual Convention. Louisville, KY: 1990. (audiotape)
119. Farrell, *Inventing the American Way of Death,* pp 162-63.
120. New research indicates length of AIDS virus survival after patient's death. *YB News.* Youngstown, OH: Nomis Pub, January 1993, pp 2A+.
121. *The Director.* 1992;64(3):6.
122. Fredrick JF: The vital public health function of embalming, part 3. *De-Ce-Co Magazine.* 1969;62(June):6+.
123. Fredrick JF: The vital public health function of embalming, part 1. *De-Ce-Co Magazine.* 1969;62(February):4+.
124. Beck-Sagué CM, Jarvis WR, Fruehling JA, et al: Universal precautions and mortuary practioners: influence on practices and risk of occupationally acquired infection. *J Occupational Med.* 1991;33:874-78.
125. OSHA: Occupational exposure to bloodborne pathogens; final rule—29 CFR 1910.1030. *Federal Register.* 1991;56(235):64004-182.
126. Inman, *Cremation Liability,* 1990. (audiotape)
127. New Jersey's Funeral Director License.
128. LeDoux M: Readers Forum. *Mortuary Management.* 1992;79(7):11-12.
129. Smith SS: The impact of AIDS cases on funeral service practices. *The American Funeral Director.* 1992;115(9):44-46.
130. Sawyer D: Cavity treatment. *The Dodge Magazine.* 1991;83:1.
131. State of Arizona, *A Performance Audit,* 1983
132. Beck-Sagué, Jarvis, Fruehling, *J Occupational Med,* 1991.
133. Turner SB, Kunches LM, Gordon KF, Travers PH, Mueller NE: Occupational exposure to human immunodeficiency virus (HIV) and hepatitis B virus (HBV) among embalmers: a pilot seroprevalence study. *American Journal of Public Health.* 1989;79:1425-26.
134. Ibid.
135. Carr J. As quoted in: Mitford, *American Way of Death,* pp 82-83.
136. State of Arizona, *A Performance Audit,* 1983.
137. Editors of Consumer Reports: *Funerals—Consumer's Last Rights.* New York: WW Norton, 1977, p 96.
138. Feinberg IM: *Funeral Service Journal.* As quoted in: Mitford, *American Way of Death,* p 82.
139. Mitford, *American Way of Death,* p 66-67.
140. Strub CG, Frederick LG: *The Principles and Practice of Embalming.* 4th ed. Dallas, TX: Frederick, 1967, p 136.
141. Pine, *Caretaker of the Dead,* p 96.
142. Strub, Frederick, *Principles and Practice of Embalming,* p 133.
143. Farrell, *Inventing the American Way of Death,* p 10.
144. Ibid., p 160.

145. Greenhill T: *Art of Embalming.* 1705. As quoted in: Gittings, *Death, Burial and the Individual,* p 104-105.
146. Pine, *Caretaker of the Dead,* p 96.
147. Tuckerman H: The law of burial and the sentiment of death. *Christian Examiner.* 1856;61:345.
148. Lamm M, Eskreis N: Viewing the remains: a new American custom. *J Religion and Health.* 1966;5(2):137-43.
149. *Book of Genesis* 50:26.
150. Mayer, *Embalming,* pp 23-57.
151. Glob PV: *The Bog People—Iron Age Man Preserved.* (trans. by Bruce-Mitford R). Ithaca, NY: Cornell Univ Press, 1969, multiple pages.
152. Shakespeare W: *Hamlet.* Act V, scene 1, lines 159-65.
153. Mayer, *Embalming,* pp 23-57.
154. Ibid.
155. Herodotus: *History.* Book IV, verse 71.
156. Mayer, *Embalming,* pp 23-57.
157. Mendelsohn, *Ciba Symposia,* 1944.
158. Litten, *English Way of Death,* p 37.
159. Ibid., pp 32-56.
160. Grabuschnigg, Rous, *Beitrage zur Gerichtlichen Medizin,* 1990.
161. Gittings, *Death, Burial and the Individual,* p 104-105.
162. Mayer, *Embalming,* p 33.
163. Geddes GE: *Welcome Joy: Death in Puritan New England, 1630-1730.* (Ph.D. Thesis) Riverside, CA: Univ of California, 1976, pp 209-10.
164. Litten, *English Way of Death,* pp 32-56.
165. Franklin J, Sutherland J: *Guinea Pig Doctors.* New York: William Morrow, 1984, p 35.
166. Evans WED: *The Chemistry of Death.* Springfield, IL: Charles C Thomas, 1963, p 78.
167. Grabuschnigg, Rous, *Beitrage zur Gerichtlichen Medizin,* 1990.
168. Barber P: *Vampires, Burial, and Death: Folklore and Reality.* New Haven, CT: Yale Univ Press, 1988, p 41.
169. Litten, *English Way of Death,* p 44.
170. Mendelsohn, *Ciba Symposia,* 1944.
171. Habenstein, Lamers, *History of American Funeral Directing,* p 216.
172. White TM, Sandrof I: The first embalmer. *The New Yorker.* November 7, 1942, pp 43-46.
173. Mayer, *Embalming,* p 42.
174. Boatner MM: *The Civil War Dictionary.* New York: David McKay, 1988, pp 263-64.
175. Davis WC: *First Blood—Ft. Sumter to Bull Run.* Alexandria, VA: Time-Life Books, 1983, pp 62-69.
176. Johnson EC: A brief history of U.S. military embalming. *The Director.* 1971;41:8-9.
177. Carson SL: The Civil War mortician. *The American Funeral Director.* 1970;93(4):28-32.
178. Johnson, *The Director,* 1971.
179. Mendelsohn, *Ciba Symposia,* 1944.
180. Sawyer DW: *Embalming Techniques—Restoration After Organ Donation.* (lecture) National Funeral Directors Association Annual Convention, Louisville, KY: 1990. (audiotape)
181. Habenstein. As quoted in: Pine, *Caretaker of the Dead,* p 120.
182. Mayer, *Embalming,* p 207.
183. Ibid., p vii.
184. Mayer R: *Embalming Techniques—Transplants and Trauma.* (lecture). National Funeral Directors Association Annual Convention. Baltimore, MD: 1989. (audiotape)
185. Adams, *The Dodge Magazine,* 1992.
186. Ibid.
187. Sawyer D: Embalming stillborns and infants. *The Dodge Magazine.* 1983;75:1-3.
188. Adams, *The Dodge Magazine,* 1992.
189. Evans, *Chemistry of Death,* p 65.
190. Adams, *The Dodge Magazine,* 1992.
191. Mayer, *Transplants and Trauma,* 1989. (audiotape)
192. Farrell, *Inventing the American Way of Death,* p 161.

193. Mayer, *Transplants and Trauma,* 1989. (audiotape)
194. Ibid.
195. Ibid.
196. Ibid.
197. Ibid.
198. Mayer, *Embalming,* p 97.
199. Adams, *The Dodge Magazine,* 1992.
200. Sanders RC: Professional cosmetology. *The Dodge Magazine.* 1992;84:3:10-11+.
201. Sawyer, *Restoration After Organ Donation,* 1990. (audiotape)
202. Ibid.
203. Ibid.
204. Mayer, *Transplants and Trauma,* 1989. (audiotape)
205. Mitford, *American Way of Death,* pp 66-67.
206. Mayer, *Embalming,* p 53.
207. Nathan H: A simple method of embalming human cadavers by intracardiac injection. *Acta anatomica.* 1970;77:155-59.
208. Sawyer D: Cavity treatment. *The Dodge Magazine.* 1991;83:1.
209. Ibid.
210. Mayer, *Embalming,* p 53.
211. Ibid., p 18.
212. Ibid., p 79.
213. Williams MJ: *The Funeral Director's and Embalmer's Role in Medical Technology.* (lecture) National Funeral Directors Association Annual Convention. Louisville, KY: 1990. (audiotape)
214. Mayer, *Embalming,* pp 7-8.
215. Williams, *Medical Technology,* 1990. (audiotape)
216. Linos A, Blair A, Cantor KP, Burmeister L, VanLier S, et al: Leukemia and non-Hodgkin's lymphoma among embalmers and funeral directors. *J National Cancer Institute.* 1990;3:66.
217. Hayes RB, Blair A, Stewart PA, Herrick RF, Mahar H: Mortality of U.S. embalmers and funeral directors. *American J Industrial Med.* 1990;18:641-52.
218. Partanen T: Formaldehyde exposure and respiratory cancer—a meta-analysis of the epidemiological evidence. *Scandinavian J Work, Environment & Health.* 1993;19:8-15.
219. Yager JW, Cohn KL, Spear RC, Fisher JM, Morse L: Sister-chromatid exchanges in lymphocytes of anatomy students exposed to formaldehyde-embalming solution. *Mutation Research.* 1986;174:135-39.
220. Holness DL, Nethercott JR: Health status of funeral service workers exposed to formaldehyde. *Arch Environmental Health.* 1989;44:222-28.
221. Penno T: Compliance connection. *The Director* 1992;63(8):40-42.
222. Williams, *Medical Technology,* 1990. (audiotape).
223. Finkelstein J, McCully W, MacLaughlin D, Godine JE, Crowley W. The morticians' mystery: gynecomastia and reversible hypogonadotropic hypogonadism in an embalmer. *N Engl J Med.* 1988;318:961-65.
224. Sawyer, *Restoration After Organ Donation,* 1990. (audiotape)
225. Mayer, *Embalming,* p 63.
226. Ibid, pp 63-65.
227. Arbuthnot HF: Bamford F & the Duke of Wellington, eds: *The Journal of Mrs Arbuthnot 1820-1833.* London: Macmillan, 1950.
228. Oatfield, *Embalming,* pp 112-42.
229. Peter W: *'Flicted Arm Pete.* Recorded March 18, 1966. On Jackson B, ed: *Get Your Ass in the Water and Swim Like Me! Narrative Poetry From the Black Oral Tradition.* Somerville, MA: Rounder Records, 1966.
230. Gordon R: *Great Medical Disasters.* New York: Dorset Press, 1983, p 204.
231. Howard Belkoff (funeral director): Interview. Lakewood, NJ: March 2, 1993.
232. Mayer, *Embalming,* p 97.
233. Ibid., p 106.
234. Troutman R: *Cremation Liability.* (lecture). National Funeral Directors Association Annual Convention. Baltimore, MD: 1989. (audiotape)

235. Grabuschnigg, Rous, *Beitrage zur Gerichtlichen Medizin*, 1990.
236. Froede R: Personal communication. Armed Forces Institute of Pathology, July 1992.
237. Evans, *Chemistry of Death*, p 66.
238. Editors of The American Heritage Dictionaries: *Word Mysteries and Histories*. Boston: Houghton Mifflin, 1986, pp 229-30.
239. Polson CJ, Brittain RP, Marshall TK: *The Disposal of the Dead*. Springfield, IL: Charles C Thomas, 1962, p 8.
240. Evans, *Chemistry of Death*, p 64.
241. Habenstein, Lamers, *History of American Funeral Directing*, p 8.
242. Ragon M: *The Space of Death: A Study of Funerary Architecture, Decoration, and Urbanism*. (Sheridan A: trans) Charlottesville, VA: Univ Press of Virginia, 1983. Originally published as *L'espace de la mort: Essai sur l'architecture, la décoration et l'urbanisme funéraires*. Albin Michel, 1981, p 8.
243. Symonds JA: *Renaissance in Italy: The Age of Despots*. Quoted in: Hastier, *Dead Men Tell Tales*, p 24.
244. Haestier, *Dead Men Tell Tales*, p 24.
245. Mehta G: *Karma Cola: Marketing the Mystic East*. New York: Simon & Schuster, 1979, pp 94-95.
246. Morrison J: Crypt of the economic miracle. *American Way*. October 1, 1992, pp 36-39.
247. Ragon, *Space of Death*, p 9.
248. Litten, *English Way of Death*, p 33.
249. Polson, Brittain, Marshall, *Disposal of the Dead*, p 6.
250. Kates BC: The crypts of the Capuchins. *The American Funeral Director*. September 1971, p 22.
251. Ragon, *Space of Death*, pp 164-65.
252. Augé L: *Les Tombeaux*. Paris: Hachette, 1879. Cited in: Ragon, *Space of Death*, p 165.
253. Baudrillard J: *L'echange symolique et la mort*. Paris: Gallimard, 1976. Cited in: Ragon, *Space of Death*, p 165.
254. Puckle BS: *Funeral Customs—Their Origin and Development*. London: T Werner Laurie, 1926, p 159.
255. Hill RB, Anderson RE: *The Autopsy—Medical Practice and Public Policy*. Boston: Butterworths, 1988, p 167.
256. Ibid.
257. Giacometti L, Chiarelli B: The skin of Egyptian mummies. *Arch Dermatol*. 1968;97:712-16.
258. Garrison FH: *An Introduction to the History of Medicine*. 3rd ed. Philadelphia, PA: Saunders, 1924, pp 50-52.
259. Herodotus: *History*. Book II, verse 85-88, in *Loeb Classic Library*, Cambridge, MA: Havard Univ Press, 1921.
260. Mayer, *Embalming*, p 26.
261. Koosman, *Cultural Variations in Funeral Practice*, 1989. (audiotape).
262. Ibid.
263. Ibid.
264. Evans, *Chemistry of Death*, p 67.
265. Bahn PG: The making of a mummy. *Nature*. 1992;356:109.
266. Evans, *Chemistry of Death*, p 68.
267. Giacometti, Chiarelli, *Arch Dermatol*, 1968.
268. Hunter D: *Papermaking*. New York: Knopf, 1932, 1947. Cited in: Oatfield, *Embalming*, p 113.
269. Twain, Mark: *Innocents Abroad*.
270. Donnelly I: *Atlantis, the Antidiluvian World*. New York: Harpers, 1882, p 81. Cited in: Oatfield, *Embalming*, p 113.
271. Haestier, *Dead Men Tell Tales*, p 26.
272. Ibid., p 27.
273. Ibid., p 26.
274. Embalming. In: *The New Encyclopaedia Britannica*. vol 4 Chicago: Encyclopaedia Britannica, 1987, p 468.
275. Dricks V: Preserve yourself through eternity. *Green Bay* (WI) *Press-Gazette* October 17,

1993, p A4.
276. Weiss R: Looking good—forever. *Health.* Nov/Dec 1992, pp 30-31.
277. Strub, Frederick, *Principles and Practice of Embalming,* pp 469-500.
278. Grabuschnigg, Rous, *Beitrage zur Gerichtlichen Medizim,* 1990.
279. Mayer, *Transplants and Trauma,* 1989. (audiotape)
280. Strub, Frederick, *Principles and Practice of Embalming,* p 233-36.
281. Ibid., pp 469-500.
282. Daniel, *Analysis of the Funeral Rule,* 1989, p 10.
283. Kubasak, *Cremation and the Funeral Director,* p 89.
284. Central Area Motivation Program: *Consumer Action Project Survey.* Cited in: *Federal Register.* 1982;47(186):42269.
285. *Federal Register.* 1982;47(186):42275.
286. Funeral Rule Section 453.5(a)(1)-(2). *Federal Register.* 1982;47(186):42303.
287. Polson, Brittain, Marshall, *Disposal of the Dead,* p 286-87.
288. Consumer Reports, *Funerals,* pp 91-93.
289. Weed LA, Baggenstoss AH: The isolation of pathogens from tissues of embalmed human bodies. *Am J Clin Pathol.* 1951;21:1114-20.
290. Ives E: The Sanitary Use of Embalming. (unpublished Doctoral thesis.) 1959. Cited in: Consumer Reports, *Funerals,* p 97.
291. Polson, Brittain, Marshall, *Disposal of the Dead,* p 13.
292. NFDA: 1991 Survey—How do you compare?. *The Director.* November 1991, pp 42-44.

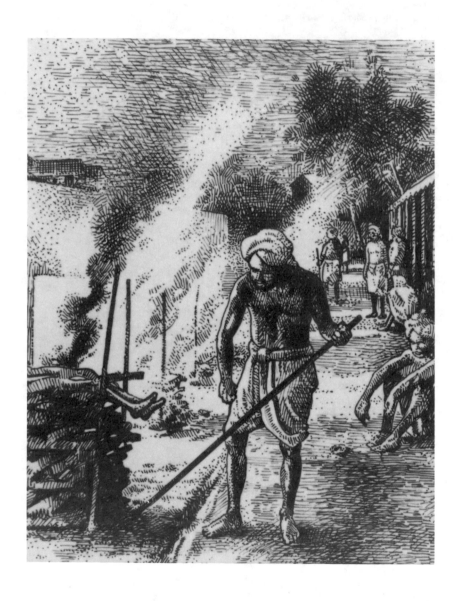

Cremating plague victims in Bombay, India. Original drawing published by *Harper's Weekly*, New York, 1899.

# 6: THE ETERNAL FLAME

*Cremation, an ancient method of corpse disposal and an integral part of some religions, is becoming an increasingly popular method of corpse disposal in the United States and around the world. How is the body cremated? What are the mystical, religious, legal, and psychological aspects of cremation? What can happen to the "ashes" after cremation, and what are some alternative methods people have used to dispose of cremated remains?*

## A. WHAT IS CREMATION?

Cremation is a process that reduces a corpse and its container to ashes and small bone fragments. The application of intense heat, and subsequent evaporation, converts the body to its basic components, idealized as "ashes to ashes, dust to dust."

More technically, cremation uses intense heat to rapidly burn (oxidize) the body. The body contains bones (chiefly calcium phosphate), water (70-80 percent of non-bone tissue), and carbon-based soft tissues. The intense heat used during cremation evaporates the water, burns the soft tissues, and for an average-sized adult, reduces the bones to 4 to 8 pounds of ash and fragments.[1]

Richard Selzer describes the process nicely:

> The good fellow slides you into the oven, and ignites the fire. If you are burned in your casket, an exhaust fan sucks away the wood ash, until there is only your body. He observes through a peephole at the back of the oven. Now he turns off the exhaust, and lets the flames attack the body. Three hours later, at two thousand degrees Fahrenheit, it is done. The oven is turned off.[2]

With the oldest cremation technique, the pyre, bodies were placed atop a wood pile which was then set ablaze. This method, used in ancient times, is still used in many parts of Asia and other remote areas of the world. In modern pyre cremations, attendants continually add fuel to the fire until the flames completely consume the body. Pyre cremations are necessarily public and often major social events.[3]

In Western countries, bodies to be cremated are usually placed in cardboard or wood containers and burned over several hours in specially designed furnaces called crematoriums or retorts. Early crematoria, such as Professor Gorini's at Woking, England, had a coke-burning furnace at one end, separated by a vertical partition from the cremation chamber at the other end. Once the fire was going, the body was put in the chamber and the partition was removed.

If the partition was not removed, the process was called "coking." Coking reduced the body to a hard, brittle substance called *coke* by applying flameless heat. This method took too long and left too much residua, so is no longer used.

Modern crematoria have inner linings of refractory material backed by heat-insulated bricks, all enclosed by steel plates.[4]

## B. WHAT IS DIRECT CREMATION?

In direct cremation, the body is incinerated without embalming, viewing or a ceremony. Multiple variations exist to suit individual family needs. California has led the direct cremation movement, although until 1971 direct cremation did not exist in the state. In that year, Thomas Weber started the Telophase Society, a San Diego business designed to meet the needs of those wanting a simple cremation, without the trimmings. In an effort to close Telophase down, the funeral industry raised multiple legal barriers. This finally ended when the California legislature passed a law requiring direct cremation companies to employ licensed funeral directors. While this marginally raised Telophase's costs, it legitimized the new industry.

During this period, Charles Denning began a similar business in San Francisco—the Neptune Society. These two "societies," not to be confused with memorial societies, are profit-making businesses. They are, however, significantly less expensive than traditional funeral homes, if only because they do not try to sell unwanted goods or services. The Neptune Society has fared very well, quickly dominating the California market and becoming the national leader in direct cremations, partly because of Denning's own showmanship. Dressing in nautical attire and sporting a Colonel Sanders-type goatee, he gleefully referred to himself as "Colonel Cinders," and told the media that people had better uses for their money than to pay it to "undertakers" for a "tin can" (casket) to put them in a "hole in the ground." The Neptune Society signed people up for memberships at $10 to $25 each, with a relatively low fee to be paid for cremation, paperwork, and the distribution of ashes when needed. Of approximately 17,000 direct cremations in California in 1988, the Neptune Society did about 12,000.[5]

## C. HOW LONG HAS CREMATION BEEN USED?

Man has used cremation to dispose of the dead since prehistoric times. Stone Age man cremated his dead in Northern and Eastern Europe and in the Near East. Ancient Australians cremated their dead as long as 20,000 years ago after covering the body with red ochre. Iron Age Palestinians cremated some of their dead, often placing the remains in the simple storage jars they used in daily life.[6] Ancient Babylonians also cremated their dead. They wrapped the corpses in combustible materials and then encased them in clay coffins around which they built the funeral pyres.[7]

The Bible first mentions cremation in the story of the disposal of the corpses of Saul and his sons. After their bodies were removed from the wall of Beth-shan where the Philistines had fastened them, they were taken by the Israelites to Jabesh for cremation,[8] burying the remaining bones under a tree.[9] This cremation, however, was unusual for the Israelites, since ancient Jews usually reserved cremation for criminals.[10] It may have been done to discourage further desecration of these soldiers' bodies. Interestingly, Saul killed himself during battle, although his sons died fighting.

The Bible also mentions the Valley of Gehenna (*Geh ben Hinnom*), a name that became synonymous with Hell, where children were supposedly sacrificed to Moloch, the Phoenician god of fire.[11] Yet scientists from Hebrew University have recently discovered that this valley, lying just west of Jerusalem's walled city, actually contained the ancient Phoenician city of Ahziv. A crucible and nearby bones provide convincing evidence that the city was home to an early crematory, rather than the site of human sacrifice.[12]

The Greeks began cremating their dead around 1,000 B.C., and by Homer's time it had become the customary method of corpse disposal. The Greeks believed that cremation would quell outbreaks of plague, prevent enemies from molesting their dead on the battlefield, and liberate the souls of the deceased.[13] According to Greek myth, Achilles, to fulfill his duty to his dead friend Patroclus, publicly cremated the body even though the gods tried to stop him.[14] Greeks often cremated bodies of the wealthy by using a covering of leaves ignited with butterfat—a method that was both efficient and socially proper. The remaining boney fragments were anointed with oil, gathered with the ashes and buried in urns.[15] The bodies of lesser citizens, however, were often incompletely consumed by the flames and it became an insult to describe someone as "half-burned."[16] (Did this eventually translate into being "half-baked?")

The Romans, following the example of Remus, a mythic founder of Rome, adopted cremation about 750 B.C. With cremation being the honorable method of corpse disposal, Romans reserved earth burial for murderers, suicides, and individuals who died after being struck by lightning (since they were thought to be cursed by Jupiter). They also buried infants who had not yet developed teeth so that the essential ingredient of resurrection in the undeveloped teeth would not be destroyed, as it might be by cremation.[17] For similar reasons, the Egyptians never cremated their dead. They believed to do so destroyed all prospects of an afterlife.

First century A.D. Romans built their funeral pyres of fast-burning pine logs, stuffing the holes between logs with sweet-smelling gums for aroma, and decorating the pyre with cypress branches. They placed the uncoffined body atop the pyre and the chief mourner, with head averted, torched it. To honor the deceased, gladiators often fought while the body burned. After the body had burned, mourners collected the bones, washed them with milk, and placed them in perfumed cinerary urns. This closely parallels Virgil's (70-19 B.C.) description of Misenus' elaborate cremation in the *Aeneid*:

> Then the wept-for limbs
> Upon the couch they lay, and over them
> Cast purple robes, the well-known raiment: some,
> Sad service, bowed them to the heavy bier,
> And, eyes averted, their ancestral wont,
> Applied the torch and held. The heaped gifts blaze—
> Frankincense, viands, and bowls of streaming oil.
> When sank the embers, and the flame was stilled,
> The remnant of the thirsty dust they drench
> With wine, and Corynaeus gathered up,
> And in a brazen casket hid, the bones.[18]

Excessive in all things, Nero reportedly used more myrrh, incense, and fragrant oils to cremate one of his wives than was produced in all of Arabia that year.[19] Julius Caesar (100-44 B.C.), after being murdered, was given a hero's funeral, including an almost *ad lib* cremation:

> [The people] tore away the benches and tables out of the shops round about, and, heaping them altogether, built a great funeral pile, and having put the body of Caesar upon it, set it on fire, the spot where this was done being moreover surrounded with a great many temples and other consecrated places, so that they seemed to burn the body in a kind of sacred solemnity.[20]

Due in part to the increasing expense, Romans used cremation only for patricians from the end of the Republic (31 B.C.) through the second century A.D.

The Germans also have an ancient tradition of cremating their dead. The Teutons used cremation as a religious rite, as exemplified in the legends of Siegfried on his funeral pyre. Some old German chronicles indicate that Attila the Hun was cremated while fully armed and sitting on his horse (although others state that he had an elaborate secret burial).[21,22]

Scandinavians began to cremate their dead in the Middle Bronze Age after the custom was introduced from Central Europe. Early Norse legends relate that the Aesir raised Balder's funeral pile on board a ship, laid his body on it, and committed the blazing vessel to the waves.[23] Tenth century A.D. visitors to Scandinavia wrote that Vikings first buried corpses, but soon disinterred them and placed the bodies on ships that they set ablaze. Depending on the wealth and power of the deceased, they would place clothing, weapons, dead animals, and even sacrificed servants on board. As fire consumed the ship and its contents, it was set adrift. Scandinavians continued to primarily use cremation for corpse disposal until around the eleventh century A.D., when Christianity abolished the long-held practice.[24] (See Section Z, *What do religions say about cremation?*)

People in Bronze Age Britain began cremating their dead when the pre-Christian European tradition was imported by way of Britanny. Cremation soon became the predominant form of corpse disposition in southwestern England and Wales. It was less popular in northern England.[25] Cremation in Britain has given us the word "bonfire" which initially described a pyre on which to burn a corpse's bones (*bone-fire* or *bane-fire* in Scotland).

Cremation followed Buddhism to Japan in A.D. 552, with the first recorded Japanese cremation being that of a Buddhist priest in A.D. 702.[26] As elsewhere, cremation was first accepted by the aristocracy, and then by the general population. In A.D. 647, a Japanese imperial ordinance further encouraged the wealthy to cremate their dead by banning elaborate funerals. It is thought that the first Japanese emperor to have been cremated was Emperor Jito (A.D. 645 to A.D. 702). The Japanese greatly expanded their use of cremation after an 1867 law required it for all corpses who had died from a contagious disease (a common cause of death at that time). To more easily control sanitation and land use,[27] large Japanese cities eventually required all corpses to be cremated.

The Russians also have a tradition of cremating their dead, as attested to by Ibn Haukal, a tenth-century Arab traveller who described a cremation at Kiev. Suggesting some cultural intolerance, a Russian said to him: "As for you Arabs, you are mad, for those who are the most dear to you, and whom you honour most, you place in the ground, where they will become a prey to worms, whereas with us they are burned in an instant and go straight to Paradise."[28]

By the fifth century A.D., as Christianity supplanted ancient traditions, burial completely replaced cremation in Christian Europe. It continued to exist only in remote areas, but even there cremation was finally abolished. By the nineteenth century, burial had become the most prevalent means of corpse disposal.

## D. WHY DID OUR ANCESTORS CREMATE BODIES?

Cremation derives from ancient religio-mystical sources.

Primitive man feared the dead as well as the "undead," who, they believed, could return to their corpse and harm the living. Cremation effectively destroyed the body, and thus eliminated any threat to the living from the dead. Nomadic tribes, who believed that they had to periodically offer gifts at a deceased person's grave to appease his spirit, used cremation to eliminate the gravesite. They were thereby spared supernatural hazards.[29]

The ancients also believed cremation helped the dead avoid evil spirits, and provided them with heat and warmth in the next world.[30] Herodotus, for example, related the tale of Melissa's ghost who appeared to Periander saying she was cold, since her clothes had been buried rather than burned. To remedy this, city leaders stripped the women of Corinth of their clothes and burned them to provide clothing to Melissa's spirit in the hereafter.[31]

Cremation also thwarted the seemingly dangerous process of decomposition and protected the body from mutilation by animals or humans.

Soldiers cremated their dead to prevent enemies from mutilating those corpses that could not be returned home for burial. It was said, "To be gnaw'd out of our graves, to have our sculs made drinking bowls, and our bones turned into pipes to delight and sport our Enemies, are Tragicall abominations, escaped in burning Burials."[32] Following cremation, the soldier's ashes were usually repatriated with appropriate honors.

From earliest historic periods cremation has also been used to prevent the introduction or spread of plagues. This was why Percy Bysshe Shelley, the famous English poet, was cremated after he drowned in a boating accident off the coast of Italy in 1822. His body washed ashore ten days after the drowning and was quickly buried in the sand. Although legend says otherwise, the Tuscans dug him up and cremated his body because their Quarantine Law required burning anything washed up from the sea to avoid the spread of plague. While a health officer burned the body on a collection of driftwood and pine logs, Shelley's friends added frankincense, salt, wine and oil to the pyre in a romantic remembrance of the ancient rites. Despite these spices, Lord Byron could not tolerate the smell and left saying, "Don't repeat this with me. Let my carcass rot where it falls." Friends recovered Shelley's heart from the still-hot embers, preserved it in alcohol, and eventually interred it in Bournemouth, England.[33,34] His ashes were taken to the Protestant cemetery of Rome, to be near Keats.[35]

Cremating the dead was also fostered by the belief that souls were transported to paradise by means of fire.[36] Native Americans on the Pacific coast and elsewhere used cremation because, as they said, "Unless the body is burnt the soul will never reach the land of the dead...In the hot smoke it rises up to the shining sun to rejoice in its warmth and light; then it flies away to the happy land in the west."[37] They may also have used cremation to prevent the dead from being disinterred by animals. Two crude containers thought to contain cremated Indian remains were found in Connecticut in 1974.[38]

American frontiersmen also occasionally used cremation. A fictional example is Robert Service's description of the cremation of Sam McGee:

> The Northern Lights have seen queer sights,
> But the queerest they ever did see
> Was that night on the marge of Lake Lebarge
> I cremated Sam McGee.[39]

Some people also used cremation to save the expense and bother of burial. In 1824, before any modern European began to formally advocate cremation, an Edinburgh woman created a stir when she cremated her own stillborn infant, placing it on a blazing fire and reducing it to ashes. When the police questioned her about this illegal act, she replied that "she resorted to cremation to save the fash [bother] and expense of burial."[40]

## E. HOW DID MODERN SOCIETY REINSTITUTE CREMATION?

European interest in cremation was revived in the late nineteenth century. Physicians were the earliest modern proponents of cremation because they believed that it caused less pollution and fewer public health problems than did burials.

In 1869 Dr. Brunetti, in Italy, conducted the first scientific experiments on modern cremation methods.[41] Simultaneously, the International Medical Congress of Florence was urging all nations to promote cremation. In 1872, Italy's cremation movement gained momentum when individuals opposed to the Catholic Church's monopoly on burial sites aroused public sentiment against traditional burials.

An organized European cremation movement began in 1874 when Queen Victoria's surgeon, Sir Henry Thompson, established The Cremation Society of England and gained momentum when Germany built the first modern crematory at Gotha in 1878. England's first crematorium was built in 1879 at Woking, but because of Church and government reluctance to permit human cremation, the public was not permitted to cremate their dead until the courts ruled it to be legal in 1884.[42]

An unusual series of events led up to this court case. Dr. William Price, an eccentric 84-year-old Welsh physician, sired a son, Iesu Grist (Jesus Christ) Price. When the boy died at 5 months of age (probably a "crib death"), Dr. Price attempted to cremate the body, wrapped in napkins, on a cask of paraffin oil. He intentionally picked a conspicuous time and place to perform the cremation—on Sunday evening in full view of people leaving church services. The crowd was livid. They rescued the child's body from the flames and chased Dr. Price home, where his mistress held the crowd at bay with a shotgun until the police saved his life by arresting him. Dr. Price defended himself before the Winter Assizes at Cardiff, obtaining the verdict that cremation was legal, provided that it did not become a nuisance to others. After he had kept his son's remains under his bed for eight weeks, authorities finally allowed him to cremate the body. After siring two more children, Dr. Price died in 1893, and his body was cremated in front of about six thousand people and a coterie of police.[43] (See illustration, p 244.)

During the late nineteenth century, English police often had to provide protection during cremations. This did not encourage its widespread use and in 1885 only three bodies were cremated. England did not incorporate cremation as a method of body disposal into statute until 1902. By 1905, crematoria operated in Britain, performing 604 cremations that year. (Today, because of the scarcity of land for burial, sixty percent of England's dead are cremated.) Between 1887 and 1906, nearly every European country erected at least one crematorium.[44]

In Paris, between 1874 and 1887, proponents of cremation (mostly physicians) actively lobbied authorities to approve cremation. In 1880, they founded the Society for the Propagation of Cremation. On November 15, 1887, the Chamber of Deputies passed a law permitting cremation, and the first French crematorium opened. The crematorium, built by Formigé, was equipped with two gas and two oil-fired ovens, the former being used only for the remains of hospital dissections. As occurred elsewhere, the crematory's first "customer" did not arrive for two years.[45]

In Australia, as elsewhere, physicians were pre-eminent in the cremation movement and medical arguments were used to promote cremation. Dr. John Le Gay Brereton, a mid-nineteenth century proponent of cremation in Australia, argued that the flesh "was riddled with disease, stained with sin, and foul with heredity."[46] Yet the Legislative Council of New South Wales repeatedly defeated a Cremation Bill, introduced by Dr. John Mildred Creed, who was both a legislator and an officer of the New South Wales branch of the British Medical Association. Cremation became legal, however, when Britain legalized it in the late nineteenth century, since at that time Australia was still governed by the English common law system.[47]

At the turn of the century, Australians in Sydney circulated a pamphlet, *Short Reasons for Cremation*, that graphically described "twelve arguments in favour of cremation:"

1. Land in and around Sydney is too valuable to be used as a graveyard.
2. This fact will some day be realised, and the corpses moved further afield. It is not pleasant to think that the bodies of our dear ones may thus some day be tampered with.
3. Land once used for burial purposes may well be contaminated for centuries to come, and be the cause of much ill-health to future generations.
4. Disease germs breed freely in the earth. Every human body contains those disease germs. Therefore *every corpse buried in our midst constitutes a direct menace to the public health.*
5. Cremation does quickly and cleanly exactly what earth burial does slowly and by a process too disgusting to bear thinking of.
6. Cremation is as cheap as earth burial, and as it entails no charge for maintenance and there is no freehold to be purchased, it is, in the long run, very much cheaper.

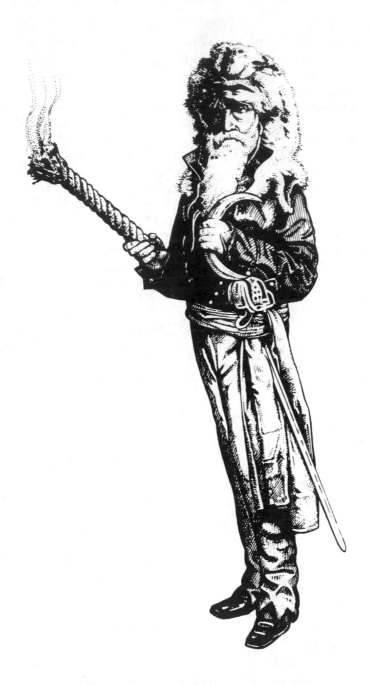

Dr. William Price, an early British cremation advocate.

7.   It furthermore eliminates the danger of seeing that most distressing spectacle—a neglected grave.
8.   The cremation ceremony is more dignified and infinitely less barbaric than the ceremonial which earth burial involves.
9.   Cremation entails no danger of pneumonia from standing beside an open grave on a cold winter's day.
10.  *Cremation eliminates all danger of being buried alive.*
11.  Cremation makes possible a return to the delightful old custom of making one's final resting place within the precincts of a church.
12.  Cremation means that one's friends are not compelled to travel long distances to figure at a dismal and distressing ceremony. They would, of course, not be asked to be present at the actual cremation, but merely to attend a short service afterwards, in the course of which the ashes would be laid to rest.[48]

The first U.S. citizen intentionally cremated was Colonel Henry Laurens, an influential South Carolinian who had presided over the Continental Congress of 1777-78 and had been a member of George Washington's military staff.[49] As Col. Laurens had requested, upon his death in 1792 he was enfolded in 12 yards of tow-cloth and burned until he was "entirely consumed." His ashes were placed in the family graveyard. It was not until 1873, however, that the United States first held meetings to formally discuss cremation. By 1876, nine American scientific articles had been published on the topic and Dr. Francis Julius Le Moyne, a noted abolitionist and free-thinker, had built the first U.S. crematory in Washington, Pennsylvania. Later that year (December 6), Baron de Palm, a German nobleman thought to be somewhat eccentric, was cremated at Le Moyne's crematory in an invitation-only ceremony covered by the national press. Although several noted individuals were subsequently cremated at Le Moyne's crematory, including Le Moyne himself, by 1900 the crematory had only had forty-two customers and was closed down.[50] It is now a National Historic Landmark.

The original American cremation advocates were not subtle. An early U.S. pro-cremation pamphlet, for example, graphically described the choice "between incineration which disposes the body in one hour in a beautiful glow of heat, and earth burial which prolongs the process through 14 to 20 years of loathsome decay."[51]

In 1881 the United States Cremation Company was established and four years later it opened the more successful Fresh Pond Crematory in Queens, New York. Scarcely a year later *The Modern Cremdtist*, the first cremation journal, was founded in Lancaster, Pennsylvania. Between 1876 and 1884 were only 41 cremations in the United States, but by the end of 1900 more than 13,000 had been performed.[52] In 1913, with more than 40 crematories in operation, the Cremation Association of America (CAA, later to become the Cremation Association of North America, CANA) was formed to coordinate and promote the cremation business. Illustrating the public health and sanitation rationale for cremation often cited in times past, CAA's first president, Hugo Erichsen said, "Every crematist must be a missionary for the cause, and embrace every suitable occasion to spread its gospel, the glad tidings of a more sanitary and more aesthetic method of disposing of our beloved dead."[53]

## F. WHY DO MODERN PEOPLE USE CREMATION?

The reasons for modern cremation are well described by Richard Seltzer, who wrote, "Man is pompous in the grave, splendid in ashes...A smaller package to mail...Cremation is tidy."[54]

The Consumer's Union suggests four reasons why cremation is growing increasingly popular in the United States: (1) Cremation usually costs less than interment; (2) there is a marked decrease of cemetery space; (3) modern cremation methods are clean, quick and efficient; and (4) there is more religious tolerance, even encouragement, of cremation than in the past.[55]

Americans, among others, waste large land areas on cemeteries. The amount of land used annually for burials in the United States (not counting the land used for space between graves, roadways, crypts, and administrative facilities) approximates two square miles, as can be seen by the following calculation:

(4 x 8 ft) = typical grave plot

2 million people die in United States each year

More than 85% of deaths are followed by in-ground burial.[56]

4 ft x 8 ft x 2 million deaths x 85% = 54,400,000 sq. feet =

1, 249 acres = **APPROXIMATELY 2 SQUARE MILES**

This means that with the same rate of death and burial, over the next 230 years new graves will take up a land area equal to the size of Los Angeles. George Bernard Shaw understood this when he said:

...dead bodies can be cremated. All of them ought to be; for earth burial, a horrible practice, will some day be prohibited by law, not only because it is hideously unaesthetic, but because the dead would crowd the living off the earth if it could be carried out to its end of preserving our bodies for their resurrection on an imaginary day of judgement (in sober fact, every day is a day of judgement).[57]

Another reason to cremate a corpse might be to hide a murder. No one knows how often cremation has been used to hide criminal acts, but murderers have been convicted after unsuccessfully attempting to cremate their victims. As C. J. Polson said, "No matter how remote the risk of concealment of crime by cremation may or may not be...the fact remains that cremation effectively destroys all trace of violence and, radio-active substances excepted, of poisoning."[58] He mentions that exception because of a case in which a body containing Thallium, a highly toxic radioactive metal used in poisons, was cremated. The substance was subsequently found in the cremains and helped convict the killer.[59]

That may be one reason that the "Model Cremation Law" designed by the Cremation Association of North America (CANA) specifies both that "a Crematory Authority [operators of a crematory] shall not accept unidentified human remains," and that "human remains shall not be cremated within forty-eight (48) hours after the time of death, as indicated on the regular medical certificate of death...unless such death was a result of an infectious, contagious or communicable and dangerous disease, and such time requirement is waived." It goes on to say that, "In the event such death comes under the authority of the coroner or medical examiner, the human remains shall not be received by the Crematory Authority until authorization to cremate has been received in writing from the coroner or medical examiner or the county in which the death occurred."[60] Parts of Canada (including Ontario) also require waiting 48 hours after death before cremation.

There may be psychological reasons for cremation as well. Philippe Ariès describes cremation as a manifestation of enlightenment and modernity. He suggests that the actual motivation for cremation is that it is the most radical means of disposing of and forgetting about the body—of nullifying it. Cremation expresses the finality of death to the mourners, since the body through which they related to the person no longer exists.[61] Mourners also benefit from knowing that the disposition is quick and clean, rather than slow and foul as is decomposition after burial.[62]

The mourners' psychological response, however, could be quite different. Puckle suggested that in the early days of modern cremation "a natural horror of fire [was] the first obstacle to be overcome if cremation [was] to become a general practice."[63] The opposite could also be said, however, since cremation can actually short-circuit the mourning process or enhance the guilt felt in a hostile relationship through its total destruction of the body.

As modern cremation developed, some rather odd ideas were advanced. Early European advocates of scientific cremation suggested that society might use burning bodies as fuel, and then collect the by-products for other uses.[64] With the exception of the Nazi concentration camps, no society has accepted these practices. Today, even the mention of such a theory is abhorrent and would assuredly slow the public's acceptance of cremation.

Finally, medical schools generally use cremation to dispose of the tissues dissected from bodies during anatomy courses. The removed tissues are not separated, but cremated *en masse*. The schools often separately cremate the residual boney skeleton and body parts, and may return the ashes to relatives, if requested. Unless a special request is made, however, it is possible that the remains may not be returned to relatives for up to two years.[65]

## G. WHO USES CREMATION?

Three-fourths of the world's population has a legal right to dispose of their dead through cremation. Some countries where cremation is legal, however, have no crematoria.

Since World War II, countries with high population densities and shortages of public land, such as Japan and England, have had the greatest increase in cremations. In England, cremation has become the primary method of body disposal, with their average crematory performing twenty cremations a day.[66] By 1980, 60% of the dead in England and 75% in Japan were cremated. In the past the use of cremation in Japan varied by region, with burial preferred in Shinto-dominated areas and cremation nearly universal in large metropolitan areas.[67] Currently, 96% of Japan's deceased are cremated.[68] In Russia, cremation and burial occur in equal proportion.[69]

## TABLE 6.1: Percentage of Cremations by U.S. Region and Culture

| | | |
|---|---|---|
| Pacific States | (AK, CA, HI, OR, WA) | >38% |
| Southern States | (AL, KY, MI, TN) | < 3% |

| | |
|---|---|
| Japanese-Americans | 53% |
| Anglo-Americans | 29% |
| African-Americans | 5% |
| Mexican-Americans | 5% |

Adapted from: Kalish RA, Reynolds DK: *Death and Ethnicity—A Psychocultural Study*. Los Angeles, CA: Ethel Percy Andrus Gerentology Center, Univ of Southern CA, 1976, pp 47 & 152.

The Cremation Association of North America (CANA) reports that in 1992, 18% of all dead in the United States were cremated.[70] This is a sharp increase from 1988 when just over 15% of the 2,169,773 United States deaths were cremated (332,183 cremations), and a dramatic increase from 1970 when only 4.6% of U.S. deaths were cremated.[71] In contrast, by 1988 Canadians were cremating nearly 31% of their dead, and by 1989, about 35% of all corpses in Ontario, Canada, and 85% on Victoria Island were cremated.[72,73] In the United States, the use of cremation varies greatly by region and by local culture (Tables 6.1 and 6.2).

In the Midwest, some small, ultra-traditional cities and towns cremate only 2-3% of their dead, while the rate rises to 60% in locales populated by Westerners and ethnic groups that routinely use cremation, such as Thais, Indians, Cambodians, Laotians, Vietnamese, and Koreans. Japanese-Americans claim cremation has two advantages: it allows them more time to select an appropriate spot to deposit the remains, and it allows easier transportation of the remains if the family later wants to relocate.[74]

---

**TABLE 6.2: Number and Percentage of Dead Cremated Annually in Selected U.S. States: 1989\***

|  | # of Cremations | % of Deaths Cremated |
|---|---|---|
| Nevada | 4,628 | 50.89% |
| Hawaii | 3,365 | 50.16% |
| Washington | 15,808 | 43.50% |
| Colorado | 8,712 | 40.03% |
| California | 82,252 | 37.82% |
| Kentucky | 1,342 | 3.95% |
| Tennessee | 1,577 | 3.32% |
| West Virginia | 554 | 2.85% |
| Alabama | 932 | 2.49% |
| Mississippi | 433 | 1.78% |

\* The District of Columbia, Mississippi, New Hampshire, North Dakota, South Dakota, Vermont, and Wyoming each have fewer than four crematories.

Adapted from: *Cremations and % of Deaths*. Chicago: Cremation Association of North America, 1989.

---

CANA expects the U.S. rate of cremation to exceed 22% of all deaths by the year 2000 and to reach nearly 27% by 2010. In some areas of the country, the percentage of bodies cremated is expected to double during the next ten years (Table 6.3).

The average U.S. funeral home arranges for or performs 27 cremations annually. In 1990, each crematory in the United States handled an average of 362 cremations. In spite of an expected increase in the number of crematories, by 2010 each is expected to handle 398 cases per year. Comparable figures for Canada are 571 cremations per crematory in 1990, a figure projected to rise more slowly to 584 by 2010, when Canadians expect that more than 50% of their dead will be cremated.[75,76]

Persons preferring cremation in the United States are generally younger professionals and those not actively practicing a religion. Mainstream Protestants are more likely to elect cremation than Catholics, Jews or Fundamentalists.[77] Geographical distance from one's family roots also predisposes to choosing cremation.

It is usually the deceased, rather than the family, who primarily desires cremation. Within the demographic group who elect cremation, it is usually men who cremate their wives' bodies. Neither men nor children are usually cremated.[78] Interestingly, a preference for cremation instead of burial is not usually based on the wish for a ceremony, the desire to keep costs low, or a concern for land conservation.[79]

The cremation of famous people has increased acceptance of the procedure. It is likely that when Nelson Rockefeller, the former Vice President and New York governor, and Michael Landon, the noted television celebrity from *Bonanza* and *Little House on the Prairie,* were cremated, many people reconsidered their attitudes toward the procedure.

---

## TABLE 6.3: Expected Rise in U.S. Cremations: 1990-2010

|            | *1990* | *2010* |
|------------|--------|--------|
| California | >40%   | >50%   |
| Florida    | 34%    | 43%    |
| New York   | 14%    | 25%    |

Adapted from: *Cremation Rates: 1985-1989, 100 Top U.S Metros.* Chicago: Cremation Association of North America, 1989.

---

In Scandinavia, although the rate of cremation is generally high, Lapland, above the Arctic Circle, has the highest rate. In Lapland, the land remains frozen up to ten months of the year and bodies that are not cremated must be stored for burial until the ground thaws.[80] This actually presents no problem, since bodies destined for burial can be frozen outdoors until the ground softens.

In China, the world's most populous country, cremation was fashionable only in large cities before the Communist Revolution. The official Communist position stated that the elaborate traditional funerals, common in the countryside, should be replaced by cremation—at least for those who were not prominent government officials. Ashes could be stored adjacent to the cemetery or crematorium, but they would be discarded unless retrieved by relatives within five years. By the 1970s, cremation was nearly universal in large cities, but in smaller cities, towns and villages only 13% of corpses were cremated. A subsequent decrease in cremations caused the government to issue new regulations in 1985 requiring cremation in all densely populated areas, those areas that had a shortage of arable land, or where there was easy access to a crematorium. The penalty for violation was loss of burial subsidies for the individual and there were additional penalties for entire work units.[81]

## H. CAN ANY BODY BE CREMATED?

Any *body* can be cremated, but many items *in* our bodies do not burn. Dental gold, prostheses, metal plates, and metal sutures or screws cannot be destroyed by cremation. Although pacemakers do not burn, those with lithium batteries *explode* when cremated.[82] Most funeral directors remove pacemakers before cremation to eliminate this hazard. They normally discard the device unless the family requests that it be given back. While cremated tooth fillings emit so much mercury that health authorities are investigating them as toxic air pollutants,[83-85] bodies with some radioactive isotopes, such as those administered in diagnostic and therapeutic medical procedures, may be cremated. The crematorium must keep special records and must not handle an excess amount of radioactive material per year.[86]

All small pieces of metal from the body or container are normally removed with an electromagnet before the ashes are even removed from the oven. If a piece of jewelry or other memento is to be interred with the cremains, it is added to the urn after cremation. Removing dental gold, however, is generally not worth the cost, since the gold in dental work constitutes only about two percent of the alloy, with three gold crowns being worth only about $35.[87,88] In rare cases, however, such as at the now-closed Pasadena Crematorium, unscrupulous personnel made hundreds of thousands of dollars from ripping gold crowns from the massive number of cadavers they received for cremation.[89]

Bodies do *not* have to be embalmed before they are cremated. However, funeral directors may pressure families to embalm the body prior to cremation. The Cremation Association of North America (CANA) states that "the factors of time, health, possible legal regulations and religious beliefs might make embalming prior to cremation either appropriate or necessary."[90] This is an exaggeration. Embalming a body prior to cremation primarily procures business and fees for the funeral director. Unless there is to be an open-casket funeral or viewing prior to cremation, or if the law requires embalming to transport a body across state or international lines prior to cremation (which is *not* always the case), embalming is just an expensive desecration of the body. Yet the Federal Trade Commission (FTC) found that funeral directors told 23% of people selecting cremation funerals that embalming was required by law if the body was not cremated quickly. (Actually, people usually have 24 hours to bury, cremate, embalm, or refrigerate a body; any of these are acceptable.) Another 4% of respondents were told that embalming was required by their funeral home and 4% were told that it was *always* required by law.[91]

Refrigeration is a more suitable method of preserving a body prior to cremation than embalming and, if necessary, can be used for months. This is the method used by Telophase, a direct cremation business based in southern California.

Only bodies with the proper documents can be cremated. Most states require that a licensed funeral director be involved in a cremation, supposedly to prevent public health problems or the misuse of a crematorium by criminals. These funeral directors or the crematory directors require the family or other party responsible for the body to sign an "authority to cremate" document. This is a service contract and normally names the deceased as well as the survivor ordering the cremation. It also lists the funeral home's or crematory's policies on holding the body prior to cremation, the disposition of cremated remains, the disposal of noncrematable items, and any other procedures. In general, directors also require a death certificate, cremation permit (certificate of disposition of remains), and permission from the next-of-kin. If the body is transported by someone other than a funeral home employee, a permit for this is also usually required.

Finally, most crematories will only cremate bodies that are in good financial standing. A crematory may be unwilling to cremate a body unless the bill is prepaid. In one recent case, the Evans Mortuary in Richmond, Texas, refused to cremate George Bojarski's body because his son could not pay the entire bill in advance. Having already picked up the corpse, the funeral home deposited Mr. Bojarski's body at his son's front door. "His head was right in the entrance of the doorway," his son said. "I was in shock." Another funeral home later cremated the body without charge and a grand jury indicted Newell Evans for "abuse of a corpse."[92,93]

## I. IS A CASKET OR COFFIN REQUIRED FOR CREMATION?

No. A body need not be in either a casket or a coffin to be cremated in the United States or Canada. However, all crematoria require the body be in a strength-tested container made of combustible material, and individual crematoria can require more than this.

The U.S. Federal Trade Commission's (FTC) Funeral Rule requires that funeral directors who offer direct cremations: (1) must not say that state or local law requires a casket for direct cremation; (2) must disclose, in writing, the right to buy an unfinished wood box (a type of casket) or an alternative container for direct cremation; (3) must provide in writing a description of the available alternative containers, and (4) must provide an unfinished wood box or alternative container.[94] (see Appendix G)

A non-standard box used for cremations is officially an "alternative container," according to the FTC. The funeral industry uses the term "alternative container" pejoratively in an attempt to sell higher-priced, but unneeded, merchandise. Their attitude was well summed up by Michael Kubasak, a Southern California funeral director (author of *Cremation and the Funeral Director*), when he said, "Of the 332,000 cremations performed in 1988, approximately 250,000 of these cremations were performed without the deceased being in *a decent container*. The potential for improving this situation is significant. Seventy-five percent of any market is worth pursuing."[95] It is not surprising, therefore, that the FTC found that 7% of individuals involved in funerals using cremation were told that caskets were required. Another 11% were told that an unfinished box (essentially a coffin) was required. Only one-half of them were told that a casket was *not* required. Of this group, 38% never did use a container, 11 percent used caskets, 11% used unfinished wood boxes, and 27% used some other type of container (usually the standard cardboard container furnished by funeral homes and crematories).[96]

CANA's official position is that "the body is cremated in the same enclosure in which it arrives at the crematory."[97] Many crematories use an uncovered cremation "tray" with sides about four- to six-inches high, for bodies arriving without a container. Most crematories, therefore, require that a body be in some type of covered box. If a cardboard box is used to transport the body, a sheet of wood under the body ensures the box's rigidity.

Rare among crematory operators, the Neptune Society of Northern California requires human remains for cremation to be wrapped in a muslin shroud and plastic liner. Only on specific request will they cremate bodies in caskets or alternative containers, and they never cremate a body in a metal casket.[98]

When a family desires a viewing or funeral service before cremation, many funeral homes will supply a rental casket for that purpose. They can then use an inexpensive container for the actual cremation. Some funeral homes, however, don't find this profitable and refuse to offer caskets as anything other than one-time-use items.[99]

Some other countries also have been eliminating a casket requirement for cremations. For example, since 1991, caskets or coffins are no longer required for cremation in the Netherlands. However, caskets are still required for any other type of body disposal.[100]

## J. CAN ANY CASKET OR COFFIN BE CREMATED?

No. A casket or rigid container used for cremation must be combustible and must fit into the oven.

The container, according the CANA, must also "be strong enough to assure protection of the health and safety of the operator" and must "meet reasonable standards of respect and dignity."[101] Cardboard boxes supplied by most funeral homes suffice. Wooden caskets also work well, although they may increase the size of the urn needed, since their ashes will also be inurned. Most casket manufacturers now mark appropriate caskets as "suitable for cremation."

It is dangerous, however, to cremate fiberglass or plastic caskets, or plastic-reinforced wooden caskets. These substances release toxic gasses that can coat the crematory retort and explode. Polystyrene caskets are not completely reduced to ashes.

The Federation of British Cremation Authorities requires that any coffin for cremations be less than 7-feet long, 28-inches wide and 22-inches high. The coffins can only contain enough metal to ensure safe construction, and this metal must have a high iron content. The lining of these coffins may not contain excessive sawdust or cotton-wool, and no metal, rubber or pitch can be used as a sealant.[102]

CANA opposes the use of non-rigid containers, such as body bags (plastic or canvas). They claim this opposition stems from health and safety reasons, although public service agencies, including the military, routinely handle bodies in body bags over long periods of time and distances with no adverse results. Some funeral directors object that it is difficult to get bagged bodies into a crematory retort. Yet some crematories have had no difficulty maneuvering bodies wrapped only in a sheet. They employ a technique similar to that used for pizza ovens—simply sliding the body off a board with a jerking motion. (Unlike pizza oven operators, though, they don't have to retrieve much in the way of finished product.)

Some crematoria even accept metal caskets. They say that since the metal (except some very lightweight metals) will not be consumed by the flames, it is easier to collect the cremated remains without getting them intermixed with residue from the container. If metal caskets are used, their tops must be opened or removed during cremation, and the crematory may charge extra for disposing of the burned casket. Many crematories object to using metal caskets because they tend to scratch and gouge the walls of the retort.

Some cremation containers are quite unusual. Gypsies once burned the bodies of their kings and queens, along with all of their possessions, in their own wagons. On the island of Bali, corpses are burned in coffins carved into the shape of animals. The animals designate the social status of the dead person: half-elephants and half-fish for ordinary people, deer for soldiers, cows for noblewomen, bulls for noblemen, and winged lions for kings or very holy priests.[103]

## K. WHAT AND WHERE ARE CREMATORIES?

Crematories contain the ovens or retorts in which cremations occur. Some crematories not only cremate bodies, but also cremate some medical wastes, including hazardous, contaminated and infectious items. If this service is offered, regulations may limit where the crematory can be built.

Most crematories are owned by and located in cemeteries, although some cemeteries do not want crematories on their grounds, since they generate increased traffic and require refrigeration facilities and a special staff. Some funeral homes have crematories, although many are also reluctant to install crematories on their premises because of the 750 to 1,500 square feet of space needed for the oven, family viewing area, and staff operating areas. In addition, the process generates heat and noise, and the smokestack may not be a welcome addition to the funeral home's neighborhood. The ideal site for a crematory would be in an industrial park—but few families would view that location amiably. Most, therefore, are located near funeral homes or cemeteries. A few crematory-columbaria are separate operations.

Crematories usually have chapels for funeral services. Similar to the standard chapel in a funeral home, it differs only in that there is a hole in the wall through which the body can pass to the "committal chamber" (anteroom to the crematorium). In some crematory chapels the body may be rolled or lowered into the committal chamber. The committal chamber is normally decorated like the chapel, since family members or executors may wish or be required to watch as the coffin is placed in the furnace. Crematoria also usually contain a *columbarium* within which urns with ashes can be interred. They may also have a *Garden of Rest, Garden of Remembrance* or *Memorial Garden*, where ashes can be strewn or interred, memorials can be placed, or visitors can meditate undisturbed.

By 1990, the United States had approximately 1,000 crematories and Canada had 113. More than 38% of U.S. crematories are in the Pacific states. CANA estimates that by the year 2000, the United States may have as many as 1,800 crematories and Canada 217. However, the high cost of complying with the new OSHA regulations and the federal Clean Air Act may result in fewer crematories being built.[104]

## L. WHAT ARE COLUMBARIA?

In Western society, cremated remains are commonly placed in a columbarium, which may be an entire building, a room, a wall, or a column with a series of niches for urns. Other societies have placed urns in graves (Assyria and elsewhere), in large jugs on supports (Etruscans), in catacombs (parts of Italy, Greece and Rome), in cells beneath special hills called *mogotes* (Zapotecs of Mexico and Mosquitos of Nicaragua), or on home altars (modern Buddhist countries).[105]

In modern columbaria, the niches (recessed compartments) may have an open front protected by clear, stained, tinted, frosted or etched glass or have a front closed with a bronze, marble, or granite facing. For niches with glass faces, inscriptions are usually on the urns and the columbarium managers may have restrictions on the types of urns used. For niches with opaque facings, the inscription is on the niche covering. Depending on their location, niches can cost as much as burial plots do. While the cost of the niche usually includes "perpetual care," some columbaria may charge for upkeep separately. Some crematories also provide inexpensive permanent storage for urns in large vaults.[106] Columbaria exist at nearly all crematoria and in many cemeteries. Ashes can also be kept at home (a practice that may connote necrolatry).

An early modern columbarium, built in France by Formigé, was opened in 1887. The building, containing 25,000 niches, has two underground stories and two stories opening onto the garden; 15,000 of the niches are occupied. The ashes of Isadora Duncan, among others, reside here.[107]

At the end of the nineteenth century, Americans built San Francisco's historic Neptune Society Columbarium. Well designed by British architect Bernard J.S. Cahill (it withstood both the 1906 and 1989 earthquakes), it was built in 1898 amidst multiple cemeteries and within one block of a crematorium. When the cemeteries were moved in the mid-1930s, the columbarium survived only because it had been declared a memorial and claimed under the Homestead Act. But the building was left to decay until 1979. By that time it leaked badly, had mushrooms and other flora growing in the walls and niches, had gaping holes everywhere, and its grounds were overgrown. In 1981 the Neptune Society of Northern California renovated the columbarium, the largest one on the West Coast—and the only such building in San Francisco. The building now stands on a three-acre parcel in San Francisco's Richmond District, the last remnant of a cemetery founded by the Independent Order of Odd Fellows in 1865.

The building has been beautifully restored to its previous elegance, including $3 million stained-glass Lefarge windows, although a few niches have been left in disrepair to show visitors how they looked. The columbarium is studded with personalized niches decorated with teddy bears, tree stumps, stagecoach chests, milk jugs, and antique tobacco jar urns. The columbarium offers guided tours (every Saturday; otherwise open to the public daily, 9 a.m. to 1 p.m.) that often draw huge crowds, as do their candlelight masses, chamber music concerts, plays, ballets, exhibitions and memorials. Recently, a couple even had their wedding there, a quartet recorded an album, and one voting precinct used it as their polling place in the November 1992 election. The price for permanent housing here is high: $1,800 for a top-floor "community" niche; $7,000-$12,000 for a lower floor; and $60,000 for an elite semicircular window niche.[108,109]

One of the world's most famous columbaria (although it has had more notable uses) is Moscow's Kremlin Wall. Leonid Borisovich Krassin's ashes were the first to be placed in the wall after he died in 1926 while serving as Soviet envoy to England. As was said at the time, "The ashes and memorial tablets of our leaders will redeem the wall of the fortress built to protect tyrants."[110]

Recently an enormous columbarium opened in the Hong Kong hills, containing, within its 200,000 square feet, 28 memorial halls, a five-tiered pagoda, three giant Buddhas, a Chinese garden with a turtle pond, and a Swiss-made cable car. The columbarium can hold 43,000 remains. Prices for a one-cubic-foot niche range between $1,300 and $12,000. This helps to reimburse the owner who has had expenses of his own, including having to pay "direct charity" to neighbors to alleviate their fear of ghosts.[111]

A columbarium opened for military personnel and dependents in 1980 at the Arlington National Cemetery. Originally built with 5,000 niches, it will eventually expand to 50,000 niches. Each niche is sealed with a marble plaque inscribed with the name, highest military grade, and years of birth and death of the inurned. As with the niche itself, there is no cost to the family for the plaque. The cost of cremation, urn and transportation are the family's responsibility. Unlike military burial, requirements for inurnment are quite liberal. Those who qualify include any member of the armed services who died while on active duty, any former member of the armed forces whose last service ended honorably, certain reserve and ROTC members who die on active duty (including training), American members of allied forces whose last service ended honorably, certain commissioned officers of the National Oceanic and Atmospheric Administration or U.S. Public Health Service, and the spouse (or surviving spouse who remains unmarried at time of death) or an unmarried minor or dependent adult child of any eligible person. One niche is normally assigned to each family at

257

the time of death. Verification of eligibility and arrangements for inurnment are handled by the Office of the Superintendent, Arlington National Cemetery, Arlington, VA  22211-5003; (703) 697-3250/3255. Verification normally takes at least two working days. Cremated remains can be brought to the cemetery or shipped to the Superintendent's office via the Postal Service (registered) or commercial carrier. The cemetery staff will arrange for military honors at the inurnment if they are requested by the next-of-kin.[112]

While many columbaria are quite elaborate, people rarely visit urns as they do graves. In general, as Ariès points out, "cremation excludes a pilgrimage."[113] For those cultures in which ancestor worship is important, portable columbaria are now available. Multiple generations of cremains can be stored in these columns, which can be moved when a family changes residences.

## M.  WHAT KIND OF CEREMONY ACCOMPANIES CREMATION?

Relatives can arrange nearly any type of ceremony to accompany a cremation. Obviously, if they want a traditional funeral with the body present, it must occur before the cremation. The ceremony can take place in a funeral home, a church, or at the crematorium. If it is at the crematorium, the funeral often ends with the body passing out of the funeral area directly into the retort's anteroom. Many Christian burial services can proceed as with an inhumation, needing only to change the word "body" to "ashes," as in "commit his *ashes* to the ground, earth to earth, dust to dust."

Alternatively, relatives and friends may hold a memorial service after cremation, when the ashes are inurned in a columbarium niche or when they are scattered or buried.

Not everyone is pleased with the standard modern Western cremation ceremony. One English funeral historian disdainfully notes,

> Few funerals now take place in church. Too often one is asked to meet at the crematorium, and what then ensues is dismal: an unaccompanied funeral car glides noiselessly under the *porte-cochère*, the coffin is transferred to a stainless steel 'hors-d'oerve' trolley and wheeled into the chapel, which looks more like a waiting-room in a university college hospital than a dignified setting for the disposal of the dead. Ten minutes later, to the accompaniment of slurred canned music, the curtains jerk their way noisily round the catafalque as the coffin sinks slowly through the floor...to the furnace below.[114]

## N.  WHAT ARE CREMATION RITUALS IN SOME OTHER COUNTRIES?

Cremation rituals vary across the world because of limited resources, religious customs, and social norms.

In Tibet, partly due to the scarcity of wood, only the most exalted members of the community, such as high Lamas, are cremated. (Dried cow dung, a common material for fires in that region, is not considered either appropriate or adequate for cremations.) Cremations usually occur in closed ovens after which the ashes are mixed with clay and molded into tiny pagodas. Priests then distribute these pagodas in heaps across the countryside. Occasionally, Tibetans use open pyres for cremations, after which they bury any remaining bone fragments.[115]

In Mongolia, cremation has not been commonly used, since it is both time and resource intensive. When it is used, a ring of stones is built surrounding an open pyre. A member of the funeral party who is about the same age as the deceased lights the fire. After cremating the corpse, they usually send the cremains to one of seven holy sites or a temple for safekeeping.[116]

Hindus traditionally use cremation to dispose of corpses. The public cremation of Mrs. Indira Gandhi, the former prime minister of India, gave the world a view of this ceremony. Her uncoffined body was carried to the burning *ghats* where it was cremated. Her ashes were then strewn on the Ganges.

The Hindu cremation ritual begins with a funeral procession led by a man with a fire kindled in the deceased's home, carried in a black earthen pot. Nothing may get between this fire and the corpse. If the procession goes near the Ganges River, the mourners immerse the body in the river before they place it on the funeral pyre. After a priest performs a brief disposal ceremony, the mourners cut the winding sheet and smear the body with *ghi* (clarified butter). The chief mourner, usually a son or grandson, uses the fire in the pot to light a torch. He uses this torch to ignite the pyre, at the foot of a dead woman or at the head of a dead man.

As the flames spread, the mourners march around the pyre without looking into the fire. The priest then intones: "Fire, you were lighted by him, so may he be lighted from you, that he may gain the regions of celestial bliss. May this offering prove auspicious."[117] If the skull fails to spontaneously shatter from the heat, the mourners smash it, since the person's spirit is thought to flee into the skull during cremation, and must be released. At one time, perhaps as much for economic as religious reasons, living widows "voluntarily" accompanied their dead husbands onto the funeral pyre in a now-banned practice termed *Suttee* or *Sati*. Hindus traditionally bury rather than cremate ascetics, lepers, and children under 2 years of age.[118]

The non-Hindu Toda tribe of southern India uses a unique form of cremation. They ritually slaughter a sacred buffalo and place the deceased's body near the buffalo's head. Relatives then cover the corpse in cloth and place the body on a bier next to the funeral pyre, where they lay gifts on the body. They light the 3-foot high pyre by friction for men, or with an already-blazing rag for women. They then swing the body over the flames three times to symbolize destruction of the gifts, so that it becomes appropriate for the living to retrieve these valuables. Before they cremate the body, mourners cut off a lock of hair. A month later, they slaughter another bull and a raise a new pyre. They combine the remains from the first cremation (more than in a modern crematorium) with the lock of hair and other offerings and cremate them. They then ceremoniously bury what remains.[119]

In Thailand, the traditional ceremony for a king's cremation is conducted one year after death, by which time the body has been thoroughly dried out. For the cremation, mourners place the body on a 300-foot-high sandalwood catafalque with the heir to the throne igniting the pyre. They then collect the ashes, mix them with clay, and distribute them as souvenirs to the assembled crowd.[120] A similar and only slightly less lavish ceremony has been traditionally conducted on Bali.[121]

The Japanese, who have the highest rate of cremation among industrialized nations, do not have ostentatious crematoria. Japanese crematories have been described as looking "much like the waterworks of an American town of ten thousand inhabitants."[122] On the day of or the day after the cremation, a family member (usually a woman) goes to the crematory to perform the "honorable bone-gathering." She receives the cremated remains, takes them home, and about a week later either delivers them to the temple or erects a tombstone, and prepares the family cemetery plot for their burial.[123]

## O. CAN MY FAMILY OBSERVE THE CREMATION?

Yes, but don't expect the crematory to be overjoyed about allowing people to witness the cremation. Many retort anterooms are crowded and the crematory may not have an adequate method for observing the actual cremation.

What if you only want to be there to see the body put in the chamber? The cremation industry frowns on this. Speaking of cremation, Kubasak patronizingly said, "Some of the technical aspects...are as complicated as aspects of surgery and involve procedures for which the ordinary layperson has no basis of technical understanding or psychological preparation. It is possible, therefore, that a layperson might misunderstand or misinterpret what is happening and may knowingly or unknowingly transmit inaccurate information to others."[124]

Yet George Bernard Shaw, who witnessed his mother's cremation did not feel that way, saying:

> A door opened in the wall; and the violet coffin mysteriously passed out through it and vanished as it closed. People think that door the door of the furnace; but it isn't. I went behind the scenes at the end of the service and saw the real thing. People are afraid to see it; but it is wonderful. I found there the violet coffin opposite another door, a real unmistakable furnace door. When it lifted there was a plain little chamber of cement and firebrick. No heat. No noise. No roaring draught. No flame. No fuel. It looked cool, clean, sunny, though no sun could get there...Then the violet coffin moved again and went in, feet first. And behold! The feet burst miraculously into streaming ribbons of garnet-colored lovely flame, smokeless and eager, like pentecostal tongues, and as the whole coffin passed in it sprang into flame all over; and my mother became that beautiful fire.[125]

A more practical reason for limiting access to the working areas of the crematory is concern about legal liability. The combination of family members, a very hot oven, heavy equipment, and possibly more than one corpse in a tiny area could conceivably lead to injuries. Some crematories dissuade observers by charging a hefty fee to those family members who wish to observe the procedure.

It is interesting that in Japan, where cremation is the norm, there are large galleries opposite the ovens so that relatives can watch the body being committed to the flames.

## P. WHAT HAPPENS TO THE BODY DURING CREMATION?

Dr. Evans, a physician and anatomist, described a cremation quite graphically in his book, *The Chemistry of Death*:

> The coffin is introduced into the furnace where it rapidly catches fire, bulges and warps, and the coffin sides may collapse and fall, exposing the remains to the direct effect of the flames. The skin and hair at once scorch, char and burn...The muscles slowly contract, and there may be a steady spreading of the thighs with gradually developing flexion of the limbs...Occasionally there is swelling of the abdomen before the skin and abdominal muscles char and split; the swelling is due to the formation of steam and the expansion of gases in the abdominal contents. Destruction of the soft tissues gradually exposes parts of the skeleton. The skull is soon devoid of covering, then the bones of the limbs appear, commencing at the extremities of the limbs where they are relatively poorly covered by muscle or fat, and the ribs also

become exposed. The small bones of the fingers, wrists and ankles remain united by their ligaments for a surprising length of time, maintaining their anatomical relationships even though the hands and feet may fall away from the adjacent long bones. The abdominal contents burn fairly slowly, and the lungs more slowly still...The brain is specially resistant to complete combustion...Eventually the spine becomes visible as the viscera disappear, the bones glow whitely in the flames and the skeleton falls apart.[126]

## Q.  HOW LONG DOES IT TAKE TO CREMATE A BODY?

The first cremation in the LeMoyne crematory required over 48 hours to preheat and cool down the oven and four hours to cremate the body. In the most modern of today's gas-fired crematories, the equipment can cremate a body within one-half hour, requires virtually no preheating, and needs only one hour for cooling between cremations. Most crematories, however, still require 2½ to 3 hours for the entire process. The size of the body, the type of container, and the type of crematory affect the cremation time.

While most modern crematories (termed "pathological incinerators" by the Environmental Protection Agency) use natural gas heat, some still use electricity, propane gas or oil. Modern units have burners located on two sides and below the body. Efficient cremation without smoke production requires an initial temperature of about 1,100°F to 1,300°F, but the chamber temperature may actually rise to over 1,700°F during the cremation process.[127] Some crematoria may register chamber temperatures of from 2,000°F to 2,500°F, especially if a cremation recently took place in that oven.[128] This heat is generated not only from the gas, but also from the burning coffin and body. A 140-pound body in a 90-pound wood coffin generates over 800,000 BTU, so that external heat is ideally needed only at the start and at the end of a cremation.[129] Most retorts, however, do not decrease the temperature to compensate for the additional heat emitted by the burning body and container.

Complete combustion also needs air. Smoke from incomplete combustion in a crematorium can be greatly reduced if an adequate amount of air is added to the burning mixture. Yet obese bodies still emit heavy black smoke and flames when cremated. The exact amount of air required depends on the state of the body, the components of the coffin, and the temperature at which the crematorium is operated. All new crematories are built with afterburners and scrubbers to prevent air pollution. All of these factors affect the cremation time.

## R. WHAT IS LEFT AFTER CREMATION?

Cremated remains, often called cremains, consist principally of boney residua (sixty percent of bone is inorganic [nonburnable] material), since the lighter ash from a wooden casket or cardboard container is largely broken down by the heat. The "ashes" are mostly small, clean white bone fragments. One seventeenth-century observer was startled by how little of the body actually remained after cremation:

> How the bulk of a man should sink
> into so few pounds of bones and ashes,
> may seem strange unto any who considers
> not its constitution, and how slender
> a masse will remain upon an open and urging
> fire of the carnall composition.[130]

The color of the cremated remains, or "cremains," varies. Gray to white coloration represents differences in the exposure of the material to heat. Yellow represents unburnt trabecular bone (bone with an internal latticework).[131] Occasionally, some fragments may be slightly yellowed from zinc in the coffin (rare), green from iron (about 1% of cremations), or pink from copper, perhaps in 'gold' wedding or signet rings, other jewelry, dental fillings, or gold injections for arthritis (15% to 20% of cremations).[132]

When a metal casket has been used, the ashes are removed from it by hand and then by vacuuming, and the casket is discarded.

The Cremation Association of North America says that adult cremains weigh between three and nine pounds. Others have found they average 7.4 pounds (men) and 5.8 pounds (women).[133]

Some crematoria deliver the residua as is, while others first grind up the bone fragments. In England, cremains are routinely pulverized, but in the United States the practice is less common unless the "ashes" are to be scattered. To process the cremains, crematory operators once had to pass them through a hand-operated laboratory grinder. Most modern crematoria now use electric processors to quickly pulverize residual bone fragments to the size of sugar crystals. Some processor manufacturers guarantee that all cremated remains passing through their machines will fit into a 167-cubic-inch capacity container; the normal minimum urn size is 175-cubic inches. A very small portion of the cremains may be irretrievably lost in this pulverization process.[134]

The Neptune Society of Northern California clearly describes what the potential customer should expect:

> When the cremated remains are removed from the cremation chamber, they often contain recognizable bone fragments. For this reason, all cremated remains will be mechanically processed

263

(pulverized) so as to make them unrecognizable as bone fragments in accordance with the requirements of California law. This process may cause inadvertent or incidental commingling from the residue of previous cremations. These granulated particles will be virtually unrecognizable as human remains."[135]

*Mortuary Management* recently warned funeral directors and crematory operators that they can expect legal problems from discussing "the pulverization and sifting of bone to produce the so-called ashes the survivors expect to be given."[136] However, CANA advises them to disclose this process to relatives.[137]

## S. ARE THESE REALLY MY ASHES?

In most cases, yes. Most funeral homes and crematories follow a protocol that enables them to correctly and continuously identify a body from the time they receive it until the remains are released to the family. Crematories use either a stainless-steel tag on the body or a plastic tag on the cremation chamber that stays with the cremains.

Usually, only one body at a time is placed in each oven. CANA's "Model Cremation Law" specifies that the "simultaneous cremation of the human remains of more than one person within the same cremation chamber is forbidden, unless the Crematory Authority shall have received specific written authorization to do so from all Authorizing Agents [relatives] for the human remains." It goes on to say that "upon completion of the cremation, and insofar as is possible, all of the recoverable residue of the cremation process shall be removed from the cremation chamber."[138] So much for the ideal. As Walter Birkby, a noted forensic anthropologist said, "Inappropriate handling of cremains has produced a corresponding increase in civil litigation."[139]

Examples of such litigation abound. The Harbor Lawn-Mount Olive Mortuary and Memorial Park in Costa Mesa, California, paid $14 million to settle a suit by 25,000 people who claimed their relatives' bodies were cremated en masse, rather than separately.[140] Another southern California firm, the Pasadena Crematorium, which was luridly described in the book, *A Family Business*, routinely packed nine to fifteen bodies into each oven, which was about the size of the interior of a typical American sedan. After pulverizing all remaining bone fragments with two shot-puts and a small cement mixer, they dumped the ashes into large containers. Operators often added white powder to make the mixture attractive to relatives before they dole them out by weight—three-and-a-half pounds for a woman and five to seven pounds for a man.[141]

In 1992, a widow sued The Neptune Society of Los Angeles for giving her cremains that were labeled as being those of her husband, but weren't.

The Society finally found Dallas William's body four months later in a mortuary refrigerator. No one knows whose ashes she originally received.

Other California crematoria have been known to have routinely performed "multiple cremations," in which two or more bodies were cremated at once to increase cost efficiency. One settlement of more than $15 million involved a California funeral home that was alleged to have "mishandled, mutilated, commingled, multiply cremated, and otherwise disrespectfully, improperly, and illegally cremated the remains of the decedents entrusted to them" during a seven-year period.[142]

In 1989, California Judge Sheldon Grossfield announced a partial settlement of $27 million for the 5,000 families duped by a professional cremains scatterer who was unceremoniously piling the ashes on his farm rather than scattering them from the air as promised.[143] Several officials who were responsible for overseeing the California funeral industry resigned when the state failed to pursue these breaches of industry standards.

In another incident, a Connecticut family was understandably distressed when their their loved one's cremains sailed into Long Island Sound, still in the original box. The cremains had not been scattered (the identification was still inside), and no holes had been punched in the box so it would sink.[144]

In Florida, a large and growing number of funeral directors have been sued by families over the improper handling of cremated remains. As the *National Law Journal* recently said, "Cremation litigation is lurid and often lucrative."[145]

In another Florida case, a Mr. Smith made arrangements for cremation with Telophase, a cremation society, stipulating that his ashes not be scattered at sea. When his widow went to collect his ashes, she was given an unlabeled container. While she was scattering the ashes at sites they had previously selected, she was surprised to find dentures among the cremains—her husband did not wear dentures! Telophase admitted that they had given Mrs. Smith the wrong ashes and that Mr. Smith's ashes had been scattered from an airplane *at sea*. The Florida Appellate Court gave Mrs. Smith $250,000 in compensatory damages and $250,000 in punitive damages (reduced from the original award of $1.2 million).[146]

This litigious trend appears to be increasing. The American Association of Retired Persons reports that one crematory was cited for salvaging jewelry and dental gold from some bodies and selling it without authorization.[147] Ron Brown, owner of Arizona Cremation and Burial, and Brown's Colonial Mortuary in Phoenix, Arizona, was accused of mixing cremated human and animal remains. In some cases where families wanted rapid cremation services, he gave them animal ashes rather than those of their loved ones. He was also said to have dumped ashes in vacant lots or irrigation canals rather than scattering them in the desert as promised. He settled his two-year court battle by agreeing to temporarily surrender his funeral director's license, sell his crematory, never operate a crematory again, and pay a $25,000 fine. The Arizona Board of Funeral Directors and Embalmers suspended his license in 1991.[148]

Forensic anthropologists now analyze cremated remains to discern the identity of cremated individuals. In one case, a family was given their mother's cremains, and three years later received another set of cremains purported to be their mother's. The latter cremains had somehow made their way to a local school system's warehouse. Which was their mother's cremains? One, both or neither? Forensic scientists used variations in the weight, material, and color of the cremains to make their determination. Bits of metal indicated the person in one box had worn a pacemaker (only the wires were cremated), and that the person in the other box had a dental bridge. The family, believing the second box contained their mother's cremains, returned the first container to the crematory—and filed suit. It was settled out of court.[149]

Russell Troutman, a lawyer who writes for the cremation industry, suggests five ways cremation liability can be reduced:

1. *Proper identification* of the body and cremated remains. He suggests that a family member or responsible party be required to identify the body up to the point where it enters the retort, while recognizing that there are problems associated with having a non-employee in the cremation area. Written procedures, conforming to state laws, should detail ways to avoid co-mingling remains and deal with improper actions by a referring funeral home.
2. Disposal of *non-crematable objects* such as jewelry, pacemakers and orthopedic devices in a uniform manner with family approval. He cites one case where an employee returned cremains to the family with a metal bar from prior bone surgery sticking out of the urn. Uniform procedures would avoid this.
3. Agreement as to proper *disposition of the cremains*. One crematorium kept a woman's ashes on a shelf for seven years while her widower made pilgrimages to put flowers on the grave where he thought the ashes were buried. In that case the funeral home got off cheaply by supplying him with a free funeral when he died. It is vital to know who has a right to the remains and what will be done if they are not received by the rightful party.
4. Clearly understood plans for the *routing of remains* to the proper party. There have been many cases where the cremains were sent to the wrong person or the wrong address.
5. And, perhaps most importantly, *proper authorization for the cremation*. The person authorizing the cremation must give

266

informed consent to all of the procedures, including "processing" or "pulverization" of the bone fragments.

What Mr. Troutman does not say is whether this same type of detailed consent should be given for those choosing embalming and burial.[150]

## T. WHAT IS TYPICALLY DONE WITH THE ASHES?

Cremated remains are usually scattered, or placed in urns (inurned) which are then kept in columbaria, at home, or are buried. Unlike a corpse, the ashes of a cremated body, the "cremains," will remain stable without care indefinitely, and can be disposed of in many ways. Ernest Morgan, a spokesman for the memorial society movement, said, "Modern cremation is a clean, orderly process for returning human remains to the elements...The ashes are clean and white and may be stored indefinitely or mailed by registered mail and some express services for distant interment."[151]

Not all disposal methods are legal in all jurisdictions, but it is unclear why, since cremains pose no public health threat. It is impossible, however, to stop anyone who wants to dispose of ashes nearly anywhere. In fact, cremation itself is considered the final disposition of a corpse in the United States, meaning that the cremains need neither be buried nor entombed. This returns control over a loved one's disposition to the family.

At least fifty percent of all cremains in the United States are not placed in columbaria, mausoleums or graves. Many people mail cremains elsewhere for scattering or safekeeping. CANA recommends that cremains *not* be mailed in the reinforced cardboard boxes in which families sometimes receive them. They recommend instead that people use triple-layered packing when shipping cremains by U.S. mail or other transport companies.[152] In response to a letter in Ann Lander's column, one postal worker in a town with a National Veterans Cemetery wrote, "we see a lot of those cardboard boxes come in for burial at the cemetery. Most of the boxes are not very sturdy, nor are they well sealed. It is not uncommon for us to handle several boxes a week that were so poorly wrapped they were almost empty." When one such box arrived nearly empty, a supervisor said that he would "just go home and clean out the fireplace" to refill the box.[153]

Note that UPS and Federal Express will not carry cremated remains. This is not due to any squeamishness on their part, but merely from a policy of not transporting anything they cannot replace if it gets lost or damaged.[154,155]

Many people carry ashes on airplanes to the site where they will inter or scatter them. Anyone thinking of travelling by air with cremated remains should know, however, that they can be immediately identified under the X-ray machine. How? Cremains look like sand under the radiographic "eye." When security agents spot cremains, what happens depends on the person at the machine. Many will merely let them pass, since carrying cremains on board is perfectly legal—the cremation was the legal disposal of the body.

## U. MAY I BURY THE ASHES?

Yes. Ashes may be buried on private property or in a cemetery. Also, nothing prevents people from burying cremains on their own property.

Many cemeteries and memorial parks provide outdoor areas, generically labeled "urn gardens," for interment of cremated remains. These plots generally, but not always, cost less than gravesites. It may cost even less in the cemeteries that permit the cremated remains of more than one person to be interred in a single adult space. They charge an opening and closing fee to bury each urn, however.

Some cemeteries require buried urns to be placed within larger boxes, called urn vaults. Since urns don't decompose and cremains pose no conceivable public health risk, the only reason for this requirement appears to be to generate more income. One interesting phenomenon demonstrating the funeral industry's ability to keep up with changing fads, is that they now offer urn vaults that can expand to fit the larger, more elaborate urns some people are buying.

Some crematories with their own cemeteries refuse to bury ashes for six months after cremation, in case the relatives change their minds and want the ashes back—which sometimes happens.[156]

## V. WHERE MAY THE ASHES BE SCATTERED?

Ashes are usually scattered into lakes and streams, in favorite parks, on mountaintops, or at sea (sometimes out of an airplane).

As early as 1887, at the dawn of modern cremation, a man who died in Pittsburgh, Pennsylvania, had his ashes scattered in the middle of the Atlantic Ocean, by the steamship *Elbe's* captain. For this ceremony, the captain required "all passengers to dress in nautical costume and to stand at attention."[157] Some professional scatterers take along survivors or clergy, some take pictures of where the ashes were strewn, and some send information back to the family about the conditions during the scattering (such as altitude, wind velocity, and geographic location).

The publisher of the *Advance News* in Ogdensburg, New York, died on April 20, 1975, after arranging for his paper to publish these instructions to his attorney:

> ...I would like to have my remains cremated, one half buried with Janet in the Ogdensburg cemetery and the other sent to Colorado. I want half of my ashes scattered from an airplane over the Sangre de Christo Range in the West Mountain Valley of Colorado just at sunset when the setting sun has turned that

magnificent blood-red which the Spanish explorers described as "Sangre de Christo" or "Blood of Christ." The section where I would like to have my ashes scattered is at the peaks back of the Canda Ranch, where I spent several very happy summers when I was a boy.[158]

Until recently, California (as well as Alaska, Indiana and Washington) had a law prohibiting private scattering. Authorities, however, were never keen about enforcing these misdemeanor laws. California repealed its law only with great public effort and despite massive lobbying by the funeral profession. According to CANA, only two states continue to restrict scattering of cremated remains. California now restricts scattering ashes on some land areas and Washington limits the size of the bone fragments that can be scattered. California, however, has also recently restricted some professional scattering after relatives sued an air delivery service, saying they spread the cremains over a vacant lot rather than dispersing them over public areas as they had requested.

When scattering cremains by air, it is recommended that they first be reduced (pulverized) to no more than a one-eighth-inch diameter. Larger pieces could give the funeral industry another customer if they hit someone. One pilot who scatters cremated remains from the air noted, "It crosses everybody's mind that it might be nice to, well, float around...Not all the ashes fall to the ground, you know. There are tiny particles that maybe fly forever."[159]

Funeral homes and professional scatterers will scatter ashes at sea in many seaboard states. In California, many cremation companies, including the Neptune and Telophase Societies, will not only perform the cremation, but also dispose of the ashes at sea. The professional scatterers say they conform with regulations and complete all necessary paperwork for the Environmental Protection Agency. The U.S. Navy and U.S. Coast Guard will also perform this service (if a ship and personnel are available) for eligible retirees and dependents. Occasionally these sea scatterings become real parties.

One San Francisco bar owner, learning that he had cancer, planned a yacht-cruise party featuring a jazz band and a blues group for the Saturday after he died. During the cruise, his friends were to scatter his ashes. He handed out invitations to about 100 friends, saying "I'm having a party. I just don't have a date on it yet." Another man has planned a breakfast cruise for his friends during which they will scatter his ashes. His wife, however, plans to have her ashes scattered from a hot air balloon. "She's always wanted to take one of those balloon trips, but she's afraid of heights."[160]

"Scattered" may not be an agreeable word to everyone. The British Anglican Church states that ashes should be "strewn," which seems, to them, more civilized.[161] In Britain, families are rarely present during the

269

scattering, although the crematory keeps a record of where ashes were strewn so families can visit.[162] In France, dispersal of cremains is illegal.[163]

The funeral and cremation industries, as represented by CANA, are frantic over losing income due to the personal disposal of ashes. Some of their members have gone so far as to develop their own "cemetery gardens," also called "scattering gardens," where ashes can be scattered without being disturbed. Typically, the cremains are placed in a three-foot hole and covered. They generously point out that "often the individuals whose cremated remains have been scattered in the garden are identified on a special memorial plaque, marker or artwork in the garden, or memorialized in a Book of Memories or Remembrance displayed in a building on the cemetery grounds."[164]

## W. WHAT ARE URNS AND CREMATION MEMORIALS?

People often store cremains in small jars called urns and purchase memorials to commemorate the deceased. The Cremation Association of North America (CANA) puts out a brochure ironically titled, "Cremation is not the end...". The funeral industry uses this booklet to sell urns, niches and other "memorialization" commodities. Crematories usually deliver ashes to relatives in a "temporary container"—a box made of cardboard, plastic film or other material. These containers normally cost between $15 and $20. These boxes, securely sealed and identified with the deceased person's name, can be used for shipping, although they normally are first placed within a more secure and rigid container. If relatives have not purchased an urn before cremation, or if the crematory receives no other instructions, they will deliver the cremains in the cardboard box, much to the chagrin of the uninitiated.

The typical urn has a capacity of 175- to 300-cubic inches, large enough for most adult remains. According to Robert Inman, past president of CANA, a normal adult's cremated remains will fit, "if properly processed," into a 200-cubic inch container, and only rarely, as in the case of a professional basketball player, will a 300-cubic inch container be needed.[165]

In ancient times, urns of different cultures or for different social classes were made of, among other things, terra-cotta, stone, crystalline rock (porphyry), alabaster, bronze, silver, gold, or ceramic ware.[166] The simple horizontal rectangular urn used today is often made of metal, porcelain, or wood, and is typically 6 5/8-inches high, 8¼-inches wide, and nearly 4-inches deep.[167] Urns can cost less than $100 or many thousands of dollars, depending on the type. A columbarium in Hartsdale, New York, has a set of priceless Ming vases and a Wedgwood urn behind their glass front, and San Francisco's Neptune Society Columbarium has cremains inurned in, among other things, a milk pitcher, a tobacco humidor, an ice bucket and a sailing trophy.[168-170]

"Boutique" urns are also available. As cremation has become more common, urns have become fancier. Many crematoria now stock decorated and elaborately designed marble, bronze, glass, pewter and plastic urns; some urns come with matching picture frames, presumably to hold portraits of the deceased. San Francisco's Ghia Gallery, a death boutique, sells wearable urn jewelry so relatives can wear their loved one's ashes. Spouses sometimes purchase these mementos and they have become fashionable among San Francisco's gay community.[171] The Gallery also sells the "Living Urn," a terrarium containing a niche for a bag of cremains.[172] When using a commercial columbarium's niche, relatives must consider whether a custom urn's size and shape will fit it.

In Britain, families often commemorate the deceased with a plaque at the base of a rose bush. Cemeteries charge families about £100 to rent the bush and plaque for 10 years; the rental can be renewed at the end of that time. Another way they commemorate the deceased is to buy a plaque or curbstone in the cemetery, for about £40, with the person's name engraved on it. The space for these memorials is also rented for ten years; if the rental is not renewed at the end of this time, the name is sandblasted off and it is readied for a new inscription. Finally, as in the United States, families can buy engraved memorials in a "book of remembrance." The person is listed on the page corresponding to the date of death. On the anniversary of the death, the book is opened to the appropriate page.[173]

## X. WHAT UNUSUAL DISPOSITIONS HAVE BEEN USED FOR CREMAINS?

Cremains are not always disposed of in a "normal" manner. In ancient times, Asychis, a king of Egypt, held the urns containing the ashes of his subjects' ancestors hostage to compel them to pay their taxes.[174] An interesting, albeit somewhat macabre tale is that of Artemesia, wife of Mausolus, king of Caria, who, to assuage her grief at his loss, drank some of his ashes mingled with wine.[175]

More recently, police suspect some Florida cocaine addicts may have been accidentally inhaling cremains. When thieves burgled a Boynton Beach, Florida man's home, they took only the grayish-white powder he kept in a cardboard box. While the powder looked similar to cocaine, it was actually the cremated remains of his sister, Gertrude.[176]

Occasionally, keeping ashes has become an obsession. One man preceded his wife to "the grave" by 15 years. She had his body cremated. Rather than securing his ashes in one location or scattering them in a favorite place, she carried his urn with her wherever she went—for 15 years! In a bid for even more permanence, a famous artist, rather than interring or scattering his cremains, had his ashes mixed with oil paints and had his portrait painted from a picture for his family to keep.[177]

In a twist on the typical scattering of ashes, a landscaper in Des Moines, Iowa, loads hunters' cremains into shotgun shells and fires them in an area where the deceased loved to hunt. He also performs whatever memorial service the family requests.[178] Some people ask their friends to do this service for them, as did Chuck Roberts of Lawsonville, North Carolina, whose pals loaded up their shotguns with shells filled with his cremains and fired them in a volley. Said one friend, "He had odd ideas at times and he loved a good joke."[179] Yet they probably are unaware that many years before they thought of it, British architect Sir Clough Williams Ellis had his cremated remains scattered over his village by means of a number of specially packed fireworks.[180]

In Northern California, a former forest ranger who was also part Native American had relatives put his cremated remains into a large boulder. Then they used a helicopter to drop it near a favorite backcountry site. The boulder, with directions for hikers painted on it, sits near an intersection of hiking trails, so he could "still do his job, even after death." Hikers affectionately call the rock the Grandfather Stone.[181]

One example of fanciful cremains disposition was that of New York's James M. O'Kelley who, in 1901, invented an egg-like "Navohi" that was supposed to use the gasses given off by the body during cremation to fuel the cremains *into space*. Recently, an actual proposal by a Florida group "to launch cremated cremains into space never got off the ground."[182]

Deviating from all civilized norms and typical of their barbarity, Nazi death camp officials had the ashes of those cremated in their ovens turned into fertilizer and soap, and spread over the roads in wintertime. All other cultures have shown more respect for cremains.

In some cultures, keeping the ashes of dead ancestors at one location serves as a valued family memorial. But when families move, even around the world, they often take the ashes of their ancestors with them. In some Eastern cultures, scattering an ancestor's ashes is the height of sacrilege. In the Netherlands, a 1991 law for the first time permitted cremains to be kept in the home. This law, in development since 1971, was in response to a growing number of Hindus living in Holland.[183] In Japan where the ashes of ancestors are worshipped, a widow will use chopsticks to pick any remaining bones out of the cremains after her husband's cremation. She stores them in a jar. The practice is called *kokubetsu shiki*, translated as "the fine old custom."[184]

## Y. ARE THERE PROBLEMS WITH CREMATION IN FOREIGN COUNTRIES?

The "problems" with cremation in foreign countries come in two forms: either cremation will be mandatory unless the body is shipped out of the country, or more commonly, cremation may be very difficult to accomplish. As mentioned previously, cremation is virtually mandatory in England and Japan because they have no room for new cemeteries. In most countries, however, cremation can be hindered by social, bureaucratic, or logistical barriers.

Local laws and religious restrictions may make cremation difficult or impossible in many predominantly Catholic or Moslem countries. Not only these countries, but also more secular nations have bureaucratic rules requiring that a person, during life, must have documented a wish for cremation. The U.S. National Funeral Director's Association (NFDA) recommends that if a person desires cremation, a statement should be carried with the passport reading, "I direct that upon my death, whenever it may occur, that my body be cremated (if such a facility is available and permitted by law of the country) and the cremated remains (indicate disposition—burial or return to the United States)."[185] A more inclusive approach may be simply to carry advance directive documents (living will, durable power of attorney for health care) that include this information.

In many countries, the lack of crematoria increases the cost and difficulty of obtaining cremation services, since the body may have to be transported a long distance to the crematorium. Further complicating the procedure, in some countries the nearest crematorium may be across an international boundary. Costs quoted by foreign crematoria will normally include the funeral service, cremation fee, documentation, an urn, and a casket, when used. Urns in foreign countries will generally be metal boxes, sealed glass jars, or metal-lined wooden boxes, plastic or ceramic containers.

## Z. WHAT DO RELIGIONS SAY ABOUT CREMATION?

Religions vary widely in their acceptance of cremation. While some require it, others ban it completely (Table 6.4).

Cremation is an integral part of Buddhist and Hindu religious practice. Exactly why Hindus adopted cremation is uncertain. Theories range from the religious (cremation is a gesture of purification and a means of releasing the soul from a corrupted body) to the philosophical (it is a symbol of the transitory nature of any particular life and a means to achieve total anonymity in death) to the social (it reduces the public health risk from a corpse and doesn't clutter up an already-crowded country). The ancient Hindu *Rig-Veda* includes a funeral hymn beseeching the fire god to offer safe conduct to the deceased and the Hindu *Grihya-Sutras* says, "On this day I shall go to my father and fulfill the sacrament of the cremation."[186]

Other religions support, or at least tolerate, cremation. Many mainstream Protestant denominations, including the Episcopal church, support cremation. This follows the Church of England's position which actively supports cremation and officially approved the scattering of ashes in 1944. The Church reasoned as did Lord Shaftesbury, who perceptively asked if the Church banned cremation, "What would in such a case become of the Blessed Martyrs?"[187] The Unitarian/Universalist church strongly supports cremation, while Reform Judaism supports a person's expressed wish to be cremated. Christian Scientists take no position.

Many religious prohibitions to cremation exist. Orthodox Jewish tradition, supported by biblical precedent and Talmudic teachings, forbids cremation and generally refuses to allow burial of cremated remains in a Jewish cemetery. This stems in part from the Old Testament, where cremation was used to dispose of the bodies of executed criminals and for public health reasons, such as to dispose of large numbers of bodies after battles or catastrophes. Biblical Jews considered other uses of cremation a form of idolatry.[188] So strict is the ban that the family of a cremated individual is now absolved from mourning. Conservative Jews are not as staunchly opposed to cremation, but generally follow this prohibition, based as much on the experience of the Holocaust as from religious dicta. Conservative Rabbis, however, may officiate at funeral services even if they know that the body will later be cremated. Conservatives also permit cremains to be buried in their cemeteries.

## TABLE 6.4: Religious Attitude Toward Cremation

| REQUIRE | DISAPPROVE | ALLOW |
|---------|------------|-------|
| Buddhism | Armenian Orthodox | Christian Spiritualists |
| Hinduism | Mormons | Church of England |
| | Plymouth Brethren | Churches of Christ |
| | Roman Catholic | Congregational Church |
| | Russian Orthodox | Episcopal Church |
| | | Jehovah's Witness |
| | | Judaism (Reform) |
| | | Methodist |
| DISALLOW | | Moravian |
| Baptist Society | | Seventh Day Adventist |
| Free Presbyterian Church | | Unitarian/Universalist |
| Islam | | |
| Judaism (Orthodox/Conserv) | | NO POSITION |
| Shintoism | | Baptist Church |
| Zoroastrianism | | Christian Scientists |
| | | Lutheran |

The early Christian church followed Jewish tradition, seeing cremation as a pagan (essentially Graeco-Roman) rite. Writing at the time when Romans and early Christians were at odds over the practice of cremation, Minucius Felix wrote:

> ...it is easy to understand why they curse our funeral pyres and condemn cremation; just as if every body, although withdrawn from the flames, were not reduced to dust as the years roll on, just as if it makes any difference whether our bodies are torn to pieces by wild beasts, swallowed up in the sea, covered with earth, or destroyed by fire. Any kind of burial must be a punishment to them, if they have any feeling after death. If they have not, cremation must be regarded as a beneficent remedy in the rapidity of its effect.[189]

Yet it has been said, "If the Christians of the first centuries no longer feared that they would go to join the shades who wandered on the bank of the Styx, they were still pursued by the superstitious dread that they would have no part in the resurrection of the flesh if their bodies did not rest in the grave."[190] Early Christians also shunned cremation for a more practical reason. Christians were still being persecuted during the period when the sect was developing its rituals, and cremation pyres attracted too much attention to be safe. Eventually, the Church used cremation as a posthumous excommunication rite.[191]

In 1886, the Catholic Church banned cremation when the Italian cremation movement fomented an anticlerical and irreligious rebellion against Church authority. Under Canon law, cremated remains could be denied Christian burials and the deceased could be excommunicated. Since the ban on cremation was based not on theological grounds, however, the Church pragmatically (but against considerable resistance) reconsidered its position when, after World War II, an increasing number of Catholics began cremating their dead. In 1963, the Second Vatican Council agreed to allow priests to conduct funeral services before cremation with specific permission from their diocese. The Church now allows cremated remains to be buried in consecrated ground, unless the desire for cremation was based on a denial of Christian dogma. The Church, however, continues to prefer earth burial and still urges its members to "religiously maintain" the custom of burial. Bishops must instruct their flock not to choose cremation except for serious reasons.[192]

Eastern Orthodox churches forbid cremation, as do some Protestant denominations, such as the Missouri Synod of the Lutheran Church, the Evangelical churches, and fundamentalist sects. Muslims also forbid cremation, requiring burial so that the preservation of the body will give consolation to the soul. The Church of Jesus Christ of the Latter Day Saints

(Mormon) feels that nothing should be done to destroy the body, but leaves body disposal to family discretion. Though the practice is not encouraged, the Church will honor the deceased's wish for cremation.[193]

In some instances religious objections to cremation may succumb to secular pressures. One early English cremation proponent related that when an old acquaintance died, he left instructions that his body be cremated. The deceased's son-in-law, a clergyman, refused to allow the body to be cremated because of his and his wife's religious views. When informed, however, that the deceased's will stipulated that the cremation society would receive £10,000 (a very large amount of money at that time) if his body was buried, they reconsidered. The body was cremated.[194]

## AA. WHAT IS THE FUNERAL INDUSTRY'S RESPONSE TO CREMATION?

The funeral industry, according to Kubasak, has responded to cremation in three ways: (1) with the "ostrich" approach, pretending that cremation does not exist; (2) with the "big-foot" approach (tried unsuccessfully in California) that attempts to suppress cremation, especially direct cremation; and (3) with the "active interest" approach, in which the industry tries to "develop new ways to incorporate cremation within the scope of traditional funeral service."[195] He describes how funeral directors can very successfully use "active interest" to steer people requesting direct cremation towards more expensive and elaborate services. Think "used-car salesman."

The funeral industry first responded to the threat of direct cremation by questioning the philosophical basis for cremation and opposing it on principle. As Kubasak says, "We became the enemy of cremation and low cost disposal...most funeral directors erroneously interpreted a request for cremation to mean *no ceremony, no embalming, no viewing, no casket...we* refused to listen to what the public was trying to tell us."[196] More graphically, he says, "We reacted to talk about cremation as though it were a social disease. If death was a taboo subject for polite conversation, cremation was the black plague coming to haunt us."[197]

Has the funeral industry changed? Successful funeral homes that operate in areas with direct cremation businesses now make "cremation-oriented families" welcome, assuring them that the funeral home can also serve their needs. They then use hard-sell tactics (under the theme of "service") to push unwanted goods and services on these "prospects" (their term).[198]

"Hard-sell" is a harsh term, but it fits. Kubasak proudly points to his own funeral business where, using these tactics, he has had more than a 300 percent increase in "prospects" purchasing ceremonies to accompany cremations, and a nearly 600 percent increase in the purchase of caskets or containers in less than a decade.[199] One technique he uses is to require a family member to identify the corpse to be cremated. This individual viewing requirement "generally provides an occasion to explain the benefits of viewing...once the family identifies the deceased, the benefits of viewing become obvious and many inquire about regular visitation."[200] Robert Inman, while president of CANA, endorsed Kubasak's methods and strongly urged members to buy Kubasak's book.[201]

Embalming would appear to be a difficult service to sell to prospects intent on cremating their loved ones. Kubasak gets around this by selling most families a "basic care" option at about one-third the cost of embalming. For this price, all that is done is "positioning the deceased, disinfecting the mouth and eyes, combing the hair and wrapping the body in a plastic gown and sheet."[202] Not content with that profit (for so little effort), he also requires refrigeration for bodies held more than 8 hours. The cost for these two services totals about sixty-five percent of the cost for embalming.[203] This provides even more profit than selling the more complex embalming services.

Funerals may also be difficult to sell, given the non-traditional and often non-practicing religious nature of those seeking cremation services. The funeral industry gets around this by using the word "ceremony." As Kubasak proudly declares, "The word ceremony does not cause people to shudder or become defensive..[and]..very few people select 'plain vanilla' in funeral services. We offer much more than thirty-one flavors."[204]

Finally, in a chapter titled, "Merchandising Cremation Products," Kubasak gives a 15-step process for using an "arrangement conference" to persuade families that they need more and increasingly expensive services. He details all of the objections these "prospects" might make and offers advice on how to deftly steer them as close to a traditional funeral package as possible. The patina of "service" cannot hide the ooze coming off these pages. Unfortunately, the book is marketed by the NFDA and is widely read by those in the industry. (In defense of the honest funeral and crematory directors, including some who helped prepare this book, they are not all used-car salesmen. One funeral home in Santa Fe, New Mexico, for example, supplies free caskets and services for burials of children 6-years old and younger. This, however, is unusual.)

## AB. HOW MUCH DOES CREMATION COST?

Families can save money by using cremation, especially if they cremate the body immediately and hold a simple memorial service rather than a full-blown funeral. There are three types of cremation, each with an increasing cost: (1) no preparation of the body, with no viewing or funeral, and cremation in a simple wooden or cardboard box (direct cremation); (2) cremation soon after death with a subsequent memorial service; and (3) all normal funeral arrangements carried out, with or without embalming or an open casket, and with cremation substituting for burial.

The least expensive cremations (with or without formal funeral services) are usually available through local memorial societies. These societies sell memberships for about $30, and upon a member's death, they generally charge an additional $500 to $600 to handle all arrangements, including the necessary authorizations and scattering of the ashes. Unlike direct cremation businesses, memorial societies arrange to have the services performed at this low price (through force of their numbers) by licensed funeral and crematory operators.[205] Some memorial societies even assist families who wish to do all of the transportation and the preparations themselves.[206]

Memorial societies exist throughout the United States and Canada and stem from a movement that started in 1939. Most legitimate operations are members of the Continental Association of Funeral and Memorial Societies. Commercial ventures masquerading as memorial societies can be "unmasked" by checking to see if they are members of such a national group, by questioning excessive membership fees, and by being wary if they try to sell anything.[207]

Commercial firms specializing in direct cremations are a moderately expensive choice. These firms, such as California's Neptune Society, Telophase Society, and Ghia Gallery have undergone a constant barrage of funeral home- and cemetery industry-instigated lawsuits, administrative barriers, and statutory entanglements designed to make them reduce or eliminate direct or inexpensive cremations. These obstructionist techniques have been repeated in other states with high cremation rates, such as Florida and New York.

The most expensive cremations are those in which families make their own arrangements through regular funeral homes.

Aside from the cost of the body's container and for using the crematory, funeral professionals estimate that their other costs for each cremation, including personnel, insurance, and advertising, total $75. How do they recoup their costs and make a profit? According to the funeral industry, the average charge for direct cremations when the family provides the container is $824. (It is $886 when the funeral home provides the container.)[208] Industry experts claim, however, that funeral homes can charge as little as $300 for a cremation and still make a profit. In 1987 the Federal Trade Commission found that consumers actually paid an average of $1,054 to funeral homes for cremations and related services.[209] As the AARP says, "After many years of resistance, most funeral directors and cemeteries now gladly handle cremations. But their new attitude is linked largely to the realization that cremations can lead to the sale of other highly profitable goods and services."[210]

What expenses do crematories have? Crematories cost $50,000 to $75,000 for the furnace, building modifications to accommodate the oven, and ancillary tools and equipment. In addition, the natural gas or electricity for each cremation costs about $35 to $50.

According to CANA, "The basic charge for just cremation is somewhat less than traditional burial. However, with so many items of service available to the family both in the funeral service before and in the mode of disposition after, it's not possible to make an accurate comparison."[211] To increase their profit margin, some California crematoria now charge an average of $150 for family members to observe the cremation.

Costs to the family in addition to the actual cremation, include the urn, $50 and up, the body's cremation container (if any), a columbarium niche or cemetery grave, an urn vault (if required), professional ash scattering, transportation (body and ashes), refrigeration until cremation (if required), and any funeral or memorial services. These can each vary tremendously in price, depending on the type of disposal, area of the country, and other services desired.

Cardboard cremation containers in the United States cost between $8 and $15 wholesale, and retail for $15 to $350.[212] Particle-board caskets can also be used. These average $50 to $70 wholesale and between $100 and $350 retail.[213] The American Association of Retired Persons, however, reports retail prices for these items ranging up to $1,000![214]

If a death occurs in a foreign country, cremation will normally be the least expensive method of disposition, if there is an available crematory. The costs in foreign countries, however, vary widely, with cremation in the Sudan costing $60, while in France it costs $1,500.[215] After cremation, ashes may be carried home or sent by mail.

Paying for cremation services may be a problem. Since many insurance companies do not directly pay crematories, some crematoria require payment at the time of service. Others will wait for insurance reimbursement.

## AC. REFERENCES

1. DeSpelder LA, Strickland AL: *The Last Dance.* Palo Alto, CA: Mayfield Pub, 1983, p 185.
2. Selzer R: *Mortal Lessons: Notes on the Art of Surgery.* New York: Simon & Schuster, 1987, p 138.
3. Abercrombie JR: *Palestinian Burial Practices From 1200 to 600 B.C.E.* (Ph.D. Thesis, Univ of Pennsylvania) Ann Arbor, MI: Univ Microfilms International, 1979, p 44.
4. Polson CJ, Brittain RP, Marshall TK: *The Disposal of the Dead.* 2nd ed. Springfield, IL: Charles C Thomas, 1962, pp 140-41.

5. Kubasak MW: *Cremation and the Funeral Director—Successfully Meeting the Challenge.* Malibu, CA: Avalon Press, 1990, p 13.
6. Abercrombie, *Palestinian Burial Practices,* p 34.
7. Carlson L: *Caring for Your Own Dead.* Hinesburg, VT: Upper Access, 1987, p 24.
8. *I Samuel* 31:12,13.
9. Tegg W: *The Last Act: Being the Funeral Rites of Nations and Individuals.* London: William Tegg & Co, 1876, p 357.
10. Abercrombie, *Palestinian Burial Practices,* p 190.
11. *Jeremiah* 7:31.
12. Gehenna:No altar but crematorium. *Prodigy News Service.* March 19, 1993. (Quoting *Scientist.*)
13. Habenstein RW, Lamers WM: *The History of American Funeral Directing.* Milwaukee, WI: National Funeral Directors Association, 1985, p 20.
14. Homer: *The Iliad.* Book 23. In: *Great Books of the Western World.* vol 4. Chicago: Encyclopaedia Britannica, 1952, p 163.
15. Tegg, *The Last Act,* p 41.
16. Kastenbaum RK, Kastenbaum B, eds: *Encyclopedia of Death.* Phoenix, AZ: Oryx Press, 1989, p 58.
17. Pliny. Quoted in: Walker GA: *Gatherings From Grave Yards.* London: Longman & Co, 1839. Reprinted by Arno Press, New York, 1977, p 16.
18. Virgil: *Aeneid.* Book VI, lines 219-29. In: *Great Books of the Western World.* vol 13.
19. Carlson, *Caring for Your Own Dead,* p 125.
20. *Plutarch's Lives: Marcus Brutus.* In: *Great Books of the Western World.* vol 14, p 810.
21. Haestier R: *Dead Men Tell Tales: A Survey of Exhumations, From Earliest Antiquity to the Present Day.* London: John Long, 1934, p 21.
22. Cook WS: Cremation: From ancient cultures to modern usage. *Casket and Sunnyside.* 1973;103(1):42+.
23. Basevi WHF: *The Burial of the Dead.* London: Geo Rutledge & Sons, 1920, p 55.
24. Habenstein, Lamers, *History of American Funeral Directing,* p 49.
25. Mackenzie DA: *Ancient Man in Britain.* London: Blackie & Son, 1932, pp 109-10.
26. Carlson, *Caring for Your Own Dead,* p 25.
27. Cook, Cremation, *Casket and Sunnyside,* 1973.
28. *The Mythology of the Eddas.* pp 538-39. *Translations of the Royal Society of Literature Second Series.* vol 12. Quoted in: Mackenzie, *Ancient Man in Britain,* p 110.
29. Puckle, BS.: *Funeral Customs—Their Origin and Development.* London: T Werner Laurie, 1926, p 211.
30. Bendann E: *Death Customs: An Analytical Study of Burial Rites.* New York: Alfred A Knopf, 1930, p 50.
31. Herodotus: *History.* Book V, verse 92, section 7.
32. Browne T: Hydriotaphia. 1658.
33. Puckle, *Funeral Customs,* pp 214-15.
34. Trelawny EJ: *The Last Days of Shelley and Byron.* London:1858.
35. Haestier, *Dead Men Tell Tales,* p 67.
36. Mackenzie, *Ancient Man in Britain,* p 109-10.
37. Glob PV : *The Bog People—Iron-Age Man Preserved.* (Bruce-Mitford R, trans) Ithaca, NY: Cornell Univ Press, 1969, p 145.
38. Carlson, *Caring for Your Own Dead,* p 26.
39. Service RW: "The Cremation of Sam McGee." *Collected Poems of Robert Service.* New York: GP Punam's Sons, 1940, p 33.
40. Gordon A: *Death is for the Living.* Edinburgh: Paul Harris, 1984, p 51.
41. Puckle, *Funeral Customs,* p 220.
42. *Regina v. Price* 12 Q.B.D. 247.
43. Griffin JP: Eccentric or visionary—Dr. Price of Llantrisant. *J Royal Soc Med.* 1991;84:229-32.
44. Puckle, *Funeral Customs,* p 220.

45. Ragon M: *The Space of Death: A Study of Funerary Architecture, Decoration, and Urbanism.* (Sheridan A: trans). Charlottesville, VA: Univ Press of Virginia, 1983. Originally published as *L'espace de la mort: Essai sur l'architecture, la décoration et l'urbanisme funéraires,* Albin Michel, 1981, pp 99-100, 285.
46. Brereton JLG. Quoted in: Cooke S: Death, body and soul: the cremation debate in New South Wales, 1863-1925. *Australian Historical Studies.* 1991;24:323-39.
47. Cooke S: Death, body and soul: the cremation debate in New South Wales, 1863-1925. *Australian Historical Studies.* 1991;24:323-39.
48. Cremation Society of Australia: *Twelve Arguments in Favour of Cremation.* Undated. (Adaptation of the eight *Short Reasons for Cremation.* Originally published by Cremation Society of England.) Quoted in: Cooke, *Australian Historical Studies,* 1991.
49. Cook, Cremation, *Casket and Sunnyside,* 1973.
50. Habenstein, Lamer, *History of American Funeral Directing,* p 296.
51. Holmes HM: *Incineration of the Dead.* Lansing, MI: self-published, pp 3-5.
52. Habenstein, Lamer, *History of American Funeral Directing,* pp 296-97.
53. Erichsen H: *Proceedings of the First National Convention.* Detroit: Cremation Association of America, 1913. As quoted in: Habenstein, Lamers, *History of American Funeral Directing,* p 298.
54. Selzer, *Mortal Lessons,* p 137.
55. Editors of Consumer Reports: *Funerals—Consumers' Last Rights.* New York: WW Norton, 1977, p 158.
56. Daniel TP: *An Analysis of the Funeral Rule Using consumer Survey Data on the Purchase of Funeral Goods and Services.* Washington, DC: Federal Trade Commission (FTC), February 1989, p 6.
57. Shaw GB: Quoted in: Mitford J: *American Way of Death.* New York: Simon & Schuster, 1963, pp 162-63.
58. Polson, Brittain, Marshall, *Disposal of the Dead,* p 119.
59. *Regina v. Young* (1972) St. Alban's Crown Court.
60. Cremation Association of North America (CANA): *Model Cremation Law.* Chicago, IL: CANA.
61. Ariès P: *The Hour of Our Death.* New York: Oxford Univ Press, 1981, p 577.
62. Gorer G: *Death, Grief and Mourning in Contemporary Britain.* London: The Cresset Press, 1965, p 45.
63. Puckle, *Funeral Customs,* p 210.
64. Ibid., p 216.
65. Morgan E: *A Manual of Simple Burial.* Burnsville, NC: Celo Press, 1966, p 85.
66. Koosman S: *Cultural Variations in Funeral Practice.* (lecture). National Funeral Directors Association Annual Convention. Baltimore, MD: 1989. (audiotape)
67. Kalish RA, Reynolds DK: *Death and Ethnicity—A Psychocultural Study.* Los Angeles: Ethel Percy Andrus Gerentology Center, Univ of Southern CA, 1976, p 152.
68. Kubasak, *Cremation and the Funeral Director,* p 143.
69. Koosman, *Cultural Variations,* 1989. (audiotape)
70. Odds & Ends: People Patterns. *Wall Street J.* December 21, 1992, p B1.
71. Cremation Association of North America: *North American Cremation Statistics, 1970-1988.*
72. Cremation Association of America (CANA): *Cremations and % of Deaths.* Chicago, IL: CANA, 1989.
73. Inman R: *Cremation Liability.* (lecture). National Funeral Directors Association Annual Convention. Louisville, KY: 1990. (audiotape)
74. Kalish, Reynolds, *Death and Ethnicity,* p 47.
75. CANA, *Cremations and % of Deaths,* 1989.
76. Inman, *Cremation Liability,* 1990. (audiotape)
77. Kubasak, *Cremation and the Funeral Director,* p 25.
78. Dempsey D. *The Way We Die: An Investigation of Death and Dying in America.* New York: MacMillan, 1975, pp 178-79.

79. Adams JA: Project understanding: A national study of cremation. *Research Record.* 1986;3:73-96.
80. Habenstein RW, Lamers WM: *Funeral Customs the World Over.* Milwaukee: National Funeral Directors Association, 1963, p 405.
81. Watson JL, Rawski ES, eds: *Death Ritual in Late Imperial and Modern China.* Berkeley, CA: Univ of California Press, 1988, pp 289-307.
82. Carlson, *Caring for Your Own Dead,* p 27.
83. Out with their teeth! *The Forum.* 1992;58(9):12.
84. Mills A: Mercury and crematorium chimneys. *Nature.* 1990;346:615.
85. Künzler P, Andrée M: More mercury from crematoria. *Nature.* 1991;349:746.
86. Ludwig J: *Current Methods of Autopsy Practice.* Philadelphia, PA: WB Saunders, 1972, p 251.
87. Carlson, *Caring for Your Own Dead,* p 28.
88. Englade K: *A Family Business.* New York: St. Martin's, 1992, p 55.
89. Ibid.
90. Cremation Association of North America (CANA): *Cremation Explained: Answers to Questions Most Frequently Asked.* (pamphlet). Chicago, IL: CANA, 1986.
91. Market Facts: *Report on the Survey of Recent Funeral Arrangers.* Washington, DC: FTC, April 82, 1988, pII-12.
92. No cash, no ashes: Body returned. *USA Today.* October 14, 1992, p A4.
93. Landers A: Funeral home 'dumps' body. *Temple* (TX) *Daily Telegram.* January 10, 1993, p 2B.
94. Federal Trade Commission: *Funeral Industry Practices; Trade Regulations Rule.* 16 *CFR* Part 453. *Federal Register.* September 24, 1982;47(186):42277.
95. Kubasak, *Cremation and the Funeral Director,* p 137.
96. Market Facts: *Report on the Survey of Recent Funeral Arrangers.* Washington, DC: FTC, April 82, 1988, pp II-11, 12.
97. CANA, *Cremation Explained,* 1986.
98. Neptune Society of Northern California (NSNC): *Disclosures Regarding the Cremation Process.* (leaflet). San Francisco, CA: NSNC, undated, distributed in 1993.
99. Kubasak, *Cremation and the Funeral Director,* p 71.
100. van der Woude J: De Wet op de lijkbezorging en de verpleegkundige. *TVZ.* 1991:12:402-404.
101. CANA, *Cremation Explained,* 1986.
102. Polson, Brittain, Marshall, *Disposal of the Dead,* p 139.
103. Puckle, *Funeral Customs,* various pages.
104. Inman, *Cremation Liability,* 1990. (audiotape)
105. Auboyer J: Rites and Ceremonies: Ceremonial and Ritualistic Objects. In *The New Encyclopaedia Britannica.* vol 26 (Macropaedia). Chicago: Encyclopaedia Britannica, 1987, pp 868-76.
106. Editors of Consumer Reports, *Funerals,* p 174.
107. Ragon, *Space of Death,* pp 99-100.
108. Dolan C: In the bad old days, dead people could often be found at the polls. *Wall Street J.* October 28, 1992, p B1.
109. Interview with Emmitt Watson: caretaker and historian, Neptune Society Columbarium. San Francisco, CA: May 18, 1993.
110. Inman, *Cremation Liability,* 1990. (audiotape)
111. Brauchli MW: Columbarium owner finds cash can cure local fear of ghosts. *Wall Street J.* November 17, 1992, p A1.
112. Grycznski, ES, Tolleson LJ, Audie EH: *Taps—A Guide to Military-Oriented Burial.* Alexandria, VA: Retired Officers' Assn., 1990, pp 12, 14.
113. Ariès P: *Western Attitudes Toward Death.* (Ranum PA, trans). Baltimore, MD: Johns Hopkins Press, 1974, p 91.
114. Litten J: *The English Way of Death: The Common Funeral Since 1450.* London: Robert Hale, 1991, p 3.
115. Habenstein, Lamers, *Funeral Customs the World Over,* p 81.

116. Ibid., p 90.
117. Ibid., p 122.
118. Pallis CA: Death. In: *The New Encyclopaedia Britannica.* vol 16 (Macropaedia). Chicago: Encyclopaedia Britannica, 1987, pp 1030-1042.
119. Habenstein, Lamers, *Funeral Customs the World Over,* p 134-42.
120. Puckle, *Funeral Customs,* p 213-14.
121. Habenstein, Lamers, *Funeral Customs the World Over,* p 329-44.
122. Ibid., p 59-60.
123. Ibid.
124. Kubasak, *Cremation and the Funeral Director,* p 79.
125. Shaw GB: Lawrence DH, ed: *Collected Letters, 1911-1925.* vol 3. Max Reinhardt, 1985.
126. Evans WED: *The Chemistry of Death.* Springfield, IL: Charles C Thomas, 1963, pp 84-85.
127. Polson, Brittain, Marshall, *Disposal of the Dead,* p 137.
128. DeSpelder, Strickland, *The Last Dance,* p 185.
129. Polson, Brittain, Marshall, *Disposal of the Dead,* p 137.
130. Brown T: *Hydriotaphia, or Urne Buriall.* London: 1658.
131. Murray KA, Rose JC: The analysis of cremains: a case study involving the inappropriate disposal of mortuary remains. *J Forensic Sciences.* 1993;38:98-103.
132. Dunlop JM: Traffic light discoloration in cremated bones. *Med Sci Law.* 1978;18:163-73.
133. Holck P: *Cremated Bones: A Medical Anthropological Study of an Archeological Material on Cremation Burials.* Antropologtiske Skrifter nr. 1, Anatomisk Institutt, Universitetet i Oslo, 1968. Cited in: Murray, Rose, *J Forensic Sciences,* 1993.
134. Inman, *Cremation Liability,* 1990. (audiotape)
135. NSNC, *Disclosures Regarding the Cremation Process.*
136. Inman, *Cremation Liability,* 1990. (audiotape)
137. Ibid.
138. CANA, *Model Cremation Law.*
139. Birkby WH: *The Analysis of Cremains.* Presented at the 43rd annual meeting of the American Academy of Forensic Sciences. Anaheim, CA: Feb 18-23, 1991.
140. Englade, *A Family Business,* p 130.
141. Ibid., pp 49-51.
142. Settlement proposed for class action. *The American Funeral Director.* 1992;115(4):18-19.
143. Inman, *Cremation Liability,* 1990. (audiotape)
144. Carlson, *Caring for Your Own Dead,* p 32.
145. Inman, *Cremation Liability,* 1990. (audiotape)
146. *Smith v. Telophase National Cremation Society* 471 S 2nd 163.
147. American Association of Retired Persons (AARP): *Cemetery Goods and Services.* (brochure). Washington, DC: AARP, 1988, p 8.
148. State Funeral Board suspends man accused of mixing remains. *Tucson (AZ) Citizen.* May 26, 1993, p 2D.
149. Murray, Rose, *J Forensic Sciences,* 1993.
150. Troutman R: *Cremation Liability.* (lecture). National Funeral Directors Association Annual Convention. Baltimore, MD: 1989. (audiotape)
151. Morgan E: *A Manual of Death Education & Simple Burial.* Burnsville, NC: Celo Press, 1977, p 48.
152. Inman, *Cremation Liability,* 1990. (audiotape)
153. Landers A: Funeral home's action shock to the bereaved. *Tucson (AZ) Citizen* April 23, 1993, p 2C.
154. Inman, *Cremation Liability,* 1990. (audiotape)
155. Federal Express main shipping office: Phone Interview. Tucson, AZ: April 23, 1993.
156. Inman, *Cremation Liability,* 1990. (audiotape)
157. Coffin MM: *Death in Early America: The History and Folklore of Customs and Superstitions of Early Medicine, Funerals, Burials, and Mourning.* Nashville: Thomas Nelson, 1976, p 140.

158. *Advance News.* Ogdensburg, NY: April 1975. As cited in: Coffin, *Death in Early America,* p 141.
159. Editors of Consumer Reports, *Funerals,* p 173.
160. Dolan C: Burying tradition, more people opt for 'fun' funerals. *Wall Street J.* May 20, 1993, p A1+.
161. Polson, Brittain, Marshall, *Disposal of the Dead,* p 154.
162. Koosman, *Cultural Variations,* 1989. (audiotape)
163. Ragon, *Space of Death,* p 287.
164. CANA, *Cremation Explained,* 1986.
165. Inman, *Cremation Liability,* 1990. (audiotape)
166. Auboyer, Rites and Ceremonies, 1987.
167 Editors of Consumer Reports, *Funerals,* p 171.
168. Ibid., p 174.
169. Dolan, *Wall Street J,* May 20, 1993.
170. Watson E: Interview. (caretaker and historian) Neptune Society Columbarium. San Francisco, CA: May 18, 1993.
171. Ghia, Alex (Owner of Ghia Galleries): Interview. San Francisco, CA: January 23, 1992.
172. Ibid.
173. Koosman, *Cultural Variations,* 1989. (audiotape)
174. Walker GA: *Gatherings From Grave Yards.* London: Longman & Co, 1839. Reprinted by Arno Press, New York, 1977, p 16
175. Tegg, *The Last Act,* p 357.
176. Di Paola J: Burglars leave TV, take cremated remains in apparent belief that they were cocaine. *Arizona Daily Star.* Tucson, AZ: June 4, 1993, p 13D.
177. Ghia, Interview, January 23, 1992.
178. Shotgun funerals spread sportsmen's ashes. *Arizona Daily Star.* Tucson, AZ: February 18, 1991, p A4.
179. Final volley. *USA Today.* April 30, 1993, p 3A.
180. Litten, *English Way of Death,* p 121.
181. Ghia, Interview, January 23, 1992.
182. Dolan, *Wall Street J,* May 20, 1993.
183. van der Woude, *TVZ.* 1991.
184. A Japanese Custom. *The American Funeral Director.* 1992;115:6.
185. Inman, *Cremation Liability,* 1990. (audiotape)
186. Bendann, *Death Customs,* p 46.
187. Lord Shaftsbury. As quoted in: Mitford, *American Way of Death,* p 163.
188. *Talmud,* Avodah Zarah 1:3. Cited in: Rosner F: *Modern Medicine and Jewish Ethics.* 2nd ed. New York: Yeshiva Univ Press, 1991, p 342.
189. Felix M. As cited in: Rush AC: *Death and Burial in Christian Antiquity.* Washington, DC: Catholic Univ of America Press, 1941, p 236.
190. Leblant. Quoted in: Cumont F: *After Life in Roman Paganism.* New Haven, CT: Yale Univ Press, 1922, pp 68-69.
191. Jackson PE: *The Law of Cadavers and of Burial and Burial Places.* New York: Prentice-Hall, 1937, p 9.
192. Editors of Consumer Reports, *Funerals,* p 166.
193. Habenstein, Lamers, *Funeral Customs the World Over,* p 719.
194. Richardson, Sir Benjamin. Quoted in: Puckle, *Funeral Customs,* p 223.
195. Kubasak, *Cremation and the Funeral Director,* p 4.
196. Ibid, p 15.
197. Ibid, p 16.
198. Ibid, p 21+.
199. Ibid, p 69.
200. Ibid, p 87.
201. Inman, *Cremation Liability,* 1990. (audiotape)
202. Kubasak, *Cremation and the Funeral Director,* p 90.
203. Ibid.

204. Ibid, p 93.
205. AARP, *Cemetery Goods and Services,* p 7.
206. Editors of Consumer Reports, *Funerals,* p 182.
207. Morgan E: *A Manual of Simple Burial.* Burnsville, NC: Celo Press, 1966, p 19.
208. National Funeral Directors Association (NFDA): 1991 Survey: How do you compare? *The Director.* November 1991, pp 42-44.
209. Daniel, *Analysis of the Funeral Rule,* February 1989, p 7.
210. AARP, *Cemetery Goods and Services,* p 7.
211. CANA, *Cremation Explained,* 1986.
212. Ghia, Interview, January 23, 1992.
213. Ibid.
214. AARP, *Cemetery Goods and Services,* p 7.
215. Morgan, *Manual of Simple Burial,* 1966, p 62.

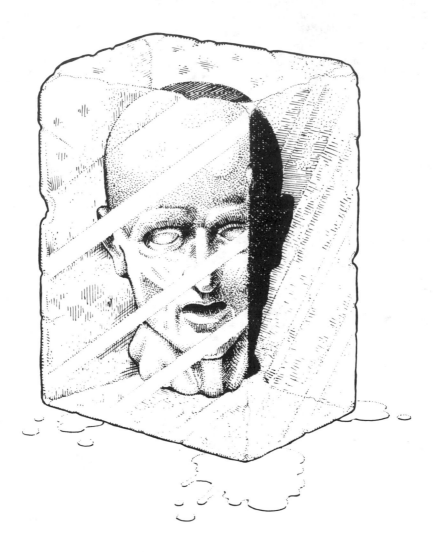

# 7: SOULS ON ICE

287

*Is cryonic suspension of whole bodies and dead heads ("corpsicles") a scam or a realistic option? Do reputable scientists believe there is any chance that cryonauts can be revived in the future? Will frozen bodies be subjects for future research or will they simply be allowed to thaw? Who is undergoing cryonic preservation now and how much does it cost?*

## A. WHAT IS CRYONIC SUSPENSION?

Cryonic suspension or solid-state hypothermia is the process of freezing and maintaining a dead human at an extremely low temperature, in the hope that the body may be resuscitated after medical science improves.

This dream is not new. In 1773, Benjamin Franklin wrote, "I wish it were possible from this instance to invent a method of embalming drowned persons, in such a manner that they may be recalled to life, however distant."[1]

The modern idea of preserving dead bodies for future repair is credited to a science fiction story, *The Jameson Satellite,* written by Neil R. Jones in 1930.[2] Other authors and film-makers have since used plots involving cryonic preservation, among them F. Pohl's *Age of the Pussy Foot* (1970), in which the main character emerges from a "sleep freeze" in A.D. 2527 and must face a changed world; Woody Allen's movie, *Sleeper* (1973); Robert Altman's *Quintet* (1979); Fred Schepisi's *Iceman* (1984) which addresses some of the moral dilemmas of cryonics; Les Mayfield's *Encino Man* (1992); and Marco Brambilla's *Demolition Man* (1993).

Robert C. W. Ettinger popularized the concept of cryonic preservation with his book, *The Prospect of Immortality* (1964), in which he suggested that freezing was the easy part of the process and could be accomplished with present technology. He believed that the complicated process of thawing could be worked out at a later time. He stated that "Most of us now breathing have a good chance of physical life after death—a sober, scientific probability of revival and rejuvenation of our frozen bodies."[3] Ettinger felt that "No matter what kills us, whether old age or disease, and even if freezing techniques are still crude when we die, *sooner or later* our friends of the future should be equal to the task of reviving and curing us."[4]

Ettinger was aware that freezing destroys the body's tissues, dehydrating them and causing considerable cellular and subcellular damage. He optimistically preached that future technology would overcome these problems. So, with a leap of faith, the first cryonic society was established in New York in 1965 as a result of the book. The next year a Life Extension Society Conference was held in Washington, D.C..[5]

In 1965, two bodies were *almost* frozen, but circumstances prevented it. The first was of a woman dying of heart disease in Springfield, Ohio. Her family wanted to cryonically freeze her after death and had actually set up the equipment. Yet the hospital in which she was dying refused to allow the procedure in their facility after an all-night meeting of its Board of Directors.[6] While Ettinger, who had arrived to assist in the procedure, was willing to freeze the woman's body outside of a hospital, the process was further stymied when relatives pressured the woman's husband to opt instead for burial.[7] The second near-cryonaut was a 44-year-old scientist, Danridge M. Cole, who unexpectedly died from a heart attack. Since the family was not prepared to immediately begin cryonic preservation, they decided, despite the pleadings of Robert Ettinger, to bury Cole's body.[8]

The first corpse to be intentionally "frozen" with the idea of restoring it to life after medical science advanced was that of Professor James H. Bedford, a 73-year-old retired psychology professor, land investor and cryonics adherent, who died on January 12, 1967. His body was cooled while preservatives were injected over a four-hour period.[9,10] ("Dr. Harold Greene," sometimes cited as the first body preserved is actually a pseudonym one author used in a book describing the preservation of Professor Bedford's corpse.)[11,12] Bedford's freezing received widespread publicity, including an article in *Life* magazine. (This article was preempted by coverage of the fire that killed three Apollo astronauts, so only a small fraction of *Life* issues had the cryonics feature.) Later, it was feared that Bedford would be the first one thawed when some of the nitrogen gas in his cryogenic tank boiled-off. Not so—he remains frozen in California.[13]

Another early freezing with significant media attention was that of Steven J. Mandell, a 24-year-old New York City aeronautical engineering student who died on July 28, 1968 of "enteritis and adrenal failure." Knowing his health was only "fair," he joined the Cryonics Society of New York as a student member just eight months before his death.[14] After he died, his body was stored in a $4,000 liquid nitrogen capsule at -320°F (-196°C). When Mandell's life insurance company refused to pay off on his policy (he had concealed his terminal illness to obtain coverage), his mother bore the cost of maintaining his cryonic capsule, first at the Washington Memorial Park Cemetery in Coram, New York, and later in Chatsworth, California. While in California, however, the capsule was inadequately monitored and Mandell's corpse thawed.[15]

None of the above cryonauts have, as yet, been reanimated. And, of the first seventeen corpses cryonically preserved, only James Bedford remains frozen today; more recent cases have fared somewhat better.[16]

A science writer, Charles Platt, who has arranged to be cryonically frozen, describes the procedure as "being turned into a Popsicle."[17] Perhaps the term "corpsicle" would be more appropriate, or as some people say, "thermally challenged." Despite his cynicism, he elected to have his corpse frozen because it is "the ultimate gesture of defiance."[18] (Subsequently he withdrew from the organization and terminated his arrangements to be cryonically preserved.)[19] Most cryonics adherents feel that "the prospect of ultimately succeeding at this medical longshot and bold bet on human achievement is emotionally exciting on many levels."[20] However, a noted scientist who studies the freezing of organisms, cryobiologist David Pegg, has been quoted as saying that cryonic suspension preserves "meat, not living cells."[21] Even Ettinger, accepting the possibility of failure, wrote "Clearly, the freezer is more attractive than the grave, even if one has doubts about the future capabilities of science. With bad luck, the frozen people will simply remain dead, as they would have in the grave."[22]

## B. WHAT IS THE SCIENTIFIC VIEW OF CRYONIC PRESERVATION?

Opinion among scientists is divided over the feasibility of cryonic preservation. Those who deal with conventional medicine and cryobiology tend to be pessimistic, while those in such fields as computer science and nanotechnology (a new field that studies atomic- and molecular-level manipulation of matter) are more favorable.

Much of the mainstream scientific community, including those scientists who work in the area of cryobiology, views cryonic preservation as science fiction at best, and a cruel hoax at worst. When Robert Ettinger's book, *The Prospect of Immortality,* the bible of cryonics, first appeared in 1964, the reviewer for the respected journal *Science*, said:

> One may take this kind of thing seriously or one may not. If one does, the book can only be considered the work of an utterly confused optimist...There is absolutely no evidence that low temperature storage and recovery procedures will be possible in the near future with live human beings, let alone dead ones...Perhaps the author has been pulling our legs. Maybe it's science fiction after all.[23]

Another scientist evaluated Ettinger saying, "R.C.W. Ettinger is referred to as 'Professor' by his followers in their publications...He is also introduced as 'Professor' during his frequent radio and TV appearances. One should remember that the medicine men who traveled the old west selling *snake oil* as a healing elixir for all disease also called themselves 'Professor'...so the title may be most appropriate."[24]

The major scientific organization for cryobiologists, The Society for Cryobiology, categorizes cryonic suspension (also known simply as *cryonics*) as unethical, and denies membership to anyone involved in "any practice or application of freezing deceased persons in the anticipation of their reanimation."[25] Arthur Rowe, Ph.D., of the New York University School of Medicine provides a more vivid description saying, "Believing cryonics could reanimate somebody who has been frozen is like believing you can turn hamburger back into a cow."[26] "After the circulation stops, all the cells of the body die," says David Pegg, a noted cryobiologist from the University of Cambridge, England. "They are structurally disorganized and there is no way of bringing them back to life."[27] "The flaw in the cryonics argument," says John Baust, Ph.D., of the State University of New York in Binghamton, "is the leap between tending to the living and raising the dead. You can't bring dead people back to life. Resurrection falls into the domain of religion, not into the realm of what is scientifically feasible."[28]

Summarizing mainstream science's position, James Southard, Ph.D., of the University of Wisconsin, said, "It's misleading to take $100,000 from a person and say you'll wake them up in 100 years."[29] Robert Prehoda added, "The false promise of cryogenic salvation is an exceedingly cruel deception for many people."[30]

Other scientists, however, are considerably more optimistic about cyonics' possibilities, with some even raising the possibility that *not* freezing the dead could be a moral error. The well-known Arthur C. Clarke (respected both as a scientist and a science-fiction writer), believes cryonic preservation may work. Clarke has said, "Although no one can quantify the probability of cryonics working, I estimate it is at least 90 percent—and certainly *nobody* can say it is zero!"[31] James B. Lewis, Ph.D., a molecular biologist, commented that "the argument of the cryobiology community that preservation is absurd is not correct, because the functional damage caused by freezing is irrelevant to the question of whether cryogenically preserved individuals could be reanimated with radically advanced technology."[32] In the first medical article on cryonics, Ralph C. Merkle, Ph.D., of Xerox PARC, Palo Alto, California, said, "The damage done by current freezing methods is likely to be reversible at some point in the future...Restoration of the brain down to the molecular level should eventually prove technically feasible." In the same article he suggested that "it would be tragic if [cryonics] were to prove feasible but was little used."[33]

## C. CAN ANY BODY BE FROZEN?

Any body that can be arterially embalmed (with blood vessels intact so preservative solutions can be infused) can theoretically also be frozen, although very few actually undergo cryonic preservation.

Currently in the United States, a body can only undergo cryonic preservation after a person is pronounced legally dead. Once dead, a body is subject first to the legal requirements of an autopsy, if one is required under the circumstances. If an autopsy is done, vital organs are removed, often including the brain, so subsequent reanimation after cryonic suspension becomes even more unlikely.

Since few cryonic preservation facilities exist, death away from such a facility also limits one's ability to be frozen. Most people dying far from cryonics facilities will not have timely access to trained technicians who can render "cryonic first aid," including the initial cooling and administration of cryonic preservatives. The Alcor Life Extension Foundation (12327 Doherty Street, Riverside, CA 92503) does, however, publish a pamphlet, titled *Cryonics, The Home Town Way,* that can aid local cryonics adherents in designing their plans for freezing a body in outlying areas. It can also guide morticians who are willing to participate in the process.[34]

Bodies begin to decompose quickly after death, thus the effectiveness of cryonic preservation clearly decreases when the time from death to freezing is inordinately long. Therefore, cryonic procedures are usually done on an emergency basis. In fact Alcor has volunteer cryonic suspension "emergency response teams" in Southern and Northern California, Florida, Indiana, and New York City. They also have a cooldown/temporary storage facility in London, England. There are also two other cryonics organizations in the United States providing "suspension services," Trans Time (associated with The American Cryonics Society and The International Cryonics Foundation), in Oakland, CA, and the Cryonics Institute (associated with The Immortalist Society), Oak Park, MI.[35,36]

A client expected to die at home or in a cooperating health care facility may have cryonic preservation technicians waiting at the bedside for death to occur. Since the technicians can begin their cooling techniques immediately upon the subscriber's death, these patients should theoretically be cooled much faster than those dying in non-cooperating facilities or without technicians at the bedside.

People enrolled in cryonic suspension programs wear stainless-steel identification necklaces or bracelets and carry wallet cards. These IDs provide an emergency number for medical personnel to call if the enrollee dies unexpectedly. They also provide cryonic stabilization information for medical personnel, although it is doubtful that most health care professionals would use it.

Medical personnel often obstruct cryonics technicians, usually because they see cryonics as a scam perpetrated on grieving families. Their resistance to the procedure may stem from pressure they see exerted on the family by cryonics organizations to shun autopsy and organ donation.[37] Medical reluctance to assist cryonics technicians increases when they are asked to continue cardiopulmonary resuscitation (CPR) on a cadaver while the technicians administer cryonic preservatives and cool the body with crushed ice.

## D. HOW IS A BODY FROZEN?

Once the cryonics technicians get control of a corpse, they reinstitute cardiopulmonary resuscitation and as quickly as possible put the body on a heart-lung machine, similar to that used in an operating room. Attaching a body to this machine, however, takes considerable time, even in the most expert hands. Technicians must not only set up this complicated device, but also insert catheters into the large (femoral) artery and vein in the groin. Cryonicists say that under optimal circumstances a body can be on the machine within thirty minutes after death. Circumstances are rarely optimal.

Once the body is attached to this machine, technicians rapidly cool the blood, and then the body, to 59°F (15°C) in as little as fifteen minutes. Technicians then administer drugs which supposedly reduce damage from decreased oxygen going to the tissues, such as calcium channel blockers, blood thinners, and free radical inhibitors. All of these medications have shown experimental evidence of protecting tissues, and one, the calcium channel blocker nimodipine, is used in some patients with brain injuries. (Calcium channel blockers alter the pathways through the cell wall and are commonly used as heart medications.) Cryonicists watch the brain during this process through a hole made in the skull. They place a temperature probe through this hole when the bypass is done.[38]

They then submerge the body in a bath of silicone oil for 36 to 48 hours, cooling it to a temperature approximating that of dry ice (-108°F/-78°C). When the body reaches this temperature, it is wrapped in two precooled sleeping bags, placed inside a protective aluminum pod, and is lowered into a unit filled with liquid nitrogen. The body gradually cools over 24 hours to -321°F (-196°C).[39]

When cooled down, the body is transferred to a storage container, called a *dewar*, filled with liquid nitrogen. British Professor James Dewar devised this type of double-walled vacuum storage vessel in 1898 to handle and store liquid hydrogen. Each custom-made cylinder weighs about a ton, stands nine-feet high, and can store one or two bodies. Constructed like large Thermos[R] bottles and filled with liquid nitrogen, they are fragile and difficult to transport. The neck of the flask is plugged with a plastic foam stopper.[40]

If death occurs at a location where technicians are not available, cryonicists suggest that a cooperative mortician administer cryonic "first aid" by replacing the blood with a commercial solution used to preserve organs for transplant. He should then pack the body in ice and transport it to the cryonic organization for "permanent" cryopreservation. Once the body arrives at the main facility, it is placed on a heart-lung bypass machine by opening the chest and attaching tubes to the main heart vessels. The temporary preservative is replaced with glycerol and sucrose (sugar) over a two- to four-hour period and the freezing is then completed by the usual methods.

Advocates of cryonically preserving the entire body, or "whole body suspension," as opposed to "brain freezing," feel that this procedure (1) preserves all of the individual's biological structures, preventing a possible identity crisis if a person's mind is reawakened in another body; (2) may reduce the time in cryonic suspension since whole bodies may be easier to reanimate than heads alone; (3) avoids the societally unacceptable notion of decapitation associated with neuropreservation; (4) often begins early enough after clinical death so that many organs may be viable; and (5) preserves parts of the body scientists can use as a reservoir of information to aid in the reanimation or regeneration process.[41]

## E. COULD I JUST HAVE MY BRAIN FROZEN?

Yes. In fact, radical advocates of cryonics would prefer to euthanize and cryonically preserve the brains of patients just before clinical death, and even earlier in those with a degenerative brain disease, such as Alzheimers. They say that "an extreme example of inappropriate care from a cryonics standpoint would be so-called 'supportive' care of patients with dementias that progressively erode brain structure, such as Alzheimer's disease or multi-infarct dementia."[42] Whether people have been killed and then cryonically frozen is uncertain, but cryonics advocates say that "unfortunately, it is not yet legally possible to suspend patients during the initial stages of these diseases, when it would be most productive to do so."[43]

If cryonicists kill a person by decapitation or with cryonic preservatives, however, all U.S. jurisdictions now consider it homicide. Thomas Donaldson, a mathematician, computer-software scientist, and an Alcor Life Extension Foundation member suffering from a malignant brain tumor was refused permission to "achieve cryogenic suspension of his head, premortem, before his relentlessly advancing brain tumor destroys the quality and purpose of his life, reduces him to a vegetative state, and makes futile his hope for reanimation." The cryonicist, Carlos Mondragon, a friend of Donaldson's, was told by the court that if he participated, he would be "committing a homicide, or alternatively, aiding and advising a suicide." The court further said "a third person will simply kill Donaldson and hasten the encounter with death. No statute or judicial opinion countenances Donaldson's decision to consent to be murdered or to commit suicide with the assistance of others."[44]

The court did say it was permissible for Donaldson to take his own life to "experience a dignified death rather than an excruciatingly painful life...It is one thing to take one's own life, but quite another to allow a third person assisting in that suicide to be immune from investigation by the coroner or law enforcement agencies."[45]

Donaldson also sought to prevent the coroner from performing an autopsy for medicolegal reasons, if indicated after his death, saying that an autopsy would "destroy his chance of reanimation." The court did note that "the legal and philosophical problems posed by his predicament are a legislative matter rather than a judicial one."[46]

294

When cryonicists do "neurosuspension," they open the chest, isolate the blood vessels supplying the head, and inject cryopreservatives and cooling solutions through these vessels to preserve the brain. They then remove the head by cutting the neck at shoulder level (about the sixth cervical vertebra) and place it in a silicone oil bath with dry ice for about 24 hours, cooling it to -109°F (-78°C). Next, they place the head in a "neurocan" and cool it to -321°F (-196°C) with liquid nitrogen over about 10 days. Unlike whole-body dewars, containers for head preservation are commercial cryogenic units normally used to preserve plant and animal materials. These units, used to store up to 10 heads, weigh 1,200 pounds and stand four-feet high.[47]

Once the head is preserved, the rest of the body is cremated. By the end of 1992, Alcor Life Extension Foundation was storing twenty-six frozen cryonauts, many of whom had only their heads "on ice."[48] All of the cryonically preserved heads and bodies are thought to have been declared dead *before* they were preserved, although there was initially a legal dispute about one case.[49]

Advocates believe that neurosuspension:

1. Preserves all that is unique about an individual;
2. Allows a body to be regenerated or transplanted to support the brain;
3. Requires sophisticated cellular and molecular repair techniques to be successful;
4. Leads to faster cooling than whole body suspension;
5. Costs less than whole body suspension; and
6. Allows preserved heads to be more easily transported if necessary, than whole bodies.[50]

Ettinger, in fact, suggested that reanimated individuals might do better with all or most body parts replaced by improved mechanical components, thus becoming *cyborgs*. He described the possibility of "improved" humans, such as a scientifically-designed aquaman, a flying man, a super soldier with natural body armor and the ability to sting, shock or breathe fire, individuals resistant to cold, heat, and drought, and ultimately, humans with universal consciousness.[51] He also suggested that "sports" would again become intentionally lethal since athletes would only have to protect their brains; the rest of the body could be replaced.

Even cryonics adherents understand how queasy people become when they hear that a loved one's head will be removed for preservation. They therefore encourage the individual to explain the process to relatives. As Stephen Bridge, Alcor Life Extension Foundation's president wrote to cryonics society members, "And you probably think that WE should explain Neurosuspension to them also, right? ('And then we perform the cephalic isolation.' 'The what?' 'We cut off little Freddie's head, ma'am.' 'AAA-CKK!')"[52]

## F. HOW SECURE WOULD MY FROZEN BODY BE?

Trusting in cryonic eternity has been hazardous to numerous potential cryonauts, particularly in the early days when organizations were unstable. A few cryonics organizations have ceased operations, leaving untended frozen corpses in their wake. Other cryonic companies went bankrupt and never froze clients with whom they had contracts. Even the Cryonic Society of California, the pioneering company that froze James Bedford in 1967, went bankrupt and nine of its corpsicles thawed when liquid nitrogen levels fell in their dewars. Bedford's relatives, however, maintained his body until it was transferred to Alcor Life Extension Foundation in Riverside.[53,54,55]

Alcor Life Extension Foundation, the major U.S. cryopreservation organization, claims that its facility for body storage protects the stored bodies and heads against vandalism, fire and earthquake damage. They place their cryonic containers inside a steel-reinforced concrete vault, and claim to have around-the-clock on-site personnel and a warning system to notify off-site personnel of any potential emergency. The greatest dangers (aside from already being dead), are nitrogen leaks from the containers. In one case, two brothers sued the Cryonic Society of California and a subsidiary, Cryonic Interment, for $10 million because their dead mother's body was accidentally allowed to thaw. They won a substantial amount of money.[56]

Alcor Life Extension Foundation does tell clients that in the event of an emergency, "including legal or financial emergencies," patients in whole-body suspension may be converted to the less-expensive neurosuspension (head only).[57]

## G. WHAT ARE THE PROSPECTS OF SUCCESSFULLY REVIVING A CRYONICALLY FROZEN BODY?

None at this time. Even devout cryonics advocates admit that the necessary science and technology to revive a cryonically preserved body are still in the realm of science fiction.

In 1981, *The Book of Lists* forecasted that by 1992 the first cryonically preserved individual would be successfully reanimated.[58] Yet 1993 has come and gone without a successful reanimation, and it is clear that none will happen any time soon. Some people have estimated the chance of successful reanimation of a cryonically preserved body (at least with present scientific and medical knowledge) to be one percent.[59] That may be a very generous estimate. While an embryo's undeveloped tissues and cells can be successfully implanted after being frozen, this is very different from reviving a biologically much more complex, not to mention unhealthy, person.

Early successful open-heart surgery involved rapid cooling of the body, and submersion in cold water has allowed some drowning victims to survive and return to normal function after more than one hour underwater. Human bodies have been intentionally cooled to temperatures as low as 48°F (9°C) for short periods of time and then revived.[60] Before the advent of heart-lung bypass machines, intentional cooling during heart surgery was used, as pioneered in 1951 by Pierre Huguenard of the Hospital Vaugirard in Paris.[61]

Sensational results from hypothermia have also occurred accidentally. In one dramatic case, Warren Churchill, a 60-year-old University of Wisconsin fish researcher accidentally fell into the icy (41°F/5°C) water of Lake Wingra, in April 1975. By the time he was rescued, his breathing had stopped and his heartbeat was barely noticeable. His body temperature had dropped to 61°F (16°C) by the time he got to the hospital two hours later. He survived without any brain damage. (Normal body temperature is 98.6°F (37°C).) These events, however, do not freeze the body's tissues and cells. When a cell freezes, the cell's mechanisms and wall are badly damaged.

Freezing not only damages individual cells, but entire organs as well. At temperatures below -202°F (-130°C), the liver, kidneys, heart, brain, lungs, spleen and other tissues simply crack. Cryopreservatives that are used actually exacerbate this process. This might not occur if bodies could be preserved at higher temperatures, but the need to curb costs and to use relatively simple and reliable technology presently limits human bodies to being stored at -321°F (-196°C).[62,63] Advocates, however, have faith that genetic and molecular manipulation techniques, now only in their infancy, will eventually allow successful reanimation.

Cryonicists routinely dismiss the damage done to brain cells from even a few minutes of oxygen deprivation at normal temperatures. At least with presently available technologies, cryonicists cannot cool the brain and spinal cord fast enough to preserve them intact. It would be unfortunate if cryonic preservation restored people to life with severe brain damage. Even the Alcor Life Extension Foundation, an ardent advocate of cryonics, admits in an obvious understatement, that "a serious scientific uncertainty of cryonic suspension today is possible memory and identity loss due to imperfect brain preservation."[64]

While some simple cells can easily be restored to life after freezing, it is unclear whether complex cells, entire organs or complex organisms such as people, could be reanimated—even under hypothetically perfect conditions. Different types of cells require different thawing conditions to survive freezing. To avoid cell damage during reanimation, even different types of cells next to one another in a single organ may need different thawing techniques. This may be due, in part, to the presence of ice outside of the cells forming or reforming at different rates during warming or cooling.

Even the size of organs plays havoc with freezing and thawing. A kidney, for example, has about 10 *trillion* times the volume of a single cell. And if a kidney is to work like a kidney after being thawed, its cells cannot be separated to optimize the rate at which each cell type freezes or thaws. The result is that complex cells and organs do not survive cryonic preservation with their functions intact.[65]

The only hope for cryonic reanimation lies in the repair of molecules and individual cells, including a cell repair technology that could identify billions of injured cells and repair or replace them. This technology would not only have to repair cells damaged by the original disease, but also repair the damage inflicted to body tissues by the freezing process. So far, however, these techniques are in the far-distant world of science fiction.

For successful reanimation, cryonicists are betting on *nanotechnology,* an infant discipline that combines science and engineering. Nanotechnology, first hypothesized by the Nobel-physicist Richard Feynman, extends the realm of current molecular biology to machines so small that they use individual molecules as tools and are fitted with cell-sized computers.[66]

Reanimation scenarios also anticipate successful brain transplants—without indicating whose body will be used. Elements of cryonic preservation, therefore, seem to combine *Star Trek's* science fiction with Dante's *Inferno.* Cryonicists however, emphasize that no macabre body snatching will be necessary since new bodies will be built from the ground up, as necessary.

The real questions one must ask are, "what constitutes a 'person'?" and "what should one ideally expect from reanimation after cryonic suspension?".

Personality, memories and abilities reside within the brain, specifically the cortex or outer portion of the brain. If the brain that contains this information is destroyed suddenly, as with a major head injury or a massive stroke, or slowly, through the progression of Alzheimer's disease or other types of dementia, does the "person" even remain? No, say most ethicists, legal and religious experts, and state statutes. Even cryonics adherents believe there are certain "identity-critical" brain structures without which a reanimated person would not be himself. The problem is, no one has any clue as to what these structures are.[67] It stands to reason, then, that if the brain is destroyed during life, cryonics will not preserve the "person," although an attempt may be made to preserve the body. Why preserve the body? Is it for experimentation, to benefit cryonics organizations, or to preserve future museum specimens?

One author has suggested that "like those ancient Egyptians who placed their faith in mummification, the cryonicists, rather than becoming the first immortalists, are more likely to be museum curios of the future."[68] Cryonicists say that even that is better than disintegration.[69]

## H. WHAT PROBLEMS WOULD THERE BE IF I WERE REANIMATED?

If a cryonaut could be reanimated, many questions remain unanswered. Would the reanimation process be horribly painful, would there be irreparable brain damage, or might the cryonaut be a freak in an advanced society? Ettinger spoke of "eventual rescue—revival, repair, rejuvenation and *improvement*."[70] Prospective cryonauts must *really* believe that enormous scientific advances will occur and that a future society will willingly expend its resources for the cryonaut to experience a second chance at life. (Of course, historians and anthropologists may feel compelled to attempt to revive a "living relic.") Even if cryonauts get this chance, will they want to enter a society that is markedly different from the one they left behind?

A more practical consideration for those considering cryonic preservation is whether their cryogenically preserved bodies or heads will be considered "fair game" for future researchers. We may feel reasonably secure about our current protections against inhumane or unconscionable research—but are we as confident about future societies? Certainly if scientists ever attempt human reanimation, bodies and heads now being cryonically preserved will necessarily be the subjects of the first tests. Current cryonic organizations explicitly state that "the results of being suspended cannot be guaranteed...Cryonic suspension is still an unproven procedure with many uncertainties. Problems exist on both social and technical levels."[71] Yet as proponents point out, many scientific advances that we now take for granted, such as airplanes, television, space travel, and computers were once considered impossible.[72]

Society may also face serious questions in the unlikely event that human reanimation becomes practical. Isaac Asimov suggested three social and personal problems with cryonic preservation that cannot be overcome: (1) prolonged life would become boring; (2) preserving old leaders would petrify society by recycling the "old dogs;" and (3) massive cryonic preservation might prevent our species from evolving into a better species before it becomes extinct.[73] Some writers have described cryonics as "a bad idea whose time has *not* come."[74] Yet proponents suggest that rather than thinking of cryonics as a "door to the future, it might be described as an emergency exit from a burning building."[75] In these situations, they say, "our primary concern should be making it to safety, not stopping to muse about our ability to adapt to that safety while flames are licking at our heels."[76]

## I. HOW RICH WOULD I BE IF I WERE REANIMATED?

The Reanimation Foundation, based in Liechtenstein, offers an Individual Reanimation Account (IRA) for potential cryonauts. With a minimum balance of $10,000 (in 1991) deposited through a Swiss bank, the investor stands to get a tidy sum—assuming both that the investor is reanimated and that the Foundation is still operating. The Foundation's brochure suggests that if the investor reawakens 100 years after cryopreservation, an investment of $100,000 at an interest rate of 8% would net $219,976,130. It goes on to say that the money would really be worth more than this, since more advanced technologies will be able to be purchased at lower costs.[77] Perhaps more financial scams will also be available. What about inflation? Who gets the money if reanimation does not occur or is unsuccessful? No one is saying.

## J. WHAT ARE RELIGIOUS & LEGAL ATTITUDES TOWARD CRYONICS?

Religious figures have only sporadically commented directly about cryonic preservation. Ettinger suggested that cryonics appeals to the humanistic "life affirming" nature of Christianity and Judaism.[78] Although an early Catholic proponent of cryonic preservation had a funeral Mass with consecration of the capsule after she was frozen,[79] the Church has remained skittish about the new "science."[80] Some proponents have argued that Christians should view successful cryonic preservation merely as extended life rather than as a scientific resurrection.

Similarly, although Steven Mandell had an Orthodox Jewish funeral in connection with his cryonic suspension, subsequent Jewish thought about cryonics has been less favorable. Rabbi Solomon B. Freehof, writing in the *American Reform Responsa,* says that since it is clearly prohibited in Jewish law to do anything to either hasten or delay a death which cannot be prevented by modern medicine, cryonics would be permissible only "if there were a trustworthy remedy already available for the disease, and this remedy involved freezing...If there is only speculation that some day a remedy might be discovered...that is contrary to the spirit of Jewish law."[81]

Secular law is equally skeptical about cryonic preservation. Although some medical examiners have investigated cryonics organizations, most states have remained silent on the matter of disposal of bodies by cryonic preservation. California bureaucrats have not viewed cryonics kindly. The California Department of Health Services refused a permit to dispose of human remains to the Alcor Life Extension Foundation. The state's contention was that cryonic suspension was not a legal method of disposing of human remains under current statutes. Although a superior court judge granted the permit, the state continued the appeal process through 1992, when the suit was finally quashed by the California Court of Appeals.[82,83]

In the Canadian province of British Columbia, however, a 1990 law prohibits the sale of human cryonic suspension services.[84] Although frozen bodies do not present a public health hazard, authorities want legal restrictions on cryonic preservation to limit what they see as a fraudulent enterprise. Since the chance of reanimation is nil, they believe cryonics organizations are simply bilking people of their money.

One unanswered legal question is whether a patient who is cryonically preserved before the moment of clinical death is legally dead. Leonard Tushnet explored this issue in his science fiction story, "In re Glover," but allowed the body to thaw because of a disruption in power to the preservation tank, before the question was resolved—an "act of God."[85] It is inconceivable, however, that a modern court would consider a cryonically preserved body or head alive. To do so would raise societally disruptive questions such as the duty of society to aid in cryonic preservation. Some cryonicists counter sarcastically, "better just declare them dead than raise delicate issues!"[86]

Legal issues would also have to be addressed, such as the proper distribution of the estate and insurance benefits, the status of a surviving spouse to remarry (what would " 'til death do us part" mean?), and the consummation of contracts with the "non-dead" individual. Other legal questions that should be of paramount importance to the potential cryonaut are who decides when to attempt to revive the body, and when are any heirs or descendants notified about a potential revival? Also, a point Ettinger raised, but failed to successfully answer is, would these former cadavers be citizens if they were reanimated?[87] No one has good answers, and the proponents of cryonics say somewhat simplistically that the law, as well as societal mores, will just have to be changed.

## K.  WHO ARE CRYONAUTS?

Actually, there are no cryonauts—at least not yet. A cryonaut, however, would be an individual, successfully reanimated after cryonic suspension, who rejoins society. Who, though, are members of cryonic societies, the potential cryonauts?

Generally, potential cryonauts are non-religious, apolitical, have above average education, and are in the lower- to middle-income bracket. Most are also unmarried, white males.[88] Many are devotees of science fiction for whom cryonics is a substitute for religion. Some cryonics adherents, unwilling to subscribe to the afterlife promised by many organized religions, "opt for cryonic preservation as a type of materialistic, active mastery over their own destinies."[89] For example, the motto of the Cryonics Society of New York was "Never say die."[90]

The best-known supposed cryonaut was actually never frozen. Many people believe the rumor that Walt Disney's corpse was cryonically preserved; it wasn't. Rather, his body was quietly cremated and the ashes inurned at Forest Lawn Cemetery.[91]

Cryonics has been described as a "cult." As as in other cults, "the true-

KENNETH V. ISERSON

believers are expected to completely subordinate all outside interests to the movement."[92] In support of this concept, Ettinger himself wrote:

> This is not a hobby or conversation piece: it is the principal activity of this phase of our lives; it is the struggle for survival. Drive a used car if the cost of a new one interferes. Divorce your wife if she will not cooperate. Save your money; get another job and save more money.[93]

In keeping with a cult tradition, some cryonics adherents marry each other. One woman, however, after finding out that her husband would probably be thawed at the same time she was, decided to forego preservation as not worth the effort![94] Most members think that reanimation will occur within a century and expect to find an improved society upon awakening.[95] The number of cryonics adherents, although small, seems to be growing at an increasing rate. Membership in largest cryonics group, Alcor Life Extension Foundation, went from 29 paid members in 1983 to 353 in 1993. Most of their members reside in California (147), New York (31), Florida (25), Arizona (12), and Nevada (12).[96] Alcor had 26 bodies or heads cryonically preserved as of April 1993.[97] In 1992, one group froze three patients in a single month.[98]

Some people become cryonics society members when they find they are dying. And, although Alcor actively discourages suicide, some members have intentionally dehydrated themselves to hasten their death and supposedly improve the quality of the cryopreservation.[99]

## L. HOW MUCH DOES CRYONIC PRESERVATION COST?

Cryonics is very expensive. The 1993 *minimum* fee at Alcor Life Extension Foundation, a cryonics organization near Riverside, California, was $120,000 for whole-body suspension. About $28,000 of this fee was for the suspension procedures and the balance was for long-term care. An additional minimum $10,000 fee was charged to those outside of the continental United States. The price for neurosuspension was raised to $50,000 on January 1, 1994, with about $19,000 for the suspension procedure and the balance for long-term care.[100]

Nearly all those currently in cryosuspension were already Alcor Life Extension Foundation members when they died. Membership in Alcor currently costs $100 as an application fee plus $324 per year (half-price for students). People who appear competent, can sign the appropriate papers, and pass financial scrutiny can even become members on their death beds. If they are not competent, yet family members wish for the body to be cryonically preserved, they may be accepted for cryonic preservation as non-members, but a with surcharge of $25,000. This fee is used for legal defense if other relatives later appear and challenge the procedure.[101] The

Foundation charges additional fees if the cryonics team must standby at a dying patient's bedside, if long-distance transport is required, or if a Foundation-supplied nurse provides care at home for a dying patient. Additional standby fees alone normally average about $15,000.[102]

Many people pay for cryonic preservation by using life insurance policies. With Alcor Life Extension Foundation, the person names the Foundation as the beneficiary of a policy covering at least the minimal fee for the services they desire. Such policies cost about $540 per year in premiums for a policy that will pay for neurosuspension (at 1991 prices).[103] Cryonics organizations are more than pleased to help arrange this insurance policy. A major question to be considered is if insurance companies will want their money back if cryonauts are revived? Another consideration is whether, after reanimation, people will be able to afford treatment for their originally lethal medical condition.

Finances are serious business in the cryonics movement. When Andrew D. Mihok died of a heart attack in 1968, the New York Cryonics Society quickly froze him. However, when his widow was unable to pay for long-term freezing and storage, he was quickly defrosted and given a military burial.[104] If a person pre-pays for cryonic suspension but the procedure is not possible due to the individual's place or method of death, some organizations permit secondary beneficiaries to be cryonically preserved in their place. People must arrange this at the time they enroll.[105] Money is not normally refunded if cryonics is not used.

Is cryonics too expensive, especially if it is a hoax? One writer compared it with other unusual human behavior concerning the dead, saying, "Some amused observers contend that $10,000 spent on the cryogenic preservation of a corpse is no more wasteful, or useful, than a comparable sum spent on a bronze casket."[106]

## M. REFERENCES

1. Franklin B: Quoted in: Wallis CL: *Stories on Stone.* NY: Oxford Univ Press, 1954, p 240.
2. Jones NR: The Jameson Satellite. *Amazing Stories.* Radio-Science, July 1931. Reprinted in Asimov I, ed: *Before the Golden Age—A Science Fiction Anthology of the 1930s.* London: Robson, 1974, pp 43-64.
3. Ettinger RCW: *The Prospect of Immortality.* New York: Doubleday, 1964, p xxi.
4. Ibid., p 1.
5. Smith GP: *Medical-Legal Aspects of Cryonics: Prospects for Immortality.* Port Washington, NY: Associated Faculty Press, 1983, p 16.
6. Prehoda RW: *Suspended Animation.* Philadelphia, PA: Chilton Book, 1969, pp 111-12.
7. Ettinger RC: Letter. *Freeze-Wait-Reanimate.* 1965;13:4.
8. Prehoda, *Suspended Animation,* pp 111-12.
9. Kurtzman J, Gordon P: *No More Dying—The Conquest of Aging and the Extension of Human Life.* Los Angeles: JP Tarcher, 1976, pp 199-217.

10. Smith, *Medical-Legal Aspects of Cryonics,* pp 9-11.
11. Nelson RF: *We Froze the First Man.* New York: Dell, 1968.
12. Perry M: Personal communication. October 23, 1993.
13. Dempsey D: *The Way We Die.* New York: MacMillan, 1975, pp 189-91.
14. Cryonic suspension of Steven J. Mandell. *Cryonics Reports.* 1968;3(9):162-66.
15. Perry M: Suspension failures: the dark side of cryonics history. *Cryonics.* 1992;13(2):5.
16. Ibid.
17. Platt C: Confessions of a cryonicist. *OMNI.* February 1, 1992, p 28.
18. Ibid.
19. Platt C: Letter. *Cryonics.* 1993;14(10):4-5.
20. Wowk B, Darwin M: *Cryonics—Reaching for Tomorrow.* 3rd ed. Riverside, CA: Alcor Life Extension Found, 1991, p 47.
21. Ibid., p 40.
22. Ettinger, *Prospect of Immortality,* p 6.
23. Goldman DE: The American way of life? *Science.* 1964;3631:475-76.
24. Prehoda, *Suspended Animation,* p 110.
25. Society for Cryobiology: *Society By-Laws, Sec 2.04.* Denial of Membership and Discipline of Members.
26. Rowe A: As quoted in: Wowk, Darwin, *Cryonics,* p A40.
27. Pegg DE: As quoted in: Wowk, Darwin, *Cryonics,* p A39.
28. Baust, J: As quoted in: Wowk, Darwin, *Cryonics,* p A40.
29. Southard J. As quoted in: Wowk, Darwin, *Cryonics,* p A40.
30. Prehoda, *Suspended Animation,* p 108.
31. Clarke, AC: Letter. In: Wowk, Darwin, *Cryonics,* p A41.
32. Lewis J: Letter to Christopher Ashworth. dated January 22, 1988. CA Sup Ct, Riverside, CA, Case no. 191277. Appendix of Declarations, February 1, 1988.
33. Merkle RC: The technical feasibility of cryonics. *Medical Hypotheses.* 1992;39:6-16.
34. Bridge S: *Cryonics, The Home Town Way: Practical Planning For A Cryonic Suspension In Your Own Area.* (pamphlet). Riverside, CA: Alcor Life Extension Found, June 1989.
35. Merkle, *Medical Hypotheses,* 1992.
36. Anderson P: *Affairs in Order.* New York: MacMillan, 1991, p 56.
37. Wowk, Darwin, *Cryonics,* pp 27-28.
38. Ibid., pp 31-37.
39. Ibid.
40. Ibid.
41. Ibid.
42. Ibid, p 28.
43. Ibid, p 26.
44. *Donaldson vs. Van de Kamp,* 4 Cal. Rptr. 2d 59, 60 (Cal. Ct. App. 1992).
45. Ibid.
46. Ibid.
47. Wowk, Darwin, *Cryonics,* pp 27-28.
48. Bridge S: Financial Changes. *Cryonics.* 1993;14(4):6+.
49. *Saul Kent v. Raymond L. Carillo, et. al.,* Superior court of the State of California, County of Riverside, Docket No. R191277.
50. Wowk, Darwin, *Cryonics,* p 36-37.
51. Ettinger RCW: *Man Into Superman.* New York: St. Martin's Press, 1972, pp 43-87.
52. Bridge S: Details make the difference. *Cryonics.* 1993;14(4):14-15.
53. Anderson, *Affairs in Order,* p 56-57.
54. Perry M: They froze the first man. For the Record. *Cryonics.* 1993;14(4):3-6.
55. Perry, Suspension failures, *Cryonics,* 1992.
56. Perry, They froze the first man, *Cryonics,* 1993.
57. Wowk, Darwin, *Cryonics,* p 37.
58. Wallechinsky D, Wallace A, Wallace I: *The Book of Lists.* New York: Bantam, 1981, pp 162-63.
59. Georgakas D: *The Methuselah Factors—Strategies for a Long and Vigorous Life.* New York: Simon & Schuster, 1980, pp 288-89.

60. Niazi SA, Lewis FJ: Profound hypothermia in man: Report of a case. *Annals of Surgery.* 1958;147:264-66.
61. Kurtzman, Gordon, *No More Dying,* pp 199-217.
62. Federowicz MG, et al: Postmortem examination of three cryonic suspension patients. *Cryonics.* 1984;5:16.
63. Kroener C, Luyet BJ: Formation of cracks during the vitrification of glycerol solutions and disappearance of the cracks during rewarming. *Biodynamica.* 1966;10:47-52.
64. Wowk, Darwin, *Cryonics,* p 43.
65. McGrath JJ, ed: *Low Temperature Biotechnology: Emerging Appliations and Engineering Contributions.* New York: American Soc Mechanical Engineers, 1988, p 11.
66. Feynman R: There's plenty of room at the bottom. In: Gilbert HD, ed: *Miniaturization.* New York: Reinhold, 1961, pp 282-96.
67. Wowk, Darwin, *Cryonics,* p 22.
68. Georgakas, *The Methusala Factor,* pp 288-89.
69. Perry M: Personal communication. October 23, 1993.
70. Ettinger, *Man Into Superman,* preface.
71. Wowk, Darwin, *Cryonics,* p 38.
72. Ibid, pp 38-40.
73. Asimov I: The Price of Life. *Cavalier Magazine.* January 1967.
74. Dempsey, *The Way We Die,* p 191.
75. Wowk, Darwin, *Cryonics,* p 46.
76. Ibid.
77. For the return trip: Firm offers IRA for the cryogenic. *The American Funeral Director.* 1991;114(3):16.
78. Ettinger, *Man Into Superman,* p 208.
79. Ibid., p 258.
80. Smith, *Medical-Legal Aspects of Cryonics,* p 18.
81. Freehof SB: Freezing bodies for later revival (cryobiology). In: Jacob W, ed: *American Reform Responsa.* vol 1. New York: Central Conf of American Rabbis, 1983, pp 277-78.
82. Platt C: Questions and answers about cryonics. *OMNI.* 1993;15(4):41-46.
83. *Mitchell v. Roe,* 9 Cal Rptr. 2d 572 (Cal. Ct. of App., July 7, 1992).
84. *British Columbia Cemetery and Funeral Services Act.* para 57. 1990.
85. Tushnet L: *In re Glover.* In: Sargent P, ed: *Bio-Futures: Science Fiction Stories About Biological Metamorphosis.* New York: Vintage Books, 1976, pp 39-53.
86. Perry M: Personal communication. October 23, 1993.
87. Ettinger, *Prospect of Immortality,* pp 102-103.
88. Perry M: Personal communication. October 23, 1993.
89. Bryant CD, Snizek WE: The cryonics movement and frozen immortality. *Society.* 1973;11(1):56-61.
90. Dempsey, *The Way We Die,* pp 189-91.
91. Poundstone W: *Big Secrets.* New York: Morrow, 1985, pp 2119-224.
92. Prehoda, *Suspended Animation,* p 108.
93. Ettinger RW: *Cryonics Reports.* 1967;2(9):6.
94. Ettinger, *Man Into Superman,* p 100.
95. Bryant, Snizek, *Society,* 1973.
95. Ryan D: An update on membership growth. *Cryonics.* 1993;14(4):9-14.
97. Bridge, Financial Changes, *Cryonics,* 1993.
98. Platt, *OMNI,* 1993.
99. Whelan R: Beginnings of winter. *Cryonics.* 1993;14(4):16-19.
100. Bridge, Financial Changes, *Cryonics,* 1993.
101. Telephone information from Alcor Foundation. April 15, 1993.
102. Ibid.
103. Wowk, Darwin, *Cryonics,* pp A27-A37.
104. Bryant, Snizek, *Society,* 1973.
105. Wowk, Darwin, *Cryonics,* pp 53.
106. Prehoda, *Suspended Animation,* p 109.

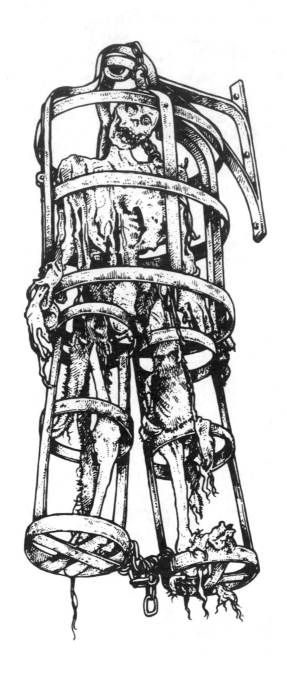

The gibbet.

# 8: WAYWARD BODIES

A. What happens to bodies exposed to the environment?
B. Will the "worms crawl in"?
C. Do other animals eat corpses?
D. How long does it take for an exposed body to turn to dust?
E. Will embalming prevent decay?
F. May I be buried at sea?
G. How are bodies buried at sea?
H. What happens to a body interred in water?
I. Are bodies buried at sea eaten by fish?
J. Must a boat be used for a water burial?
K. Why do dead bodies float?
L. What will happen to bodies adrift in space?
M. Why steal corpses for anatomical study?
N. Why else were corpses stolen?
O. How were corpses stolen?
P. How were graves protected?
Q. Who were some infamous body snatchers?
R. Was corpse stealing common in the United States?
S. What happened to captured grave robbers?
T. When were "grave-robbed" bodies not dead?
U. Are corpses still stolen?
V. May I be buried in foreign soil?
W. How and why are corpses transported across international borders?
X. How are bodies or ashes transported into the United States?
Y. How are bodies or ashes transported by air?
Z. Are there problems transporting bodies or ashes across state lines?
AA. Will I be an archaeological find?
AB. References

*What happens when dead bodies do not find a final disposition in a grave or as cremated remains? What happens to bodies exposed to the environment, buried at sea, robbed from their graves, and taken for archaeological study? What might happen to dead bodies in space? How can the bodies of people who die in distant places be transported or cremated?*

## A. WHAT HAPPENS TO BODIES EXPOSED TO THE ENVIRONMENT?

Exposed corpses normally decompose, although researchers are only now learning how this occurs. Since 1980, the Anthropology Research Facility of the University of Tennessee in Knoxville has been studying the natural decay process using the bodies of homicide victims, bodies donated to science and unidentified bodies. Researchers discovered that bodies actually decompose at different rates, depending upon multiple factors (Table 8.1). They have also found that bodies go through four stages after death: fresh, bloating, decay, and dry—that vary depending upon various environmental factors.[1]

Although the studies may appear ghoulish, they have given forensic pathologists a baseline from which to determine the time and nature of death when bodies are found.[2] *Quincy* would have been lost without this information.

Temperature and access to the body by carrion insects and carnivores have the greatest effect on a body's decay rate. Warm temperatures accelerate decomposition and freezing temperatures drastically slow the process, primarily by promoting or reducing activity by scavengers.

In warm to hot weather, a body completely exposed to the elements takes only two to four weeks to be reduced to a skeleton. Carrion insects and carnivorous animals, stimulated by warm weather, play a large role in this destruction. Anything that protects a body from these invaders slows decomposition.

Burying a body or even wrapping it in a plastic covering and leaving it on the ground will protect it from carrion insects and carnivores. Shallow burials are also protective, but much less so than deeper burials. When buried at depths of 1 or 2 feet (0.3 or 0.6 meters) bodies may be reduced to skeletons in a few months to a year, while those buried only slightly deeper, at 3 or 4 feet (0.9 or 1.2 meters) may take many years to skeletonize. It appears that the speed with which a corpse will decompose primarily depends on how many and what types of critters are able to get to the body.[3]

Warm temperatures also hasten decomposition by the body's natural enzymes. Enzymes (chemical catalysts) are found in many of the body's cells, and in the digestive juices that help break down food while the body is alive. In warm bodies, these enzymes continue to work after death, destroying

308

## TABLE 8.1: Variables Affecting Decay Rate of the Human Body

| *Variable* | *Effect on Decay Rate[*]* |
|---|---|
| Temperature | 5 |
| Access by insects | 5 |
| Burial and depth | 5 |
| Carnivore/rodent access | 4 |
| Trauma (penetrating/crushing) | 4 |
| Humidity/aridity | 4 |
| Rainfall | 3 |
| Body size and weight | 3 |
| Prior embalming | 3 |
| Clothing | 2 |
| Surface body rests on | 1 |

[*] Subjective criteria, with "5" the most influential factor.

Adapted from: Mann RW, Bass WM, Meadows L: Time since death and decomposition of the human body: variables and observations in case and experimental field studies. *J Forensic Sciences.* 1990;35(1):103-111.

tissues in a process called autolysis. When a person dies from an illness with a high fever, this process accelerates and the stomach or lower esophagus can perforate within a few hours after death, spreading enzymes and digestive juices throughout the abdomen.[4]

Conversely, cold weather slows decomposition, primarily by slowing the activity of carnivorous insects. While insects, especially flies and their maggots, normally ravage an exposed corpse, cold temperatures slow or stop this carnage. Below about 45°F/5°C, flies are not very active and are less likely to visit a body and lay eggs. Below freezing (32°F/0°C), any fly eggs and all maggots outside of the corpse die. If eggs have been deposited within the body, however, the maggots will give off enough heat to survive and will continue to feed even in freezing weather. They produce so much heat, in fact, that when a pathologist opens a portion of a frozen corpse where maggots are feeding, steam vapors rise from the body. The larger carnivores, such as birds and mammals, also are slowed by cold weather.

Cold weather also slows or stops the other mechanisms through which bodies decompose. (The normal mechanisms of decomposition are discussed in Chapter 2, *What will happen to my body when I die?*) Extreme cold inactivates the body's enzymatic breakdown (autolysis) and slows bacterial activity (putrefaction). Corpses in freezing conditions may, therefore, not decay. However, their skin changes from its natural color to orange or black, usually embellished with patches of mold.

"Iceman" is an extreme example of low temperatures halting decomposition. "Iceman" is the body of a Stone Age hunter discovered by a tourist in September 1991 on the Similaun glacier in the Oetztaler Alps (hence his local nickname, *Oetzi*), 10,500 feet above the Italian-Austrian border. This 30-year-old mountaineer met his demise by falling into a crevasse about 5,300 years ago, or more than three millennia before Christ was born! Not only was his body preserved, including the elaborate tattoos on his back and knees, but so were his leather clothes, an arrow quiver, 14 arrows and a copper axe. He currently lies frozen at the University of Innsbruck, Austria, while scientists investigate his corpse amidst scientific and political haggling.[5] In 1994 the body will be returned to Italy as a tourist attraction, although the Austrians are already inundating tourists with "Oetzi" momentos.[6]

Fresh-frozen corpses are still being accidentally produced, even in the heart of our modern society. In 1992 an 84-year-old Swedish woman died while sitting on her balcony in the Stockholm suburb of Traneberg. After she sat there for two months, her neighbors decided that something was wrong when she didn't go inside, even during blizzards. Authorities speculate that she died on New Year's Eve while watching the city's fireworks. They found her body to be very well preserved in that extremely cold climate.[7]

## B. WILL THE "WORMS CRAWL IN?"

In bodies left unprotected from the elements, "worms" will indeed make their grand appearance and help nature return them to dust. The "worms," however, are normally maggots, and rather than "crawling in," they arrive airmail. Forensic entomologists now use insect evidence to determine the time of death and help identify murderers.

Maggots were once thought to be a type of worm, and many writers throughout the ages commented on the effect of "worms" on the corpse. (See Chapter 15: *Say It Gently: Words, Sayings and Poetry About the Dead.*) Shakespeare, among others, described man simply as "worms' meat."[8] Similarly, the *Book of Job (24:20)* records that "The worms shall feed sweetly on him." The best known description of these "worms," however, was first penned in 1795 by M.G. Lewis, who wrote, "The worms they crept in, and the worms they crept out, And sported his eyes and his temples about."[9] This was modernized by British soldiers during the Crimean War (1854-1856) and by unknown multitudes thereafter, so that one twentieth-century version of the song goes:

310

Did you ever think when a hearse goes by,
That you may be the next to die?

They take you out to the family plot,
And there you wither, decay and rot.

They wrap you up in a bloody sheet,
And then they bury you six-feet deep.

And all goes well for a week or two,
And then things start to happen to you.

The worms crawl in the worms crawl out,
The ants play pinochle on your snout!

One of the worms that's not so shy,
Crawls in one ear and out one eye.

They call their friends and their friends' friends too,
They'll make a horrid mess of you!

And then your blood turns yellow-green,
And oozes out like whipping cream.
[Spoken] Darn, me without a spoon!

Your eyes fall in your teeth fall out,
Your liver turns to sauerkraut.

So never laugh when a hearse goes by,
For you may be the next to die.[10]

Yet, as might be expected, it was Edgar Allan Poe who epitomized the gruesomeness of a moldering corpse by writing of the dreadful "Conqueror worm," in *Ligeia*:

But see, amid the mimic rout,
  A crawling shape intrude!
A blood-red thing that writhes from out
  The scenic solitude!

It writhes!—it writhes!—with mortal pangs
  The mimes become its food,
And the seraphs sob at vermin fangs
  In human gore imbued.[11]

Insects, however, do not just happen upon a corpse, but appear to be attracted by a "universal death scent." What causes this scent has yet to be determined, but it seems to powerfully summon the insect population which can recognize microscopic quantities of odor-producing chemicals.[12] Although people cannot detect the odor from a newly-dead body, flies, especially fleshflies (*Sarcophagidae*) and blowflies (*Calliphoridae*), swarm to the odor from as far away as two miles. In wooded areas, especially where there have previously been dead animals or humans, they begin to land on a corpse within seconds, and within one hour some species may produce maggots.[13,14] Even in areas without prior bodies, they land on exposed corpses within the first few hours (wrapping or burning a body delays this).[15] In the open air these flies quickly lay thousands of eggs in a body's mouth, nose and ears. If the body has suffered a penetrating or crushing injury (e.g., gunshot wound), a large number of flies land on the wound area, causing the body to decompose faster than normal.[16] When they are finished feeding, they leave the body, only to be replaced by beetles who come to feed on the drying skin. Beetles are subsequently replaced by spiders, mites and millipedes which feed on the insects already there or on the body itself. Catts and Goff describe four roles for arthropods around a corpse:

1. Necrophages: the species feeding on corpse tissue (Often *Diptera* and *Coleoptera*).
2. Omnivores: species that feed on both the corpse and associated fauna (ants, wasps, and some beetles).
3. Parasites and Predators: species that feed on both the corpse and other arthropods. Some species are parasites in the early larval stage and become predaceous later.
4. Incidentals: species that use the corpse to extend their normal habitat, such as spiders, centipedes, pill bugs, and some mites.[17]

Not only do insects swarm over an exposed corpse in great numbers, but they also arrive in a very precise sequence depending upon the body's location and condition. This has given rise to a new field, forensic entomology. Since the exact feeding pattern varies with a body's location, the time of death, and the climate, forensic entomologists are often able to determine the date of death very accurately—even a decade later.

On several occasions criminals have been convicted after committing a "perfect crime"—just because of some dead insects.

The first recorded episode of insects revealing a killer occurred in thirteenth-century China, where an individual had been slashed to death in a rural village. When no one confessed, authorities ordered all of the villagers to lay down their sickles. The murderer was identified when flies swarmed to only his sickle, an apparently clean implement that still retained small traces of the victim's flesh and blood.[18] Insects were also used to identify the killer in England's famous Lydney murder trial, when the time of death, as determined from insect evidence, invalidated the killer's alibi.[19]

More recently, insect evidence helped Tacoma, Washington police track down the killer of a man found dead from a gunshot wound in a room completely sealed from the inside. Entomological investigators found two generations of maggots in the body, allowing them to determine that the death had occurred a little more than three weeks before the body was found. (Depending on local factors, it generally takes one generation about three weeks to reach adulthood). By dating the death, police were able to discover that a man had fired a gun during a party at a nearby house, and had accidentally killed the victim.[20]

Police in Wisconsin and Hawaii have also used insect evidence to place suspects with victims at the time of death, and one murderer was convicted when his story about coming home to find his girlfriend dead and the windows open did not match the insect evidence. The body was not infested with insects as it would have been if the windows had really been open since her death.[21] In another "perfect" crime, a Florida murderer dumped the body of his victim in a swamp during one of the few days when mayflies were active. His alibi collapsed when investigators found mayflies on his car radiator.[22]

Insect evidence can also help free the innocent. The first European case using forensic entomology was in the mid-nineteenth century. It led to the acquittal of a French couple accused of murdering an infant whose mummified remains were discovered behind the mantelpiece in their home.[23] In a Hungarian case, a ferryboat captain was sentenced to life imprisonment for murdering a postmaster aboard his vessel. After serving eight years in prison, he was exonerated when a forensic entomologist proved that the insect larvae in the corpse had to have been laid before the captain ever boarded his vessel.[24]

Intentionally exposed bodies are not the only ones subject to the ravages of the insect world. Recently, a California family was temporarily storing the body of their oversized relative in a cemetery shed until the grave could be widened. They were aghast to find the casket swarming with ants. The cemetery then had to hire a funeral home to take on the task of laying these wayward ants to rest before they buried the body.[25]

## C. DO OTHER ANIMALS EAT CORPSES?

Carnivores and rodents also help destroy exposed corpses. Carnivores, including dogs, coyotes, wolves, and foxes, eat the body's soft tissues, especially the face and hands. They also prefer the spongy parts of the arm and leg bones, pelvis and backbone. Dogs and coyotes eat exposed human corpses in a definite order (Table 8.2) and often carry the bones long distances to their dens to continue feeding.[26] Mice and rats generally feed on the soft tissues of the face, hands, and feet, on the abdominal organs, and on the small bones of the hands and feet.[27] The farther away from human habitation a corpse lies, the greater the chance that a carnivore will feed on it, although even Lassie might take a bite from a corpse should one show up in her neighborhood.

At one time fire departments throughout the United States had Dalmatians ride with them as mascots. This practice, however, declined rapidly once fire trucks began to routinely accompany ambulances to accident scenes. When they noticed that "Spot" had an affinity for the flesh of victim's bodies, the firemen decided that neither their public image nor their stomachs could tolerate their dogs' atavistic eating habits. "Spot" was retired and no longer rides the engines.

## D. HOW LONG DOES IT TAKE FOR AN EXPOSED BODY TO TURN TO DUST?

An unembalmed adult body buried six-feet deep in ordinary soil without a coffin normally takes ten to twelve years to decompose down to the bony skeleton; a child's body takes about half that time. Burial depth and soil temperature vary the decomposition rate. The rate of decay is the same in different-sized adult corpses and those of men and women. Clothing on exposed bodies may speed up decay, since it provides the shade maggots seek.[28] Given approximately the same temperature, body size, clothing, and other factors, a body in water (without fish or reptiles) decomposes four times faster, and a body in air eight times faster, than when buried.[29]

In 1868, a British surgeon examined a series of 350-year-old graves to see how the bodies had fared. Francis Haden studied the bodies buried at the St. Andrews, Holborn, burial ground while they were being disinterred to make way for a viaduct. Only putrid, unrecognizable contents remained of the bodies buried in still-intact wooden or lead coffins. When the coffins were no longer intact or the bodies had been buried without coffins as in the plague pit, nothing remained except a few bones. As he said, "the body itself had disappeared, and 'earth to earth' had been accomplished."[30] More recently, a group of dental researchers found that the skulls of younger adults remain intact longer than those of older people, no matter how long they have been buried.[31]

Scottish lore held that a "grave was ripe" for twenty years after burial, meaning that it was likely that more than bones would turn up if the grave were reopened before that time. Since the Scots frequently reused gravesites, this maxim was well-founded. It applied, however, mainly to unembalmed bodies that were buried in wooden coffins or without any containers. This informal guideline was eventually incorporated into the Burial Grounds Act.

Environmental conditions can delay decomposition.

Desert climates with low humidity not only decrease or obliterate fly and maggot activity, but can also halt other forms of decomposition. Very dry climates may cause a body to naturally mummify, converting its skin and tendons to a leathery or parchment-like wrapping surrounding the bones, while the organs decay by autolysis and putrefaction.[32] Paradoxically, heavy

## TABLE 8.2: Stages of Carnivores Feeding on Exposed Human Corpses

STAGE 1: Front of the chest eaten and one or both arms removed. The facial tissues are often eaten away.

STAGE 2: Both legs eaten and possibly removed.

STAGE 3: Only the bones of the spine remain connected. Virtually all of the flesh is gone.

STAGE 4: All body parts devoured. The bones or fragments of bones are widely scattered.

Adapted from: Haglund WD, Reay DT, Swindler DR: Canid scavenging/disarticulation sequence of human remains in the Pacific northwest. *J Forensic Sciences.* 89;34:587-606.

rainfall also slows fly activity, including egg laying. Maggot activity, however, continues—but with fewer maggots.[33]

When bodies are exposed to cool moist soil, the soft tissues may decay slowly and turn into adipocere ("fat-wax"), a cheesy, grayish-white mass produced when the body's proteins convert to fat. This state of decomposition may last for many years, since adipocere inhibits the action of putrefactive bacteria.[34]

The "Bog people" who have been found for centuries throughout Europe represent a similar type of preservation. While soil acidity alone does not affect decomposition, the combination of the acid water and the almost-total absence of air occurring in former bogs has tanned the skins of, and helped to preserve these unusual corpses.[35] An 1837 Danish almanac says of this odd phenomenon, "There is a strange power in bog water which prevents decay. Bodies have been found which must have lain in bogs for more than a thousand years, but which, though admittedly somewhat shrunken and brown, are in other respects unchanged."[36] In the last two hundred years, more than 150 preserved bodies of men, women and children, many 5,000 years old, have been discovered in Danish peat bogs alone. Some of these bodies still show evidence of having been murdered or ritually sacrificed, as was said of the infamous Queen Gunhild:

Now you lie naked, shrivelled and foul
With a bald skull for a head
Blacker far than the oaken stake
That wed you to the bog.[37]

Bog people are not confined to Europe. One Florida bog has yielded up the remains of nearly two hundred 8,000-year-old Native Americans. The combination of a lack of oxygen, minerals which inhibited bacterial and fungal growth, and alkalinizing plant life within the bog has preserved these ancients' brain DNA which scientists are now studying. They hope to unearth secrets about the history, medical diseases, and susceptibility to disease of these ancients, and to better define the interactions among prehistoric American peoples.[38]

Except for these unusual cases, however, bodies exposed to the environment will generally be reduced to skeletons relatively quickly. How fast the boney skeleton turns to dust ranges from months to millennia.

### E. WILL EMBALMING PREVENT DECAY?

Yes, no and maybe.

Yes, because intense embalming prevents decay for many years—even occasionally for centuries. Embalming, however, is rarely done thoroughly enough to slow decay of the entire body. Embalmers normally concentrate on the parts of the body that mourners see, such as the face, neck and hands. Body parts that are covered by clothing normally receive much less attention. (For more detail on embalming, see Chapter 5, *Beauty in Death*.)

An embalmed body exposed to the environment decomposes differently than a non-embalmed body, in part because insects dislike embalming chemicals. Embalmed bodies decompose first in the buttocks and legs, perhaps because the chemicals do not reach these areas in sufficient amounts. The last areas to decompose are the face, chest, arms and hands, although they do shrivel from dehydration.[39]

Anyone seriously interested in slowing a body's decay must get a better-than-average embalming job. They can inform the embalmer that they will be checking on the condition of a loved one's body over the next year. One man who did periodically inspect the condition of his mother's body after it had been interred in a mausoleum, found that the body was badly decomposed after a supposedly excellent embalming job. He sued the funeral home—and won.

### F. MAY I BE BURIED AT SEA?

Yes. Sea burials are possible, but they may be rather expensive and difficult to arrange, depending upon what you desire. Civilian "sea burials" are offered in the United States through funeral homes in California, Maine, North Carolina, Florida, and New York. However, these "sea burials" usually mean scattering cremated remains at sea, rather than whole-body interment. Scattering cremains at sea can often be performed for a small sum ($40 to $100) if the ashes are sent to the company. If they hold a memorial service aboard the boat, however, the cost may be over $1,000.[40]

Scatterings at sea are also done from airplanes. Stories abound concerning airplane scatterings that have gone awry. The typical scenario involves a novice "scatterer" who attempts to dump the ashes into the sea from the small window of a private plane. Unfortunately, unless the pilot slows down the plane, the force of the wind blows the ashes back into the plane, covering both the passengers and the cockpit.

Whole-body interment at sea, though unusual in the civilian sector, is available through at least one company in New York, one in North Carolina, and the Neptune Society. According to Sea Services, Inc., in New York, these interments cost $8,000 to $10,000, with the fee covering both the funeral home preparation of the body and the sea burial. Sea Services allows only one visitor to witness a whole-body sea burial since they usually inter the corpse from a relatively small boat, far out to sea (in international waters), resulting in an uncomfortable ride in the normally rough seas. Companies that perform either scatterings or whole-body sea burials conform to state and federal requirements and will complete required Environmental Protection Agency reports. The paperwork includes a description of the exact location of the burial so that if a fisherman dredges up a body, as occasionally happens, it can be identified from records of known sea burials.[41]

With an understanding funeral director, sea burials can be arranged almost anywhere there is a seacoast. One California woman, for example, wanted to be buried at sea in a hand-carved canoe. She could not obtain a local sea burial, however, because whole-body interment is illegal in California waters. When she died, her mortician put her body and a canoe in a U-Haul[R] truck and drove it to Oregon. He launched the funeral canoe from a fishing vessel about 15 miles off the coast. The total cost was about $4,000.[42]

According to the Retired Officers Association, the U.S. Navy offers burials at sea or sea scattering of cremated remains to those eligible for a military burial. They can do this, however, only if they have a ship and personnel available when and where the burial will take place. There is no cost to the family except for preparation of the body and its transportation to the designated ship's port. The U.S. Coast Guard performs the same service for retirees or spouses of retirees.[43] Unfortunately, these arrangements cannot be made in advance and the agencies involved may require a request in writing at the time of death. To contact the Navy, write or call the Casualty Assistance Branch, Code NMPC-122, Department of the Navy, Washington, D.C. 20370; (202)694-2926. For the Coast Guard, write or call the Commandant, U.S. Coast Guard Headquarters, (G-PS-1) Trans Point Bldg., 2100 Second Street, Room 4402, Washington, D.C. 20593-0001; (202)267-1845.

If this method of disposition is used, the Retired Officers Association recommends that a memorial headstone be obtained from the Veterans Administration (VA Form 49-1330) and erected in a national cemetery. This preserves the spouse's right to also be buried in a national cemetery, and is itself an old military tradition.[44]

While whole-body sea burials are uncommon, they are a legitimate method of body disposal. U.S. courts have held that sea burial, when necessary, is both legal and acceptable. One state court said that "A decent committal of the body to the deep in accordance with the custom in such matters ordinarily discharges the duty which the law imposes."[45]

## G. HOW ARE BODIES BURIED AT SEA?

Burial at sea has traditionally meant either sliding a corpse ceremonially off the side of a ship or placing a body on a ship that is set adrift. Nowadays, sea burial has also come to mean scattering cremated remains over the ocean. No matter what the method, sea interment has always had special meaning for various societies and religions.

The ancient Romans feared dying in shipwrecks, since their bodies would then end up in the sea rather than being buried in the ground. As a result, they believed, they might have to wander along the river Styx for a hundred years before entering the land of the dead.[46]

While most religions do not comment on sea burials, Jewish tradition bans sea burials except in crisis conditions. They even permit the usually prohibited custom of embalming if it is necessary to keep the body intact until it reaches land.[47]

Early Europeans often equated water burial with the myth of the god-hero who sailed away with a promise to return. This led to elaborate sea burial ceremonies. Wealthy Vikings, for example, were usually cremated with their ships. Accounts from the tenth century A.D. describe bodies being taken from temporary graves to their ships, that were then set ablaze. Depending upon the wealth and power of the individual, clothing, weapons, dead animals, and even sacrificed servants were also placed on board. David Dempsey describes a modern variation of this theme in his account of a multimillionairess who gave her loyal yacht captain the sea burial he wanted by sinking his body off the Florida coast inside the yacht he had commanded.[48]

Less heroic was the use of water burials in southeastern France during one of the great plagues of the Middle Ages. Faced with an increasing number of corpses, and knowing that both burial and cremation take time and effort, "in Avignon the Pope saw himself obliged to consecrate the Rhône, so that the corpses could be thrown into it without delay, when the churchyards were no longer sufficient."[49]

Some modern cultures also perform sea burials. The Badjaos, or sea gypsies of the Philippines for example, weight their dead with boulders or metal blocks and throw them into the sea along with their favorite possessions, such as fishing nets, hook-and-lines, or paddles.[50]

Deaths aboard ships usually warranted a sea burial. The following are three descriptions of sea burials in different eras. In 1652, Captain John Smith (of Pocahontas fame) wrote that a surgeon's duty after a sea battle was to "winde up the slaine, with each a bullet or weight at their heads and feet to make them sinke; and give them three Gunnes for their funeral."[51]

A nineteenth-century writer described a shipboard burial in the British Navy:

> The deceased is prepared by his messmates for his 'deep sea grave;' who, with the assistance of the sailmaker, in presence of the master-at-arms, sew him up in his hammock, putting a couple of shot at his feet. The body is then carried aft, and placed upon the after-hatchway, or on the half-deck, with the Union Jack thrown over all...When all is ready, the chaplain (the captain, or any of the officers) reads the service for the dead. On coming to the passage, 'we therefore commit his body to the deep,' one of the sailors disengages the flag, and the others launch the grating [on which the body rests] overboard; the body, loaded with the shot at one end, glances off the grating, and plunges at once into the ocean...After the funeral the grating is hauled on deck.[52]

A similar tale was told by Irene "Greenmouse" Edwards, a nurse whose patient, a young nun, tragically died on a civilian British ship in 1929.

> A part of the deck-rail had been removed, and in front of this stood a trestle. Lucy's body, sewn up in green canvas, was brought down in a lift. The sailors placed her body on the trestle and draped a Union Jack over it. The padre, surgeon and officer stood on one side, we stood on the other. The sailors stood on each side close to the trestle. When the committal service began the ship's engines were stopped and the man-overboard flag hoisted. The ship glided silently over the Arabian sea while the padre read the service. When he came to the words '...we commit her body' I closed my eyes. The trestle was tilted and the body slipped from under the flag into the sea.[53]

Lord Byron, who probably observed sea burials, gave a poet's description saying, "like a drop of rain, He sinks into thy depths with bubbling groan/ Without a grave/ unknelled, uncoffined, and unknown."[54]

Bodies buried at sea by Western cultures are normally sewn into canvas bags, weighted and slid into the ocean. Only rarely are they enclosed in coffins, and if they are, it is usually only in a box made of spare planks; a box is harder to sink than a shrouded body.

While sea burial was common in both the British and American navies during the eighteenth and nineteenth centuries, French and Spanish sailors "buried" their dead in the gravel ballast in the ship's hold until they returned to port, so the bodies could be interred in a church cemetery.[55] For the U.S. Navy's Pacific Fleet, the acquisition of Hawaii, Guam, and the Philippines at the turn of the century decreased their use of sea burials, since bodies could be buried or embalmed at these sites and then transported home.[56]

## H. WHAT HAPPENS TO A BODY INTERRED IN WATER?

A corpse interred in water becomes an ugly, smelly mess.

Bodies exposed to water decompose approximately four times faster than in earth,[57] and if the water is warm or polluted, the corruption occurs much faster. The corpse's decomposition may be accelerated when it is damaged while drifting along the bottom, by cuts from boat or ship propellers, and even from spear gun wounds in some coastal or inland waters.

Insects also get into the act. Bodies that float near land for even a few minutes will have maggot infestations in all body cavities.[58] Aquatic insects may also feed on the body, but these insects seem to accidentally happen onto the body rather than being attracted by the odor. (Forensic scientists are investigating whether aquatic insects can be used to estimate the time a body was immersed in water.)[59]

If a body rests in water for only a short time, especially if the water is cold and contains minimal fish life, a variety of changes can occur. If it is near the shore or rests near a sandy bottom, sand may wash into the mouth and throat, sometimes forming a hard cast. The skin of the palms and soles initially becomes very wrinkled, called "washerwoman skin" by pathologists, looking similar to a person's hands and feet after spending too much time in a swimming pool or bathtub.[60] If the body is submerged in cool (less than 70°F or 21°C) to cold (less than 40°F or 4.4°C) water for as little as one to three weeks, the corpse's tissues convert to adipocere, a compound that stops the activity of bacteria. The preservation from cold water was exemplified by two bodies trapped for five years in a car that sank in Lake Superior outside of Duluth, Minnesota. The very cold water produced extensive adipocere formation and well-preserved internal organs.[61]

After being in water for hours to days, a corpse's skin becomes white, soft, and extremely unpleasant to sight and smell. In warmer water, the decomposition advances rapidly, with the skin quickly loosening, darkening and becoming stained with blood. The body bloats and the eyes protrude—the typical "floater." Eventually, the corpse decomposes and becomes part of the environment, as the Hindu *Rig-Veda* recognized: "Go unto the waters, if you are placed there. You must establish the plants with your flesh."[62]

At one time pathologists autopsied "floaters" with gunpowder burning in the morgue to mask the smell. They now put tincture of benzoin on their surgical masks or freeze the bodies for at least four hours to reduce the odor. (Benzoin or similar substances are also used by disaster workers while they search for bodies decomposing under earthquake rubble, at airplane crashes, and in similar catastrophes.)

Occasionally, bodies lost at sea become objects of amusement. In Truk lagoon, a world-famous wreck-diving site in the South Pacific, the bones of Japanese sailors were often retrieved as souvenirs by divers or used as props in underwater pictures. This practice stopped in the late 1980s when the Japanese sent a professional diving team to retrieve the remains and bring them back to Japan.

## I. ARE BODIES BURIED AT SEA EATEN BY FISH?

Yes. If fish are present to help consume the body, decomposition accelerates a hundred-fold. Fish, crabs and small marine animals quickly begin to feed on the soft parts of a corpse's face. The eyelids, lips and ears are the first to go, and then the eyes, nose and mouth. Dr. Carr, former Chief of Pathology at San Francisco General Hospital has said that bodies floating in the cold waters of San Francisco Bay routinely have "shrimps at the orifices."[63]

In some areas of the sea, large fish are scarce, so it is the smaller animal life that feeds on the remains. These small creatures, however, are quite efficient. Evidence of this was seen during the recent exploration of fourteen World War II warships recently found undisturbed in 3,000 feet of water fifty years after the bloody naval battle around Guadalcanal. As Robert Ballard, the undersea explorer, said, "All that's missing are the bodies of the thousands of sailors."[64]

Larger animals feed on the torso and extremities, with sharks typically removing pieces 8 to 10 inches across. Throughout history, sharks have been found with recognizable body parts in their stomachs, perhaps due in part to the shark's very slow digestion time (8 to 21 days). According to Dr. Joseph H. Davis, Chief Medical Examiner for Dade County, Florida, one shark was caught off the Florida coast with an entire human leg in its stomach—from the hip to a sneaker-clad foot.[65]

In one notorious Australian case, a shark that had recently been captured and put into an aquarium for public viewing suddenly regurgitated an entire human arm and hand. This "famous Shark Arm mystery" was eventually solved by matching the fingerprints and a tattoo on the arm with those of a missing person. An Australian court, however, ruled that one arm a homicide does not make—the case was never prosecuted for want of the rest of the body.[66]

Fish do seem to be finicky eaters. Yet occasionally, when through accident or intent embalmed bodies are buried at sea, fish generally avoid them. Although these bodies decompose faster than they would after an earth burial, fish do not like the odor they emit, so bacterial activity and the physical action of the sea cause most of their decomposition.

## J. MUST A BOAT BE USED FOR A WATER BURIAL?

Many cultures which used water burials did not bother with boats, but simply tossed bodies into the water from the shore. Ancient Ethiopians, in a pragmatic gesture, threw their dead into lakes so the deceased's body could give back to the fish the nutrients the person took from them while alive.[67] In Melanesia, some corpses, especially those of commoners, were thrown into the sea, either at the deceased's request or to save friends and relatives the trouble of arranging for a burial.

In the Middle Ages, particularly during the Inquisition in Germany, the Iron Maiden, a spike-lined sarcophagus, was used to cause a tortuous death. Pragmatically, the device was often suspended over a river after its use, so that when it was opened the body simply dropped into the water.

Many Indians still traditionally consign corpses to their sacred Ganges River. In the past, during deadly cholera epidemics, entire corpses were thrown in the river, spreading the disease and leading to the production of still more corpses. But today, only ashes or bones are consigned to the river, signalling the end of the mourning period. However, since many corpses do not completely burn in the Hindu open-air pyres, the Ganges still receives many large portions of unburned bodies. To rid the river of this pollution, the Indian government developed special snapping turtles. These 70-pound turtles were bred to eat only dead human flesh, not live bathers. They each consume one pound of flesh a day, and the hope is that they will keep the Ganges clear of this postmortem pollution.[68]

In Tibet, the bodies of the poor, beggars, lepers and babies are still routinely thrown into rivers and streams. Their weighted bodies are often put into the water intact. Some, however, are dismembered before they are cast into the water, to speed the body's disappearance.[69,70]

## K. WHY DO DEAD BODIES FLOAT?

Corpses that are purposely interred in the ocean with proper preparation will generally sink, since they are weighted. But those that are accidentally or haphazardly interred (accidents, drownings, foul play) may float for a while if there is enough air in their clothing to lend sufficient buoyancy. Once the body sinks, it resurfaces when enough gas forms during decomposition to lift what remains. Once it resurfaces, it will sink again only after enough flesh decomposes to let the gas escape.

Bodies in cold water, especially those in inland waters, may not resurface for months since putrefaction is slowed. In warm water, which accelerates the gas-producing bacterial putrefaction, resurfacing may occur in only a few days. (Water temperature at the bottom of a lake, however, even during the hottest part of the summer, may be very cold.) If a body is trapped among debris, rocks or plant life, or in a vehicle, it may never resurface.

With most properly prepared bodies, weights counteract any tendency to surface as they do with the 'cement boots' traditionally used by organized crime. However, if the weights are insufficient to overcome the buoyancy of gasses produced in the decomposing body, it may surface. In one case, a body weighted down with a 145-pound cast-iron generator housing floated to the surface, despite the weight being 5 pounds heavier than the body.[71]

If a body resurfaces, it will normally be in a face-down position, and the back of the body that is exposed to air will occasionally mummify in the form of adipocere, while the front becomes a skeleton.[72] This is, however, not always the case.

A nineteenth-century ship's physician, Dr. Clarke, reported that "one day leaning out of the cabin window, by the side of an officer who was employed in fishing, the corpse of a man, newly sewed in a hammock, started half out of the water, and continued its course, with the current, towards the shore. Nothing could be more horrible: its head and shoulders were visible, turning first to one side, and then to the other, with a solemn and awful movement, as if impressed with some dreadful secret of the deep, which, from its watery grave, it came upwards to reveal."[73] Dr. Clarke further quotes a contemporary physician who said, "in a certain stage of putrefaction, the bodies of persons which have been immersed in water, rise to the surface, and in deep water are supported in an erect posture, to the terror of uninstructed spectators. Menacing looks and gestures, and even words, are supplied by the affrighted imagination, with infinite facility, and referred to the horrible apparition."[74]

## L. WHAT WILL HAPPEN TO BODIES ADRIFT IN SPACE?

No one knows for sure.

Based on the nature of space and the factors that cause a body to decompose, however, one would suspect that a human corpse in space would decay just like any other body as long as it was sealed under an atmospheric pressure approximating that of Earth. No spacecraft, however, is completely airtight; each is rated by the speed at which it loses its internal atmosphere. If a body were to be rapidly exposed to the near-vacuum of space, it would disintegrate or very possibly explode. If it were slowly exposed to the vacuum, it would remain in deep freeze, while being exposed to variable amounts of radiation. The normal mechanisms which cause a body to decompose, autolysis, putrefaction, and exposure to insects and animals, would fail to disturb an ice-cold body in deep space. The only change would be a gradual drying of the body—creating a freeze-dried mummy. Thankfully, the National Air and Space Administration has not yet had to deal with this issue, and its spokespeople want neither to be quoted nor to be named when discussing this topic.

## M. WHY STEAL CORPSES FOR ANATOMICAL STUDY?

Corpses were stolen primarily to supply medical schools with cadavers for anatomical dissection. This mainly occurred in Great Britain and areas of the United States where for many years no legal method existed for providing all medical schools with an adequate supply of bodies for anatomy classes.

As physicians and surgeons in Britain began seriously studying anatomy using the human body, the law grudgingly supplied a few specimens. Beginning in 1540, English surgeons received four criminals' corpses a year for "anatomies."[75] In 1694 surgeons in Edinburgh, Scotland, also were allowed a small legal supply of bodies for anatomical dissection. The doctors got the corpses of those who died in prison, executed prisoners, foundlings who died before entering school or a trade, and unclaimed stillbirths.

Anatomists highly valued these few legal anatomical corpses. The barber-surgeons normally gave liberal Christmas gratuities to the public hangman to assure that their supply of bodies continued.[76] Many condemned criminals, however, went to extraordinary lengths to prevent their corpses from being dissected, resulting in frequent struggles over the possession of remains in the streets and under the gallows. Relatives sometimes succeeded in keeping bodies away from the anatomists.

In 1751, the Scots passed a law decreeing that the bodies of executed murderers should either be publicly dissected or hung in chains or gibbets. (A gibbet was a narrow metal cage that kept the corpse upright while it rotted. See illustration, p 306.) After that, the postmortem anatomical study of one's body may have seemed a more acceptable option for executed murderers.

Even though medical students often prevailed in getting the bodies they were legally allotted, the number of corpses available to them proved woefully inadequate. For example, during the early 1800s there were an average of 900 medical students in Edinburgh, ideally requiring nearly 1000 cadavers annually. (The lack of preservation methods required several cadavers per dissecting group per class.) English schools fared no better. In 1826 for example, the 701 students at the twelve London schools of anatomy dissected only 592 bodies.[77] The medical schools felt they needed more cadavers.

Not getting cadavers from legal sources, many medical students turned to grave robbing and the medical schools turned to grave robbers to supplement their cadaver supplies. As medical schools proliferated at the beginning of the nineteenth century, so too did the number of body snatchers or "resurrection men," who robbed fresh graves to supply anatomy schools with material for dissection. (These men who literally "raised the dead," were also called fishermen, snatches, grabs, and sack-em-up-men.) Their job, as described by Ambrose Bierce, was to be "a robber of grave-worms. One who supplies the young physicians with that with which the old physicians have supplied the undertaker."[78]

In what was probably more than just a coincidence, Edinburgh University appointed its first Professor of Anatomy, a Mr. Elliott in 1704. The first reports of body snatching in that city came six years later. As Ambrose Bierce noted, in that period graves were "a place in which the dead are laid to await the coming of the medical student."[79]

The U.S. also saw its share of grave robbing (see *Was grave robbing common in the U.S.?*).

Early medical professionals needed to study anatomy to get their degrees, to stay proficient in their skills, and to avoid malpractice. After one practitioner was heavily fined in 1823 for diagnosing a dislocated shoulder as a shoulder sprain, an editorial in the January 25, 1824 *Lancet* said,

> Of that verdict we do not complain. It is perfectly right to visit such gross ignorance with severe punishment; but what we do complain of is—the ridiculous anomaly of first making laws to punish medical practitioners if they do not possess a knowledge of their profession, and subsequently passing other laws which deprive them of the only source from whence it is possible that knowledge can be obtained.
>
> If dead bodies can not be procured, it will be impossible for the pupils to learn anatomy, and without anatomy, neither surgeons nor physicians can practice with the least prospect of benefiting their patients.[80]

Both professors and medical students often participated in body snatching. Professors such as Dr. Andrew Moir, founder of the Aberdeen School of Anatomy in Scotland and Robert Liston, the noted Edinburgh surgeon, often accompanied their students to cemeteries on body raids. This was primarily for adventure since they did not need to participate. Medical students, however, were sometimes required to supply their own cadavers for anatomy, and students in Aberdeen's medical school who would not participate in obtaining corpses were fined. Some medical students became so good at body snatching that they turned professional, using their gruesome skills to finance their schooling.[81]

Anatomists also robbed some graves to obtain rare specimens. Some bodies, especially those of giants, dwarfs and others with unusual shapes, were taken to study and exhibit, rather than to simply be dissected. John Hunter, one of England's most famous anatomists, for example, arranged to have the body of Irish circus giant Charles O'Brien stolen. Although the 8-foot 2-inch O'Brien had dreaded the thought of being dissected after death and arranged to have his body buried at sea, Hunter had other ideas. When the giant died in 1763, Hunter bribed the funeral escort with more than £500 (an extraordinary amount since most corpses sold for £10 or less). The escort replaced the body with stones in the coffin.[82] They gave the body to Hunter who quickly dissected it and boiled it down to its skeleton. The mounted skeleton could be seen in a glass case facing visitors as they entered the Hunter collection of the Royal College of Surgeons until 1941 when German bombers destroyed much of the building. Body snatchers also retrieved the bones of Sir Walter Scott's character, the "Black Dwarf," in reality David Ritchie, for anatomical study ten years after he died.

The bodies of ordinary people, however, constituted most of the corpses stolen to be anatomical cadavers. Eventually the anatomists and their practice of consorting with grave robbers became so well known that their names were widely published.

Thomas Hood, an English poet, provided a description of what happened to one woman's corpse, as related by her ghost in his poem, *The Invisible Girl, or Mary's Ghost*. The names of the anatomists he used were actually those of famous surgeons and anatomists who have left their names in the annals of medicine (e.g., Dr. Bell of Bell's Palsy and Sir Astley [Cooper] of Cooper's Ligament and Fascia). In fact, Dr. Bell supposedly bought, unknowingly, the house in which "Mary" had lived and where her ghost was said to still reside, to use as his anatomy school. He was able to purchase it very cheaply.[83]

> Twas in the middle of the night,
> To sleep young William tried,
> When Mary's ghost came stealing in,
> And stood at his bedside.
>
> O William dear! O William dear!
> My rest eternal ceases;
> Alas! my everlasting peace
> Is broken into pieces.
>
> I thought the last of all my cares
> Would end with my last minute;
>
> But tho' I went to my long home,
> I didn't stay long in it.

The body-snatchers, they have come,
    And made a snatch at me;
It's very hard them kind of men
    Won't let a body be!

You thought that I was buried deep,
    Quite decent-like and chary,
But from her grave in Mary-bone,
    They've come and boned your Mary.

The arm that used to take your arm
    Is took to Dr Vyse;
And both my legs are gone to walk
    The Hospital at Guy's.

I vow'd that you should have my hand,
    But fate gives us denial;
You'll find it there at Dr Bell's,
    In spirits and a phial.

As for my feet, the little feet
    You used to call so pretty,
There's one, I know, in Bedford Row,
    The t'other's in the city.

I can't tell where my head is gone,
    But Doctor Carpue can;
As for my trunk, it's all pack'd up
    To go by Pictord's van.

I wish you'd go to Mr P.
    And save me such a ride;
I don't half like the outside place,
    They've took for my inside.

The cock it crows—I must be gone!
    My William, we must part!
But I'll be yours in death, altho'
    Sir Astley has my heart.

Don't go to weep upon my grave,
    And think that there I'll be;
They haven't left an atom there
    Of my anatomie.[84]

    Body snatching lived on even after the Anatomy Act of 1832 provided a ready supply of bodies for anatomical dissection. Fifty years after the Act was passed, a group of Aberdeen medical students, emulating their forebears, rowed eight miles to Perterculter to snatch a body. They saw their feat as an adventurous prank.[88]

## N. WHY ELSE WERE CORPSES STOLEN?

Corpses have also been stolen to profit from valuables in the grave, to provide materials for bizarre rites, and to ransom.

Some body snatchers robbed graves primarily to sell the bodies for anatomical study, but simultaneously retrieved jewelry and metallic fillings from the corpses, and when they couldn't sell the bodies, they recovered the body's fat to make candles.[86] Ben Crouch, the infamous body snatcher, began his career following the troops during Britain's French and Peninsular campaigns. Under the guise of a troop provisioner he extracted teeth from dead soldiers to sell at a profit. At that time human teeth were highly valued for their use in dentures.[87] Indeed, teeth were almost as valuable as whole bodies were. Although porcelain teeth were invented in 1776, they were rarely used until the early 1800s. In those times, when dentistry was crude and false teeth common, the molars were often made of ivory, and the front teeth, because of their durability and color, came from cadavers. One body snatcher who entered a subterranean vault got away with £60 worth of teeth, leaving behind the rest of the bodies.[88] American body snatchers, however, apparently did not participate in this particular aspect of the trade.

It is also claimed that some people stole corpses for unusual rites. Archaeologists know that the use of dead baby parts for witchcraft became a major problem in ancient Rome.[89] Early recipes in witchcraft and sorcery often required thumbs, fingernails, little finger joints, or knots of virgin's hair—which had to be collected from the dead.[90] John Weever, in his book *Ancient Funeral Monuments* said witches "search into the graves and sepulchres of the dead, to mutilate, dismember, and cut off, certaine parts of the carcases therein inhumed, and by those pairings and cuttings, together with certaine horrid enchantments, charmes and spels, to bring to passe strange, diabolicall conclusions."[91] Shakespeare even penned a chant to be used to prevent this practice in *Cymbeline*:

> No exorciser harm thee!
>   Nor no witchcraft charm thee!
> Ghost unlaid forbear thee!
>   Nothing ill come near thee!
> Quiet consummation have:
> And renowned be thy grave![92]

Shakespeare was also evidently afraid that his own body would be disinterred for unusual reasons. His epitaph reads:

Good frend, for Iesus sake forbeare
To digge the dust encloased heare.
Bleste be ye man [that] spares these stones,
And curste be he [that] moves my bones.[93]

The English made it a felony to steal dead bodies for use in witchcraft in 1604,[94] but repealed the law in 1736.[95]

Some body snatchers practiced corpse-kidnapping for ransom, with varying success. In 1876, a gang of counterfeiters attempted to steal Abraham Lincoln's body to trade for a jailed compatriot, master engraver Ben Boyd. With Lincoln's wooden coffin half out of its sarcophagus, the body snatchers, led by "Big Jim" Kinealy, were interrupted by Pinkerton detectives. In 1901, to prevent further desecration of the grave, Lincoln's coffin was embedded in steel and concrete six feet beneath the tomb's floor.[96] This type of burial, called *cementation*, is rarely used outside of organized crime circles.

In the late 1870s, thieves stole the body of a New York millionaire, T.A. Stewart. The body snatchers asked for $25,000 to return the body. The money was not paid and the body was never recovered.[97]

The most celebrated English case of corpse-kidnapping was that of Alexander William Lindsay, the Fifth Earl of Crawford and Balcarres. Thieves stole his corpse in 1881, although it had been interred in three coffins, one of which was sealed in lead, and placed within the Dunecht Vault, a tomb of massive granite under a chapel. The thieves demanded £6,000 to return the body. No ransom was paid and the body was subsequently found in a shallow grave.[98]

Such body thefts markedly affected the populace, as seen by a comment in the 1882 *Arizona Daily Star*: "Ghouls are doing more than the New York Cremation Society to encourage cremation. The robbery of Stewart's grave in this country and that of the Earl of Crawford in England have produced a profound impression upon the minds of prominent people everywhere, but less conspicuous cases of the same kind of outrage are of frequent occurrence...Were cremations effected more scientifically and conveniently, undoubtedly the number of persons directing that their dead bodies be burned would greatly increase."[99]

Corpse-kidnapping was not confined to the United States and Britain. About the same time as the theft of Stewart and Lindsay's bodies, Argentinean thieves stole the corpse of a wealthy woman, agreeing to return it if her family paid $2 million. The resolution of this case was never revealed.

## O.  HOW WERE CORPSES STOLEN?

Body snatchers jealously guarded their trade practices, and only minimal information exists about how they actually retrieved corpses. In general though, they got good information about which grave to attack, worked fast and, where possible, left no mark of having been there.

Grave robbers often obtained information on which graves to sack from gravediggers or church sextons. On occasion, the body snatchers supplemented this information by accompanying the body to the grave in the guise of a mourner. Gravediggers were particularly helpful since they appreciated being paid twice for the same grave, and reopening the grave for body snatchers was physically much easier and often paid more than initially digging the grave for the parish church. Usually, however, body snatchers worked quickly and in small groups, without outside assistance.

To rob a grave, they first located the head end of the grave they wanted. This was usually easy in Christian graveyards where bodies were interred with their feet facing east.[100] Then, using short, dagger-shaped wooden spades to speed digging and to avoid the chink of metal against stone, body snatchers removed the corpses from their graves, often in less than 15 minutes. They illuminated their work area with shaded lanterns, and sometimes even erected tents or lean-tos over the area while they worked.

Skillful body snatchers did not reopen the entire grave. According to Sir Astley Cooper:

> A hole was dug down to the coffin only where the head lay—a canvas sheet being stretched around to receive the earth and to prevent any of it spoiling the smooth uniformity of the grass. The digging was done with short, flat, dagger-shaped implements of wood, to avoid the clicking noise of iron striking stones. On reaching the coffin, two broad iron hooks under the lid pulled forcibly up with a rope, broke off a sufficient portion of the lid to allow the body to be dragged out; and sacking was heaped over the whole to deaden the sound of the cracking wood. The body was stripped of the graveclothes, which were scrupulously buried again; it was secured in a sack; and the surface of the ground was carefully restored to its original condition—which was difficult, as the sod over a fresh-filled grave must always present signs of recent disturbances. The whole process could be completed in an hour, even though the grave might be six-feet deep, because the soil was loose, and the digging was done impetuously by frequent relays of active men.[101]

Dr. Henry Lonsdale, a nineteenth-century Scottish anatomist, described one method of body snatching with which he was familiar: "In the disinternment [sic] of bodies considerable force was required, and this was mainly exerted round the neck by means of a cord and other appliances. Now, withdrawing the contents of a coffin by a narrow aperture was by no means an easy process, particularly at dead of night and whilst the actors were in a state of trepidation; a jerking movement is said to have been more effective than violent dragging."[102] The process became somewhat easier when, during epidemics, three or four coffins were buried simultaneously in the same grave. Then, although they had to completely uncover the grave, resurrectionists could extract several specimens at once. These body snatchers, as well as the anatomists, however, ran the risk of contracting deadly diseases from handling these fresh bodies.

Francis Clerihew, in a fictionalized account of his own experiences, described handling the body during a body snatching in, "My First Resurrectionist," published in *Aberdeen Magazine*, Spring 1831:

> Slowly we dragged the dead man up; and just as we got him to the surface out flashed the moon, full on his wan, discoloured face. His dull glassy eyes were wide open, and, as I thought, leered knowingly on me; his blue lurid lips were drawn back, and showed his white teeth; his arms hung dangling to the ground, and his head rolled about on his shoulders. In a trice he was stripped of the graveclothes, tied neck and heels, and bundled into the sack. We pitched him over the wall, and two of my comrades set off with him to the gig, while Peter and myself remained to fill up the grave.[103]

After removing the body, professional body snatchers took care to tidy the grave so that it appeared undisturbed. This precaution was not due to any compassionate regard for the family, but to avoid alerting the village and having them place guards around new graves.

Once retrieved, corpses were carried off in sacks, orange baskets and tea chests. Some professionals "dispensed with the usual sack, put the body, doubled up, into a square green-baize cloth, tied the crossed corners, and left their burden in some half-built house, or out-of-the-way spot, all night."[104] Authorities retrieved one young woman's body from body snatchers, and reported that the "arms were tightly corded to the body with the hands resting on the shoulders; her legs were bent backwards to the thighs and both firmly tied round the body; another cord was put through behind the knee joints and tied round the neck, and in this state she had been neatly sewn into a small bag, looking like a bundle which anyone might carry by hand without suspicion."[105]

The next morning, appearing to be a porter, the resurrectionist usually carried his package undetected through the crowded streets. One foolish medical student hid a body in a flour sack in his father's bakery. When it was discovered, not only did it ruin his father's business, but the student also went to jail.[106]

331

Body snatchers often targeted paupers' corpses because they were easy to disinter. Paupers' corpses were either buried in mass graves or shallow graves, so grave robbers had to do less work to get them and so could quickly be away from the cemetery and out of potential danger. One body snatcher, giving testimony to a governmental committee in 1828, said: "I like to get those of poor people buried from the workhouses, because, instead of working for one subject, you may get three or four; I do not think, during the time I have been in the habit of working for the [anatomy] schools, I got half a dozen of wealthier people."[107]

Grave robbing was big business. Body snatcher Ben Crouch, testifying before a British governmental investigative commission, claimed he had once disinterred 23 bodies in four nights. Another, Joseph Napier, listed the bodies retrieved by his gang for the working year 1811-1812:

|  |  |  |
|---|---|---|
| To the London schools | 305 adults | 44 smalls |
| Exported to Edinburgh | 37 adults | |
| Bodies unused | 18 adults | |
| Totals | 360 adults | 44 smalls |

"Small" bodies were those under 3-feet in length, and were sold by the inch. They were generally classified as "large-small," "small," and "foetus." Napier's gang stole 783 corpses in just two years.[108]

Summing up the entire process and the trade of body snatching, Ruth Richardson says:

> Corpses were bought and sold, they were touted, priced, haggled over, negotiated for, discussed in terms of supply and demand, delivered, imported, exported, transported. Human bodies were compressed into boxes, packed in sawdust, packed in hay, trussed up in sacks, roped up like hams, sewn in canvas, packed in cases, casks, barrels, crates and hampers; salted, pickled or injected with preservative. They were carried in carts and wagons, in barrows and steam-boats; manhandled, damaged in transit, and hidden under loads of vegetables. They were stored in cellars and on quays. Human bodies were dismembered and sold in pieces, or measured and sold by the inch.'[109]

## P. HOW WERE GRAVES PROTECTED?

At one point body snatching in Great Britain became so rampant that people went to great lengths to protect their own corpses and those of loved ones.

A common protection was to post guards over many new graves, especially those with bodies that anatomists would relish, until enough time had passed for natural decomposition to make the body useless—normally four to six weeks. In some areas this grave watch was organized into communal watching societies, such as the North Quarter Friendly Churchyard Guard Association of Glasgow. In 1823 the Association had 2,000 members who, by being posted in rotating teams of watchers, were supposed to foil both grave robbers and all attempts to bribe their members into assisting these blackguards.[110]

Even after guards began to be posted at night to protect fresh graves, however, the resurrectionists continued to have success. They would strike during daylight or at dawn, when the guards were sleepy or drunk. Occasionally they did foil inexperienced body snatchers, as when guards shot one Cincinnati, Ohio medical student through the eye while he was trying to steal the body of a recently buried young woman.[111]

In 1798, Robert Southey (later to be England's Poet Laureate) wrote "The Surgeon's Warning," which described a surgeon's dread on his deathbed of being "resurrected" and anatomized, and which gave directions on how to protect his corpse:

> All kinds of carcases I have cut up,
>     And the judgement now must be!
> But brothers, I took care of you,
>     So pray take care of me!
>
> I have made candles of infants' fat,
>     The sextons have been my slaves,
> I have bottled babes unborn, and dried
>     Hearts and livers from rifled graves.
>
> And my 'prentices will surely come
>     And carve me bone from bone,
> And I, who have rifled the dead man's grave,
>     Shall never rest in my own.
>
> Bury me in lead when I am dead,
>     My brethren, I entreat.
> And see the coffin weigh'd, I beg,
>     Lest the plumber should be a cheat.
>
> And let it be solder'd closely down
>     Strong as strong can be, I implore,
> And put it in a patent coffin,
>     That I may rise no more.[112]

The surgeon's preparations did not suffice, as the poem continued:

They laid the pick-axe to the stones,
  And they moved them soon asunder,
They shovell'd away the hard-prest clay.
  And came to the coffin under.

They burst the patent coffin first,
  And then they cut through the lead.
And they laugh'd aloud when they saw the shroud
  Because they had got at the dead.

And they allow'd the sexton the shroud,
  And they put the coffin back,
And the nose and knees they then did squeeze
  The surgeon in a sack.

So they carried the sack a-pick-a-back,
  And they carved him bone from bone.
But what became of the surgeon's soul,
  Was never to mortal known.[113]

Another surgeon and anatomist, Philip Syng Physick, who died in 1837, took better precautions to avoid the grave robbers (although few British resurrectionists remained after the 1832 passage of the Anatomy Act). He left instructions that his body should be kept wrapped in flannel blankets in his heated bedroom, until it was decayed. Only then was it to be interred in a sealed lead coffin. The attendants for his corpse were to be only two women, presumably in the mistaken assumption that no women were involved in the resurrectionist's trade.[114]

Other methods used to foil grave robbers included: (1) raising the graveyard wall; (2) putting tough material, such as heather, in a grave's fill dirt to make digging difficult; (3) digging very deep graves; (4) placing gunpowder on top of the grave to blow up anyone disturbing it; and (5) putting a gun with a tripwire on a grave. As late as 1878, one company in Columbus, Ohio was selling "torpedo coffins" with pipe bombs attached to them that would blow up if someone tampered with the grave.[115] None of these methods met with great success.

More effective protection for corpses was achieved through the use of heavy mort-stones, often 10-inches thick and at least as long and as wide as a coffin, that were laid over the coffin before filling the grave. Another successful barrier was the use of mortsafes or cages. These coffin-shaped iron grills, often weighing a ton or more, were lowered over the coffin using a block-and-tackle. The grave was then filled around them. After about six weeks, when the body would no longer be of use to body snatchers, the grave was reopened, the mortsafe removed and the grave refilled. The mortsafe was then used for other graves. A more radical solution was building morthouses, structures in which coffins of the newly dead were secured for up to three months before burial. These protective methods preserved some bodies from the resurrectionists, who, by being resourceful, were always able to secure others.

## Q. WHO WERE SOME INFAMOUS BODY SNATCHERS?

British body snatchers developed infamous reputations. In the first three decades of the nineteenth century, people lived in fear of professional body snatchers such as the notorious "Corpse King," Ben Crouch, who anatomists hired to teach their students the art of corpse stealing. Only slightly less ominous were the various surgeons and anatomy professors who ruled over legions of lesser-known body snatchers. The most famous body snatcher of all, however, was Mr. Jerry Cruncher, a fictional character in Charles Dickens' *A Tale of Two Cities* (1859).

Body snatchers and their handlers developed inflated egos, and had no moral scruples. Many did not even hide the fact that they trafficked in corpses. In 1828, Sir Astley Cooper, President of the Royal College of Surgeons in London, boasted to a Select Committee investigating how anatomical subjects were obtained that: "There is no person, let his situation in life be what it may, who, if I were disposed to dissect, I could not obtain."[116] He was subsequently dubbed the "King of the Resurrectionists," and used the body-snatchers' services liberally. His love for the art led him to dissect corpses in anatomical theatres at St. Thomas' Hospital, Guy's Hospital, and even in his own home. Nevertheless, he testified that professional body snatchers "are the lowest dregs of degradation. I do not know that I can describe them better; there is no crime they would not commit, and, as to myself, if they should imagine that I would make a good subject, they really would not have the smallest scruple, if they could do the thing undiscovered, to make a subject of me."[117]

Not to be outdone in this ghoulish enterprise, one noted Edinburgh body snatcher, "Merry" Andrew Merrilees, robbed his own sister's grave (after scaring away his occasional compatriots) and sold her body to the anatomists.[118]

Not all body snatchers were infamous, however. Some were famous. Well-known physicians were often involved in the enterprise. Such medical luminaries as Abernathy, Bell, Cooper, and Monro, whose names still grace surgical and anatomical literature, were resurrectionists. So were the first six presidents of the New York Academy of Medicine, and the founder of Bellevue Hospital.[119] One grave-robbing physician, Dr. Thomas Sewall, whose Massachusetts medical practice and reputation were destroyed by his nocturnal avocation, went on to found the predecessor to the George Washington University School of Medicine.[120]

## R. WAS CORPSE STEALING COMMON IN THE UNITED STATES?

With the proliferation of U.S. medical schools in the eighteenth and nineteenth centuries, stealing corpses for anatomical dissection gradually increased. In contrast to Britain, however, the practice continued in some states well into the twentieth century.

In the early United States, not only obtaining cadavers, but anatomical dissection itself, was illegal, although it was required to become a physician (an early Catch-22). However, two famous Boston physicians, Drs. John Collins Warren and Joseph Warren, overcame the problem when they "founded a super-secret little group of resurrectionists [body snatchers] who called themselves the Spunkers, [a term] that could have been derived from a Scotch [sic] term for will-o'-the-wisps: elusive, night-haunting flames that delude wayfarers and cannot be traced...Spunkers adopted the code of the ancient Spartans, who allowed their young boys to steal but taught them that the real crime was in getting caught."[121] (Despite his years with the Spunkers, one participant, William Eustis, later became governor of Massachusetts.)

John Collins Warren's father, a professor of anatomy, was dismayed at first when he found that his medical-student son had begun stealing corpses. The discovery came after John had nearly been caught snatching the body of "a stout young man" from Boston's North Burying-ground. "When my father came up in the morning to lecture, and found that I had been engaged in this scrape, he was very much alarmed; but when the body was uncovered, and he saw what a fine healthy subject it was, he seemed to be as much pleased as I ever saw him."[122]

The public feared grave robbing and sometimes vented their outrage in riots, such as one that occurred in New York in 1788. When the *New York Packet* disclosed that bodies had been snatched from the graveyards of two prestigious churches, Trinity and Brick Presbyterian, the city exploded. A mob ransacked Columbia Medical School and harassed numerous city physicians. By the time troops restored order, several rioters lay dead.[123] Attempting to cause another riot and to discredit the new Franklin Medical College, someone planted a body behind the school. The plot, however, was foiled.[124]

In a quieter denunciation of anatomists, an epitaph from the Maple Grove Cemetery in Hoosick Falls, New York, suggests that the physician-anatomists will get their due.

> Ruth Sprague, dau of Gibson
> and Elizabeth Sprague, died
> Jan. 11, 1846, aged 9 yrs., 4
> mos., and 18 days. She was
> stolen from the grave by

Roderick R. Clow and dissected
at Dr. P.M. Armstrong's office
in Hoosick, New York, from
which place her mutilated
remains were obtained and
deposited here.
Her body dissected by fiendish Men,
Her bones anatomized,
Her soul, we trust, has risen to God,
Where few physicians rise.

Although 85 U.S. medical schools existed prior to the Civil War, only Connecticut (1824), Massachusetts (1831) and New York (1854) had passed "anatomy acts" to supply these schools with sufficient legal cadavers for dissection.[125] By the time New York passed its law, grave robbers were emptying 600 to 700 graves around New York City annually to supply anatomical specimens.[126] Yet other state legislatures could not bring themselves to pass such laws. As one Pennsylvania physician wrote in 1867, "Your committee found the legislative mind opposed to the passage of our Act, and it became necessary to explain its virtues with becoming care, for it was called a 'Ghastly Act' with more temper than wisdom, by leading representatives."[127]

By 1878, however, U.S. medical students needed about 5,000 cadavers a year for anatomical study.[128] Without a legal supply of cadavers, the schools resorted to rampant grave robbing.

Well-known medical schools routinely dealt with professional resurrectionists in most areas of the United States throughout the nineteenth century. One resurrectionist, William Cunningham of Cincinnati, Ohio, had a thriving business with the Ohio Medical College and even sold his own body to them before his death.[129] His skeleton still graces their (University of Cincinnati College of Medicine) museum. Another, George Christian, operated his body-snatching and body-shipping business out of the Surgeon General's Office in Washington, D.C.[130] In 1882 the *Philadelphia Press* exposed an organized ring of grave robbers including not only professional "resurrectionists," but also doctors and cemetery overseers, who had been supplying bodies to several schools, including the Jefferson Medical College.

Body snatchers commonly haunted cemeteries in close proximity to medical schools. Legend says, for example, that few bodies remain in the several graveyards near the University of Maryland School of Medicine in Baltimore. Ironically, one of these supposedly empty graves is that of Edgar Allan Poe, the author of *The Premature Burial*. (Actually, however, since his remains were only moved to that cemetery from a more ignominious resting place in 1875, it is unlikely that either his bones, or those of his wife or

337

mother-in-law that also rest there, have been stolen.)[131]

Letters from the 1870s show that cadavers were shipped (illegally) from the University of Maryland's Medical School to the medical school at Bowdoin College, Maine; from the Cincinnati area throughout the Midwest; and from the Washington, D.C. area to many medical schools, including the University of Virginia and the University of Michigan.

The participants in these transactions worried about how the corpses were shipped. They wanted to ensure that their enterprise would not be discovered and that the bodies would arrive intact. As a cover, they often labeled boxes containing bodies as "pickles." Yet the shipments did not always go well, as evidenced by a letter from a University of Michigan anatomy professor to George Christian, a convicted body snatcher:

> Boxes have come, or rather barrels. Do not send barrels; they always get the heads knocked in, and excites suspicion if they do not, as the subjects shake about so. The best way to pack is in a tight box three feet by two, or near that dimension, the subject having the legs and thighs flexed and head resting on chest. Sawdust packed about prevent odor and the subject from shaking about in the box. Two can be put in a single box a little larger than the one I describe. You may keep on sending until I am done work at $25 each for good ones...The express averages about $7 a subject...[132]

Even when the Johns Hopkins Medical School opened in 1893, they could not start teaching anatomy because they had no cadavers to dissect. As one Hopkins anatomy professor wrote, "The problem now changed from teaching anatomy to obtaining cadavers for a new school...We postponed work until the 16th and then the 17th [from November 15 when class was supposed to begin], and late in the evening, a subject was mysteriously left in the basement. The next day, one came from the state, and a few days later, another appeared in the basement."[133] It was only in 1898 that Johns Hopkins was able to obtain enough bodies through legal channels. Despite passage of Maryland's Anatomy Act, the six other Baltimore medical schools were still struggling to get bodies at the start of the twentieth century. Maryland's medical schools supposedly obtained their last body from extralegal sources in 1899.[134]

Most graves robbed for anatomical cadavers were those of the poor, black or powerless. As was said by Harriet Martineau in 1835, "In Baltimore the bodies of coloured people exclusively are taken for dissection, because the whites do not like it, and the coloured people cannot resist."[135] This attitude persisted. H.L. Mencken, describing the attitude of poor blacks in late nineteenth-century Baltimore wrote that none would allow himself to be taken to the University of Maryland Hospital as long as they were conscious, because of the medical students "who never had enough cadavers to supply their hellish orgies, and were not above replenishing their stock by sticking a knife into a patient's back, or holding his nose and forcing drink out of the black bottle down his throat."[136]

Paupers were also the primary victims in Philadelphia, where the Board supervising the poorhouse commented that " 'the colleges must have subjects' and should grave robbers be barred from the almshouse, they would plunder church cemeteries and other private burial grounds."[137] This led people to irreverently call this supervisory group the Board of Buzzards.[138] Before the Civil War, southern medical schools used black, rather than white, bodies almost exclusively for dissection. They hired (or in one case at the Medical College of Georgia, bought) black porters to obtain these black cadavers.[139]

Occasionally the rich, famous, and powerful would also end up on the dissecting table. In 1859, students at the Winchester (Virginia) Medical College obtained the body of Owen Brown (the son of abolitionist John Brown of Harper's Ferry fame), who was killed during a raid on Hall's Rifle Works.[140] In 1876, the University of Minnesota's medical school received the body of a member of the James-Younger gang, who was killed attempting to rob the Northfield, Minnesota bank.[141] In 1878 a search party found the body of Congressman John Scott Harrison at the Ohio Medical College in Cincinnati (now the University of Cincinnati College of Medicine). The departed Congressman was the son of the late President William Henry Harrison and the father of future President Benjamin Harrison.[142] Congressman Harrison's body had been procured under a contract with professional grave robber, Dr. Henri Le Caron (AKA Charles O. Morton), and his wife. This theft actually prompted many states to pass laws that increased the legal supply of bodies for medical-student dissection.[143,144]

Grave robbers flourished even in rural America. In 1888, the *Meyersdale Commercial*, a weekly newspaper in western Pennsylvania, described the plague of body snatchers that had descended on the town. They estimated that in only two years, about 200 bodies had been stolen in the area before a major body-snatching ring was shut down by federal officers. The motivation, of course, was economic. As one captured grave robber said, "It may be against the law, but it seems a pity to waste so much material when a subject will bring $25 in cash. What's the use of letting him waste away in the ground? People have feelings about it, but if they don't know that the grave is empty, they are just as well off and we are a great deal better off."[145]

At least two cases similar to Burke and Hare's also occurred in the United States. (see *When were "grave-robbed" bodies not dead?*) On February 15, 1884, the bodies of the occupants of a one-story log cabin could not be found after it burned to the ground in Cincinnati. Investigators suspected that the bodies had found their way to the Ohio Medical College. After some prodding, Dr. Cilley, the demonstrator in anatomy, remembered the bodies of the elderly man, middle-aged woman and 11-year-old child he had received from two known resurrectionists the night of the fire. A subsequent autopsy on these bodies showed they had died from head injuries. Reminiscent of Edinburgh's Dr. Knox, Dr. Cilley responded to a *Cincinnati Post* reporter's questions about the incident by stating, "I will say that it is possible that persons are murdered and brought to the college and sold to us. We never ask any questions, and our suspicions are never aroused by wounds as they may be caused by the handling." Asked the reporter, "Then all these people who so mysteriously disappear may many of them land in medical colleges?" "It is possible," he replied.[146]

In 1886, Emily Brown, an elderly Baltimore woman fond of alcohol and drugs, was murdered by two men, one of whom was a porter in the dissecting room at the University of Maryland Medical School. They took her body there pretending to be funeral directors with an insolvent "client" and received $15. The school's staff, suspicious of how the still-warm, fully dressed, and bloodied body was obtained, notified police. Authorities caught and convicted the culprits; the ringleader was hanged.[147]

Corpse stealing in the United States continued unabated into the twentieth century. In December 1902, a major body-snatching ring was uncovered in Indianapolis. According to the *Medical Standard*, "Twenty-five persons have been indicted for 'body-snatching' or complicity in this gruesome business, among them several physicians connected with the local medical colleges. Some fifteen graves have been found empty and several bodies have been traced to medical schools and identified. It is estimated that in the neighborhood of one hundred bodies have been removed from their supposed last resting places by this gang."[148]

By 1913, twelve states still had no laws whereby medical schools could legally obtain bodies for dissection. Two of these states, Alabama and Louisiana, had medical schools (including Louisiana State University and Tulane) that could not obtain legal cadavers for anatomical study. North Carolina and Tennessee's (Duke, Vanderbilt) laws only allowed the dissection of the paltry number of prisoners that died in jail each year. Decreasing the number of available cadavers even farther, the bodies of ex-Confederate soldiers and their wives were exempted from dissection in Mississippi and North Carolina, and in the latter state, "the body of no white person [could] be sent to a Negro medical college."[149]

Even when anatomy laws were passed, officials would often refuse to send bodies to the medical schools. Into the 1920s grave robbers were still selling bodies to Nashville's four medical schools, with the surplus going to Iowa City.[150]

## S. WHAT HAPPENED TO CAPTURED GRAVE ROBBERS?

Body snatching was a relatively safe career in England until the 1820s, when public sentiment turned ugly. Although body snatching was greatly feared by the populace, jail was not a common penalty, since the law considered stealing a corpse a very minimal offense. Corpses were not regarded as "property" under English law, in part because stealing property had long been punishable by death.[151] (While stealing a human body was not a crime in Britain in the early nineteenth century, during the same period it was a capital offense to steal the body of a sheep, pig, calf, ox, or fowl. Even receiving a stolen animal's body resulted in transportation to Australia.) Therefore, the only way family members could prosecute a grave robber was if they owned the land where the graveyard stood (extremely rare) or if the coffin, grave clothes, or other valuables were stolen along with the corpse.[152,153] Most grave robbers, therefore, took great care only to remove the naked body. The *London Times* in 1794 urged the Archbishop of Canterbury to encourage Parliament to make robbing a churchyard a capital offense (he didn't).[154]

Occasionally, however, captured body snatchers were thrown into rivers, whipped, shot and beaten. One young Scottish doctor was so badly beaten during a body raid near Aboyne, Aberdeenshire, that he was crippled for life. A Glasgow medical student fared even worse. He snagged a tripwire on a spring-loaded gun set over a grave and was killed instantly. His two companions, not being able to leave him, propped his body between them and tied his ankles to theirs, "walking" him home. They then placed him in his bed and claimed he was a suicide.[155] Other students barely escaped with their lives. Two medical students caught while robbing a grave in 1832 at Inveresk, a village near Edinburgh, asked that they be jailed, since it was safer than facing the outraged citizenry, who later tried to storm the jail. The students survived.[156]

On another occasion, a medical student transporting a packaged body foolishly took a cab to his medical school. He was horrified when, instead, the cab stopped in front of the police station, the cabman saying, "My fare's a guinea, sir, (an outrageously high fare) unless you would like to be put down here."[157]

In the 1820s, the public became incensed by the notoriety surrounding body snatching, the gruesome details of importing bodies, and finally, the capture of murderers who killed people to sell their bodies as anatomical specimens. Rioters burned down the homes and offices of anatomists suspected of receiving stolen bodies and lethal measures to protect graves became more common.

One Glasgow anatomist who later founded Bellevue Hospital in New York, Dr. Granville Sharp Pattison, was forced to flee to America after he was disgraced when authorities found fresh bodies in his home. He subsequently sold his extensive collection of 1,000 sugar-cured anatomical specimens to the University of Maryland. (All but a few were later destroyed in a fire.) According to Dr. Pattison, anatomists also had their anatomical specimens "salted in the summer and hung up and dried like Yarmouth herrings," to preserve them.[158]

Another physician-resurrectionist, Dr. Joseph N. McDowell, barely escaped capture by the mob—in a most unusual way. The mob had him trapped in his anatomy building with a corpse he had just unearthed. Just then, " ...in the dark, the ghost of his dear, departed mother came to his rescue and bade him stretch out on the dissecting table from which he had just removed the cadaver. This he did, frantically pulling a sheet over his head just as the angry crowd swarmed into the room. They peeked under the sheet and remarked upon the freshness of this corpse. McDowell wrote, "I thought I would jump up and frighten them, but I heard a voice, soft and low, close to my ear, say 'Be still, be still.' " The mob left and McDowell survived.[159]

The official penalties for grave robbing in the United States were also minimal, as a letter written to the *Zanesville* (Ohio) *Daily Courier* during debates over the passage of Ohio's Anatomy Law points out:

> Surely, it is time something were done by the legislatures of our country to put a stop to this business. The punishment now for robbing a grave is little, if any, heavier than for robbing a hen-roost. Eastern nations have an imaginary demon, which they conceive preys upon the bodies of the dead, that they call a Ghoul. But our ghouls are no imaginary demons. They walk about among us in broadcloth and kid gloves; physicians and surgeons, with lawyers to defend them, when caught at their obscene work; nice young men, who clerk in stores during the day, take their girls to places of amusement in the evening, and then replenish their depleted pockets by invading the cemeteries, putting hooks through the jaws of our deceased friends, sacking and carting away the bodies, and selling them to Professors of Anatomy for $25.00 a piece! This is horrible; but it seems to be true. The whole business of body snatching is becoming a systematized profession; and it will continue to branch out, and become a more prosperous profession, so long as the petty punishment for the offense is a poor six months in the county jail.[160]

## T. WHEN WERE "GRAVE-ROBBED" BODIES NOT DEAD?

Many stories exist about grave robbers who came across "corpses" which had been buried but were not dead. Evidence on grave stones, in church records, and elsewhere verify some of these episodes. (See Chapter 2,

*Are there real cases of premature burials?*) One fictional account that has subsequently been repeated with multiple variations, was published in the 1846 book, *Marietta or the Two Students, A Tale of the Dissecting Room and Body Snatching.* The tale revolves around the body of a young woman procured by grave robbers and brought to a medical school. One medical student, reluctant to dissect such a beautiful woman, exchanged his ring with hers and instructed that she be reburied. Instead, the body was re-sold to another medical student experimenting with electricity. To his surprise, he brought the corpse back to life. The story concludes with her later meeting and marrying the first medical student.[161]

While this story centers on the accidental use of a "live" cadaver, obtaining bodies for anatomical study became so profitable in the early nineteenth century that the living rather than the dead became intentional targets. One Irish woman offered her 2-month-old healthy son to a surgeon for dissection for £7; she had turned down the offer of £5 from another surgeon. She also offered her 13-year-old son, "whom," she said, the surgeon "could kill or boil or do what he liked with." The doctor reported her to authorities.[162]

The most notorious group to switch from body snatching to murdering individuals to sell their bodies for anatomical cadavers was Edinburgh's Burke and Hare.

William Burke and William Hare, along with Hare's wife, Margaret, and Burke's mistress, Helen McDougal, murdered sixteen men, women and children over a nine-month period in 1828 and sold their bodies for dissection. They killed most of their victims by holding their mouths and noses closed while pressing on their chests. They used this method so that their victims would die without showing any external evidence of violence that the anatomists might question. To this day, their murderous technique is still called "burking."

All of their victims were bought by the anatomist, Dr. Robert Knox, for between £8 and £14. While Knox later denied knowing how Burke and Hare obtained their bodies, the citizens of Edinburgh thought otherwise, penning this ditty:

> Down the close and up the stair,
> But and ben wi' Burke and Hare.
> Burke's the butcher, Hare's the thief,
> Knox's the man who buys the beef.[163]

A children's rhyme goes even further:

> Hang Burke, banish Hare,
> Burn Knox in Surgeons' Square.[164]

They were arrested in 1828 and all but McDougal were tried for the crimes. Hare turned King's evidence, was released from prison and disappeared,

McDougal fled to Australia, and Margaret Hare fled to Belfast, Ireland. William Burke was hanged in 1829. Unrepentant to the end, he demanded payment for the last body he delivered so that he could buy a coat and waistcoat. As he said, "since I am to appear before the public, I should like to be *respectable*."[165] His body, like those of his victims, was dissected.

In passing sentence, the Lord Chief Justice said,

> In regard to your case, the only doubt that has come across my mind is, whether...your body should not be exhibited in chains, in order to deter others from like crimes in time coming. But taking into consideration that the public eye would be offended with so dismal an exhibition, I am disposed to agree that your sentence shall be put into execution in the usual way, but accompanied by the statutory attendant of the punishment of the crime of murder—viz., that your body should be publicly dissected and anatomized, and I trust that if it is customary to preserve skeletons, yours will be preserved in order that posterity may keep in remembrance your atrocious crimes.[166]

Both his execution and his anatomized body were viewed by over 30,000 people. His skeleton is still displayed in the anatomical museum at Edinburgh University. Unlike his victims, however, his skin was tanned into leather and used to make wallets and tobacco pouches.[167] Knox continued his surgical career, although public sentiment can be inferred from Robert Louis Stevenson's short story, *The Body Snatcher*, in which "Professor K___'s" anatomy assistant says, "They bring the body, and we pay the price...Ask no questions for conscience' sake."[168]

Burke and Hare were not the sole practitioners of this crime, though. In 1831, Thomas Williams and John Bishop, after supplying between 500 and 1000 disinterred corpses to London anatomy schools, tired of body snatching and turned to obtaining corpses that were "fresher." They, along with John May, killed at least three people to sell the bodies to the anatomists. They murdered their victims by first disabling them with narcotic-laced rum and then suspending them head first into a well until they died. Bishop and Williams were convicted and hanged for murdering a young Italian boy, Carlo Ferrari, whose body was taken to King's College Hospital for dissection. Bishop and Williams' bodies were in turn dissected by the Royal College of Surgeons. May was exiled to Australia.[169,170]

Scotland's only "Resurrectionist Women," Helen Torrence and Jean Waldie, were hung in 1752 for stealing and killing an eight-year-old child, John Dallas. The pair had actually planned to wait until the sickly lad died, but as he did not cooperate quickly enough for them, they killed him. The pair, who were prostitutes and alcoholics, sold the body to an anatomist for a paltry sum and a drink of whiskey.[171]

## U. ARE CORPSES STILL STOLEN?

Yes. Corpse stealing still exists in the United States, and murder to obtain anatomical cadavers occurs elsewhere in the world.

Bodies in the United States are now often "snatched" in an unusual manner. The *New York Times* reported in 1975 that undertakers' agents often appropriate unclaimed bodies, saying they are long-lost friends and claiming the body for burial. This practice imitates the old body snatcher's method of sending the "grieving widow" into the workhouse to claim a body. These modern agents then collect a portion of the state burial allowance for the poor as kickbacks from cooperating undertakers. As one modern body snatcher was quoted as saying, "Nowadays, it's all white-collar work. Respectable. It's like you're doing a service because instead of digging them up, you're helping to put them away in style."[172] This modern body snatching has dropped the number of unclaimed bodies so precipitously that New York medical schools have had to pay expensive transportation costs to import anatomical cadavers from Wisconsin and California.

Relic hunters are now the most common actual grave robbers in the United States. In late 1991, the Arkansas Historic Preservation Program announced a toll-free phone number to report any disturbance of an historic or prehistoric grave that was not on official burial grounds, including those of Native Americans, Civil War casualties, pioneers and slaves. Other states are considering similar measures.

"Corpse-kidnapping" also still occurs. In early 1992, for example, several people broke into the mausoleum of the Ransom Olds family (of automobile fame) in Lansing, Michigan, and stole five urns containing cremated remains and an infant's casket. The thieves carefully cut through a stained-glass window and unlocked the dead-bolt to gain entry. Ransom's crypt was not disturbed and no payoff was publicly requested.[173]

Tragically, the crimes associated with Burke and Hare are not merely historical oddities; murdering people to use their bodies as anatomical cadavers still occurs.

In February 1992, watchmen at the medical school of the Free University of Barranquilla, Columbia, lured 24-year-old Oscar Hernandez onto campus and tried to bludgeon him to death to sell his body as an anatomical specimen. Feigning death, he waited for his attackers to depart and then fled to the police. When police arrived at the school, not only did they find 11 bodies and parts from 22 others, but they also found one badly beaten man still alive awaiting his death. A University security chief, Pedro Viloria, was arrested for clubbing at least 50 people to death and selling their bodies to the Institute. Each fresh body sold for $200, with the checks drawn on the University account. The security chief claimed he acquired the bodies at the direction of the Institute's director, and investigators have said that the city's police were actually running the operation. Their "murder-for-medicine ring" mainly preyed on the poor people who earned their livings by collecting salvageable items from the trash bins of this Caribbean city of one million people. The Barranquilla Legal Medical Institute was part of one of Columbia's oldest and most prestigious institutions of higher learning, the privately run Free University. The Institute was immediately closed.[174]

## V. MAY I BE BURIED IN FOREIGN SOIL?

Maybe, but the rules will be different from those in the United States.

Even if an individual wants to be buried in a foreign country, religious restrictions or simply a lack of burial space may make burial there impossible. Japan and England, for example, have too little land to devote much room to graveyards. Their citizens are generally cremated. In countries with strong biases against different religions, "infidels" may not be allowed burial. Even where burial of foreigners is permitted, the way the body is prepared and the subsequent costs may give cause for concern, since they may not correspond to practices in the United States.

Embalming is commonly practiced in the United States, but is rare elsewhere in the world. Even where embalming is practiced, the term may mean different things. While "embalming" in the United States means an injection of disinfectant and preservative chemicals into the arteries and body cavities, this is not what it means in all other countries. "Embalming" may mean randomly injecting disinfectant chemicals into body cavities, simply wrapping the body in a sheet saturated with chemicals, or placing chemical-saturated cotton into random body incisions. In many countries, the law requires that embalming be done by physicians who have variable interest and skill in the procedure. As the president of the European Association of Thanatologists said, "Doctors are busy people, so they may inject five mils [a teaspoon] of formaldehyde into a corpse and say, 'that's embalmed.' "[175] Their charge for the service seems to bear no relationship to their success.

Quotes for funeral and burial expenses in other countries often do not include services that might be considered routine in the United States. Persons making funeral arrangements should inquire about what services are included and about any charges for extra services. "All-inclusive" burial charges in foreign countries normally include all ground transportation, the funeral services, and the use of a grave. A few also include a small engraved headstone, but embalming is never included in the quoted costs.

Of greatest interest, however, should be the length of time the deceased will have use of the grave. Graves outside of the United States and Canada are often rented for 20 to 30 years. Survivors should consider what will be done with the body when the grave lease is up at any gravesite that is not obtained "in perpetuity." In contrast, once the body is buried in a foreign grave, the law usually prohibits disinterrment for from one to twenty years. In some cases, especially when local law allows relatively rapid disinterment and repatriation of the body, graves may be rented for as few as 2 to 3 years.

If funds are not available for burial or transportation of the body or a body is not claimed, local officials will dispose of the body in accordance with local law.

## W. HOW AND WHY ARE CORPSES TRANSPORTED ACROSS INTERNATIONAL BORDERS?

While people in many cultures wish to be buried near their homes or loved ones, transporting bodies across international boundaries can be quite complex, and very expensive, with the rules varying greatly depending upon the countries involved. Many of the regulations go back to the days of steamship transportation, when it took weeks or even months to ferry a body from one country to another. Today, of course, the actual travel time is measured in hours or days, but most of the rules have not been changed.

Increasingly, people are dying far from home. Yet a constant cross-cultural wish is to be buried near friends and family.

In Western cultures, the wish to be buried in one's native country was first expressed in *Genesis 47:30:* "But I will lie with my fathers, and thou shalt carry me out of Egypt, and bury me in their burying-place." The ancient Greeks routinely cremated the bodies of important persons who died abroad and brought their ashes home to receive their normal funeral honors. During the Peloponnesian War they extended this custom to returning the bones of Athenian soldiers to their homes. Australian aborigines have traditionally been even more specific about where they bury their dead. Those in the Victoria area bury their dead at the exact spot where they were born.

Returning the dead to their "native land," however, did not always necessarily mean the person had ever been to that country in life. Early African and South American peoples transported remains long distances to bury them in a traditional homeland, and descendents of the Spanish Conquistadors sent bodies "home" to Spain for burial for centuries after the Spanish conquest of South America. Similarly, many Jews still return their dead to Israel for burial, nearly two millennia after the Diaspora. And, no matter where they lived, Chinese have traditionally sent their dead back to China for burial.[176] For all of these groups, returning these bodies solidifies ties with their cultural heritage, as well as with the people left behind.

Occasionally, people have clearly not wanted their bodies to be transported to their native lands. Such was the case with Lord Byron, who wrote in 1819, that "I am sure my bones would not rest in an English grave, or my clay mix with the earth of that country. I believe the thought would drive me mad on my deathbed, could I suppose that any of my friends would be base enough to convey my carcass back to your soil."[177] Although he died in Greece, he was buried in Newstead Abbey in England.

Approximately 5,000 non-military Americans die while travelling abroad each year, and many Americans who have retired and are living in foreign countries also wish to be buried in the United States. (Interestingly, they die from the same causes as in the United States: chronic diseases, suicides, homicides, and injuries—mainly automobile accidents and drownings, even in less-developed countries.)[178] Americans typically feel the need to inter their dead in home soil. After World War II, the U.S. government transferred 225,000 dead back to America for reburial. This attitude is typified in a famous American ballad (and Robert Louis Stevenson's epitaph):

> It matters not, I've oft been told,
> Where the body lies when the heart goes cold,
> Yet grant, oh grant, this wish to me:
> Oh bury me not on the lone prairie.[179]

The rules for transporting corpses across international borders can be complex. One of the main stumbling blocks is that few countries agree on funerary standards concerning health precautions, packaging, shipping, and documentation. Most countries cannot even agree on common definitions, such as what constitutes a casket. An exception is many South American countries that adhere to a uniform set of rules.

While the rules concerning transport of a body out of the United States say only that the shipment must conform to the requirements of the receiving country, this can be a major obstacle. The National Funeral Director's Association (NFDA) reports that many of the requirements for transporting bodies to or from foreign countries are unreasonable or unnecessary.[180] Some countries have nearly impossible regulations such as requiring bodies "to be surrounded by powdered charcoal or peat dust."[181] Others require that the body be placed in three nested boxes for shipment. Still others specify that bichloride of mercury, arsenic and carbolic acid be used in preparing the body for shipment—all of which are illegal in the United States. The NFDA has the requirements for over 100 countries on file, and member morticians can access this information. The experience of NFDA members has been, however, that countries modify or revise regulations without notice, especially the fees. Current requirements can usually be obtained from the receiving country's embassy or consulate. In some cases, officials can alter requirements to make them more acceptable.

Even the European Community met stiff opposition when they tried to pass their "Intra-Community Transfer of Human Remains" bill. Even after they abandoned plans for a standardized Euro-coffin and a single "passport for corpses," the multitude of bizarre and conflicting laws in member countries could not be reconciled. Italy's requirements, the most restrictive, require that a body be shipped inside a double coffin, one with a thick zinc lining and separated by charcoal from the other, made of hardwood with tongue-and-groove corners.[182]

More typical requirements are those for shipping human remains to England (as of mid-1993):

1. A burial permit and a transit permit.
2. One certified copy of the death certificate.
3. A letter certifying that the body has no contagious disease.
4. An embalmer's affidavit.
5. A letter from the funeral home stating that the casket contains only the remains of the deceased.
6. A casket contained in a sealer.
7. An airtray (outer shipping container). (No consul legalization, fee or inspection is required.)

Another example is Israel's requirements. The bodies of American Jews are often sent to Israel for burial. Howard Belkoff, a New Jersey funeral director who handles many of these shipments describes the procedure:

> Israel requires bodies to be shipped in a wood casket lined with zinc (called an "Israeli shipper"). The body has the traditional washing and dressing, and then is placed in a "disaster pack," a heavy rubber bag. The funeral director then pours two bottles of arterial or cavity embalming fluid over the body, puts a piece of dry ice over the area of the person's appendix (right lower part of abdomen) and puts it into the wooden shipper that is nailed closed. When the body gets to Israel, they remove the bag from the box and bury the body only in the bag (Israelis do not normally bury their dead in boxes). The wooden casket is then broken up and used to make stools for other mourners (*shivah benches*).[183]

What happens when the requirements are not met? The receiving country will often not accept the body and ship it back to the sender—at the sender's expense. To be certain that all current rules are being followed, experts recommend that in each instance the consulate for the receiving country be contacted to verify the current requirements and that when necessary, a consular official should personally band or place a wax seal on the shipping container.

## X. HOW ARE BODIES OR ASHES TRANSPORTED INTO THE UNITED STATES?

Returning ashes to the United States is very simple. It requires only (1) a marker on the container stating that they are cremated remains; (2) an official death certificate; (3) a cremation certificate; (4) a certificate from the crematorium stating that the container holds only the cremated remains of the deceased; and (5) a permit to export (if required by the country where the shipment originates).

United States regulations for returning bodies are also relatively straightforward. In fact, the most difficult part of getting corpses back to the United States is meeting the local requirements in the country of death.

Many foreign countries have elaborate requirements for shipping a body out of their country. Dr. William Forgey, in his *Travelers' Medical Resource,* claims that over 300 steps, involving 100 or more contacts in two or more countries, may be required to ship a corpse back to the United States.[184] If a person dies under suspicious circumstances, especially if the death is the subject of a court case, they may not release the body until the judicial process is complete. This could take months or years.

Most foreign caskets approved for returning bodies to the United States are woo

den, with metal liners that can be soldered shut. They can be quite expensive. Survivors may want the body embalmed so they can have a viewing or open-casket funeral on the corpse's return to the United States. American-style embalming from professional embalmers, however, rarely exists outside of Britain, former British colonies, former American protectorates, and southern France. Elsewhere physicians often perform the embalmings, with varying outcomes. Where embalming is unavailable, the body may be packed in sawdust or charcoal with a disinfectant such as zinc sulfate powder before the metal liner is sealed. By the time the body returns to the United States, no embalmer may be able to make it viewable.

The U.S. State Department estimates that it normally takes 10 to 15 days following death for a body to be returned from western European countries and considerably longer from other parts of the world.[185] Transportation time from primitive areas may be markedly extended, since containers in which to transport the body may have to be custom-made.

There may be a few complications of which the State Department is unaware. As Howard Belkoff, a New Jersey funeral director describes it:

> Normally to get a body back from Spain, a common destination of U.S. tourists and expatriates, the family sends $2,500 to the U.S. consulate official. Some of that money goes to obtain permits from *nearly every town* between the site of death and the airport. (The rest of the money is used for transportation costs and other

official documents.) It usually takes about two weeks for a body to be returned from Spain to the U.S. When the bodies return to the U.S., they are always in an advanced state of decomposition. The best the mortician can do is open the casket (that has been soldered closed) with a can opener and soak the remains in embalming fluid.[186]

Kathryn Coe, an Arizona State University anthropologist related her personal trials in trying to get her father's body back to the United States:

My father died of a heart attack while we were sailing near the Galapagos Islands, 600 miles off the coast of South America. It took six hours (while doing CPR) to get him to the nearest island with a doctor; tragically, our resuscitative effort was of no help. The local carpenter made a crude coffin which we loaded on a ferry to another island. From there we would board a military flight to the mainland. (There was only one tourist flight a week at that time). The airplane was full of officers and their floozies—young, overly painted girls who were obviously not wives. I am certain that none of them knew that the crudely made wooden box they were sitting on and using as a cocktail table held the body of our beloved husband, father, brother, and grandfather. I can see them to this day with their bright red, yellow, green, and purple dresses, silk stockings, high heels, and provocatively crossed legs, draping themselves over his coffin, smiling wisely and too often. They also used its flat surface for their cocktail glasses and overfilled ashtrays. We were too dazed to protest. Besides, my father probably would have found it all to be very funny. When we got to Quito, Ecuador, it took about four days to complete all of the U.S. embassy requirements to return a body to the United States. After all of this, my father's casket, with its mandatory lead covering, weighed ten pounds more than Braniff Airlines' weight limit, so they refused to fly him home. (Since my father was really thin, all adult bodies must have weighed too much to fly home.) Later that day, after bribing Ecuatoriana Airlines to accept the overweight cargo, we headed home. If we were to do it over again, we would have buried him at sea. He loved the sea and its hero tales. It would have been a fitting burial.[187]

Airlines often require a person to accompany an air-shipped corpse. This individual's airfare may be costly. To avoid this, experts suggest obtaining travel insurance before a trip. Such insurance often not only covers costs but also supplies an ombudsman to help make complicated arrangements with foreign governmental agencies and funeral and transport services.

351

Bereavement fares, half-price fares available without prior purchase restrictions for those people accompanying a body or traveling to a funeral, were generally available from all U.S. carriers until mid-1992. At that time United, American, Northwest and USAir stopped offering this discount; Delta offered a meager 10% discount.[188] Not exactly a compassionate move. (TWA and Continental still offered the regular bereavement fare discount.) By the end of 1992, most carriers had reinstated the fares, but at only 17% below the lowest unrestricted fare. The requirements necessary to prove that one qualifies for these fares vary among the airlines. These requirements, and fares, are subject to change at the airlines' whim. Many foreign carriers never offered any bereavement discount, although Air Canada and Canadian International currently do. American Airlines offers a door-to-door delivery service for cremated remains between the crematorium and the recipient of the remains.

If the person making funeral arrangements needs a passport to get to the country where the death occurred, special arrangements can be made through the U.S. State Department's Citizens Emergency Center (open 24-hours every day).

Once a body exits a foreign country, it only must comply with the simple rules for entering the United States. About these rules, the Centers for Disease Control and Prevention (CDC) states:

> There are no federal restrictions on the importation of human remains if death does not result from any of the following communicable diseases: cholera or suspected cholera, diphtheria, infectious tuberculosis, plague, suspected smallpox, yellow fever, and suspected viral hemorrhagic fevers (Lassa, Marburg, Ebola, Congo-Crimean, and others not yet isolated or named). If a person dies as a result of one of these diseases, the remains shall not be brought into a port under the control of the United States unless properly embalmed and placed in a hermetically sealed casket, or cremated.

> The remains must be accompanied by a death certificate translated into English to identify the remains and state the cause of death. The local mortician will comply with regulations of the local health department and the states concerning interstate or intrastate shipment.[189]

In addition, there must be (1) an affidavit stating that only the body, clothing, and necessary packing materials are in the casket; and (2) a permit for export of the body that includes the deceased's sex, race, age, and the date and cause of death.

Complying with these provisions is relatively easy, since the diseases listed are rare or nonexistent in most countries. The U.S. consular officer reports the death of a U.S. citizen to the next-of-kin or legal representative (*Report of the Death of An American Citizen;* Form FS-192/Optional Form 180). The form provides the facts concerning the death and the custody of the personal estate of the deceased. The consular official also helps to obtain private funds to pay for disposal of the body locally or for its return to the United States. Except for active-duty military personnel who die overseas, however, the consular officer will not provide funds for the burial or transportation of American citizens. In some circumstances the consular officer may act as the provisional conservator of the estate and arrange for the disposition of assets. For assistance or information from the U.S. State Department, families or funeral directors can call the Department of State Citizens Emergency Center. (Call (202) 647- 5225, Monday through Friday, 8:15 A.M. to 10 P.M. or Saturday 9 A.M. to 3 P.M. Eastern time. At other times and holidays, call (202) 634-3600 and ask for the overseas-citizens-services duty officer.) The U.S. Code of Federal Regulations for the Return of Remains to the U.S. can be found in Appendix H.

After all of this effort, hopefully, the body will get where it is going. An urban legend that has countless variations recounts the problems of one family trying to bring a dead relative back to the United States:

> A large family decided it would be fun to vacation deep in the heart of romantic Mexico. So dad packed the whole gang, including grandma, aboard their station wagon and took off. They had a fine time. But then, unexpectedly, granny died. What to do, what to do? It appears that when a United States citizen dies in Mexico, there is quite a bit of red tape and expense involved in getting the body home. Wishing to avoid all this delay, the family simply wrapped grandma up and concealed the body atop the car with camping equipment. Then a mad dash for the border followed. After six hours or so they just had to have a break and stopped at a roadside restaurant for food. When they came out, somebody had stolen their station wagon—and their granny. Neither has been seen from that day to this![190]

## Y. HOW ARE BODIES OR ASHES TRANSPORTED BY AIR?

Most bodies transported any distance within the United States, and nearly all bodies transported internationally, go by air. Cremains usually go as carryons, and most bodies needing air transportation now go as cargo in commercial airliners. But there once was an unusual alternative.

The world's first flying hearse was a twelve-passenger, one-coffin seaplane built in 1921. Passengers aboard the wooden-fabric biplane were afforded every comfort. Seated in their wicker seats, they looked out "unshatterable windows," and were provided with electric lights for reading after dark. Also on board was an "iceless Aeriole luncheon" for the passengers and crew. The funeral director followed in a two-passenger seaplane. Only for the wealthy, it is unclear how often it was used.[191]

Usually funeral homes help make air travel arrangements, both for the body and for anyone who will accompany the remains. If there is a question about the cost, especially when outside of the United States, it may be best to either contact the air carrier directly or have the U.S. funeral home make the arrangements.[192]

All major domestic and international air carriers will transport human remains; only their rules and charges differ. Airlines will normally accept bodies if they are (1) accompanied by the documentation (death certificate, burial-transit permit, burial removal permit, etc) required by the sending and receiving locations, and (2) meet the airline's standard packaging requirements.

Standard packaging requirements usually mean that the body must be wrapped in plastic, have a headrest to prevent the head from moving, have a full-length absorbing pad, and be restrained within a casket or other inner container. This inner container must be placed within a "performance tested" outer shipping container (airtray) made of rigid water-repellent material, with six handles and with the head end clearly labeled. Appropriate documentation must be attached to the exterior.

All acceptable airtrays are stamped "performance-tested" and have the manufacturer's three-digit identification number on the outside. These units must pass tests specified by the Air Transport Association, for incline impact, tilt drop, maximum load, compression, moisture repellence, exterior handle load, vibration and top surface hazardous impact. (Does the airplane have this much testing?) Some airlines will supply these outer containers on request.[193]

Although airtrays are designed for only one use, some airlines accept bodies shipped in reused airtrays. While less expensive than using a new airtray, the airline industry is replete with horror stories caused by "pre-owned" containers. On one flight, the now-defunct Eastern Airlines had an airtray leak into the baggage compartment, contaminating all of the other baggage and causing a smell throughout the plane. The smell was so bad that Eastern had to off-load passengers in an out-of-the-way airport and send in another plane to take them to their destination.[194]

Morticians know that they must place the corpse deep enough in the shipping container so that the lid does not press against the face and deform it. They must also wedge the body in tightly with packing so that it does not shift during the flight. Body orifices get extra packing to avoid excretions leaking out or attracting flies. In lieu of using a casket, the body may travel in a fiberboard shipping box if enclosed in an airtray. If the individual died from a contagious disease or the corpse was disinterred, the remains must be shipped in a hermetically (airtight) and permanently sealed casket. Carriers vary these requirements, so survivors should check with the individual airlines before shipping.[194]

Many air carriers have special toll-free phone numbers, (some with such names as AA-TRUST or DL-CARES) and special service personnel for arranging the transport of human remains. The large number of advertisements in funeral journals for the airlines' body transport services attest to the profits they make carting corpses.

Helicopters are not infrequently used to transport corpses out of wilderness areas. A former state trooper in a northern state related the following unusual story. In 1987, hunters found a body of a 40-something-year-old man in the wilderness, partly decomposed, and frozen. When the state police helicopter was sent to investigate, and to retrieve the body, the corpse's position made it impossible to put him inside for transport; so they strapped him onto the helicopter's struts. When the helicopter ran into turbulence on the return trip, the body fell off. Although they searched, they never could find it again. (Perhaps the bears got to it first.) Since the body had no identification, no relatives were ever notified.[196]

## Z. ARE THERE PROBLEMS TRANSPORTING BODIES OR ASHES ACROSS STATE LINES?

Transporting bodies within the United States has a long history, is relatively easy, and is quite common. Sending bodies "home" for burial, now part of the American psyche, began with the improvement in corpse preservation methods during the Civil War. At that time, transportation of dead officers became common, and national attention was focused on the process when, in 1865, Abraham Lincoln was slowly transported by train from Washington, D.C. to Springfield, Illinois for burial (with the coffin opened for viewing at many stops).

By 1900, there was a thriving business in transporting civilian bodies for burial. One reason for the early development of the Southern California funeral industry was that the state's transplanted population often wanted to be shipped elsewhere for burial. This required the services of the funeral director.[197]

People ship cadavers and cremated remains across the United States for several reasons: burial near a traditional home and family, use of a prepurchased burial plot, and the relatively low cost of transporting a body for burial as opposed to the cost of transporting the family to the death site. States with the highest percentage of shipments out-of-state correspond to those with the highest immigration rates: Nevada, Florida, Alaska, and Arizona.[198]

While each state has its own rules about transporting corpses, embalming is *not* usually required unless the person died from a specific contagious disease, the transport time will be inordinately long, the body has decomposed, or it has been disinterred. Contagious bodies often must also be "disinfected," but it is unclear exactly what protection this step provides. The commonly specified contagious diseases are: plague, yellow fever, smallpox, epidemic typhus, leprosy, poliomyelitis, diphtheria, Asiatic cholera, glanders and anthrax, although these diseases are either rarely seen in the United States or no longer exist anywhere in the world (smallpox). Some states, however, include any "reportable" communicable disease, which includes influenza, gonorrhea, and AIDS. Minnesota lists conjunctivitis, diarrhea, measles, mononucleosis, strep throat and pneumonia! A few states, such as Georgia, have no specific requirements.

Bodies without contagious diseases that need interstate transport must reach their destinations within 18 to 72 hours to avoid required embalming, although this too varies. Many states and carriers also require a permit to move a body. These can usually be obtained from a funeral home or the local board of health.

Bodies are normally sent by common carrier (airlines, trucking companies, railroads) that each have individual requirements. Within the United States, most bodies travel by air, and funeral directors can normally arrange for this service. If notified, many airlines provide special waiting areas and preboarding for those accompanying a body.

Amtrak also transports human remains, providing station-to-station shipment. The railroad accepts human remains in caskets enclosed in carrying cases with handles; used airtrays suffice. No special rates are available for those accompanying the body.

Some bodies travel by private vehicle and a large number of cremains travel via the postal service. When ashes are shipped by funeral directors within the United States, they are normally placed within a sturdy, pressure-resistant container, tightly sealed, and sent via a service that can track the package if it gets lost. A signature upon receipt is usually required.

Pathologists often ship parts of bodies and tissue samples to special laboratories for expert opinions or special laboratory tests that cannot be obtained locally. The pathologist arranges any necessary special packaging and handling.[199]

## AA. WILL I BE AN ARCHAEOLOGICAL FIND?

For all of history, people have marveled, without concern, at the bodies of ancient people. Cultural sensitivity, it seems, dies when no one remains to claim a relationship with the deceased. Human remains from the Stone Age, Iron Age and Bronze Age are widely displayed, although these people were the ancestors of millions now living; they cannot, however, be traced to any particular person or group. Museums commonly display human bones, entire burial sites, and recognizable bodies, such as those from the bog people of northern Europe and the iceman discovered frozen in the Alps. In fact, the better preserved one's remains, the more valuable they are to future archaeologists and paleontologists. As Ambrose Bierce said,

> Tombs are now by common consent invested with a certain sanctity, but when they have been long tenanted it is considered no sin to break them open and rifle them, the famous Egyptologist, Dr. Huggyns, explaining that a tomb may be innocently 'glened' as soon as its occupant is done 'smellynge,' the soul being then all exhaled. This reasonable view is now generally accepted by archaeologists, whereby the noble science of Curiosity has been greatly dignified.[200]

This is not only true of the ancients. Scholars and souvenir hunters have disinterred, for study and display, the remains of Romans, Celts, Greeks, Egyptians and others, some of whom are identifiable by name and lineage. The corpses and body parts of Catholic saints, exalted Buddhist priests, notable rulers and famous outlaws have also been displayed for public fascination or veneration.

Recent disinterments for display include the shrunken heads at Ripley's popular sideshows and Native American remains, including mummies, bones and other specimens from the last century that still reside in many museums. The Musée de l'Homme, in Paris displays skeletons and mummies, including Descartes' skull, shrunken heads from the Jivaro Indians, and the mummies of a Nubian foetus, a Bolivian Indian woman and child, and one from Aqsum.[201] In a departure from the norm, the natural mummies displayed in Guanajuato, Mexico and at the Capuchin monastery in Palermo, Italy are those of the area's citizens, some of whom died in this century. Increasingly, however, some countries, such as Egypt, are removing their mummies from public view.[202]

One of the largest collections of unburied human bones resides in the Smithsonian Institution's Museum of Natural History. Bones from about 33,000 individuals accumulated over more than 100 years, are stored in stacks of green drawers rising 16 feet to the ceiling along hallway after hallway.[203]

Currently, graves are being disturbed at an increasing rate by vandals, construction workers and natural events. From 1985 to 1989, 258 of the 3,386 forensic science cases (7.6%) examined in the United States by anthropology diplomates were of historic origin.[204]

In mainland China, for example, more than 25,000 tombs were plundered between 1988 and 1990 to retrieve antiquities. The growing market for the relics that were buried with bodies has produced organized gangs with sophisticated equipment who destroy gravesites and tombs to acquire their booty.[205]

In 1992, workers constructing a large federal office building in downtown Manhattan rediscovered the old "Negros Burial Ground," the oldest and largest pre-Revolutionary War African-American graveyard. Opened in the mid-1600s, it was in use until about 1790. When the workers finally stopped their construction, physical anthropologists went to work analyzing the remains. Eventually these bodies, once thought to have been buried in the most desolate acres outside of colonial New York, will be reburied.[206]

Even sea burials do not absolutely guarantee that body parts will not be found and retrieved, as has happened in some shipwrecks. Cremation provides the only certainty that an individual will not be an archaeological treasure at some future time.

## AB. REFERENCES

1. Rodriguez WC, Bass WM: Insect activity and its relationship to decay rates of human cadavers in east Tennessee. *J Forensic Sciences.* 1983;28(2):423-32.
2. Mann RW, Bass WM, Meadows L: Time since death and decomposition of the human body: Variables and observations in case and experimental field studies. *J Forensic Sciences.* 1990;35(1):103-11.
3. Ibid.
4. Spitz WU, Fisher RS: *Medicolegal Investigation of Death.* Springfield, IL: Charles C Thomas, 1973, p 18-19.
5. Bahn PG, Everett K: Iceman in the cold light of day. *Nature.* 1993;362:11-12.
6. Jaroff L: Iceman. *Time.* 1992;140(17):62-66.
7. And in Sweden: *USA Today.* March 18, 1992.
8. Shakespeare W: *Romeo and Juliet.* Act 3, scene 1, line 112.
9. Lewis MG: *Monk.* (1796) III.65 (*Alonzo the Brave,* xii). Cited in: *The Compact Edition of the Oxford English Dictionary.* vol 2. New York: Oxford Univ Press, 1971, p 3823. under "worm."
10. Words attributed to unknown British soldiers 1854/1856, and oral tradition. A version can be found in: Pankake M, Pankake J: "The Hearse Song." *Prairie Home Companion Folk Song Book.* New York: Viking Penguin, 1988; and this author's oral tradition.
11. Poe EA: "Ligeia." 1838. In: Stern P, ed: *Viking Portable Library:Poe.* New York: Viking Press, 1964, p 233.
12. Rodriguez, Bass, *J Forensic Sciences,* 1983.
13. Mann, Bass, Meadows, *J Forensic Sciences,* 1990.
14. Spitz, Fisher, *Medicolegal Investigation of Death,* p 20-21.
15. Catts EP, Goff ML: Forensic entomology in criminal investigations. *Ann Rev Entomol.* 1992;37:253-72.
16. Mann, Bass, Meadows, *J Forensic Sciences,* 1990.
17. Catts, Goff, *Ann Rev Entomol,* 1992.
18. Richards B: The maggot test: Bugs on dead bodies have tales to tell. *Wall Street J.* April 27, 1992, p A1+.
19. Simpson K: *Forty Years of Murder.* New York: Dorset Press, 1978, pp 246-54.
20. Richards, *Wall Street J,* April 27, 1992.
21. Schrof JM: Murder, they chirped. *U.S. News and World Report.* October 14, 1991, pp 67-68.
22. Ibid.
23. Bergeret M: Infanticide, momification du cadavre. Découverte du cadavre d'un enfant nouveau-né dans une cheminée ou il s'etait momifie. Détermination de l'époque de la

naissance par la présence de nymphes et de larves d'insectes dans le cadavre et par l'étude de leurs métamorphoses. *Ann Hyg Publique Med Leg.* 1855;4:442-52.

24. Nuorteva P: *Sarcosaprophagous Insects as Forensic Indicators.* In: Tedeschi CG, Eckert WG, Tedeschi LG: *Forensic Medicine: A Study in Trauma and Environmental Hazards.* vol 2. Philadelphia, PA: WB Saunders, 1977, pp 1072-95.

25. Press Clips. *The Forum.* April 1992, p 12.

26. Haglund WD, Reay DT, Swindler DR: Canid scavenging/disarticulation sequence of human remains in the Pacific northwest. *J Forensic Sciences.* 1989;34:587-606.

27. Mann, Bass, Meadows, *J Forensic Sciences,* 1990.

28. Ibid.

29. Polson CJ, Brittain RP, Marshall TK: *The Disposal of the Dead.* 2nd ed. Springfield, IL: Charles C Thomas, 1962, p 284.

30. Tegg W: *The Last Act: Being the Funeral Rites of Nations and Individuals.* London: William Tegg & Co, 1876, p 367-68.

31. van Wyk CW, Theunissen F, Phillips VM: A grave matter—dental findings of people buried in the 19th and 20th centuries. *J Forensic Odonto-Stomatology.* 1990;8(2):15-30.

32. Spitz, Fisher, *Medicolegal Investigation of Death,* p 21.

33. Mann, Bass, Meadows, *J Forensic Sciences,* 1990.

34. Spitz, Fisher, *Medicolegal Investigation of Death,* p 21.

35. Mann, Bass, Meadows, *J Forensic Sciences,* 1990.

36. Glob PV: *The Bog People—Iron-Age Man Preserved.* (Bruce-Mitford R, trans). Ithaca, New York: Cornell Univ Press, 1969, p 15.

37. Blicher SS: *Queen Gunhild.* 1841. Quoted in: Glob, *The Bog People,* p 73.

38. Williams S: Dark bogs, DNA, and the mummy. *OMNI.* 1992;14:43-44+.

39. Mann, Bass, Meadows, *J Forensic Sciences,* 1990.

40. Sea Services finds niche. *The Director.* March 1992, p 66.

41. Personal Communication: Sea Services, Inc. New York: March 1992.

42. Dolan C: Burying tradition, more people opt for 'fun' funerals. *Wall Street J.* May 20, 1993, p A1+.

43. Grycznski, ES, Tolleson LJ, Audie EH: *Taps—A Guide to Military-Oriented Burial.* Alexandria, VA: Retired Officers' Assn., 1990, p 16.

44. Ibid.

45. *Finley v. Atlantic Transp. Co.,* 220 N.Y. 249, 259, 115 N.E. 715. Cited in: Jackson PE: *The Law of Cadavers and of Burial and Burial Places.* New York: Prentice-Hall, 1937, p 66.

46. Tegg, *The Last Act,* p 45.

47. Jacob W: *Contemporary American Reform Responsa.* New York: Central Conference of American Rabbis, 1987, pp 166-67.

48. Dempsey D: *The Way We Die.* New York: MacMillan, 1975, p 169.

49. Barber P: *Vampires, Burial, and Death: Folklore and Reality.* New Haven, CT: Yale Univ Press, 1988, p 78.

50. Anima N: *Childbirth & Burial Practices Among Philippine Tribes.* Quezon City, Philippines: Omar Pub, 1978, p 104.

51. Roddis LH: *A Short History of Nautical Medicine.* New York: Paul B Hoeber, 1941, p 74.

52. Tegg, *The Last Act,* p 319-20.

53. Edwards IG: Down memory lane: burial at sea. *Nursing Mirror.* 1980;150(21):36-37.

54. Lord Byron (Gordon G): *Childe Harold's Pilgrimage.* In: Bostetter EE: *George Gordon, Lord Byron—Selected Works.* New York: Holt Rinehart & Winston, 1972, p 105.

55. Roddis, *Nautical Medicine,* p 116.

56. Johnson EC: A brief history of U.S. military embalming. *The Director.* 1971;41:8-9.

57. Polson, Brittain, Marshall, *The Disposal of the Dead,* p 284.

58. Mann, Bass, Meadows, *J Forensic Sciences,* 1990.

59. Haskell NH, McShaffrey DG, Hawley DA, et al: Use of aquatic insects in determining submersion interval. *J Forensic Sciences.* 1989;34:622-32.

60. Spitz, Fisher, *Medicolegal Investigation of Death,* p 298.

61. Cotton GE, Aufderheide AC, Goldschmidt VG: Preservation of human tissue immersed for five years in fresh water of known temperature. *J Forensic Sciences.* 1987;32:1125-30.

62. *Rig Veda.* Book 10, Hymn 16, verse 3.

63. Carr J. Quoted in: Mitford J: *The American Way of Death.* New York: Simon & Schuster,

1963, p 84.
64. Sloan G: In undersea graves of Guadalcanal warships. *USA Today.* May 10, 1993, p 3D.
65. Davis CH. Cited in: Spitz, Fisher, *Medicolegal Investigation of Death,* p 305.
66. Rathbun TA, Rathbun BC: Human remains recovered from a shark's stomach in South Carolina. *J Forensic Sciences.* 1984;29:269-76.
67. Walker GA: *Gatherings From Grave Yards.* London: Longman & Co, 1839, p 16.
68. Palmer G, exec producer: Death: The Trip of a Lifetime. Seattle, WA: KCTS-TV Public Broadcasting Station, 1993. (video production)
69. Habenstein RW, Lamers WM: *The History of American Funeral Directing.* (Revision.) Milwaukee, WI: National Funeral Directors Association, 1985, p 82.
70. Oladepo O, Sridhar MK: Public health implications of practices and beliefs in the disposal of the dead. *J Royal Society of Health.* 1985;105(6):219-21.
71. Barber, *Vampires, Burial, and Death,* p 142.
72. Spitz, Fisher, *Medicolegal Investigation of Death,* pp 307-308.
73. Clarke. As quoted in: Tegg, *The Last Act,* p 241-42.
74. Ibid., p 241-42.
75. Gittings C: *Death, Burial and the Individual in Early Modern England.* London: Croom & Helm, 1984, p 74.
76. Russell KF: Anatomy and the barber-surgeons. *Med J Australia.* 1973;1:1109-115.
77. Richardson R: *Death, Dissection and the Destitute.* London: Routledge & Kegan Paul, 1987, p 54.
78. Bierce A: *Devil's Dictionary.* New York: Dover Pub, 1958, p 18.
79. Ibid., p 50.
80. Editorial. *Lancet.* January 25,1824.
81. Adams N: *Dead and Buried?* Aberdeen, Scotland: Impulse Books, 1972, p 117.
82. Franklin J, Sutherland J: *Guinea Pig Doctors.* New York: William Morrow & Co, 1984, p 48-49.
83. Schultz SM: *Body Snatching: The Robbing of Graves for the Education of Physicians.* Jefferson, NC: McFarland, 1992, p 98-99.
84. Hood T: "The Invisible Girl." In: Gibson W: *Rambles in Europe in 1839, with Sketches of Prominent Surgeons, Physicians, Medical Schools, Hospitals, Literary Personages, Scenery, etc.* Philadelphia: Lea & Blanchard, 1841.
85. Adams, *Dead and Buried?,* p 69.
86. Haestier R: *Dead Men Tell Tales: A Survey of Exhumations, From Earliest Antiquity to the Present Day.* London: John Long, 1934, p 99.
87. Richardson, *Death, Dissection and the Destitute,* p 67.
88. Guttmacher AF: Bootlegging bodies—a history of body-snatching. *Bull Soc Med His Chicago.* 1935;4(4):353-402.
89. Soren D: Hecate and the infant cemetery of Lugnano in Teverina. (Unpublished manuscript).
90. Haestier, *Dead Men Tell Tales,* p 28.
91. Weever J: *Ancient Funeral Monuments.* 1631, p 42-43. Quoted in: Jackson, *The Law of Cadavers,* p 93.
92. Shakespeare W: *Cymbeline.* Act 4, scene 2, lines 276-81.
93. Shakespeare W.: Epitaph. In: Richardson, *Death, Dissection and the Destitute,* p 54.
94. *1 Jas. 1 c. 12* (1604).
95. *9 Geo. 2 c. 5.* (1736).
96. Adams, *Dead and Buried?,* p 135.
97. Ibid., p 133-42.
98. Ibid.
99. *Arizona Daily Star.* Tucson, AZ: October 22, 1882, p 2.
100. Montgomery HA: A body-snatcher sponsors Pennsylvania's Anatomy Act. *J Hist Med.* 1966;21:374-93.
101. Cooper BB: *The Life of Sir Astley Cooper, Bart.* London: John W Parker, 1843, p 176.
102. Lonsdale H. As quoted by:Adams, *Dead and Buried?,* p 35.
103. Clerihew: My first ressurrectionist. *Aberdeen Magazine.* Spring 1831.
104. Rodger EHB: *Aberdeen Doctors: At Home and Abroad.* Edinburgh: William Blackwood & Sons, 1893, p 220.

105. Gordon A: *Death is for the Living.* Edinburgh: Paul Harris, 1984, p 133.
106. Rodger, *Aberdeen Doctors,* p 227.
107. Richardson, *Death, Dissection and the Destitute,* p 60.
108. Napier J.Quoted by: Guttmacher, *Bull Soc Med Hist Chicago,* 1935.
109. Richardson, *Death, Dissection and the Destitute,* p 72.
110. Adams, *Dead and Buried?,* pp 72-73.
111. Baldwin JF: Grave robbing. *Ohio State Med J.* 1936;32(Aug):754-57.
112. Southey R: "The Surgeon's Warning." *Joan of Arc, Ballads, Lyrics, and Minor Poems.* London: George Routledge & Sons, 1798, pp 275-80.
113. Ibid.
114. Haviland TN: *Surgery, Gynecology & Obstretics.* 1963;117:774-76.
115. Habenstein, Lamers, *History of American Funeral Directing,* p 183.
116. Report of the Select Committee appointed by the House of Commons to inquire into the manner of obtaining subjects for dissection in schools of anatomy. *New York M & Phys J.* 1828;8:50.
117. Ibid.
118. Cole H: *Things for the Surgeon.* London: Heineman, 1964, pp 104-105.
119. Schultz, *Body Snatching,* p 49.
120. Waite FC: An episode in Massachusetts in 1818 related to the teaching of Anatomy. *New Engl J Med.* 1939;220(6):221-27.
121. Bradford CH: Countway happenings: Resurrectionists and spunkers. *N Engl J Med.* 1976;294:1331-32.
122. Warren JC. As quoted in: Schultz, *Body Snatching,* p 30.
123. Humphrey DC: Dissection and discrimination: the social origins of cadavers in America, 1760-1915. *Bull NY Academy of Med.* 1973;49:819-27.
124. Schultz, *Body Snatching,* p 56.
125. Humphrey, *Bull NY Academy of Med,* 1973.
126. Heaton CE: Body snatching in New York City. *NY J Med.* 1864.
127. Forbes WS: *History of the Anatomy Act of Pennsylvania.* 1867. In: Schultz, *Body Snatching,* pp 111-17.
128. Sozinsky TS: Grave-robbing and dissection. *Penn Monthly.* 1879;10:216-17.
129. Edwards LF: Cincinnati's "old Cunny" a notorious purveyor of human flesh. *Ohio State Med J.* 1954;50:466-69.
130. Schultz, *Body Snatching,* pp 59-62.
131. Verrastro N: Edgar Allan Poe. *The American Funeral Director.* 1991;115:62+.
132. *Evening Star.* Washington, D.C.: December 13, 1873.
133. Mall FP: Anatomical material—its collection and its preservation at the Johns Hopkins anatomical laboratory. *Bull Johns Hopkins Hospital.* 1905;16:38-39+.
134. Guttmacher, *Bull Soc Med Hist Chicago,* 1935.
135 Martineau H: *Retrospect of Western Travel.* vol 1. London: Saunders & Otley, 1838, p 140.
136. Mencken HL: *Happy Days 1880-1892.* New York: Alfred A Knopf, 1963, p 153.
137. Lawrence C: *History of the Philadelphia Almshouses and Hospitals.* Philadelphia, PA: 1905, pp 160-61.
138. *New York Times.* August 5, 1879, p 3.
139. Savitt TL: The use of blacks for medical experimentation and demonstration in the Old South. *J Southern History.* 1982;48:331-48.
140. Packard FR: *History of Medicine in the United States.* New York: Hafner, 1963, pp786-87.
141. Holtz W: Bankrobbers, burkers & bodysnatchers. *Mich Quarterly Review.* 1967;6(2):90-98.
142. Humphrey, *Bull NY Acad Med,* 1973.
143. Gindhart PS: An early twentieth-century skeleton collection. *J Forensic Sciences.* 1989;34:887-93.
144. Edwards LF: The Ohio Anatomy Law of 1881. *Ohio State Med J.* 1951;47:49-52.
145. Fuller P: Body snatchers—ghouls abounded in the late 19th century. *Tribune Review.* Greensburg, PA: 1988.
146. *Cincinnati Post.* February 22, 1884.
147. Guttmacher, *Bull Soc Med Hist Chicago,* 1935.
148. *Medical Standard.* Indianapolis, IN: 1902.
149. Guttmacher, *Bull Soc Med Hist Chicago,* 1935.

150. Truax R: *The Doctors Warren of Boston: First Family of Surgery.* Boston: Houghton Mifflin, 1968, p 313.
151. *R. v. Lynn.* 1788.
152. Bernard HY: *The Law of Death and Disposal of the Dead.* 2nd ed. Dobbs Ferry, NY: Oceana Pub, 1979, p 12.
153. *Hayne's Case,* 12 Coke 113, 77 Eng. Rep. 1389.
154. Richardson, *Death, Dissection and the Destitute,* pp 58-59.
155. Adams, *Dead and Buried?,* p 51.
156. Richardson, *Death, Dissection and the Destitute,* p 85.
157. Rodger, *Aberdeen Doctors,* p 220.
158. Adams, *Dead and Buried?,* p 75-77.
159. Flexner JT: *Doctors on Horseback: Pioneers of American Medicine.* New York: Garden City Pub, 1939, pp 223-24.
160. Edwards, *Ohio State Med J,* 1951.
161. Robinson JH: *Marietta or the Two Students, A Tale of the Dissecting Room and Body Snatching.* Boston: Jordan & Wiley, 1846.
162. Gordon, *Death is for the Living,* p 136.
163. Adams, *Dead and Buried?,* p 88.
164. Adams, *Dead and Buried?,* p 102.
165. Leighton A: *The Court of Cacus; or, The Story of Burke and Hare.* 2nd ed. London: Houlston & Wright, 1861, pp 255-56.
166. Ibid., pp 248-49.
167. Ibid., pp 268, 278-80.
168. Stevenson RL: *The Body Snatcher.* In: Stoneley P, ed: *Robert Louis Stevenson: The Collected Shorter Fiction.* London: Robinson Pub, 1991, pp 326-40.
169. Russell, *Med J Australia,* 1973.
170. Cole, *Things for the Surgeon,* pp 134-57.
171. Ibid., p 95.
172. Baker R: Undertakings. *New York Times.* 1975;124:42(Jan 12):6.
173. Puente M: Mausoleum robbery 'no prank.' *USA Today.* January 8, 1992, p 3A.
174. Gutkin S: Trash scavenger tale jolts Colombia's elite. (Associated Press) *Tucson (AZ) Citizen.* April 1, 1992, p 1+.
175. Horwitz T: Eurocrats find it's hard to bury differences over the body politic. *Wall Street J.* March 22, 1993, p B1.
176. Basevi WHF: *The Burial of the Dead.* London: George Rutledge & Sons, 1920, p 53.
177. Lord Byron (Gordon G), June 7, 1819. Quoted in: *The Oxford Dictionary of Quotations.* 3rd ed. Oxford: Oxford Univ Press, 1969, p 126-20.
178. Baker TD, Hargarten SW, Guptill KS: The uncounted dead—American civilians dying overseas. *Public Health Reports.* 1992;107:155+.
179. Stevenson RL: *Requiem.* In: Begelow CC, Scott T, eds: *The Works of Robert Louis Stevenson.* vol 8. New York: Davos Press, 1906, p 37. (also RL Stevenson's epitaph)
180 Carriers face foggy horizons. *The American Funeral Director.* 1991;115(3):20-23, 32-52.
181. Hagan J: *International Shipping Regulations.* (lecture) National Funeral Directors Association Annual Convention. Baltimore, MD: 1989. (audiotape)
182. Horwitz T: Eurocrats find it's hard to bury differences over the body politic. *Wall Street J.* March 22, 1993, p B1.
183. Belkoff H: Interview. May 15, 1993.
184. Forgey W: *Travelers' Medical Resource.* Merrillville, IN: ICS Books, 1990, p 2.6.
185. Ibid., p 2.7.
186. Belkoff,Interview, May 15, 1993.
187. Coe, Kathryn: Personal communication. November 23, 1993.
188. Airlines ending of bereavement fares adds financial burden to emotional one. *Arizona Daily Star.* Tucson, AZ: July 12, 1992.
189. CDC Regulations. Cited in: Forgey, *Travelers' Medical Resource,* p 2.7.
190. Bothwell D: *Brighten Up Monday Stories.* St. Petersburg, FL: Great Outdoors, 1978, p 13.
191. Bacr BA: The world's first flying hearse. *Casket & Sunnyside.* 1971;101:44+. (originally published in *The Sunnyside.* October 21, 1921.)

192. Carriers face foggy horizons, *American Funeral Director,* 1991.
193. Ibid.
194. Hagen, *International Shipping Regulations,* 1989. (audiotape)
195. Carriers face foggy horizons, *American Funeral Director,* 1991.
196. Interview with anonymous retired state trooper. Tucson, AZ: May 16, 1993.
197. Farrell JJ: *Inventing the American Way of Death, 1830-1920.* Philadelphia: Temple Univ Press, 1980, p 174.
198. Kastenbaum RK, Kastenbaum B, eds: *Encyclopedia of Death.* Phoenix, AZ: Oryx Press, 1989, p 37.
199. Hagen, *International Shipping Regulations,* 1989. (audiotape)
200. Bierce, *Devil's Dictionary,* p 133.
201. Ragon M: *The Space of Death: A Study of Funerary Architecture, Decoration, and Urbanism.* (Sheridan A: trans) Charlottesville, VA: Univ Press of Virginia, 1983. Originally published as: *L'espace de la mort: Essai sur l'architecture, la décoration et l'urbanisme funéraires.* Albin Michel, 1981, p 96.
202. Koosman S: *Cultural Variations in Funeral Practice.* (lecture). National Funeral Directors Assoc. Annual Convention. Baltimore, MD: 1989. (audio tape)
203. Dolnick E: Dead men do tell tales. *Wall Street J.* December 11, 1992. Bookshelf.
204. Berryman HE, Bass WM, Symes SA, Smith OC: Recognition of cemetery remains in the forensic setting. *J Forensic Sciences.* 1991;36:230-37.
205. Cohn D: Raiding China's treasure chest. *World Press Review.* 1992;39(10):48.
206. Frankel B: Black cemetery in NYC new key to colonial times. *USA Today.* September 15, 1992, p A10.

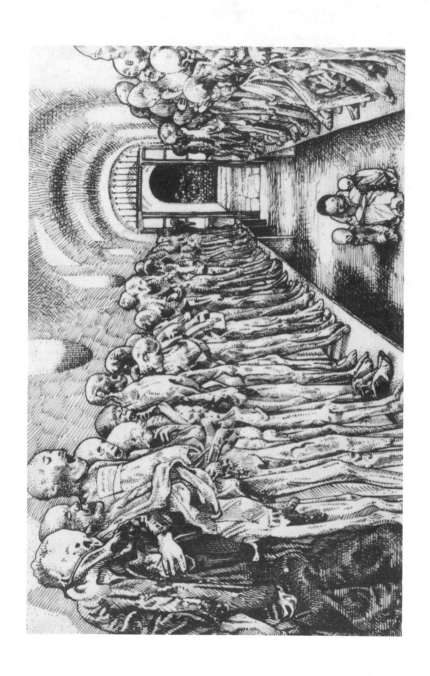

The hall of mummies, Guanajuato, Mexico.

# 9: NIGHTMARES

A. What is cannibalism?
B. When has cannibalism provided a necessary source of food?
C. How was cannibalism used to acquire powers and satisfy gods?
D. What kind of rituals honored dead relatives or enemies?
E. How was cannibalism used for revenge?
F. Has cannibalism been practiced recently?
G. Why hunt or shrink heads?
H. How is a shrunken head prepared?
I. What is stripping the flesh?
J. When else have animals been used to devour the dead?
K. Why is a body systematically dismembered after death?
L. What else was done with criminals' bodies?
M. How else are body parts used?
N. What is necrophilia?
O. What about necrophobia?
P. When have people been sacrificed to serve the dead?
Q. How were corpses supposed to help or harm the living?
R. What other unusual uses are there for dead bodies?
S. References.

*How have corpses, or their parts, been used as food, decorations, public warnings to criminals, war trophies, religious fetishes, or as sex objects? What is the reality behind many horror stories and movies?*

## A. WHAT IS CANNIBALISM?

Cannibalism is the practice of eating one's own species, in our case, human flesh. Humans have eaten the flesh of other humans since the dawn of time and the practice continues to this day.

The English word "cannibal" derives from the early Spaniards' name for the Carib Indians, based in the Antilles islands. The Caribs were fierce fighters and, reportedly, notorious eaters of human flesh. Columbus first used the name *Canibales*, but he never actually saw cannibalism. He thought the word meant "people of the great Kahn," in keeping with his belief that he had found China.[1]

Until modern times, cannibalism existed in parts of west and central Africa, Australia, New Zealand, some of the Pacific Islands, among various tribes in North and South America, and in southeast Asia. Cannibalism still occurs throughout the world because of severe hunger, and in the past some cultures used human flesh as a food supplement. Most societally accepted cannibalism, however, has been a ritualistic, symbolic activity. These rituals were associated with forming the male identity, transferring individual powers and skills, and showing respect for dead relatives or enemies. Perhaps because of a scarcity of animal protein in their diets, cannibalism has been closely tied to agrarian societies' religious or magical plant cultivation rites.[2]

Peggy Sanday found evidence of cannibalism in one-third of the 109 societies she investigated.[3] Most of these societies were from North America and the Pacific Islands; Africa and South America had fewer cannibalistic groups. She found only two cannibalistic societies in the Mediterranean area and none from eastern Europe and Asia (Table 9.1).

As it was with the Caribs, cannibalism has often been ascribed to alien groups by their enemies. When Livingstone explored Africa, for example, he was shocked to find that nearly all blacks thought whites were cannibals.

Some modern scholars caution that all "Spanish accusations [of cannibalism] must be understood within a context of 'imperial propaganda' and seen as 'self-serving,' because cannibals were the sole 'Amerindians subject to enslavement.' "[4] Other scholars dismiss English, French and Dutch claims, saying that cannibalism never existed and that there are no recorded eyewitness reports of the practice.[5] This is not true. One particularly graphic report comes from one of the first Polynesian missionaries to arrive in New Caledonia:

## TABLE 9.1: Where did Societally Approved Cannibalism Exist?*

|  | Number with cannibalism (out of number investigated) | Percent |
| --- | --- | --- |
| Pacific Islands | 11/21 | 52% |
| North America | 11/23 | 48 |
| Sub-Saharan Africa | 7/15 | 47 |
| South/Central America | 6/14 | 43 |
| Mediterranean Area | 2/13 | 15 |
| East Europe/Asia | 0/23 | 0 |

* It is not clear whether all of these cases can be substantiated.

Adapted from: Sanday PR: *Divine Hunger: Cannibalism as a Cultural System.* Cambridge: Cambridge Univ Press, 1986, p 5.

I followed and watched the battle and saw women taking part in it. They did so in order to carry off the dead. When people were killed, the men tossed the bodies back and the women fetched and carried them. They chopped the bodies up and divided them...When the battle was over, they all returned home together, the women in front and the men behind. The womenfolk carried the flesh on their backs; the coconut-leaf baskets were full up and the blood oozed over their backs and trickled down their legs. It was a horrible sight to behold. When they reached their homes the earth ovens were lit at each house and they ate the slain. Great was their delight, for they were eating well that day. This was the nature of the food. The fat was yellow and the flesh was dark. It was difficult to separate the flesh from the fat. It was rather like the flesh of sheep.

I looked particularly at our household's share; the flesh was dark like sea-cucumber, the fat was yellow like beef fat, and it smelt like cooked birds, like pigeon or chicken. The share of the chief was the right hand and the right foot. Part of the chief's portion was brought for me, as for the priest, but I returned it. The people were unable to eat it all; the legs and the arms only were consumed, the body itself was left.[6]

It is clear, however, that some reports of cannibalism were exaggerated, both out of ignorance and for their effect on enemies. The celebrated African explorer Sir Richard Francis Burton classified the ways natives looked at white men, with "stare number 12" being "the stare cannibal, which apparently considered us as items of diet."[7] Burton did not, however, ever report actually witnessing cannibalism.

## B. WHEN HAS CANNIBALISM PROVIDED A NECESSARY SOURCE OF FOOD?

Cannibalism has been used throughout history to feed starving populations, and in almost every culture cannibalism has occasionally been used for survival.[8] During the fifth and fourth millennia B.C., groups of Neolithic hunters at Fontbrégoua, France slaughtered and ate humans in the same fashion as they did sheep and wild animals. Human bones found at the site have slash marks in places similar to those made by modern butchers when they cut meat; all of the long bones were broken as if to extract marrow.[9]

In historical times, Josephus, the apostate chronicler, wrote of one cannibalistic episode just after Roman forces had taken Jerusalem following a long siege in A.D. 70:

> Famine gnawed at her vitals, and the fire of rage was even fiercer than famine. So, driven by fury and want, she committed a crime against nature. Seizing her child, an infant at the breast, she cried, "My poor baby, why should I keep you alive in this world of war and famine?...Come, be food for me, and an avenging fury to the rebels, and a tale of horror to the world to complete the monstrous agony of the Jews." With these words she killed her son, roasted the body, swallowed half of it, and stored the rest in a safe place...The whole city soon rang with the abomination. When people heard of it, they shuddered, as though they had done it themselves.[10]

Arab travelers reported towards the end of the T'ang dynasty (late ninth and early tenth centuries), that to supplement the food supply, "Chinese law permits the eating of human flesh, and this flesh is sold publicly in the markets."[11]

During the early 1400s, a cannibal clan existed in Scotland. Sawney (Sandy) Beane and his wife lived in a secluded cave on the coast of Galloway, eventually producing 14 children and 34 grandchildren. They survived by waylaying travellers and feeding on them, killing more than 1,000 people over the years. In 1435 they were caught; the evidence against them being the human arms, legs and haunches hanging neatly from the ceiling of their cave. Adults and children alike were taken to Leith and executed.[12]

Sixteenth-century New World Spanish explorers also occasionally resorted to cannibalism to survive. One incident was recounted by Cabeza de Vaca, the first European to report on the interior of Florida, Texas, New Mexico, Arizona and northernmost Mexico. Out of an initial party of 300 men, only he and three compatriots remained alive after their eight-year odyssey. According to his log, some of his party resorted to cannibalism on what they later called the "Island of Doom" (now Galveston Island, Texas) in an unsuccessful attempt at survival: "Five Christians quartered on the coast came to the extremity of eating each other. Only the body of the last one, whom nobody was left to eat, was found unconsumed...The Indians were so shocked at this cannibalism that, if they had seen it sometime earlier, they surely would have killed every one of us."[13] Only a short time later (near what is now San Antonio Bay, on Padre Island, TX) he reported: "One by one they began to die of cold and hunger...Thus the number went on diminishing. The living dried the flesh of those who died. The last to die was Sotomayor. [Hernando de] Esquivel, by feeding on the corpse, was able to stay alive until the first of March" when an Indian rescued him. He was later slain by other Indians.[14]

The Aztec Indians of Mexico sometimes used other humans as a food source. Cortés wrote that his men came across "loads of maize and roasted children which they [Aztec soldiers] had brought as provisions and which they left behind them when they discovered the Spaniards coming."[15] Fray Bernardino de Sahagún said that enemies sometimes slew Aztec merchants and ate them "with chili sauce." In societies with a protein-poor diet, such as the Aztecs', the right to eat human flesh was often an honor reserved for the most successful warriors.[16]

Queen Elizabeth I's policy toward a rebellious Ireland led to widespread famine and incidents of cannibalism. Fynes Moryson, the secretary to the Queen's Lord-Deputy in Ireland wrote in 1602, that he "...saw a most horrible spectacle of three children (whereof the eldest was not above ten years old) all eating and gnawing with their teeth the entrails of their dead mother, upon whose flesh they had fed twenty days past, and having eaten all from the feet upward to the bare bones, roasting it continually by a slow fire, were now come to the eating of her said entrails in the like sort roasted, yet not divided from the body, being as yet raw." He went on to relate that "some old women of those parts used to make a fire in the fields, and divers little children dreving out the cattle in the cold mornings, and coming thither to warm them, were by them surprised, killed and eaten."[17]

According to Jesuit observers in the mid-seventeenth century, Huron and Iroquois Indians were reduced to eating their own dead during famines. "Mothers fed upon their children; brothers on their brothers; while children recognized no longer, in a corpse, him whom, while he lived, they had called their Father."[18] In 1650 another Jesuit wrote, "Everywhere, corpses have been dug out of the graves; and, now carried away by hunger, the people have repeatedly offered, as food, those who were lately the dear pledges of love,—not only brothers to brothers, but even children to their mothers, and the parents to their own children."[19]

During this period, not only the Indians resorted to survival cannibalism. In 1608, during what came to be called "the starving time," John Smith (of Pocahontas fame) reported that surviving Jamestown Colonists disinterred the corpse of a murdered Indian, "boiled and stewed [him] with roots and herbs," and ate him. This act was eclipsed when "one among the rest did kill his wife, powdered [salted] her, and had eaten part of her before it was known; for which he was executed, as he well deserved. Now, whether she was better roasted, boiled, or carbonadoed [broiled], I know not; but of such a dish as powdered wife I never heard."[20]

Even in Victorian England some writers considered using corpses for food, thus solving the body-disposal problem while adding to the food supply. No one took them seriously.[21,22]

## C. HOW WAS CANNIBALISM USED TO ACQUIRE POWERS AND SATISFY GODS?

Some societies used cannibalism to acquire the attributes of their victims or to satisfy their gods. While most cannibals ate those of other tribes or cultural groups (exocannibalism), people in some societies have also eaten members of their own tribe (endocannibalism) to transfer social values and fertility to new generations.

Besides using corpses as a food source, the Aztecs practiced human sacrifice and cannibalism both to appease their gods and to enable those eating human flesh to commune with the gods. Historians estimate that the Aztecs sacrificed and ate up to one percent of fifteenth-century Central Mexico's population, or about 250,000 people annually.[23] On the god Totec's feast day (the first day of the second month of the Aztec's 18-month year), all captive men, women and children were sacrificed by tearing out their hearts, the "precious eagle-cactus fruit," and then rolling their bodies down the side of the pyramid so that those watching, generally the warriors, could eat them. As Father Bernardino de Sahagún wrote of the disposition of a body, "they cut him to pieces; they distributed him. First of all, they made an offering of one of his thighs to Moctezuma. They set forth to take it to him...They gave [a bowl of dried maize stew ] to each one. On each went a piece of the flesh of the captive."[24] José de Acosta, a Jesuit priest, wrote of those sacrificed in about 1520, "Being thus slaine, and their bodies cast downe, their Masters, or such as had taken them, went to take them up, carried them away; then having divided them amongst them, they did eate them, celebrating their Feast and Solemnitie...The neighbour nations did the like, imitating the Mexicans in the Customes and Ceremonies of the Service of their Gods."[25]

Cannibalism existed in secret societies of the Kwakiutl Indians of the Northwestern-U.S. coast and Canada. Their novice members, *hä'mats'a*, broke societal taboos when, possessed by the spirits of those they were to cannibalize, they ate the flesh of killed slaves and dead tribe members until they could be subdued. After this behavior, the *hä'mats'a* were socially ostracized. For four months after consuming human flesh, they could only eat using special utensils which were then destroyed; for sixteen months they could not eat warm food. In addition, for one year, they could not touch their wives, gamble or work.[26]

Individuals or aberrant groups have also used cannibalism to acquire power.

Jeremiah Johnson, the mountain man, reportedly collected and ate the livers of 247 Crow Indians during his career. Whether it was true or not, the legend alone made for a fierce reputation.

In 1912 China, a well-known rebel leader was executed in Nanking. The soldiers who killed him then extracted his heart and, using rituals from the Ming Dynasty (1368-1644), cooked it, cut it into pieces and ate it. Their purpose was to acquire this leader's courage and skill.[27]

In 1946, the World War II Joint Military Commission for War Crimes tried Lt. Gen. Joshio Tachibana (who was subsequently executed) and eleven other officers for charges including beheading an American POW and then eating "the flesh and viscera of the body."[28] In fact, as described in a statement by Major Matoba, four captured American airmen were executed on Chichi Jima in the Bonin Islands north of Iwo Jima, cooked and eaten.[29] Both Gen. Tachibana, the commanding general and Adm. Kunizo Mori, the senior naval officer on the island, helped eat the bodies.[30] The officers admitted to cannibalism, one saying, it "makes me strong."[31]

Other reports of cannibalism by Japanese troops during and shortly after World War II in Melanesia and the Philippines exist in the war crimes documents of Australia and the United States.[32] Unlike the other Allies, the Australians added "cannibalism" and "mutilation of a dead body" to war crimes violations that could be tried by their tribunals. In December 1945, a tribunal found a Japanese officer guilty of eating parts of an Australian POW's body.[33] Investigators attributed these practices to a wish to taste human flesh, madness, a view that the native people were subhuman, and a belief in the medicinal and aphrodisiac properties of the human liver.[34] The incidents of cannibalism by World War II Japanese soldiers have, however, been generally suppressed, both in Japan and elsewhere. A recent Japanese book about these incidents has engendered both public alarm and anger.[35]

A story that first appeared in the West only in 1993 was that during

China's Cultural Revolution in the late 1960s, up to several hundred "counterrevolutionaries" were publicly killed, cooked and eaten in Guangxi, a remote province in southern China. In some instances, government cafeterias displayed bodies on meat hooks, serving up portions to employees. During public displays of cannibalism, onlookers supposedly had to prove their loyalty by eating these enemies of the revolution. What information exists, however, has only been supplied by current counterrevolutionaries.[36]

Although the belief that sexual power can be acquired from cannibalism is often implicit in the act, one notorious cannibal made it explicit. In October 1992, a former office worker and Russian language teacher, Andrei Chikatilo, was convicted in Rostov-on-Don, Russia, for the killing, mutilating and eating of at least 21 boys, 14 girls, and 17 young women, though more victims are thought to have perished at his hand. This 56-year-old grandfather, known as the "Forest Strip Killer" from the place he dumped the bodies, picked up his victims at bus stops, and then used a knife, his hands and his teeth to mangle, sexually mutilate, and eat the corpses. The trial judge said that Chikatilo "gouged out the hearts or stomachs of victims, cut off fingers and noses and cut off genitals and the tips of tongues and ate them."[37] His killing spree started in 1978, and only ended with his arrest in November 1990.[38] In court, he attributed his attacks to sexual inadequacy and a Soviet system that allowed his older brother to be eaten by starving peasants during the famine in the 1930s. The judge said that the impotent Chikatilo "received sexual satisfaction after he knifed a person and saw blood, when a victim suffered."[39] "I am a mistake of nature," he said. "A mad beast."[40]

## D. WHAT KIND OF RITUALS HONORED DEAD RELATIVES OR ENEMIES?

Many cultures have used ritual cannibalism to honor the dead.

Ritual cannibalism was common in the ancient world. Herodotus (ca. 484-420 B.C.), a Greek known as the "Father of History," related that the Thracians, who lived in southern Europe, showed their grief and affection by killing and eating the bodies of various victims.[41] He also noted that the Callatians ate their fathers,[42] as did the Issedonians, a people in the very northern part of Europe, who "When a man's father dies, all the near relatives bring sheep to the house; which are sacrificed, and their flesh cut in pieces, while at the same time the dead body undergoes the like treatment. The two sorts of flesh are afterwards mixed together, and the whole is served up at a banquet."[43] The man's head was stripped of flesh, set in gold and was brought out annually for veneration. Herodotus wrote, however, that among the Massagetae peoples, the very old were not allowed to die naturally, but were killed by relatives, and their bodies were then boiled and eaten in great feasts.[44]

Some aboriginal Australians and inhabitants of New Guinea routinely ate part of a dead relative's body as an act of respect and to appease the ghost of the deceased. Everyone involved dreaded the "feast" which was accompanied by almost ceaseless vomiting, spitting, and other signs of disgust, sometimes lasting several days.[45]

In the Gimi ritual, relatives placed a dead man's body on a platform, so that he could decompose and lend his essence to the garden below. His female relatives then dragged him off the scaffold, dismembered the corpse, and carried the pieces into the normally forbidden men's hut. There they ate their portions over several days. At the end of this period they were summoned outside by the man's male relatives who distributed a portion of a sacrificed pig to each woman corresponding to the portion of the man she ate. One must wonder what power this ceremony gave the wives, since they graphically simulated the practice during their wedding ceremonies.

New Guinea tribes abandoned ritual cannibalism in the early 1960s. Unfortunately it had led to generation after generation of New Guinea tribesmen, particularly the Gimi, acquiring the devastating neurological disease, Kuru, after cannibalizing the brains of affected relatives. Since mainly women and young children participated in this practice, they were the ones afflicted by the disease. With its 20-year incubation period (a *slow virus*), Kuru was only slowly eliminated.

Ritual cannibalism was also reported among the Pawnee Indians of the American plains. One case reported that

...among the Pawnees in 1837 or 1838, [was] of a girl of fourteen or fifteen who, after being treated with great kindness and respect for six months, was put to death on April 22nd...after her body had been painted half red and half black, she was slowly roasted over a fire, and then shot with arrows. The chief sacrificer thereupon tore out her heart, and devoured it, the rest of her body being cut up while it was yet warm, placed in little baskets, and taken to the neighboring cornfield.[46]

## E. HOW WAS CANNIBALISM USED FOR REVENGE?

Diverse cultures also used cannibalism for revenge and as punishment.

Ancient Greek literature and mythology include stories of cannibalism. Among these are Homer's tale of the Cyclops Polyphemus who ate two of Odysseus' sailors each evening, the story of Chronos who ate his own children, and that of Tantalus who served up his son to the gods at a banquet. Scarier still was the tale of Atreus, who, to gain revenge for his wife's seduction, invited his brother Thyestes to a banquet where he unknowingly dined on flesh from his two sons' corpses.

This last story may have stemmed from an actual event related by Herodotus. He tells of the revenge for Harpagus killing King Astyages' grandson. After learning of the crime, Astyages killed Harpagus' son, "cut him in pieces, and roasted some portions before the fire, and boiled others."[47] He then invited the father to a banquet where he served the man his son (except for the hands, feet and head). After he was done with what he said was a very tasty meal, the basket with the rest of the boy's body was shown to the father. Very cooly, the father said that he had known exactly what he had eaten, and that since the king had caused it to happen, it was all right. He took the rest of his son's body home, presumably for burial.

Herodotus also related the story of a group of Scythians who, when scolded by King Cyaxares of Media for not bringing in meat from a hunt, conspired to make the King an unwitting accomplice to cannibalism. They killed a young boy entrusted to their care, "cut him in pieces, and then dressing the flesh as they were wont to dress that of the wild animals, serve it up to Cyaxares as game...The plan was carried out: Cyaxares and his guests ate of the flesh prepared by the Scythians, and they themselves (Scythians), having accomplished their purpose, fled."[48]

Amerigo Vespucci, reporting from the coast of what is now Brazil in 1502, said that after a battle, the native people "bury all the dead of their own side, but cut up and eat the bodies of their enemies...At certain times, when a diabolical frenzy comes over them, they invite their kindred and the whole tribe, and they set before them a mother with all the children she has, and with certain ceremonies they kill them with arrow shots and eat them. They do the same thing to the above-mentioned slaves and to the children born of them. This is assuredly so, for we found in their houses human flesh hung up to smoke, and much of it."[49]

Many native people of North America, including the Iroquois and Hurons, reportedly tortured to death and then ate captured enemies. As late as 1756 the Iroquois were still devouring captives.[50] They usually used torture to avenge the deaths of relatives killed in war, and ate the victim's heart and drank the blood to acquire his strength. One Jesuit, describing the body of a fellow priest who had been tortured to death and eaten by the Iroquois said, "Father de Breboef had his legs, thighs, and arms stripped of flesh to the very bone." Another Jesuit related how the Huron tortured and ate an Iroquois captive,

> ...fearing that he would die otherwise than by the knife, one cut off
> a foot, another a hand, and almost at the same time a third
> severed the head from the shoulders, throwing it into the crowd,
> where someone caught it to carry it to the Captain Ondessone, for
> whom it had been reserved, in order to make a feast therewith. As
> for the trunk, it remained at Arontaen, where a feast was made of
> it the same day...On the way [home] we encountered a Savage who

was carrying upon a skewer one of his half-roasted hands.[51]

The people of the Fiji Islands in the South Pacific also practiced cannibalism along with nearly constant and fierce warfare. Captain James Cook wrote of them, "These men of Feejee are formidable...on account of the savage practice to which they are addicted...of eating their enemies whom they kill in battle. We were surprised that this was not a misrepresentation. For we met several Feejee people at Tongataboo, and, on inquiry of them, they did not deny the charge."[52] Subsequently the British referred to the Fijis as the Cannibal Islands.

Training Fijians to eat human flesh began early when parents rubbed pieces of cooked victims over their infant's lips and gave them small pieces to eat. As they grew older, boys received the less desirable cuts of meat to eat. During the dismemberment of victim's bodies, the sexual organs of both males and females, referred to as "fruit," were cut off and hung up to rot on sacred trees. The head and penis of an enemy chief or important warrior was often sent back to his home as an insult. The balance of the body was divided up by social rank, with the most desirable parts going to chiefs, priests and important warriors. Hearts, thighs and upper arms were most desirable. The head, hands and feet went to the lowliest warriors; scraps went to the boys. With an especially hated captive, his ears, nose, fingers, toes or limbs were severed, cooked and eaten before he was killed. Fijians also traded the meat of cooked enemy captives for their allies' women as mates.[53]

While the victims were being cooked and eaten, men and women performed the death dance and participated in sexual orgies. Cannibalism not only flourished, but greatly increased in Fiji through the mid-nineteenth century when Europeans introduced muskets.[54]

A propensity for revenge cannibalism is still among us, as evidenced by the testimony of John F. Thanos. The murderer of two teenage boys in Oakland, Maryland, told a judge in 1992 that he still wanted to "dig these brats' bones out of their graves right now and beat them into powder and urinate on them and then stir it into a mercury yellowish elixir and serve it up to their loved ones."[55]

## F. HAS CANNIBALISM BEEN PRACTICED RECENTLY?

In the nineteenth and twentieth centuries, cannibalism has mainly been limited to isolated aberrant acts or a means of survival. A few examples exist, however, of "gustatory cannibalism."

Gustatory cannibals actually relish human flesh. While many fictional works revolve around dangers from societies of these cannibals, very few examples of true gustatory cannibalism exist. Those that do are among populations that, by virtue of available land or climate, have little access to

375

sources of animal protein.[56]

Societally approved gustatory cannibalism has mainly been reported from the South Pacific in the past two centuries. The Melanesians of Fiji, for example, referred to human flesh by the term *puaka balava* (long pig), presumably commenting on its relative taste. The Fore of eastern Papau New Guinea also equated pork and human flesh, believing that eating either would be beneficial. The Batak of Sumatra reportedly sold human flesh in their markets well into the nineteenth century, while at the same time the Maoris of New Zealand continued to feast on the bodies of those killed in battle. In Orokaiva, New Guinea, natives ate human flesh because they desired "good food." According to Peggy Sanday, "human corpses were handled as if they were animals slain in the hunt. Corpses of grown men were tied by their hands and feet to a pole and carried face downward. Slain children were slung over the warrior's shoulder in the manner of a hunter carrying a dead wallaby, with each hand of the body tied to each foot."[57]

There have also been isolated episodes of individuals exhibiting gustatory cannibalism. The notoriety these cases receive attests to their rarity.

In 1824, Alexander Pearce, an Irish felon who had been transported to Van Diemens Land, a penal colony in Australia, was hanged and "anatomized" for killing and eating a fellow prisoner, Thomas Cox, with whom he had escaped. Pearce had a piece of Cox's body in his pocket when captured, and Cox's mangled remains confirmed Pearce's cannibalistic activity. This, however, was not Pearce's first experience with cannibalism. Two years before he had killed and eaten several companions with whom he had escaped, but he had not been punished because no evidence existed. On this occasion Pearce also admitted that he had killed and eaten his companion because he had a desire for "the most delicious food."[58]

Immediately after World War II, thirty-one former Japanese soldiers hid in caves in Mindanao in the southern Philippines. Before they were captured in February 1947, they cannibalized civilians as one source of food. According to Melville Hussey, the person who recorded their confessions, they had "enjoyed eating human flesh and ate well beyond what was required to keep them from starving." The Filipino authorities tried them in September 1949; at least ten were hung.[59]

In 1981 a Japanese student, Issed Sagawa, ate his girlfriend. This incident resulted in an award-winning book, *La lettre de Sagawa*, by J-ur-o Kara.[60] Not to be outdone, in 1992, Jeffrey Dahmer, a Milwaukee chocolate-factory worker, admitted to killing, dismembering, boiling and eating 17 young men over a 13-year period. He said he ate one man's biceps after seasoning it with salt, pepper, and A-1 Sauce[R]. But his killings look minimal next to those of Fritz Haarmann, the "Hanover Vampire," who in 1924 was convicted of biting 27 young men to death and producing sausage from their flesh which he ate and sold. An accomplice picked up victims in gay bars or at dances, and experts believe more than 50 victims succumbed to the sausage pot. Haarman was executed, but his accomplice served only 12 years in prison.[61]

The most notorious gustatory (and power-motivated) cannibal on the big screen was Hannibal Lecter, the victim-devouring psychiatrist featured in *The Silence of the Lambs*. His last on-screen words were "I'm going to have an old friend for dinner."

Unlike gustatory cannibalism, modern survival cannibalism is not uncommon.

Jenness and Ballantyne reported cannibalism as late as 1900 during a period of severe famine on Goodenough Island (westernmost of the D'Entrecasteaux Islands off the eastern tip of New Guinea). "So terrible was the distress at this time that children were exchanged for food with Belebele and Kwaiaudili, where they were killed and eaten. Friends even exchanged children with one another, and in at least one instance a father murdered his own child, and all his relatives joined in the feast. It was dangerous for a child to leave his parent's side for a single moment lest he should be carried off to swell the cannibal pots."[62]

Modern Western civilization also has examples of cannibalism. In 1884 a cabin boy was killed and eaten by his comrades adrift in a lifeboat, giving rise to the landmark British legal case, *Regina v. Dudley and Stephens*.[63] Their defense indicated that this was not an uncommon practice among seafarers in lifeboats. Still, they were convicted of premeditated murder and sentenced to hang. This was later reduced to six months in jail.[64]

A large number of written accounts and several sea chanties describe seaborne cannibalism, including a passage detailing the horrors suffered by the survivors of the brig *George*, wrecked while sailing from Quebec to Greenock, Scotland with a load of timber in September 1822. The "wretched female" they speak of was a woman named Joyce Rae.

> Six days and nights with all our might
> We brav'd the foaming tide,
> The seventh day in the morning,
> The wretched female died;
> Yet still the howling tempest
> Upon our heads did burst,
> At length we drank the female's blood
> to quench our raging thirst.
> Her wrethed husband was compel'd
> Her precious blood to taste,
> But for the whole ship's company,
> The same did not long last;
> Her body then they did dissect,

Most dreadful for to view
And serv'd it out in pieces,
Amongst the whole ship's crew.
Eleven days more we did survive,
Upon this horrid food,
With nothing to supply our wants,
Save human flesh and blood.
When five more of the wretched crew
Had then resign'd their breath,
With raging thirst and hunger
Slept in the arms of death.
Full twenty one days longer
Our perils did survive,
Eating our dead companions
We kept ourselves alive.[65]

A similar, but even more gruesome episode took place when the American ship *Essex* sank after being struck by a whale on November 20, 1820.

We ranged through, no food could we get,
Confined there a long time, nothing for to eat.
Till we all cast lots to see who should die,
Which made our ship's crew for sorrow to cry.

Then lots were drawn one man was to die,
For his wife and poor children most bitterly did cry,
To kill him says the captain or take away his breath,
but to starve with hunger is a deplorable death.

Then his mess mates they killed him and cut off his head,
And all the ship's crew from the body did feed,
And at eight different times lots amongst them were drawn,
For to keep them from starving that's the way they went on.[66]

Even Napoleon's soldiers were not immune to cannibalism. When they were driven out of Russia in 1812 and had no other food, they began eating their dead comrades. As General Kreitz reported, "Hunger has compelled them to eat horses' carcasses, and many of us have seen them roasting the flesh of their compatriots."[67]

Western literature includes many tales of cannibalism. Fairy tales that contain the threat of cannibalism include *Little Red Riding Hood* and *Hansel and Gretel.* One recent black comedy, *Sweeney Todd, the Demon Barber,* told of a barber who killed customers and made them into sausage to sell and eat. This was originally written in 1847 as George Dibdin's play, *A String of Pearls, or The Fiend of Fleet Street,* based on the true story of a fifteenth-century Paris barber who killed and ate customers.

The American West also had its share of cannibals.

The most famous was the Donner Party, stranded in the High Sierras by storms in the winter of 1846-47. Thirty-six people died amidst reports of both murder and cannibalism. One survivor proudly proclaimed to a relative that their family was the only one that did not partake of human flesh.[68]

In 1874, Alferd G. Packer, the infamous man-eater of Colorado, killed and devoured his five companions as they made a dangerous winter crossing of the Rockies. Not only did he eventually admit his crime, but it was reconfirmed by a forensic pathology team in 1990. After originally being sentenced to hang, he got a second trial through a legal technicality (having been charged under a Territorial law but tried under Colorado state law) and spent 17 years in prison before being paroled in 1901.[69] Cannibalism was also rumored to have occurred during an Arctic expedition (1881-84) sponsored by the U.S. Army, led by Lieutenant Adolphus Washington Greely. Although it was a famous episode, it is unclear whether cannibalism actually transpired.

During World War II, people reportedly ate the flesh of the dead during the siege of Leningrad. Some citizens, in addition to simply eating the dead, killed others and sold their bodies for meat.[70] Dr. Franz Blaha, testifying before the Nuremberg War Crimes Tribunal also reported one incident of survival cannibalism on a crowded boxcar which arrived at Dachau from another concentration camp. The captives had been en route for two weeks without being supplied with any food or water.[71]

Japanese troops of the Eighteenth Army stationed in New Guinea in 1945, about to be overrun by Australian troops, resorted to cannibalizing indigenous people. Local eyewitnesses claimed that abundant garden produce was readily available and that the soldiers had eaten the tribesmen from fear and desperation. The timing, in the pre-harvest months, however, suggests that it may have been a survival mechanism.[72]

In 1972, survivors of an Andean plane crash admitted eating their dead companions to survive until rescued. Members of the Old Christians Club, a Uruguayan rugby team crashed in the Andes on Friday, the 13th of October. Alumni of a conservative Roman Catholic School, they had adopted English rugby as a morally uplifting sport. As described in Piers Paul Read's book, *Alive,* those who lived survived by consuming the flesh of their dead friends and relatives, even learning to enjoy and relish their new diet. Some developed a gourmet's taste for brains or lungs.[73]

At the same time, on November 8, 1972, a pilot, Martin Hartwell, crashed his plane in the Canadian Arctic during a medical transport flight. He survived by eating the body of the flight nurse who died during the crash; both Eskimo patients also died—one from the crash and the other because he refused to eat human flesh.[74]

Cannibalism has been suggested as a survival mechanism for modern societies. The film, *Soylent Green,* as well as David Sale's novel, *The Love Bite*, suggested cannibalism as a solution to the world's food shortage problem. This suggestion echoed the satire of Jonathan Swift, who in 1728, lambasted the English landlords keeping Ireland impoverished, writing, "that a young healthy child well nurs'd, is, at a year old, a most delicious, nourishing, and wholesome food, whether stewed, roasted, baked, or boiled; and I make no doubt that it will equally serve in a fricassée, or a ragoût...[and would be perfectly suitable for landlords] who, as they have already devoured most of the parents, seem to have the best title to the children."[75]

In his book, *Man Into Superman,* Robert Ettinger described a future society that grows replacement parts not only for cryogenically preserved people, but for anyone who is injured. He said, "Even *human* meat will be cheap. Yes, there will probably be 'cannibals;' some will try, and like, human flesh grown in culture."[76]

In a macabre twist on survival cannibalism, the Maricopa (Phoenix, Arizona-area) Bar Association made survival cannibalism the topic of its 1993 essay contest for sixth- through ninth-grade students. In their hypothetical problem, the student was to pretend that he was one of three junior-high-school friends who were trapped in a cave. Knowing that they could not live more than thirty days without food, they drew lots to see who would be killed so the others could survive. They were rescued thirty minutes after the victim was killed. While lawyers saw this as the classic "lifeboat dilemma," (a la *R. v Dudley and Stephens*) the childrens' parents and teachers were not amused.[77]

## G. WHY HUNT OR SHRINK HEADS?

People hunted or occasionally shrunk heads to acquire power, for religious ceremonies, to prove that an enemy had been killed, and for souvenirs. Culturally, head-hunting is associated with the belief that the head is the seat of the soul.[78]

Head-hunting and head shrinking were once common practice throughout South America and in parts of Oceania (Pacific islands). It has occurred sporadically elsewhere, including in parts of Ireland and Scotland through the Middle Ages.[79]

The best-known head-hunters (and head shrinkers; see next section) were the Jivaros (or Jibaros) of South America. For them, shrunken heads were symbols both of victory and vengeance. The mummified head had great religious significance, and tied to the belt by the hair, was worn in battle, at fiestas and when the owner was himself buried. Shrunken heads were so personal that they were never passed down to other generations.[80] The Jivaros buried the bodies of their own tribesmen only if the head was still attached. They believed that the spirit was in the head, so a headless corpse was either left exposed to the elements, or especially in the case of a chief, mummified by slowly drying it over a low fire. The internal organs were replaced with preservative herbs.[81]

Head-hunting was also practiced in the Solomon Islands, Papua-New Guinea, Sarawak (on Borneo), Indonesia, parts of India, Taiwan, among the northern tribes of Nigeria, and among the Kwakiutl Indians of the Pacific Northwest.[82] In Burma, the Wa people observed a specific head-hunting season related to their crop cycle, making it dangerous to visit this area at certain times of the year.[83] In the Malay Archipelago in Southeast Asia, the *Mayawo* took heads after battle. The chief marked the necks of enemies who were dead or nearly dead, whose heads were then removed. The Mayawo, on returning to their island, cooked the heads until only the skull remained. They then buried them as a group beneath a stone cairn at a place still known as *deulkonadinjeri*, the place of human heads. Nineteenth-century Western anthropologists collected some of these skulls for museums before they were buried.[84]

In the Philippines, head-hunting was reported by explorers as early as 1577 and was only formally abandoned by some tribes on Luzon at the beginning of the twentieth century. In parts of Micronesia, chiefs used the exhibition of the heads of slain enemies to generate income from tribe members. These mummified heads were sometimes also lent to other chiefs when they needed to raise money. The Maoris of New Zealand dried and preserved the heads of dead enemies, and early Western sailors to that area regularly acquired tattooed "pickled heads."[85]

Contrary to popular fiction, most cannibals are not head-hunters, and most head-hunters do not cannibalize the dead. Historically, when cannibalism did accompany head-hunting, it was normally a minimal, symbolic act. When head-hunting was abolished in Oceania, however, some tribes replaced it with cannibalism.

Soldiers in many cultures have a long tradition of head- (or partial head-) hunting. Herodotus mentioned ancient Asian head-hunters and evidence exists that Assyrian soldiers removed the heads of slain enemies.[86]

Ancient Chinese and Scythian soldiers regularly delivered the heads of enemies killed in battle to their leaders. This was neither for religious nor ritual purposes, but simply to prove they had accomplished their task and should be paid. The soldiers forfeited any claim to their share of the booty if they could not produce an enemy's head. The Scyths, after showing a head to their king, removed the scalp by cutting "round the head above the ears, and, laying hold of the scalp, shakes the skull out." The warrior then cleaned and softened the scalp, hanging his collection from his bridle rein as war trophies or sewing a collection of scalps together to make a cloak.[87]

Payment for "kills" was also the origin of the practice of scalping in

North America, and was introduced to Native Americans by the French, English, Dutch and Spanish colonial governments, and later adopted by white soldiers and settlers. Rather than simply scalping them, the Sioux and Cheyenne beheaded some of General Custer's dead troops at Little Big Horn and displayed the heads on stakes during the post-battle celebrations.[88]

Europe also had head-hunters into the early twentieth century. As late as 1912, Montenegrins in the Balkan Peninsula removed their enemy's heads and carried them, secured by locks of hair, on their belts. In an effort to accommodate the mores of most of the Western world which did not look kindly upon head-hunting, Montenegrin soldiers in the Balkan War of 1912-13 removed only the noses and the upper lips (including the mustaches) from their enemies, instead of their entire heads.[89] Noses were also used as a proof of "kills" by soldiers of the Japanese warlord Hideyoshi Toyotomi, who in 1597 invaded Korea. More than 20,000 noses were lopped off and taken back to Japan. They were stored in the rather understated "1,000 nose tomb."[90]

An episode of head-hunting to document war deeds also occurred during World War II, when Gurkhas, after making a series of long-range penetrations of Japanese-occupied Burma, claimed to have killed one-hundred Japanese soldiers. Their British officers were skeptical. Reportedly, after the next battle, the Gurkhas brought sacks of Japanese heads as proof.[91]

Japanese skulls were much-envied trophies among U.S. Marines in the Pacific theater during World War II. The practice of collecting them apparently began after the bloody conflict on Guadalcanal, when the troops set up the skulls as ornaments or totems atop poles as a type of warning. The Marines boiled the skulls and then used lye to remove any residual flesh so they would be suitable as souvenirs. U.S. sailors cleaned their trophy skulls by putting them in nets and dragging them behind their vessels. Winfield Townley Scott wrote a wartime poem, "The U.S. Sailor with the Japanese Skull" that detailed the entire technique of preserving the head-skull as a souvenir. In 1943 *Life* magazine published the picture of a U.S. sailor's girlfriend contemplating a Japanese skull sent to her as a gift—with a note written on the top of the skull. Referring to this practice, Edward L. Jones, a U.S. war correspondent in the Pacific wrote in the February 1946 *Atlantic Magazine*, "We...boiled the flesh off enemy skulls to make table ornaments for sweethearts, or carved their bones into letter-openers."[92] On occasion, these "Japanese trophy skulls" have confused police when they have turned up during murder investigations.[93] It has been reported that when the remains of Japanese soldiers were repatriated from the Mariana Islands in 1984, sixty percent were missing their skulls.[94]

Similar "trophy skulls" were brought back by U.S. soldiers from

Vietnam. Many were covered by graffiti, including people's names and crude aphorisms, such as "Today's pigs are tomorrow's bacon." Since collecting human parts is against Army regulations, and has been since at least World War I, skulls found by authorities were confiscated and sent to the Armed Forces Institute of Pathology.[95]

## H. HOW IS A SHRUNKEN HEAD PREPARED?

Shrinking heads has a long tradition in parts of South America. When the Spanish explorer Pizarro arrived in 1527, his men described seeing shrunken heads. The Jivaro Indians, who lived around the Pastaza, Morena and Upano-Santiago rivers in Ecuador and Peru, produced the *tsantsas*, what the modern world knows as shrunken heads. And they continued practicing this art long after other tribes had ceased to do so. *Tsantsas* were usually made from the heads of women, children, old people and warriors who were traditionally taken during formal forays to enemy camps. But the Jivaro also shrank the heads of members of their own tribe who had been decapitated by enemies.

Raphael Karsten, who explored the region in the early twentieth century, described the process of taking and preparing the heads, in his report to the Smithsonian Institute:

As soon as a Jibaro warrior has killed an enemy of another tribe he at once tries to secure his head, which he cuts off as close to the trunk as possible...During the speedy return which generally follows upon a successful attack there is not always time for the victors to at once begin with the preparation of the trophy. They first have to put themselves in safety lest the enemy pursue them. Thus it may happen that they carry the bloody head with them for a couple of days before they get an opportunity to "skin" it (*muka sukúrtinyu*). [When they can begin, they] start to take off the scalp...Along the back of the head, from the apex downward, a long cut is made with a knife, whereupon the scalp and the skin of the face is slowly and carefully drawn off from the skull, in much the same way as is done with the hides of animals for stuffing. The skinning of the face is said to be the most difficult part of this work, for here the skin does not loosen by merely drawing it off, but has to be cut from the flesh with a sharp knife. The skull and all fleshy parts that adhere to it are thrown away and the scalp obtained is further prepared. It is attached to a vine and immersed in a pot of boiling water, where it is left for a while. By boiling the scalp it is freed from microbes, contracts a little, and thickens. It is then taken out of the pot and put on the top of a stick, fixed in the ground, where it is left for a while until it has cooled.

A ring is formed of a vine which the Jibaros call *kâpi*, of the same size as the circumference of the finished *tsantsa* at the neck opening, and this ring is attached to the trophy, at first temporarily and later, as the latter assumes its final size by reduction, more firmly. By means of a needle and a thread consisting of a chambira fibre, that part of the scalp which, for the purpose of the skinning of the head had been cut open, is sewn together.

The reducing of the trophy should now begin. What is first done with it, however, has rather the character of some sort of magical ceremony. At the bank of the river three small round stones are looked for, which are heated in the fire. By means of a cleft stick one of the heated stones is taken up from the fire and put into the head through the opening at the neck...The head is kept in motion so that the heated stone rolls to and fro within it, burning off a part of the blood and flesh which is still attached to the scalp...The same procedure is repeated with the second stone, and lastly with the third stone...

The proper reduction of the trophy is brought about by means of hot sand. Some fine sand is taken from the river bank and heated at the fire in a piece of broken clay pot (*hakáchi*). When the sand is sufficiently hot it is poured into the head so as to more than half fill it. The head is kept in motion so that the sand acts uniformly upon all its parts. The object of this procedure is to remove the flesh still attached to the skin, to make the scalp thinner, and to reduce the whole trophy. This is attained by the procedure with the hot sand being repeated many times...Each time, after taking out the sand from the head, the scalp is scraped inside with a knife in order to remove from it what the sand has burned off. As the trophy dries and shrinks through this treatment the head, and especially the face, is cleverly moulded with the fingers, so that it retains its human features, becoming like the head of a small dwarf. This work is continued...for several days or even weeks...

By this treatment the Jibaros are able to gradually reduce the head to such an extent that it is not larger than an orange, or about one-fourth of its normal size, becoming at the same time completely hard and dry. Through both lips, shrunk in proportion to the rest of the head, three small chonta pins, about 5 centimeters in length and painted red with roucu, are passed parallel with each other, and round these pins a fine cotton string, which is also painted red, is wound...Lastly, the whole trophy, even the face, is dyed black with charcoal...

The Jibaros of to-day, in cutting the enemy's head and skinning it, avail themselves of knives obtained from whites, but formerly—in fact, only a few decades ago—native instruments had to be used for this purpose. The head was severed from the trunk by means of a stone axe and a big knife of hard chonta wood. Again, in stripping the skin from the skull and the face they used snail's shells sharpened against a stone, and flat pieces of split bamboo (guadua) resembling knife-blades and extremely sharp.[96]

The ceremonies surrounding the preparation of the *tsantas* takes two years—until the final feast. During this period, the hunter must dress as a penitent, wear no ornaments and no weapons, not go hunting in the forest or take part in the ordinary Jivaro occupations. He must also observe the rules of fasting for two years.[97]

Nowadays, shrunken heads can bring big dollars. In 1992, *Ripley's Believe It or Not* bought two nineteenth-century South American shrunken heads at auction for $22,000. The heads, dark-skinned and complete with hair, lip ties, and headbands, came from the Jivaro tribe.[98]

## I. WHAT IS STRIPPING THE FLESH?

People have long used animals to strip the flesh off, or excarnate, corpses. Stemming from a time before funerary rites or graves, the method is a simple, clean, efficient and ecological method of recyling the dead. Although most religions abhor excarnation, it merely represents an acceleration of the slow feeding on a body that takes place unseen after burial.

Since ancient times the Zoroastrians, or Parsees (meaning "Persians") of India have exposed corpses of their dead on *Dakhmas* (towers of silence, see illustration, p 386.) or on treetops to be devoured by vultures. As the ancients said of this practice, "There is another custom which is spoken of with reserve, and not openly, concerning their dead. It is said that the body of a male Persian is never buried, until it has been torn either by a dog or a bird of prey."[99]

This funerary practice, known as "stripping the flesh," continues to this day. According to Parsee tradition, this practice avoids polluting the sacred elements: the earth by burial, fire by cremation, and water by casting the body in the river. The fifth to eighth *fargard* of the *Venidâd*, Parsee sacred writings, detail the treatment of dead bodies and the construction of Dakhmas. *Fargard V* says, "There shall they deposit his lifeless body for two nights, or three nights, or a month long, until the time when the birds shall fly forth...in order that the corpses be attended to, the Dakhmas attended to, the impurities attended to, and the birds gorged."[100]

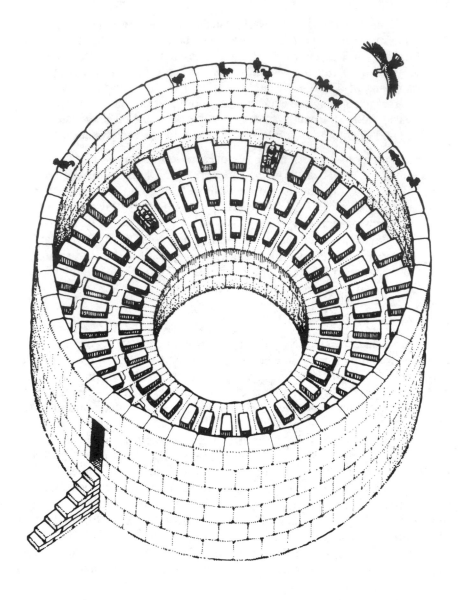

A *Dakhma*, the Parsee Tower of Silence.

The basic religious concept is the

> utter impurity of the dead and the extreme purity of and
> sacredness of earth, fire, and water. No impure thing can,
> therefore, be thrown upon any one of these elements, because it
> would spoil the good creation by increasing the power and
> influence of the *daêvas* or demons, who take possession of the
> body as soon as a man is dead. The corpse is, therefore, to be
> carried on to the barren top of a mountain or hill, and to be
> placed on stones (or iron plates), and exposed to dogs and
> vultures, so as to benefit in this way the animals of the good
> creation.[101]

After first washing, dressing and shrouding the body, Parsees move it to
the Tower of Silence in daylight. After they lay the body in the Tower, the
corpse bearers "tear off the clothes from the body of the deceased and leave
it (the body) on the floor of the Tower. ...The body must be exposed and left
partly uncovered, so as to draw towards it the eye of the flesh-devouring
birds and to fall an easy prey to them. The sooner it is devoured, the lesser
the chance of further decomposition and the greater the sanitary good and
safety."[102] Once the flesh is picked clean by vultures (usually within one
hour),[103] an attendant sweeps the sun-bleached bones into an interior shaft.
Some see this method as not only ecologically sound, but ultimately
egalitarian.

Professor Monier Williams described the towers and funerary process
for the *Times* of London, January 28, 1876:

> The Dakhmas, or Parsee Towers of Silence, are erected in a
> garden, on the highest point of Malabar hill, a beautiful rising
> ground on one side of Black Bay (Bombay, India)...But what are
> those five circular structures which appear at intervals rising
> mysteriously out of the foliage? They are simply masses of
> masonry, massive enough to last for centuries, built of the hardest
> black granite, and covered with white chunam...Towers they
> scarcely deserve to be called; for the height of each is quite out of
> proportion to its diameter. A sixth tower stands quite apart from
> the others. It is square in shape, and only used for persons who
> have suffered death for heinous crimes...Though wholly destitute
> of ornament, and even of the simplest moulding, the parapet of
> each tower possesses an extraordinary coping, which instantly
> attracts and fascinates the gaze. It is a coping formed, not of dead
> stone, but of living vultures...
>
> Imagine a round column or massive cylinder 12 or 14 feet
> high, and at least 40 feet in diameter, built throughout of solid
> stone, except in the centre, where a well 5 or 6 feet across leads

down to an excavation under the masonry, containing four drains at right angles to each other, terminated by holes filled with charcoal. Round the upper surface of this solid circular cylinder and completely hiding the interior from view is a stone parapet, 10 or 12 feet in height...

[Within this parapet is a] circle of open stone coffins divided from the next by a pathway, so that there are three circular pathways...In the outermost circle of the stone coffins are placed the bodies of males, in the middle those of females, and in the inner and smallest circle, nearest the well, those of children...

The particular funeral I witnessed was that of a child...The two [corpse] bearers speedily unlocked the door, reverently conveyed the body of the child into the interior, and, unseen by any one, laid it uncovered in one of the open stone receptacles nearest the central well. In two minutes they re-appeared with the empty bier and white cloth; and scarcely had they closed the door when a dozen vultures swooped down upon the body, and were rapidly followed by others. In five minutes more we saw the satiated birds fly back and lazily settle down again upon the parapet. They had left nothing behind but a skeleton...In a fortnight, or at most four weeks, the same bearers return, and with gloved hands and implements resembling tongs place the dry skeleton in the central well. There the bones find their last resting-place, and there the dust of whole generations of Parsees commingling is left undisturbed for centuries.[104]

When asked about the reasons for this funeral custom, the Secretary of the Parsee Puncháyal replied:

Our Prophet, Zoroaster, who lived 6,000 years ago, taught us to regard the elements as symbols of the Deity. Earth, fire, water, he said, ought never, under any circumstances, to be defiled by contact with putrefying flesh. Naked, he said, we came into the world, and naked we ought to leave it. But the decaying particles of our bodies should be dissipated as rapidly as possible, and in such a way that neither Mother Earth nor the beings she supports should be contaminated in the slightest degree. In fact, our Prophet was the greatest of health officers, and, following his sanitary laws, we build our towers on the tops of the hills, above all human habitations. We spare no expense in constructing them of the hardest materials, and we expose our putrescent bodies in open stone receptacles...not necessarily to be consumed by vultures, but to be dissipated in the speediest possible manner, and without the possibility of polluting the earth or contaminating a single living being dwelling thereon. God indeed sends the vultures, and, as a matter of fact, these birds do their appointed work much more expeditiously than millions of insects would do if we committed our bodies to the ground. In a sanitary point of view nothing can be more perfect than our plan. Even the rain water which washes our skeletons is conducted by channels into purifying charcoal.[105]

Using the Towers of Silence offers another benefit. Unlike human diagnosticians, the vultures always know when a person is not dead. They do not attack the living, who may, because of a misdiagnosis of death be placed on the Tower. If the person then awakens, the Tower is equipped with a chain a person can use to pull himself up into a position to be seen and rescued. These cases have occurred, albeit with an unfortunate aftermath. In Bombay, William Tebb observed that the Parsees did not allow "those who have returned from the Towers of Silence to intermingle among them."[106]

When Parsees emigrate to the United States, Britain and other countries that do not allow them to dispose of their dead by exposure, they use cremation.

Some ancients used tree burials, following practices similar to those of the Parsees. They exposed their dead by hanging them in trees, but stopped birds of prey from feeding upon them by enclosing the bodies in skin bags, where the bodies merely rotted.

In more recent times, the Moïs of Indochina routinely placed their dead in open coffins in trees for two years, later burying the bones. Australian aborigines also exposed their dead in trees, later placing what was left of the bodies on ant hills, and collecting the bones after they were thoroughly cleaned. Both societies have now abandoned these practices. Three Philippine tribes still use tree burial. The *T'boli* carry a corpse around his house in a pre-burial ritual and then, instead of interring the coffin, they suspend it from a tall tree. The *Subanon* wrap their dead in a blanket and suspend them from a tall tree's branch, "exposed to the savages of the forest." Only when the person died of a communicable disease will they bury the body.[107] The *Ilongots* only bury their children in trees.[108]

## J. WHEN ELSE HAVE ANIMALS BEEN USED TO DEVOUR THE DEAD?

Over at least the past three millennia, people in many cultures have used animals to devour their dead. Anthropologists call bodies that are left outside of inhabited areas, or set adrift on rivers or oceans so that animals can deal with them, "castaways."

It is thought that in ancient Egypt, as in much of ancient Africa, the bodies of dead slaves, cripples and the poor were carried into the desert to be eaten by hyenas, wolves and jackals. In areas near the Nile, the bodies became food for crocodiles.[109] Assyrian art from about the seventh century B.C. shows the eyes of the corpses of enemy Arab soldiers being plucked out by vultures. These representations are thought to have been a form of propaganda, boosting the morale back home and promoting fear in those who had been defeated.[110] Romans threw the naked corpses of dead prisoners into the street to be eaten by animals.[111]

The ancient Bactrians, who lived in part of what is now Afghanistan, not only kept dogs specifically to eat the dead bodies of friends and relatives, but also used them on the living elderly and enfeebled.[112] In a similar manner, some nomadic tribes of Central Asia cut their dead into small pieces and left them for wild animals to devour. At one time, the well-to-do of these tribes kept packs of dogs which would eat their owners' bodies upon death. If fewer than seven dogs came to feed on the body, the deceased was dishonored.[113] Yet, while the flesh was given over to the dogs, some Siberian tribes religiously honored the bones. Certain South African tribes still perform a similar act by abandoning their dead to the ministrations of the jackals.

When the tenth-century Catholic Church denied burial to various types of sinners, the chant said over a body left to rot was *"Sint cadavera eorum, in escam volatilibus coeli, et bestiis terrae"* (Give over this erring body for food to the fowls of the air and beasts of the field).[114]

Many Native American Plains tribes placed their dead on high platforms or in the limbs of trees outside the village to rot and to be devoured by animals. They did this to hasten decomposition and thus speed the soul's journey to the spirit world.[115] They dressed the body in its best clothing and sewed it into a buffalo hide or deer skin. After the tribes' exposure to white men, the body was often wrapped in a blanket. Thongs bound the wrapping at the neck, waist and feet. The sun-bleached bones were later buried in sacred ground. If a man had been killed during a raid on an enemy, the Santee Sioux sometimes sat the body facing both the enemy's country and a cooking pot containing the head of a scalped and decapitated Cree or Chippewa.[116] Among the Mandan, after the bones were stripped clean, relatives buried all but the skull, which they placed with others in a circle. Relatives came daily to the skull display.

The Naga tribes of Assam in northeastern India and the Balinesians of the south Pacific also traditionally exposed their dead on platforms. In Bali, if the body was still present after a few days, they considered that the spirits had rejected it and pushed the corpse into a ravine to be eaten by wild animals.[117]

In some parts of Central America, the corpses of important men who had committed crimes were exposed to the environment. In Victoria, Australia, when a dead tribesman had pursued an enemy in a blood-thirsty manner (a social taboo), his body was left to decay where he was slain. Similarly, while Native Alaskans broiled most corpses with oil, moss, and driftwood, those of "bad men" were left to rot.[118] In Britain before the seventeenth century, portions of hanged criminals were often left under the scaffold to be devoured by dogs.

In Tibet, where permafrost makes burial impossible, a lack of wood makes cremation impractical, and water burial is considered unsanitary, bodies are generally left to decompose away from living areas.[119] One formal method of body disposal in which birds feed on the corpse is called *Ja-Tor* or "air burial." Attendants first dismember the body with a broadsword and remove the flesh from the bones. Then they specially prepare the bones so the birds will eat them. In the 1950s, Tsung-lien Shen and Shen-chi Liu described the body of a spiritual teacher being dispatched by this method:

> The men started burning sandalwood, the aroma of which, as we learned later, aroused the birds high up among the rock caves. The men unbound the corpse and began the job, grinding the bones into bits and kneading them with barley. The birds swooped down in batches, about a hundred or so, walking and chattering noisily a good distance off...Within a half hour everything was gone. Had anything been left behind, the disciples would certainly have deemed it a bad sign. Only the bodies of the condemned, it is believed, are shunned by the birds.[120]

Then, without washing their hands, those participating in the ceremony ate a meal. When questioned, they said that "eating with unwashed hands added relish to food; besides the spirit of the dead man would be satisfied when he saw them take fragments of his mortal remains with their food without aversion."[121]

Mongolians also occasionally used formal air burial for adults, but normally abandoned corpses to be eaten by wolves, eagles or other scavengers. Central Asians commonly refer to the eagle as the "nomad's coffin." Mongolians also routinely abandon infant corpses while they leave those of children up to ten-years old in sacks at crossroads. The next Mongol to pass by opens the sack so that the spirit can be released and animals can have easier access to the corpse.[122]

## K. WHY IS A BODY SYSTEMATICALLY DISMEMBERED AFTER DEATH?

Corpses have been dismembered for religious and punitive reasons throughout the ages.

Ritual decapitation before burial dates to antiquity. Evidence from the Paleolithic era (ending about 30,000 B.C.) suggests that some of our ancestors interred only the skull, not the rest of the body. Skulls from seventh century B.C. Jericho, a city of ancient Palestine, were found in separate rooms covered by clay models of people's faces, complete with cowry shell eyes.[123] This practice, parallel to that of some agrarian people in South Asia and Oceania, suggests ritualized ancestor worship.

Other cultures dismembered some corpses to give them an honorable burial. As part of the mummification process, Egyptians removed the viscera and preserved them in four canopic jars. These jars were interred with the mummy. The Romans, in the rite of *os resectum*, ceremonially buried only a finger joint after cremating the rest of the corpse.

In biblical times, some Arab tribes dismembered warriors and sacrificial victims so that their body parts could be ritually buried in appropriate locations. They often buried parts of a brave warrior's corpse outside the north, west, south and east gates of a city to prevent invaders from entering.[124]

In medieval Europe, parts of important persons were often distributed to multiple churches for burial. During the Crusades of the eleventh to thirteenth centuries, the remains of kings, famous knights and other exalted persons dying far from home were transported to their homelands. First, however, in a process called *mos teutonicus*, the bodies were cut into pieces and the flesh removed by boiling the bones in wine or vinegar.[125] Only then were the bones wrapped in bull hides for their journey. The practice, often carried out in the side chapels of churches, was so common that in 1294 Pope Boniface VIII issued an edict that cutting up bodies to transport them for burial was grounds for excommunication.[126] Since no one paid much attention to this, Benedict XI later withdrew the prohibition.[127] When the Duke of York and the Earl of Oxford were killed at the battle of Agincourt in 1415, and again when Henry V died in Normandy in 1422, this method was used to prepare their bodies for transport back to England.[128,129] Due to Rome's continued distaste for the practice, however, it was probably butchers rather than monks who prepared their remains.

Disembowelment of English monarchs remained so common even into the seventeenth century that Queen Elizabeth I left specific orders that her body be buried intact. It is uncertain if these orders were followed.[130] Most monarchs had at least their hearts removed and placed in separate urns above the area for coffins in Westminster Abbey.[131] As late as 1701 when James II, the last Catholic monarch of England died in exile, his parish church at the Palace of St. Germain in France got part of his bowels, his head and brain went to the Scots college in Paris, and the rest of his embalmed body was interred in the priory church of the English Benedictine monks in Paris.[132]

The corpses of malefactors were also dismembered, but for less exalted reasons. Before the nineteenth century, decapitating criminals and impaling their heads on pikes around the city was not an unusual punishment. Herodotus reports that the Amathusians, a people allied with the Persians, decapitated the corpse of Onesilus, because he had laid siege to their town. They mounted the head over their gates, but were shocked to find that after it became hollow, a swarm of bees filled it with a honeycomb. Amathusian oracles then directed that they bury the head and pay homage to Onesilus as a hero.[133] To prevent a similar public display of her father's head after he was beheaded in the Tower of London in 1535, Sir Thomas More's (the "Man For All Seasons" and author of *Utopia*) daughter bribed some men to drop the head off London Bridge into a waiting boat. She kept the head with her until she died and then had it buried with her.[134] Similarly, when the British crown executed Sir Walter Raleigh (1554-1618), his wife, Elizabeth Throckmorton, reportedly retrieved his head, had it embalmed, and carried it around on a silk pillow until her own death, nineteen years later.

In 1718, at Château-Gontier, France, six-months pregnant Marie Jaguelin poisoned herself. The corpse was tried for the crimes of suicide and infanticide and then "tied to a hurdle [a low sled] and dragged upside down, the face touching the ground, through the streets and crossroads of the town, to the public square [a not uncommon 'punishment' for eighteenth-century suicides in France]; there the executioner ripped out the body of the child, which was carried to the nearby church of Saint John the Evangelist, where unbaptized newborn infants are buried, then what was left of the unfortunate Marie Jaguelin was hanged by the feet to a post for an hour, with an ignominious sign stuck to the post, then burned at the stake, and the ashes thrown to the wind."[135]

Charles Dickens described what was done with the head of a common criminal guillotined in Rome in 1845:

> The executioner was holding it by the hair, and walking with it round the scaffold, showing it to the people ... it was set upon a pole in front—a little patch of black and white, for the long street to stare at, and the flies to settle on. The eyes were turned upward, as if he had avoided the sight of the leathern bag, and looked to the crucifix. Every tinge and hue of life had left it in that instant. It was dull, cold, livid, wax.[136]

In a reversion to earlier times, during World War II the Japanese beheaded eight Malays who broke into a warehouse. They displayed the heads in the busiest part of Singapore as an example to the population.[137]

The judiciary once considered anatomical dissection an appropriate postmortem punishment for executed criminals. When Scottish surgeons received the one executed criminal's corpse the government annually allotted for anatomical study, they took it to the surgical theatre where they cut it into ten parts. The pieces were then distributed to ten surgeons who each dissected their section in front of their apprentices or paying students.

In the Barber-Surgeon's Hall in London, the site for anatomical studies, the Reverend J. Ward reported in 1661 that there were "two humane skins on the wood frames of a man and a woman in imitation of Adam and Eve put up in 1645."[138] In 1752 England passed a law similar to Scotland's, to provide anatomical specimens and dissuade crime. It was the so-called "Murder Act."

> Whereas the horrid crime of murder has of late been more frequently perpetrated than formerly...it is thereby become necessary, that some further terror and peculiar mark of infamy be added to the punishment of death...The body of any such murderer shall, if such conviction and execution be in the county of Middlesex or within the city of London...be immediately conveyed by the sheriff...to the hall of the Surgeons' Company...and the body so delivered...shall be dissected and anatomised by the said surgeons...in no case whatsoever the body of any murderer shall be suffered to be buried, unless after such body shall have been dissected and anatomised as aforesaid.[139]

Africa also saw ritual dismemberments. Pardi reports that an autopsy-like ritual was carried out on suspected witches who died among the Azande of Zaire, Sudan, and Central African Republic. If a person suspected of being a witch died,

> ... the most reliable means of trial is examination of his intestines. Since the judgement will affect his entire lineage, a man may request, prior to his death, that his oldest son or his closest blood-kin-man perform this procedure so as to clear his name. The procedure is done by incising the abdomen laterally in two places, just below the sternum and just above the penis. The duodenum is cut from the bottom of the stomach and the descending colon is cut from just above the anus. The upper end of the intestines, or duodenum, is wedged into a split branch and the branch is rotated until it has wound all the intestines out of the body. Once the intestines, usually about twenty four feet long, are all coiled upon the branch, another kinsman grasps the loose end, or colon, and walks away slowly, unrolling the coil so that the elders of the village can carefully scrutinize them for signs of witchcraft substance. When the verdict has been reached the intestines are then stuffed back into the abdomen and the body is buried. Occasionally, if the suspect has been acquitted, the intestines are first thrown in the face of the accuser or are dried and kept as evidence. The entire procedure, done at graveside, is not only public but the villagers, including the children, are encouraged to

come.[140]

## L. WHAT ELSE WAS DONE WITH CRIMINALS' BODIES?

Besides exhibiting their heads and anatomizing the corpse, judges often sentenced criminals not only to be executed, but also to have their bodies drawn and quartered (see illustration, p 397) or publicly exhibited in gibbets while they rotted.

In medieval Europe, authorities sought to deter future malefactors by publicly exhibiting the dismembered bodies of executed criminals. They often placed the offender's head, arms and legs on display, allowing dogs to devour the remaining pieces. The Edinburgh *Burgh Records* of 1583-84 ordered the Treasurer to "caus hing up at the Nether Bow and other patent pairts, the heid and certane of the legs and airmes of two men" who had recently been executed for murder. In 1584, he was ordered to "send west to Stirling the legs and arms of umquhile [formerly] David Home lately executed..."[141]

As a symbol of the enormity of their crimes, the bodies of English traitors and murderers were further mutilated after death. English law of the time described the order of punishment: "The judgement upon a traitor is, that he shall be drawn (dragged) to execution, for as much as he is not worthy to walk upon the earth: 2. His privy members cut off...which shows that his issue is disinherited with the corruption of blood...3. His bowels burned because in them he hatched the treason: 4. Beheaded: 5. Dismembered."[142]

This punishment as applied to Christopher Norton, who took part in England's Northern Rebellion and was (partially) hanged in 1570, was graphically described in the *State Trials*:

> With that the hangman executed his office: and being hanged a little while, and then cut down, the butcher opened him, and as he took out his bowels, he [Norton] cried, and said, "Oh Lord, Lord, have mercy upon me" and so yielded up the ghost. Then being likewise quartered, as the other [his uncle who Norton had just watched being executed] was, and their bowels burned, as the manner is, their quarters were put into a basket, provided for the purpose, and so carried to Newgate, where they were parboiled; and afterwards, their heads set on London Bridge, and their quarters set upon sundry gates of the city of London, for an example to all traitors and rebels, for committing high treason against God and their prince.[143]

Drawing and quartering (or an approximation) continued into modern times. Until the early twentieth century, for example, the people of Greenland customarily dismembered a criminal's body and distributed his legs. In a similar act, but for different reasons, the Eskimos of the Bering Strait region once cut corpses' arms and leg tendons to prevent their ghosts from moving; they did not, however, dismember them.[144]

Executed criminals also had their bodies sentenced to the gibbet. Used in several societies, the gibbet was a cage or post that held the corpse erect for public scrutiny. (See illustration, p 306.)

This practice began in ancient Rome, where those condemned to death were exposed on the *gemonies*, the double staircase on the facade of the prison, opposite the Forum. Exhibiting a body in this manner allowed it to rot and to be picked at by dogs and birds of prey. Afterwards the bodies were dumped into the Tiber River.[145]

In 1751, the Scots passed a law decreeing that bodies of executed murderers should either be publicly dissected or hung in chains or gibbets. The English also used the gibbet, and continued to use it until 1834. In its modern form, "The gibbet with its creaking human-scarecrow corpse occupied an important place in popular imaginative apprehension of 'justice' and judicial retribution. As an exemplary punishment it was exceeded in power only by dissection. The intention of both punishments was to deny the wrongdoer a grave."[146]

Before a criminal's body was gibbeted, it was first treated with tar to slightly slow the decomposition process.[147] Some bodies hung for years. As one judge graphically said to a rapist-murderer, your body will hang in chains "till the fowls of the air pick the flesh from your bones and the winds of Heaven bleach them white."[148] One body in Portsmouth, England, hung in a gibbet so long that the Royal Navy used it as a navigational aid. In an unanticipated sequela to this public display, Nichol Brown, who himself was executed for murder in 1754, once roasted and ate part of the leg of Norman Ross, who was a criminal hanging in an Edinburgh gibbet.[149]

The French also used a gibbet, although it differed slightly from the English version. Their gibbet consisted of stone pillars connected by wooden crosspieces. They were normally erected outside the city, near a highway where many people could view the body. If the criminal had committed the crime in another town, authorities exhibited the body there. A contemporary observer described one criminal's fate on the gibbet: "Gabriel Prudhomme, known as Massacre...hanged at Guéret on January 5, Twelfth Night's Eve, 1778...was left hanging for eighteen months and twenty-six days and fell from the gibbet only on July 26, 1779, a Tuesday."[150] When the gibbets were emptied, the bodies were left to rot beneath them, and these areas were used as rubbish dumps.

The famous gibbet of Montfaucon, in Paris, with sixteen pillars and crosspieces, was so large that forty-five criminals could be hung at once. A tourist attraction, taverns and pleasure gardens surrounded it. The French finally abolished this display in the mid-nineteenth century.

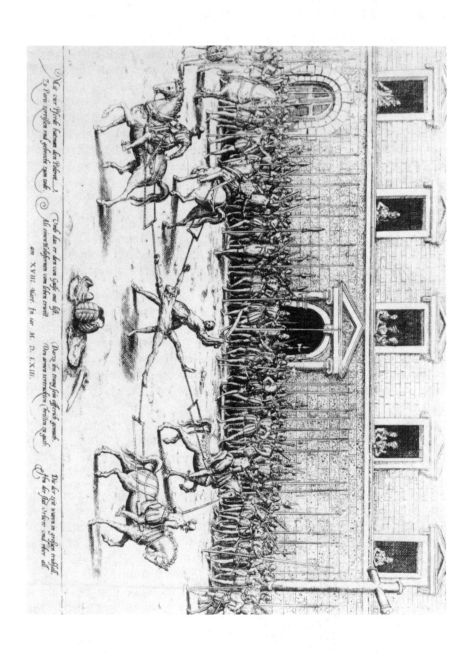

Drawing and quartering a body. (Reproduced with permission. Library of Congress.)

## M.  HOW ELSE ARE BODY PARTS USED?

People have used body parts as decorations and for implements since prehistoric times. Many of these uses stem from religious rituals and ancestor worship, as well as from practical reasons, such as the need for eating utensils. They used bones, skin, and occasionally, hair.

Both ancient Celts and Scythians used skulls as cups. The Scythians used the skulls not only of enemies, but also of relatives whom they had killed after feuds. To fashion the goblet, they sawed off the skulls below the eyebrows. The rich then covered their goblets in gold, while others covered theirs in leather. When important visitors arrived, the host took out the goblet and passed it around with a retelling of how the person had been slain.[151] Richard Selzer describes this in a way that also suggests necrophilia:

> A savage queen contrives from the skull of her young lover a wine bowl. Years later, as she lifts the kissed and polished calvarium to her lips, her old passion shudders anew, and licking an errant drop from one socket, she smiles in wild ownership.[152]

This practice was not merely ancient lore, however. Lord Byron told a friend that when a skull "of giant size and in a perfect state of preservation" was found in a nearby garden, "a strange fancy seized me of having it mounted as a drinking cup. I accordingly sent it to town, and it returned with a very high polish and of a mottled colour like tortoise-shell."[153] From this experience, he wrote his poem, *Formed from a Skull*, which included the lines,

> Better to hold the sparkling grape,
> Than nurse the earth-worm's slimy brood;
> And circle in the goblet's shape
> The drink of Gods, than reptiles' food.[154]

Ripley's museums have collections of drums made from human skulls originally used in Tibetan ceremonies to chase away evil spirits. They also have Tibetan altar bowls made from saints' skulls, and temple trumpets, flutes, necklaces and the buttons from priests' altar aprons, all made from human bone.

John Reed, who served as gaslighter in the Walnut Street Theater in Philadelphia, supposedly asked in his will that he be decapitated upon his death, and that his head be skeletonized for use in the theater's productions of *Hamlet*. He wanted his body, however, to be buried.[155]

In tantric Buddhism, skulls and leg bones arc fashioned into musical instruments for religious rituals.[156] Also, locals commonly robbed Native Americans' graves in the Southwestern United States in the 1930s, selling the contents to tourists as ashtrays. This practice came to be known as the

"Depression Industry."[157]

U.S. Marines in the Pacific routinely took parts of Japanese soldiers as souvenirs. One marine carried the severed hand of a Japanese soldier he had killed. Others routinely made letter openers from the bones of dead Japanese soldiers. One was even sent to President Franklin D. Roosevelt as a gift. He refused it. The practice became so prevalent that in September 1942, the Commander-in-Chief of the Pacific Fleet issued an order that: "No part of the enemy's body may be used as a souvenir, Unit Commanders will take stern disciplinary action..."[158]

Human skin and hair have also been used for various purposes.

Several early cultures used a lock of the corpse's hair to hang on the home to symbolize mourning. Nineteenth-century Americans took this one step farther. They routinely wove or braided a loved one's hair over fine wire to form imaginative designs which they displayed at home in shadow boxes or wore as jewelry.[159]

Scythian warriors sometimes fashioned cloaks from the scalps that they had taken in battle and used the skin from dead enemies' arms, hands, and fingers (including the nails) as coverings for their arrow quivers. On occasion, they removed the entire corpse's skin and carried it around as a trophy.[160] In a similar manner, Aztec priests sometimes wore the skins of their sacrificial victims.

In Las Vegas, Ripley's museum exhibits masks made from human skin and used for ancestor worship among the African Ekoi tribe in southeastern Cameroon. The skin on these masks, which were made until the start of the twentieth century, was taken from slaves and prisoners of war.

The French, not to be outdone by the ancients, established a tannery at Mendon, near Paris during the first French Revolution, for processing the skins of the guillotine's victims.[161]

In the nineteenth century, an American named Mahrenholz suggested tanning the skins of corpses into leather. He bought at least one skin from the widow of a workman who died in an accident. From the resulting leather he made a pair of boots and donated them to the Smithsonian Institute. William Tegg described the leather as being:

> ...remarkable for its softness and pliancy, and takes a good polish, but its wearing qualities have yet to be proved. The general impression appears to be that it is hardly adapted for rough work, such as that of sportsmen or pedestrian tourist, but for evening wear at the theatre or in the ball-room it will be found far more comfortable than boots and shoes made of ordinary leather. Some little prejudice, it is expected, will have to be overcome before the new leather is taken into general use.[162]

Early nineteenth-century French novelist Eugène Sue's mistress may have found the ultimate in body recycling. At her explicit request, a set of his books was bound in skin taken from her corpse's shoulders. These books were sold by Foyles bookshop in London in 1951 for $29. In a similar vein, it is claimed that in 1940, the Philosophical Library in Denver, Colorado, had a book, *History of Christianity*, that was bound in the skin of a Native American.[163]

One man supposedly asked Harvard's Anatomical Museum to cover two drumheads with his skin. One was to be inscribed with the Pope's "Universal Prayer," and the other with the "Declaration of Independence." A friend was instructed to beat the rhythm of *Yankee Doodle* at the foot of Bunker Hill each July 17 on these skin-covered drums.[164] No one knows if the friend complied with this bizarre request.

Nazi barbarity in using human skin to make lampshades and other ornaments is well documented. Dr. Franz Blaha, a prisoner at Dachau concentration camp, testified before the Nuremberg war crimes tribunal that "It was common practice to remove the skin from dead prisoners. I was commanded to do this on many occasions. Dr. Rascher and Dr. Wolter in particular asked for this human skin from human backs and chests. It was chemically treated and placed in the sun to dry. After that it was cut into various sizes for use as saddles, riding breeches, gloves, house slippers and ladies' handbags. Tattooed skin was especially valued by SS men...Sometimes we did not have enough bodies with good skin and Rascher would say, 'All right, you will get the bodies.' The next day we would receive twenty or thirty bodies of young people...It was dangerous to have a good skin."[165] When items made from this skin are located today, they are often buried in simple ceremonies.[166]

## N. WHAT IS NECROPHILIA?

Necrophilia is a morbid fondness for dead bodies. The word derives from the Greek, *nekros* meaning dead body, and *philo* signifying a loving attitude. Unlike the temporary devotion to a corpse sometimes seen immediately after death, necrophilia denotes an ongoing pathology that psychiatrists often link to voyeurism, sadism, the involuntarily use of obscene words, and the male fear of intimate relations with women.

Necrophilia also refers to sexual attraction for, and the performance of sexual acts with, corpses. It may result from transforming a fear of the dead into a desire for the dead—a "reaction formation" in psychiatric jargon. Although the disorder is most commonly seen in men (more than 90% of the time), it also occurs in women. Only 17% of necrophiles can be classified as psychotic. Necrophiles usually want to possess an unresisting and unrejecting partner or to "rejoin" a former lover.[167]

After reviewing 122 twentieth-century cases of necrophilia, Rosman and Resnick classified the condition into four types: (1) *necrophilic homicide,* in which a murder is committed to obtain a corpse for sexual purposes; (2) *regular necrophilia,* in which already-dead bodies are used for sex; (3) *necrophilic fantasy,* in which no actual acts are carried out on the corpse; and (4) *pseudonecrophilia,* in which a (usually inebriated) person has a transient attraction and often a sexual encounter with a corpse, but does not usually fantasize or behave in this manner.[168]

Necrophiles are usually identified when in their early 30s, although their activity may begin much earlier. Seventy-nine percent of necrophiles are heterosexual, 13% are bisexual, and 9% are homosexual. Among homicidal necrophiliacs, only 58% are heterosexual, but heterosexuals constitute 84% of pseudonecrophile killers. The sex of the corpse is normally consistent with the necrophile's sexual orientation.[169]

Necrophilia is thought to be rare, but has been recognized since ancient times. Herodotus noted that in the days of the Pharaohs, Egyptian "wives of men of rank are not given to be embalmed immediately after death, nor indeed are any of the more beautiful and valued women. It is not till they have been dead three or four days that they are carried to the embalmers. This is done to prevent indignities from being offered them. It is said that once a case of this kind occurred: the man was detected by the information of his fellow-workman."[170]

Necrophiles still often gain access to bodies through their occupations, such as morgue attendants, cemetery employees, hospital orderlies or funeral parlor assistants.[171] True or not, early European anatomists were thought by the populace to be engaged not only in dissection, but also necrophilia.

A connection between sex and the dead is well represented in art and literature. Shakespeare described Juliet as being "deflowered" by Death who had "lain" with her,[172] and intercourse with the dead occurs frequently in the works of the Marquis de Sade. The fairy tale, *Sleeping Beauty,* also invokes the classic necrophilic fantasy when the prince awakens a beautiful corpse with a kiss.

Necrophilia forms the core of Robert Dodsley's 1744 play, *The Second Maiden's Tragedy.* As Gittings describes, "The Tyrant, when the heroine chooses death rather than to submit to him, has her body removed from the tomb and hires a painter to add colour to her dead face. In fact, the painter is the hero in disguise and uses poison in his tinctures so that the Tyrant dies when he kisses her. The painter then throws off his disguise and addresses the dying villain:

> Cannot the body, after funeral
> Sleep in the grave for thee? Must it be raised
> Only to please the wickedness of thine eyes?
> Do all things end with death, and not thy lust?"[174]

Edgar Allan Poe's macabre inspiration for much of his work was clearly necrophilia. Death inspired him, and through his writings he cast an irresistible spell on mankind. His great literary concern with horror, death and love of the dead stemmed from a necrophilic-type love for his mother, who died when he was three.[175] In his famous poem, *Annabel Lee,* Poe wrote:

> And so, all the night-tide, I lie down by the side
> Of my darling—my darling—my life and my bride,
> In the sepulchre there by the sea—
> In her tomb by the sounding sea.[176]

In his macabre story, *The Premature Burial,* Poe wrote of one lover jilted first by another's marriage to his sweetheart and then by her death:

> She was buried—not in a vault—but in an ordinary grave in the village of her nativity. Filled with despair, and still inflamed by the memory of a profound attachment, the lover journeys from the capital to the remote province in which the village lies, with the romantic purpose of disinterring the corpse, and possessing himself of its luxuriant tresses.[177]

Of course, popular verse has also incorporated the bizarre practice into common humor, such as in the traditional ditty:

> There once was a fellow named Grave,
> Dead hookers he kept in his cave,
> He was heard to admit,
> I'm a bit of a nit,
> But think of the money I save.[178]

There are, however, relatively few examples of documented necrophilia outside of the recent medical literature. One notorious case in the mid-fifteenth century was that of Bluebeard, Gilles de Rais, a baron and marshal of France and a comrade in arms to Saint Joan of Arc. Before he was burned at the stake for what the church described as his "unnatural appetites," the baron murdered up to eight hundred children to masturbate against their newly dead bodies.[179]

The death of a spouse occasionally leads to necrophilia. Legend says that King Herod (73 to 4 B.C.) continued to have sex with his wife Marianne for seven years after he killed her.[180] In a more recent and better-documented case, Sir John Pryce (1698-1761) embalmed his first wife when she died and kept her in bed with him—even after he married a second time. When his second wife died, she too was embalmed and kept in the bed. His third wife, however, would have no part of this and demanded that the first two be buried and not share their marriage bed.[181] In mid-eighteenth century Europe, Jacqes Necker, Director General of Finance under Louis XVI of France, kept the corpse of his wife, Suzanne Curchod, (at her behest) at home preserved in alcohol for three months, then had it placed in the mausoleum she had built. When he died, his body was placed in the same alcohol-filled container.[182,183]

Another case of "necrophilia," known only because of its spectacular result, was cited in 1752 by Professor Louis, a noted French medicolegal expert. (Many contemporaries believed the story true, although it parallels many fictional works.) A young girl had died and was laid out for burial when a youthful monk came to watch the corpse through the night. During the night he stripped the body and had intercourse with it. The following morning, however, the girl revived; nine months later she bore a child.[184]

Necrophiliacs sometimes rob graves to perform their acts. In 1886, Henri Blot dug up the corpse of an 18-year-old ballet dancer in St. Ouen so he could have sex with it. While not caught on that occasion, he was apprehended his next time out. At his trial he was quoted as saying, *"Que voulez-vous? Chacun à son goût, le mien est pour les corps."* ("What do you want? Each to his own tastes, mine is for corpses.")

Key West, Florida was the site of a bizarre case of necrophilia that is still recounted in song and legend (and court records). In 1931, Carl van Cassel became enamored of a beautiful young woman, Maria Elena Oyoz, who was dying from tuberculosis. Although she spurned his advances while she was alive, he was not deterred. After her death, he exhumed her body and first put it in a mausoleum. Later, he took the body home, dressed it in a wedding dress, and slept with it. This went on for seven years until he was discovered. A court hearing was held, but it was clear that the law did not cover this circumstance. Near the end of his court appearance, van Cassel suddenly asked the court that since he would not be convicted, could he have the body back! The judge had the body reburied at a secret site and van Cassel disappeared.[185]

Fewer than 10 percent of necrophiles also engage in cannibalism.[186] Recently, however, Jeffrey Dahmer, Milwaukee's serial killer-cannibal, confessed to sexual obsessions, such that "My consuming lust was to experience their bodies. I viewed them as objects, as strangers."[187]

## O. WHAT IS NECROPHOBIA?

Necrophobia is a morbid aversion to corpses. Unlike the normal distaste for touching dead bodies, necrophobics develop physical symptoms, such as nausea, dizziness, chills, or other symptoms of extreme anxiety when they even think of touching a corpse. This fear existed in primitive societies, and is increasingly common in industrialized countries. William May speaks of it as "human horror before death" and believes that fleeing from a corpse is an ingrained primitive response.[188] The term *thanatophobia* generally refers only to the fear of death, although it is often used interchangeably with necrophobia.

In primitive cultures, touching a corpse is almost a universal taboo. The Kaingang of South America consider corpses so representative of virulence and danger that they often abandon them in terror. The Navaho and other Southwestern U.S. Native Americans quickly bury their deceased along with many, if not all, of its possessions. If the death occurs in a home, they abandon the building and never use it again.[189]

One popular urban legend that keeps reappearing suggests necrophobia:

> My friend from Los Angeles breathlessly announced that she could pick up a $5,400 Porsche Targa sports car for only $500. (Obviously this story is quite old.) The reason for the reduced price was that it had sat in the middle of the Mojave Desert for one week with a dead man in it; consequently, the smell of death could not be removed from it.[190]

Necrophobia recently paid off in a big way for the owner of a junkyard adjoining the McCormick Mortuary in Laguna Hills, California. Although the mortuary had a scrubber on its smokestack and complied with both California's and the Environmental Protection Agency's rules, he sued the mortuary owners for "private nuisance and trespass into thought." He claimed that he was deeply disturbed by dreams of body parts falling from the sky. The court awarded him $2 million![191]

## P. WHEN HAVE PEOPLE BEEN SACRIFICED TO SERVE THE DEAD?

People have long been killed as part of funerary and burial practices. The motives for this have been: (1) to provide for the wants of and to comfort the deceased in the afterlife; (2) to prevent the ghost from "walking;" (3) to complete the death process (since a person's personality was often believed to haunt his possessions, including his wives); (4) to grant the dead their revenge; (5) to strengthen the deceased for his future endeavors; (6) to provide company for the dead; and (7) to guide the way in the next life. Royalty often were recipients of human funerary sacrifices, and close relatives or servants often served as victims.

Both the royal graves in the Sumerian city of Ur (about 2700 B.C) and in graves of China's Shang dynasty (twelfth to eleventh centuries B.C.) contained large numbers of servants and soldiers who were buried with their masters. And in ancient Scythia, now encompassing part of European and Asiatic Russia, Herodotus wrote that persons who had attended dead kings were strangled, including the deceased monarch's concubine, cup-bearer, cook, groom, waiter, and messenger. They believed that these persons, who were so closely linked to the king, would have no purpose and their lives no meaning after the king's death. It was therefore merciful to kill them.[192] One year after the king's death, fifty of his ministers were also sacrificed and then stuffed. After death, they had their abdominal organs removed and replaced with straw, since it was felt that they had overfilled their bellies in life. Their bodies were then impaled on the bodies of dead horses and arranged around the funeral monument.[193] The human corpses were kept upright on the horses by passing stakes "through their bodies along the course of the spine to the neck; the lower end of which projects from the body and is fixed into a socket."[194]

Celts sometimes sacrificed wives, children, slaves and others at the deaths of important persons. Evidence for this comes from graves that have bodies carefully buried at a lower level, while a number of carelessly strewn bodies, some decapitated, lie nearer the surface.[195]

Ancient Greeks routinely sacrificed slaves or captives on the pyres of their eminent dead. Homer's *Iliad,* for example, describes the slaughter of twelve young Trojans who were burned with the Greek hero Patroclus on his funeral pyre.[196] The Etruscans, an Italian people who lived around the fifth century B.C., would sometimes publicly kill and dismember people to serve as a blood sacrifice for an important person's grave. In some cases, the person would be blindfolded and torn apart by war dogs.[197]

When Viking chieftains died, it was the practice to sacrifice a volunteer, usually from among the girls serving the family. Eyewitness accounts from the tenth century A.D. report that for several days after she volunteered, the girl drank, sang and copulated with multiple men who had been aides of the dead chieftain. When the chieftain's corpse was moved from its temporary grave to a tent on the ship aboard which he would be cremated, the girl was brought into the tent and laid at the side of the dead chieftain. There she copulated with up to six men, after which an old woman, the "angel of death," stabbed her in the chest while four of the men held her down and the other two strangled her with a knotted rope.[198]

In prehistoric Central America, kings were often buried with their jesters and dwarfs for amusement, a number of women for consolation, and priests to act as spiritual guides. Early Peruvians invited friends and dependents of dead men to immolate themselves and accompany them to the spirit world. In later times, llamas substituted for human victims. In ancient Japan, ten to thirty servants of dead noblemen performed *hara-kiri* so they would be available to serve their master in the afterlife. This custom continued into the seventeenth century.[199]

People were also killed during this same period not so much to serve the dead as to ensure undisturbed tombs. When Attila the Hun (d. A.D. 453) and Alaric the Goth (d. A.D. 410) died, they were both buried in elaborate tombs filled with untold riches. In both cases, when their tombs were sealed (the river Vasento was redirected over Alaric's tomb), every person who assisted in the burials was killed.[200]

Up to the late nineteenth century, the death of a king in the Congo warranted the sacrifice of twelve young girls who were buried with him. During the same period, the corpses of Ashanti kings were ceremoniously washed and dressed, with attendants killed at each stage to help them perform those tasks in another life. Some of their wives were likewise killed along with servants to perform the other chores they might need. Hundreds of freshly killed bodies accompanied the kings of Dahome to their graves, including those of their wives, eunuches, singers, drummers and soldiers.[201] Among the Azande of Zaire, spirits in a dream could demand a human sacrifice. The arms and legs of unfortunate victims would be broken and their bodies dumped in the grave of the person whose spirit was seen. As late as 1906 observers reported that they saw a king's ministers and wife killed and buried with him.[202]

Originally, human funerary sacrifices involved killing wives and very young children who could not survive without the deceased male to provide for them.[203] Into modern times, the Hottentots, as well as numerous other subsistence cultures, buried newborn babies with their mothers if they had died during childbirth or soon after. Rather than having any symbolic meaning, this practice simply recognized that there was no one to nurse the child and it would soon die anyway.[204] Sacrificing wives and children continued, however, even after societies could afford to support survivors.

When a man died among the ancient Thracians, a people who lived in southern Europe between the Black and Aegean Seas, his several wives competed for the honor of being named the one he loved the most. Herodotus wrote that "...the friends of each [widow] eagerly plead on her behalf, and she to whom the honour is adjudged, after receiving the praises both of men and women, is slain over the grave by the hand of her next-of-kin, and then buried with her husband. The others [living widows] are sorely grieved, for nothing is considered such a disgrace."[205]

In the Fiji Islands, when a chief died, at least four of his wives were strangled and interred with his corpse to keep him company. One was placed beneath his body, one above, and one to either side.[206] This type of sacrifice also occurred among other Pacific Island cultures. When Ra Nbith, the pride of the Samoans, was lost at sea, the community sacrificed seventeen of his wives. Many islanders routinely strangled the wives of commoners during their husband's funerals, since they considered it "abominable" for a wife not to follow her husband into death. In 1839, for example, when news of a massacre at Viwa arrived, eighty women were strangled to accompany the spirits of their deceased husbands. Islanders also occasionally sacrificed the deceased's mother and daughters; men were never sacrificed at a woman's death, but they were sometimes killed upon the deaths of their masters.[207]

When the Dutch first arrived in the Malay Archipelago, locals still burned the wives of a prince at his funeral, along with her female slaves.[208] Among the Natchez Indians, one or more of the chief's wives and highest officers were merely knocked out and buried with him.[209]

Wives did not always peacefully acquiesce to being the funeral sacrifice.

Hindu widows in India commonly were burned on their husband's funeral pyre in "suttee" or "sati," a rite sometimes described as self-immolation. However, women seldom ascended the piles voluntarily. Although relatives usually drugged them, some jumped off the pyre and tried to run away. They were nearly always caught, though, and returned to the burning pyre. Often, the woman was weighted down with logs or otherwise impeded from escaping when she felt the flames.[210] This act, considered virtuous by some, was abolished by British decree in 1829, although it still occurs, as with the 1987 suttee of a 25-year-old newlywed at Deorala. The origin of the practice is unclear, but was reportedly justified by Vedic texts describing ancient Hindu funerals.[211] Modern Hindu women symbolically lie upon the unlit pyre, but are helped down before it is lit.

## Q. HOW WERE CORPSES SUPPOSED TO HELP OR HARM THE LIVING?

People have long believed that corpses could help the living, through curing disease or bringing luck. Many also believed corpses could cause harm.

Perhaps the most infamous example of a belief in corpse magic stemmed from a desire for a fountain of youth. In the early 1600s, Hungarian Countess Elisabeth de Báthory bathed each morning in the blood of virgin serving girls she had killed, believing that their blood was an elixir of youth. As a very powerful and rich aristocrat, she bought the vast number of "serving girls" she needed, and later bullied the local minister into burying the blood-drained bodies. Authorities eventually caught her and sequestered her in a small room for the remainder of her life. Historians estimate that she killed and bathed in the blood of over 650 girls.[212]

People throughout the world long believed that corpses could cure multiple ailments. People used a corpse's perspiration to cure hemorrhoids and tumors, applied the still-warm corpse's hand to cure a diseased area (in early America, to a goiter or a birthmark), touched a diseased part of the body to the same part of a corpse to heal it, or ate the ashes of happily married couples or lovers as an aphrodisiac.[213,214]

The English believed that touching a still-warm corpse, especially that of a hanged criminal, cured many diseases. A visitor to England, appalled by this practice, wrote in 1799:

I observed a number of men and women carried to the scaffold to be stroked by the hands, still quivering in the agony of death, of the suspended criminals, under the notion that such an application will be of efficacy in working a cure for several complaints; amongst the rest I remarked a young woman, with an appearance of beauty, all pale and trembling, in the arms of the executioner, who submitted to have her bosom uncovered, in the presence of thousands of spectators, and the dead man's hand placed upon it. Cruel, incomprehensible superstition! Thus to outrage the good sense, the decency, and decorum of an enlightened people.[215]

Thomas Hardy also described this custom in his 1888 short story, *The Withered Arm*. Gertrude Lodge is told that she could cure her arm if she were to

...touch with the limb the neck of a man who's been hanged...Before he's cold—just after he's cut down...It will turn the blood and change the constitution...You must get into jail and wait for him when he's brought off the gallows. Lots have done it...I used to send dozens for skin complaints...in former times.[216]

A more dramatic challenge was issued by an unknown English bard:

Now mount who list, and close by the wrist
Sever me quickly the dead man's fist!
Now climb who dare, where he swings in the air,
And pluck me five locks of the dead Man's hair!

Folk tales repeatedly imbued skulls used as drinking mugs, especially those from suicides, with special powers. In the Scottish Highlands, although there was a horror of suicide, a common remedy for epilepsy was to drink water out of or to eat a (ground up) piece of a suicide's skull. Records of actual cases specified that the skull had to be fresh, and scraped clean before use. To prevent a relapse, those cured by this method were never again permitted to touch a dead body or view a funeral. This practice continued into the twentieth century.

Some societies still believe the dead can cure the living. As late as 1948, a South African court heard the case of a gravedigger who reopened the grave of a 15-month-old child and cut away part of its face with a pick-axe to make medicine. He was sentenced to six months in jail.[217]

In Jordan, remarkable healing power was attributed to the corpses of murdered or decapitated men. As one woman attested in 1959, "Barrenness can be prevented by drinking blood taken from such a man, or by stepping over his body. A wife who has prematurely ceased to bear children may become pregnant if she steps over his grave, or takes stones from the grave, puts them into water and washes herself in it. Life—new life—may be gained from the life of which a murdered man has been robbed."[218]

Common beliefs also attributed corpses with powers of protection, good luck, and medical diagnosis. A rosary made of vertebrae supposedly protected civilians from harm, while soldiers carried the finger of a dead comrade to ward off injury during battle.[219] In the Philippines, the Ilongos, Jaro, and Iloilo tribes believe the deceased's urine brings good luck in gambling. Cock fighters still vie to collect the urine to bring themselves luck.[220] Russian tradition holds that newlyweds must lay flowers on the grave of a famous person as soon as they are married so they will be granted a good life together. At some Moscow cemeteries, couples still in their wedding garb stand in line to place flowers on the graves of famous composers, military heroes, and regional celebrities.[221]

Stretching the bounds of medical practice, one eighteenth-century physician invented "divine water," supposedly with miraculous prognostic powers. The potion was a stew made from a whole man's corpse, but it only worked if the man had been in good health then died a violent death. After adding a sample of blood, urine, perspiration, or other secretions from a sick person to the liquid, one could tell if the patient would live or die.[222]

While people believed corpses could help the living, they also believed corpses could cause harm. European folk lore, for example, held that drinking a mixture of human bones and beer would cause a person to become cruel, and that touching a cadaver could halt a woman's menstruation. In Britain, the Philippines, and elsewhere a "limber corpse," one that failed to go into *rigor mortis*, was an object to be feared. In some cultures it augured another death in the family.

Many cultures also took special precautions to prevent the spirits of the dead from harming the living. Among the Oraons of Palamau, India, for example, when pregnant women died before or during childbirth, nails, needles and thorns were driven into the soles of the corpse's feet to prevent evil spirits from causing survivors trouble.

Many people believed that suicides were especially prone to harm the living after death. They often treated the bodies of suicides poorly, but explained this with the more acceptable religious justification that, as one English judge said in 1554, suicide was "an offence against nature, against God, and against the King."[223] (Yet the Bible relates giving normal burial honors to suicides, as with Ahithophel, one of Absalom's generals, who hung himself yet was "buried in the sepulchre of his father."[224])

In 1821, Thomas Hardy wrote in his notebook,

Girl who committed suicide—was buried on the hill where two roads meet: but few followed her to her unblest grave: no coffin: one girl threw flowers on her: stake driven through her body.

Earth heaped round the stake like an ancient tumulus. (This is like Mother's description to me of a similar burial on Hendford Hill when she was a child.)[225]

Burying the corpses of suicides at the crossroads supposedly confused evil spirits and diffused their influence in several directions; the stake was used to prevent the ghost from "walking." Only at the beginning of the nineteenth century could English suicides be legally buried in cemeteries, and then only between the hours of 9 P.M. and midnight.[226]

Vampire legends represent the ultimate belief that the dead cause harm. These legends exist throughout the world, including Europe, China, Indonesia, and the Philippines. Believers thought that vampires were people who had died before their time (often from suicide, murder, drowning or women dying in childbirth), who refused to remain dead, and who brought death to their friends and neighbors. As with similar superstitions, these legends stem from an ignorance of physiology and pathology, resulting in the society blaming death on the dead. Many bizarre episodes (and much entertainment) has stemmed from vampire legends.[227] But at one time, the Romanians among others, took the legends so seriously that they developed an "automatic vampire-piercing device," made of one or more sharpened stakes and driven into a grave. If the body tried to leave the grave and harm the living, it would be pierced and "killed."[228]

Even in modern times, some of these beliefs persist. Paula Cho, a physician-lawyer who grew up in Hong Kong, relates that at the end of Chinese funerals when the coffin was closed, everyone turned their back on the coffin while the mortician nailed the coffin shut. They believed that if a person looked at the coffin while it was being closed, their soul would be trapped in the box. As a child, she once peeked, and was afraid for years that her soul was trapped in the box. Perhaps it was—she just completed law school.[229]

## R. WHAT OTHER UNUSUAL USES ARE THERE FOR DEAD BODIES?

Man is an innovative creature, and never more so than when corpses are involved. Various cultures and individuals have used dead bodies as decoration and to gain military advantage. They have also given them special burials to "protect" the living, and have reproduced their images to gain immortality.

Perhaps the best known example of using human remains as decorations are the ossuaries above European cemeteries, where rows of skulls and limbs from the wretches buried in mass graves for the poor were artistically arranged. In the Capuchin Church in Rome, the walls and ceiling of the ossuary contain bones in decorative arrangements: pelvic bones form rosettes, skulls become columns, leg bones support arches, and vertebrae serve as candleholders. Similar displays, including chandeliers and ornaments made only of small bones can still be seen in other churches in Rome. At La Veille Coquette into the early seventeenth century, skeletons were posed as gardeners, carpenters and field marshals.

Corpses have found a unique artistic use in a creative-writing course at Alma College, in Alma, Michigan. The students visit cadavers undergoing anatomical dissection so they can be inspired to write about life. Taking this one step farther, the instructor once used a cadaver as a stage prop and had a writer read his works from behind the body. At one point, the writer grabbed the corpse's heart and held it above his head while he read his composition. The instructor said of this, "It was a beautiful, illuminating experience."[230]

In a type of postmortem art, people have long made effigies of the dead. The classic death mask is a wax or plaster cast made from a mold of a corpse's face. The original mold is made by oiling the face, ears, and as much of the neck as possible, and then carefully pouring on plaster or some other quick-setting material. This mold is used to produce a positive image—the death mask. If the eyes are left open when the mold is made, the mask can have glass eyes set in these holes. The mask can be painted or remain the flesh color of the plaster that was used for the mold. False eyelashes, eyebrows, and hair complete the effect.

At least since ancient Egyptian times, these masks have been used by artists to better portray their subjects after death. From the thirteenth century on, death masks have also appeared on tombs of illustrious Europeans. In medieval France and England, death masks were used for royal effigies during monarchs' funerals. Famous and infamous individuals still occasionally have death masks made. One of the most famous in recent times was Baby Face Nelson, whose mask was made after he was gunned down by the FBI.

Going somewhat farther in using corpses for art, Dr. Thomas Holmes, who claimed to be the father of modern embalming, patented a process for preserving bodies by electroplating them in 1863. This process "transforms the corpse into a beautiful statue...face and figure are covered with a shining veil, through which the familiar lineaments appear." In a more modern variation, W.F. Jones, an archaeologist, proposed encasing bodies within transparent blocks of methacrylate resin so that specimens could be exhibited. (This is similar to a method used for anatomical specimens and insects.)[231] While making formal effigies from the corpse is not a current trend (but see Chapter 5, *How does a mummy differ from an embalmed body?*), embalmers equate their practices with the making of effigies, or as they say, to "make possible to every man what once was the prerogative of kings."

Corpses have also played an active role in the military. In an effort to continue to "lead" his troops in his war with Scottish rebels, King Edward I of England, known as the "hammer of the Scots" for his ruthless suppression of rebellion, left instructions that when he died, in 1307, his bones were to be brought to the head of his army until the last Scotsman had surrendered.[232] That would have been a long wait, since his son, Edward II, quickly gave up the battle for Scotland to Robert the Bruce and returned to London to enjoy himself. Scotland did not unite with England until exactly four centuries later.

A cadaver did, however, play a key role in the outcome of World War II. Just before the Allies landed in Sicily, many tactics were used to persuade the Germans that they would land instead in Sardinia and Greece. One of the most successful ruses used the cadaver of a young pneumonia victim dressed and credentialled as a Royal Marine courier. The corpse was dropped into the sea, to simulate drowning after an airplane crash, in an area that assured that the body would be washed ashore in an area of Spain with very active German spies. The papers he carried were supposedly top secret plans to invade areas east and west of Sicily. The Germans believed the ruse and moved their troops to the wrong locations.[233]

In at least one case, a corpse was entrusted with an unusual civilian task. London's *Morning Herald* of February 14, 1829, reported that when a woman near Mansfield, England, died, her friend forgot to put letters from the dead woman's deceased son in her coffin as she had requested. The woman remained distressed until, soon after, the village postman died. The woman slipped them into his coffin, trusting that he would faithfully deliver them in the hereafter.[234]

## S. REFERENCES

1. Editors of The American Heritage Dictionaries: *Word Mysteries and Histories.* Boston: Houghton Mifflin, 1986, pp 34-35.
2. Prehistoric Peoples and Cultures. In: *The New Encyclopaedia Britannica.* vol 26. (Macropaedia). Chicago: Encyclopaedia Britannica, 1987, p 64.
3. Sanday PR: *Divine Hunger: Cannibalism as a Cultural System.* Cambridge, England: Cambridge Univ Press, 1986, p 4+.
4. Whitehead N: Quoted in Boucher, PP: *Cannibal Encounters: Europeans and Island Caribs, 1492-1763.* Baltimore: Johns Hopkins Univ Press, 1992, p 6.
5. Boucher PP: *Cannibal Encounters: Europeans and Island Caribs, 1492-1763.* Baltimore: Johns Hopkins Univ Press, 1992, p 6-7.
6. Crocombe RG, Crocombe M: *The Works of Ta'unga.* Pacific History Series No 2. Honolulu: Univ of Hawaii Press, 1968, pp 91-92.
7. Simpson AWB: *Cannibalism and the Common Law: The Story of the Tragic Last Voyage of the Mignonette and the Strange Legal Proceedings to Which It Gave Rise.* Chicago: Univ of Chicago Press, 1984, p 112.
8. Pardi MM: *Death: An Anthropological Perspective.* Washington, DC: Univ Press of America, 1977, pp 8-10.
9. Villa P: Cannibalism in the neolithic age. *Nature.* 1991;351:613-14.
10. Flavius J: Thackeray HStJ, trans: *The Jewish Wars.* Loeb Classical Library, 1926-65. New York: GP Putnam & Sons.
11. Pauthier MG, Bazin M. 1853. As quoted in: Tannahill R: *Flesh and Blood: A History of the Cannibal Complex.* New York: Stein & Day, 1975, p 45.
12. Johnson, Capt. Charles: *A General History...of the most Famous Highwaymen, Murderers, Street Robbers, &c.* London: 1734, pp 132-33.
13. de Vaca C: Covey C, trans & ed: *Adventures in the Unknown Interior of America.* Albuquerque, NM: Univ of New Mexico Press, 1961, p 60. Translated from *Relación,* 1542 & 1555; and *Comentarios,* 1555.
14. Ibid., p 74.
15. Cortes. As quoted in: Sanday, *Divine Hunger,* p 16.
16. Ibid.
17. Moryson, Fynes: *Itinerary.* London, 1617.
18. *The Jesuit Relations, 1649-50.* Quoted in Sanday, *Divine Hunger,* p 129.
19. Ibid.
20. Smith J: *Generall Historie of Virginia, New England, and the Summer Isles.* 1624. Quoted in *Annals of America.* vol 1: 1493-1754. Chicago: Encyclopaedia Britannica, 1976, p 26.
21. Curl JS: *A Celebration of Death: An introduction to some of the buildings, monuments and settings of funerary architecture in the Western European tradition.* London: Constable, 1980, p 300.
22. Parkes AE: Disposal of the dead. *Practical Hygiene.* 1873.
23. Sanday, *Divine Hunger,* p 16.
24. Sahagún B. As quoted in: Sanday, *Divine Hunger,* p 173.
25. Acosta José de: *Natural and Moral History of the Indies.* 1590. Trans in: *Purchas His Pilgrimes.* 1625.
26. Sagan E: *Cannibalism: Human Agression and Cultural Form.* New York: Harper Torchbooks, 1974, pp 14-15.
27. Puckle BS: *Funeral Customs—Their Origin and Development.* London: T Werner Laurie, 1926, p 73.
28. U.S. Department of the Navy: *Final Report of Navy War Crimes Program in the Pacific.* vol 2. Case no. 36, appendix B, pp 38-40. Submitted to the Secretary of the Navy, December 1, 1949. Cited in: Piccigallo PR: *The Japanese on Trial: Allied War Crimes Operations in the East, 1945-1951.* Austin, TX: Univ of Texas Press, 1979, pp 78-79.
29. International Military Tribunal for the Far East (IMTFE), EX 2056-A. Cited in: Kerr EB: *Surrender and Survival: The Experience of American POWs in the Pacific, 1941-1945.* New York: William Morrow, 1985, p 315.

30. Kerr EB: *Surrender and Survival: The Experience of American POWs in the Pacific, 1941-1945.* New York: William Morrow, 1985, p 259.
31. U.S. Department of the Navy: *Final Report of Navy War Crimes Program in the Pacific.* vol 2. Case no. 36, appendix B, pp 38-40. Submitted to the Secretary of the Navy, December 1, 1949. Cited in: Piccigallo, *The Japanese on Trial,* pp 78-79.
32. Brown P, Tuzin D: *The Ethnography of Cannibalism.* Washington, DC: Society for Psychological Anthropology, 1983, p 63.
33. *New York Herald Tribune.* December 2, 1945. As cited in: Piccigallo, *The Japanese on Trial,* pp 128-29.
34. Brown, Tuzin, *The Ethnography of Cannibalism,* p 65.
35. Toshi-yuki Tanaka: *Unknown War Crimes-What Japanese Forces Did to Austrailians.* Tokyo: Ohtsuki, 1993. (Japanese) (English version expected in 1994.)
36. Mabry M: Cannibals of the Red Guard. *Newsweek.* 1993;121(3):38.
37. Grisly case of serial killer grips Russia. *USA Today.* October 15, 1992, p 2A.
38. Schmemann S: 'Citizen CH.' to be tried in 53 savage murders. (New York Times news service.) In: *Arizona Daily Star.* Tucson, AZ: April 5, 1992, p C3.
39. Grisly case of serial killer grips Russia. *USA Today.* Oct 15, 1992, p 2A.
40. 'I am a mad beast.' *Newsweek.* May 4, 92, p 42.
41. Herodotus: *History.* Book 5, verse 8. In: *Great Books of the Western World.* (vol 6). 1952.
42. Brown, Tuzin, *The Ethnography of Cannibalism,* p 2.
43. Herodotus: *History.* Book 4, verse 26. In: *Great Books,* vol 6, 1952.
44. Ibid., Book 1, verse 216.
45. Pardi, *Death,* p 8-10.
46. Murdock GP: *Our Primitive Contemporaries.* New York: Macmillan, 1934, pp 399-400.
47. Herodotus: *History.* Book 1, verse 119. In: *Great Books,* vol 6, 1952.
48. Ibid., verse 73.
49. Pohl FJ: *Amerigo Vespucci: Pilot Major.* New York: Columbia Univ Press, 1944.
50. Sanday, *Divine Hunger,* p 150.
51. Knowles N: The torture of captives by the Indians of Eastern North America. *Proc Amer Philosophical Soc.* 1940;82(2):151-225.
52. Cook J: As quoted by: Clunie F: Fijian Weapons and Warfare. *Bulletin of the Fijian Museum.* no 2. Suva: Fiji Museum, 1977.
53. Sahlins M: Raw women, cooked men, and other 'great things' of the Fiji Isands. In: Brown, Tuzin, *Ethnography of Cannibalism,* pp 72-93.
54. Ibid.
55. Shepherd C: News of the weird. *Chicago Reader.* October 9, 1992, p 41.
56. Pardi, *Death,* p 8-10.
57. Sanday, *Divine Hunger,* p 6.
58. Simpson, *Cannibalism and the Common Law,* p 149.
59. Piccigallo PR: *The Japanese on Trial: Allied War Crimes Operations in the East, 1945-1951.* Austin, TX: Univ of Texas Press, 1979, pp 190.
60. Kara J: *La lettre de Sagawa.* Paris: R. Laffont, 1984. (Translated from the Japanese book: *Sagawa-kun kara no tegami.*)
61. Report of Trial of Haarman. *The News of The World.* London: December,21,1924.
62. Jenness D, Ballantyne Rev A: *The Northern D'Entrecasteaux.* Oxford: Clarendon, 1920.
63. *Regina v. Dudley and Stephens.* 1881-1885. *All England Law Reports.* p 61.
64. Simpson, *Cannibalism and the Common Law,* pp 225-70.
65. *Ballad of the Brig George.* Cornwall County Record Office, DDX 106/29. Quoted in: Simpson, *Cannibalism and the Common Law,* pp 314-15.
66. *Ballad of the Essex.* Cornwall County Record Office, DDX 106/32. As quoted in: Simpson, *Cannibalism and the Common Law,* pp 316-17.
67. Tarlé E: *Napoleon's Invasion of Russia, 1812.* London: 1942, p 244.
68. *American Experience: The Donner Party.* Seattle, WA: KTCS-TV Public Broadcasting Station, 1992.
69. Mazzulla F, Mazzulla J: *Al Packer: A Colorado Cannibal.* Denver, CO: Mazzulla, 1968, pp 6, 39.

70. Salisbury, Harrison E: *The 900 Days.* New York: Harper & Row, 1969, pp 479-81.
71. Blaha F: Testimony before Nuremberg War Crimes Tribunal. Cited in: Cary: *Eyewitness to History.* Cambridge, MA: Harvard Univ Press, 1987, p 558.
72. Brown, Tuzin, *The Ethnography of Cannibalism,* p 63.
73. Read PP: *Alive:The Story of the Andes Survivors.* Philadelphia, PA: Lippencott, 1974.
74. Tannahill R: *Flesh and Blood: A History of the Cannibal Complex.* New York: Stein & Day, 1975, pp 176-78.
75. Swift J: *Modest Proposal for Preventing the Children of Poor People in Ireland from Being a Burden to their Parents or Country, and for Making Them Beneficial to the Public.* Dublin: A Moore, 1730.
76. Ettinger RCW: *Man Into Superman.* New York: St. Martin's, 1972, p 199.
77. Bar's essay contest about cannibalism. *Tucson (AZ) Citizen.* February 25, 1993.
78. Headhunting. In: *The New Encyclopaedia Britannica.* vol 5. 1987, p 778.
79. Ibid.
80. Habenstein RW, Lamers WM: *Funeral Customs the World Over.* Milwaukee: National Funeral Directors Association, 1963, p 627.
81. Ibid.
82. Sagan, *Cannibalism,* pp 35-47.
83. Headhunting, *Encyclopaedia Britannica,* vol 5, 1987.
84. Pannell S: Travelling to other worlds: narratives of headhunting, appropriations and the other in the 'eastern archipelago'. *Oceania.* 1992;62:162-78.
85. Headhunting, *Encyclopaedia Britannica,* vol 5, 1987.
86. Ibid.
87. Herodotus: *History.* Book 4, verse 64. In: *Great Books,* vol 6, 1952.
88. Eckert WG: The forensic and medicolegal aspects of the battle of the Little Big Horn – 1876 archaeological and historical analysis. *The Inform Letter.* 1988;20.
89. Headhunting, *Encyclopaedia Britannica,* vol 5, 1987.
90. The war of the noses. *Newsweek.* October 5, 1992, p 51.
91. Tannahill, *Flesh and Blood,* p 169.
92. Fussell P: *Thank God for the Atom Bomb and Other Essays.* New York: Summit, 1988, p 46-52.
93. Bass WM: The occurrence of Japanese trophy skulls in the United States. *J Forensic Sciences.* 1983;28(3):800-803.
94. Sledzik PS, Ousley S: Analysis of six Vietnamese trophy skulls. *J Forensic Sciences.* 1991;36(2):520-30.
95. Ibid.
96. Karsten R: Blood Revenge, War, and Victory Feasts among the Jibaro Indians of Eastern Ecuador. *Bureau of American Ethnology, no. 79.* Washington, DC: Smithsonian Institute, 1923, pp 1-2, 28-30.
97. Karsten R: *Studies in the Religion of the South American Indians East of the Andes.* Helsinki-Helingsfors: Societas Scientiarum Fennica, 1964, p 158.
98. 2 shrunken Indian heads fetch $22,000. *Arizona Daily Star.* Tucson, AZ: March 9, 1992.
99. Herodotus: *History.* Book 1, verse 140.
100. Haug M: *The Parsis – Essays on their Sacred Language, Writings and Religion.* New Delhi, India: Cosmos Pub, 1978, p 325.
101. Ibid., p 240.
102. Modi JJ: *The Religious Ceremonies and Customs of the Parsees.* 2nd ed. Bombay, India: Jehangir B Karanti's Sons, 1937, pp 66.
103. Tebb W, Vollum EP, Hadwen WR: *Premature Burial and How It May Be Prevented, With Special Reference to Trance, Catalepsy, and Other Forms of Suspended Animation.* London: Swan Sonnenschein, 1905, p 168.
104. *The Times of London.* January 28, 1876. Cited in: Tegg W: *The Last Act: Being the Funeral Rites of Nations and Individuals.* London: William Tegg & Co, 1876, p 175+.
105. Ibid.
106. Tebb, Vollum, Hadwen, *Premature Burials,* pp 169-173.

107. Anima N: *Childbirth & Burial Practices Among Philippine Tribes.* Quezon City, Philippines: Omar Pub, 1978, p 110.
108. Ibid., p 70, 82.
109. Budge EAW: *The Mummy: A Handbook of Egyptian Funerary Archaeology.* London: KPI, 1987, p 336. (Reprint of 1893 edition)
110. Pallis CA: Death. In: *New Encyclopaedia Britannica.* vol 16., 1987, p 1031.
111. Tegg W: *The Last Act: Being the Funeral Rites of Nations and Individuals.* London: William Tegg & Co, 1876, p 58.
112. Ibid., p 67.
113. Ibid., p 184.
114. Jackson PE: *The Law of Cadavers and of Burial and Burial Places.* New York: Prentice-Hall, 1937, p 63.
115. DeSpelder LA, Strickland AL: *The Last Dance.* Palo Alto, CA: Mayfield Pub, 1983, p 45.
116. Habenstein, Lamers, *Funeral Customs the World Over,* p 688.
117. Ibid., pp 129, 329 30.
118. Bendann E: *Death Customs: An Analytical Study of Burial Rites.* New York: Alfred A Knopf, 1930, pp 218-19.
119. Polson CJ, Brittain RP, Marshall TK: *The Disposal of the Dead.* 2nd ed. Springfield, IL: Charles C Thomas, 1962, pp 3-4.
120. Tsung-lien shen, Shen-chi Liu: *Tibet and the Tibetans.* Stanford, CA: Stanford Univ Press, 1953, p 147.
121. Ekai Kawaguchi: *Three Years in Tibet.* Adyar, Madras: The Theosophist Office, 1909, p 388.
122. Habenstein, Lamers, *Funeral Customs the World Over,* pp 90-91.
123. Grinsell LV: *Barrow, Pyramid and Tomb.* London: Thames & Hudson, 1975, p 24.
124. Haestier R: *Dead Men Tell Tales: A Survey of Exhumations, From Earliest Antiquity to the Present Day.* London: John Long, 1934, p 279.
125. Litten J: *The English Way of Death: The Common Funeral Since 1450.* London: Robert Hale, 1991, p 37.
126. Mayer RG: *Embalming: History, Theory and Practice.* Norwalk, CT: Appleton & Lange, 1990, p 32.
127. Puckle, *Funeral Customs,* p 194.
128. Habenstein RW, Lamers WM: *The History of American Funeral Directing.* 2nd ed. Milwaukee, WI: National Funeral Directors Assn, 1981, p 67.
129. de Wavrin J: trans: Hardy W, Hardy E: *Chronicles, 1399-1422.* 1887. In: Carey, *Eyewitness to History,* p 76.
130. Bland O: *The Royal Way of Death.* London: Constable & Co, 1986, p 27.
131. Ibid., p 79.
132. Ibid., p 16, 79.
133. Herodotus: *History.* Book 5, verse 114. In: *Great Books,* vol 6, 1952.
134. Haestier, *Dead Men Tell Tales,* p 53.
135. Lebrun Fr: *Les Hommes et la Mort en Anjou.* The Hague: Mouton, 1971. Cited in: Ragon M: *The Space of Death: A Study of Funerary Architecture, Decoration, and Urbanism.* (Sheridan A: trans). Charlottesville, VA: Univ Press of Virginia, 1983, p 187.
136. Dickens C: *Pictures from Italy.* London: Bradbury & Evans, 1846.
137. Ienaga S: *The Pacific War, 1931-1945.* New York: Pantheon, 1978, p 173.
138. Ward Rev J. 1661. Quoted in: Russell KF: Anatomy and the barber-surgeons. *Med J Australia.* 1973;1:1109-15.
139. *25 Geo. II c. 37.*
140. Pardi, *Death,* p 51.
141. *Burgh Records.* Edinburgh, Scotland: 1583-84.
142. Gittings C: *Death, Burial and the Individual in Early Modern England.* London: Croom & Helm, 1984, p 70.
143. State Trials of Norton, Owen, and Stayleg. (Christopher Norton 1570.) In: Howell TB, ed: *A Complete Collection of State Trials.* 21 vols. London: 1816-31. Quoted in: Gittings, *Death, Burial and the Individual,* p 70.

144. Bendann, *Death Customs,* p 218-19.
145. Ragon M: *The Space of Death: A Study of Funerary Architecture, Decoration, and Urbanism.* (Sheridan A: trans). Charlottesville, VA: Univ Press of Virginia, 1983, p 183. Originally published as *L'espace de la mort: Essai sur l'architecture, la décoration et l'urbanisme funéraires.* Albin Michel, 1981.
146. Ragon, *Space of Death,* p 36
147. Richardson R: *Death, Dissection and the Destitute.* London: Routledge & Kegan Paul, 1987, p 35.
148. Adams N: *Dead and Buried?* Aberdeen, Scotland: Impulse Books, 1972, p 16.
149. Ibid., p 15.
150. Guibert L: *Livres de raison, registres de famille et journaux individuels limousins et marchois.* Paris: Limoges, 1888.
151. Herodotus: *History.* Book 4, verse 65. In: *Great Books,* vol 6, 1952.
152. Selzer R: *Mortal Lessons: Notes on the Art of Surgery.* New York: Simon & Schuster, 1987, p 55.
153. Bostetter EE: *George Gordon, Lord Byron — Selected Works.* New York: Holt Rinehart & Winston, 1972, p 3.
154. Ibid.
155. Coffin MM: *Death in Early America: The History and Folklore of Customs and Superstitions of Early Medicine, Funerals, Burials, and Mourning.* Nashville: Thomas Nelson, 1976, pp 82-83.
156. Hassler P: The lies of the Conquistadors. *World Press Review.* December 1992, pp 28-29.
157. Haestier, *Dead Men Tell Tales,* p 122.
158. Fussell P: *Thank God for the Atom Bomb,* pp 25-26, 51.
159. Coffin, *Death in Early America,* p 206, 211.
160. Herodotus: *History.* Book 4, verse 64. In: *Great Books,* vol 6, 1952.
161. Tegg, *The Last Act,* p 281.
162. Ibid., pp 280-81.
163. Copperthwaite DR: *A Guide to the Ripley's Believe It or Not Collection of Oddities and Curiosities.* (pamphlet). Canada: Ripley International, 1978.
164. Coffin, *Death in Early America,* p 82-83.
165. *Trial of the Major War Criminals Before the International Military Tribunal.* Nuremberg, Germany: November 14, 1945-October 1, 1946.
166. Jacob W: *Contemporary American Reform Responsa.* New York: Central Conference of American Rabbis, 1987, p 169.
167. Rosman JP, Resnick PJ: Sexual attraction to corpses: a psychiatric review of necrophilia. *Bull Am Acad Psych Law.* 1989;17:153-63.
168. Ibid.
169. Ibid.
170. Herodotus: *History.* Book 2, verse 89.
171. Rosman, Resnick, *Bull Am Acad Psych Law,* 1989.
172. Shakespeare W: *Romeo and Juliet.* Act 4, scene 5, lines 36-37.
173. Gittings, *Death, Burial and the Individual,* p 194.
174. Dodsley R: "The Second Maiden's Tragedy." 1744. In: Hazlitt WC, ed: *A Select Collection of Old English Plays Originally Published by Robert Dodsley in the Year 1744.* 4th ed. 16 vols. London: 1875.
175. Bonaparte M: *The Life and Works of Edgar Allan Poe: A Psychoanalytic Interpretation.* London: Imago Publishing, 1949.
176. Poe EA: *Annabel Lee.* 1849. In: Stedman EC, Woodbury GE, eds: *The Works of Edgar Allan Poe, Vol. X: Poems.* New York, Chas Scribner's Sons, 1914, p 42-43.
177. Poe EA: The Premature Burial. *Dollar Newspaper.* July 31, 1844.
178. Cited in interview with Don Witzke, May 1992; predates 1960. (origin unknown)
179. Bendetti J: *Giles Rais: The Authentic Bluebeard.* London: 1971. Cited in Tannahill, *Flesh and Blood,* p 67.
180. Huber Von H: Nekrophilie. *Kriminalistik.* 1962;16:564-68.
181. Litten, *The English Way of Death,* p 50-51.

182. Ariès P: *The Hour of Our Death.* New York: Oxford Univ Press, 1981, p 386.
183. Ariès P: *The Western Attitudes Toward Death: From the Middle Ages to the Present.* Baltimore, MD: Johns Hopkins Press, 1974, p 70.
184. Louis A: *Lettre sur le certitude des signes de la mort.* Paris: 1752. Quoted in: Shneidman ES, ed: *Death: Current Perspectives.* Palo Alto, CA: Mayfield Pub, 1976, p 222.
185. *CNN Headline News.* December 25, 1992.
186. Rosman, Resnick, *Bull Am Acad Psych Law,* 1989.
187. Howlett D: He wanted 'excitement, gratification.' *USA Today.* February 3, 1992, p 3A.
188. May W: Attitudes toward the newly dead. *Hastings Center Studies.* 1972;1:3-13.
189. Sills DL, ed: *International Encyclopedia of the Social Sciences.* vol 3. New York: Macmillan, 1968, p 27.
190. Brunvand JH: *The Vanishing Hitchhiker: American Urban Legends and Their Meanings.* New York: WW Norton, 1981, p 20.
191. Inman R: *Cremation Liability.* (lecture). Cremation Assoc of North America Annual Convention. Louisville, KY: 1990. (audiotape)
192. Lincoln B: *Death, War, and Sacrifice.* Chicago: Univ of Chicago, 1991, p 195.
193. Tegg, *The Last Act,* pp 270-71.
194. Herodotus: *History.* Book 4, verse 72. *Great Books,* vol 6, 1952.
195. Basevi WHF: *The Burial of the Dead.* London: Geo. Rutledge & Sons, 1920, pp 131-32.
196. Homer: *The Iliad.* In: *Great Books,* vol 4. 1952, pp 175-77.
197. Turner AW: *Houses for the Dead.* New York: David McKay, 1976, p 42-43.
198. Foszian AI: Cited in: Coon CS: *A Reader in General Anthropology.* New York: Henry Holt, 1948, pp 414-16.
199. Basevi, *Burial of the Dead,* pp 127-29.
200. Tegg, *The Last Act,* p 65.
201. Basevi, *Burial of the Dead,* p 127-29.
202. Habenstein, Lamers, *Funeral Customs the World Over,* pp 272-73.
203. Grinsell, *Barrow, Pyramid and Tomb,* pp 40-41.
204. Bendann, *Death Customs,* p 200.
205. Herodotus: *History.* Book 5, verse 5.
206. Tegg, *The Last Act,* p 204.
207. Bendann, *Death Customs,* p 199.
208. Habenstein, Lamers, *Funeral Customs the World Over,* p 341.
209. Bendann, *Death Customs,*: p 200.
210. Datta VN: *Sati: A Historical, Social and Philosophical Enquiry into the Hindu Rite of Widow Burning.* Riverdale, MD: Riverdale Co, 1988, pp 185-204.
211. *Rig. Veda.* Book 10, Hymn 18, verse 8.
212. Tannahill, *Flesh and Blood,* pp 69-70.
213. Ariès, *Hour of Our Death,* p 357-58.
214. Coffin, *Death in Early America,* p 24, 220.
215. Meister JH: *Letters Written During a Residence in England.* London: 1799, p 62. As quoted in: Gittings, *Death, Burial and the Individual,* p 68.
216. Hardy T: The withered arm. *Blackwood's Edinburgh Magazine.* January 1888.
217. *Rex v Sephuma* 1948(3) SA 982(T).
218. Granqvist H: *Muslim Death and Burial—Arab Customs and Traditions Studied in a Village in Jordan.* Helsinke-Helsingfors: Societas Scientiarum Fennica, 1965;34:22.
219. Ariès, *Hour of Our Death,* p 358.
220. Anima, *Philippine Tribes,* p 44.
221. Koosman S: *Cultural Variations in Funeral Practice.* (lecture.) National Funeral Directors Association Annual Convention. Baltimore, MD: 1989. (audiotape)
222. Ariès, *Hour of Our Death,* p 358.
223. Gittings, *Death, Burial and the Individual,* p 72.
224. *II Samuel* 17: 23.
225. Hardy T: 1821. Quoted in: Gittings, *Death, Burial and the Individual,* p 73.
226. Gittings, *Death, Burial and the Individual,* p 72-73.
227. Barber P: *Vampires, Burial, and Death: Folklore and Reality.* New Haven, CT: Yale Univ

Press, 1988, p 2-3.

228. Ibid., p 53.
229. Interview with Paula Cho, Ph.D., M.D., J.D. Tucson, AZ: June 4, 1993.
230. Kansas D: So where do mortuary instructors turn to inspire their students? *Wall Street J.* October 20, 1992, p B1.
231. Mendelsohn S: Embalming from the medieval period to the present time. *Ciba Symposia.* May 1944, pp 1805-12.
232. Fraser A: *The Lives of the Kings and Queens of England.* New York: Alfred A Knopf, 1975, p 87.
233. Mantagu E: *The Man Who Never Was.* Philadelphia, PA: JB Lippincott, 1954.
234. *Morning Herald.* London: February 14,1829. Cited in: Richardson, *Death, Dissection, and the Destitute,* p 4.

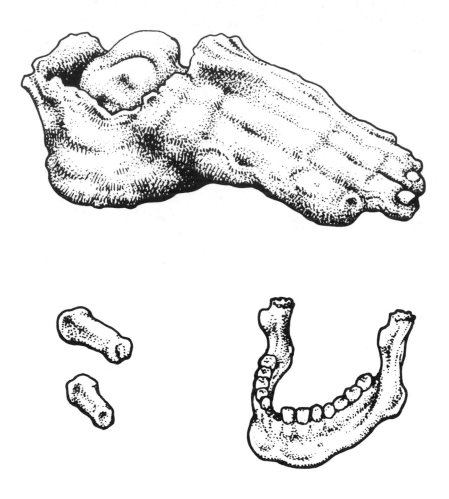

Saints' reliquaries: finger, jaw and foot.

# 10: GOING OUT IN STYLE

421

*What pomp and circumstance surrounds funerary rites, especially those of famous people? How are corpses used in ceremonies? How were they once the "life of the party" at wakes? And what strange things have happened to some corpses just because they were famous?*

## A. HOW ARE THE DEAD USED IN CEREMONIES?

Early cultures believed that dead bodies could walk and harm the living. This led to the development of ceremonies to ensure that once a corpse was disposed of properly, it could not harm the living. To assure that the spirits of the dead would never return, Scots, for example, once carried bodies "three times sunwise" around the church before burial.

Nearly all cultures have ceremonially used their dead to support varying social needs. Societies have used these ceremonies to maintain social adhesion, allow the bereaved to confront reality, establish communal rites and ceremonies, show respect for the deceased, and allow sanitary disposition of the body. Primitive societies also used the dead in ceremonies to obtain power and social control, and to maintain tradition.

Some aboriginal people of New South Wales, for example, in an attempt to acquire the power and attributes of a deceased relative, as well as to show their respect, once roasted their dead over slow fires, collecting the oils and juices from the body to rub on their own bodies. They then dried and smoked the corpse over the fire until it hardened. Eventually, it was buried.[1]

To maintain a social tradition and to show respect for their dead, the Hurons (eastern Native Americans) traditionally held a Feast of the Dead. During this ritual, families exhumed the remains of relatives who had died since the last Feast. They then cleaned their bones, dressed them in new clothes and jewelry, and carried them in a funeral procession to a central place where they would remain. There they could "live on" with others whose bones were also brought there.

In an effort to preserve the social bond as well as to honor their dead warriors, most societies have had long traditions of returning war dead once the combatants have, at least temporarily, settled their differences. This dates back to Greek and Roman times, and continues today as evidenced by the turmoil that surrounded the return of Israeli military dead from Arab hands and American dead from Vietnam and North Korea.

## B. WHAT IS "NECROMANCY?"

*Necromancy* refers to (the illusion of) raising spirits of the dead to communicate with them. Usually the spirit is asked to provide information about the future, and for other "privileged" information. People who desired knowledge and power have practiced necromancy at least since biblical times. The Bible records that Saul, even though he had previously banished necromancers from his kingdom, sought out a necromancer to ask advice of dead King Samuel's spirit. He got unexpectedly bad news from the necromancer and soon after committed suicide in battle.[2]

Necromancy has three common elements: the necromancer is usually a woman, the spirit returns only briefly, and the spirit is called upon to give advice or to perform an action.[3] While many necromancers call up imaginary spirits, the ritual to raise a real dead person's spirit traditionally requires a churchyard ceremony at midnight, as well as the physical presence of the corpse, or at the least the insertion of a tube into the grave to facilitate "communication." (Necromancers believe that raising the spirit of a suicide is extremely difficult.) Always fearful of making an error and being destroyed by a spirit they have raised, necromancers protect themselves and others when conjuring up the dead by using the cautionary phrase, "without harm to me or to anyone."[4] No necromancers are known to have died on the job—the spell must work.

## C. WHAT IS A WAKE?

*Waking* the dead is a very ancient custom that extends around the world. It refers to the practice of watching a corpse during the period between death and burial, and its length varies by custom and climate. Accounts of European wakes date back over a thousand years. Scots call this ceremony a "lykewake."

During a wake, watchers keep the dead body under surveillance for many reasons, not the least of which is to see if the deceased "wakes up." In earlier times it was also to keep stray cats, dogs and rats off the body. In Roman wakes, the corpse was usually watched for seven or eight days before interment, often with boys present to keep off the ever-present flies.[5]

Where wakes still exist, they are usually somber affairs. At one time, however, wakes provided an opportunity for a hearty party. Extravagant partying may have been the attendees' attempt to prove that, unlike the corpse, they could defy death—that they remained "alive and kicking." Maria Edgeworth, describing Irish wakes in 1810, concluded with the verse:

> Deal on, deal on, my merry men all,
> Deal on your cakes and your wine;
> For whatever is dealt at her funeral today
> Shall be dealt to-morrow at mine.[6]

Wakes were, in some ways, like the modern "viewing." Corpses were dressed in burial clothes and laid out for relatives and neighbors to pay their respects. At lykewakes, visitors were expected to use their left hands to touch the corpse on the forehead or hands, if they were to avoid dreaming of the deceased. Unlike most modern viewings, wakes often became raucous events.

In the fourteenth century, those standing watch over the corpse began enlivening their hours of tedious duty by "rousing the ghost." This included practical jokes to frighten superstitious relatives and black magic to raise the dead spirit. Indeed, attempts to raise the dead became so pervasive that the Council of York expressly forbade it in 1376, and one guild permitted its members to night-watch the dead only if they would "abstain from raising apparitions, and from indecent games."[7]

The Irish wake and its cousin in Scotland were the most notorious. Early versions included a sham duel (or, on occasion not so sham), where one combatant would mimic the voice and gestures of the deceased. This individual was "killed" and then "resurrected" by a person playing a sorcerer. The show, considered entertainment for the entire community, was fueled by liberal doses of alcohol and pancakes, the traditional food. In Ireland, bread, cheese and whiskey were distributed at midnight—and then the festivities *really* began. Throughout Scotland, the festive spread put out for the "mourners" included whiskey, porter (a dark beer resembling light stout) and tobacco for the men, and wine, biscuits, tea, bread and jam for the ladies.[8] On occasion, so much whiskey was consumed that the party goers toasted not only the memory, but also the health of the departed.

The editor of the *Records of Inverness and Dingwall Presbytery* wrote of lykewakes in 1896 that "they were more boisterous than weddings, the chamber of the dead being filled night after night with jest, song and story, music of the fiddle and the pipe, and the shout and clatter of the Highland reel."[9] While *caoine*, or weeping women, stood around the corpse, crying for the prescribed time, most celebrants routinely participated in other activities.

Common activities at wakes also included storytelling (described as *ineptae fabulae* or silly stories); the singing of love, patriotic or religious songs; playing music and dancing (sometimes with the corpse removed from the coffin to dance!); and card playing, with the corpse often dealt into the game. Wrestling and other athletic events were common, as were practical jokes, hide-and-seek and guessing games. Courtship and lovemaking were normal features of old-time wakes in Britain, Germany and Scandinavia, and lewd games and dances around the coffin were common on the European continent, especially if the deceased was a young person.[10,11]

Attempts to reduce the drunkenness, fighting and unseemly behavior at wakes usually met with little success. On one occasion in the early nineteenth century, however, to teach those assembled a lesson, a Scottish school teacher moved the corpse out of the room, replacing it with a live man covered by a sheet. The man was to rise up and scare the party goers if the wake became too rowdy. Unfortunately, he died while impersonating the corpse. This so frightened those assembled that the merrymaking at wakes did cease in that region, at least for a while.

Wakes were not confined to the British Isles. The learned monk Regino, the abbot in Lorraine, France instructed his monks in A.D. 906, that "Diabolical Songs be not sung at night hours over the bodies of the dead...Let no one there presume to sing diabolical songs nor make jests and perform dances which pagans have invited by the devil's teaching."[12] Since the custom of wakes did not persist in France, perhaps he was more successful than his British and Scottish colleagues.

In Colonial America, wakes and weddings were the two occasions when citizens felt obliged to publicly drink alcohol. As one person wrote, "Both rich and poor alike felt that the funeral arrangements were as incomplete without liquor as without a hearse or coffin. Fathers have been known to stagger to the grave, husbands to fall down and sons to be drunken at the burial of all that is dear."[13] Irish immigrants imported their tradition of rowdy wakes to the United States. One Irish wake in North Norwich, New York, in the late nineteenth century was held for two Gavin brothers who, while drunk, died when their railroad handcar crashed into a passenger train. The revelers placed the decapitated head of one of the men on a high chair with his favorite pipe hanging from his mouth. From that site he could oversee the boisterous party in his honor.[14]

A special precaution followed wakes in Pennsylvania's coal "patches." Before the burial, mourners had to ensure that the body in the coffin was the corpse, rather than a person just sleeping off the effect of his libations. During these wakes, corpses were commonly removed from their coffins to make room for inebriated mourners, since it was more comfortable to sleep in the coffin than on the floor.[15]

The former head-hunting Jivaro Indians of South America also hold wakes for dead men. With the fully dressed corpse propped upright and overseeing the activities, friends and relatives play a dice game to see who will get the dead man's possessions. Food and beer are plentiful during these festivities.[16]

The wake is taken to extremes by the Tana Toradja on the island of Sulawesi in Indonesia. During a mourning period of months to years, the corpse remains in his own home. His wife maintains a constant vigil and provides him with food. Sometime later the death is announced officially and the community begins feasting, dancing, and holding sporting events. Finally, months or years later, the naturally mummified body is placed in a coffin and buried.

Even more extreme are the wakes of the Isneg and Apayo tribes of the Philippines. These tribes never embalm their dead, and the corpse gradually rots. By the time it is buried, it has reached an advanced state of decomposition. Outsiders have commented, "From being used to it, they have of consequence developed strong stomachs. And probably a dulled sense of smell, too, that they have become immune to the stench of it all." Despite the state of decomposition, tribal custom requires the living spouse to sleep under the blanket covering the corpse until the burial.[17] A bit less drastic, the Ilongo, another Philippine tribe, simply have a custom of not bathing during the wake.[18]

The wake is increasingly avoided in industrialized Europe, but continues in the United States as "viewing the remains," or "visitations," where visitors encounter an "almost-living" person who, thanks to the benefits of embalming, waits to greet them. In the United States, it is Mexican-Americans and Japanese-Americans who most commonly have traditional wakes; only 22 percent of Anglo-Americans desire a wake. Less than one-fourth of any of these groups, however, want wakes held in their homes.[19]

Recently, along with custom funerals, joyous wakes have made a small comeback. One example (in California, of course) was that of B.T. Collins, a California state legislator and former Green Beret who died of a heart attack at age 52. He had a wake in a ballroom in Sacramento with 3,000 party goers, three bars, a buffet with an ice sculpture and a seven-piece band belting out pop tunes. In the center of the room lay his flag-draped coffin. As a friend of Mr. Collins who helped plan the event said, "I was raised Polish Catholic and [services] would always end with a blowout party with a polka band, kielbasa and vodka...Everyone would cry in the morning, but by midnight there was no pain."[20]

Some people look askance at the merriment at wakes, but as Mark Twain observed, "Why is it that we rejoice at a birth and grieve at a funeral? It is because we are not the person involved."[21]

## D. WHAT IS A VIEWING?

In the United States, the traditional Christian death rite begins with embalming the corpse, with the deceased's friends and relatives subsequently viewing the remains in a funeral home. Viewing the body may continue even during the religious funeral service several days later. There are both supporters and detractors of this practice.

Supporters believe that viewing the corpse in an open casket forces loved ones to emotionally accept the reality of death. Ann Kliman, a psychologist who consults for the funeral industry, for example, feels that with a sudden unexpected death, it is important that the family can view the body before the funeral in order to face the reality of the beloved one's death.[22]

Opponents of viewing, which is nearly always coupled with embalming, see the entire process as unseemly, undignified, wastefully expensive and unnecessary. Yaffa Draznin quotes opponents of the "grief therapy" argument as saying that it is abysmal that "no law presently exists to curb the specious claims of those who peddle grief therapy to the grieving...[It is] a theatrical production starring a theatrically made-up corpse...[making] the spiritual realities as remote as any Grade-B motion picture." She also quotes another writer who says, the American funeral "with all its vulgarity, sacrifice of spiritual values to materialist trappings, immature indulgence in privative spectacles, unethical business practices, and overwhelming abnegation of rational attitudes—has become for many students of the national scene a symbol of cultural sickness."[23] Obviously, not everyone likes these ceremonies.

After being embalmed, bodies are normally laid out for the visitation. This "wake" or waiting period before the funeral was once held in private homes, but now generally occurs at funeral homes. It can last one to four days depending upon the length of time required by distant friends and family to arrive. When a large number of mourners is expected, visitations are often structured so that lodge members, business associates, and friends are scheduled to come at different times or on different days. At least one family member is always present during visitation hours to receive condolences from visitors.

The "calling hours" or, for the more prominent, "lying in state," provide a time for family members and acquaintances to pay respects to the dead and offer condolences to the family. During visitation hours, the casket is placed in the front of the viewing room, in a niche to the side, or in an adjoining room. The casket may be open or closed; flowers may surround it.

Visitors customarily sign a guest book, go to the family to offer condolences, and then in some faiths, go to the casket to kneel or offer a prayer. Visitations are considered social, rather than religious occasions, although Pentecostal denominations often use this period to vocally and actively lament their loss. Evangelical denominations often read Scripture, say prayers and sing hymns. At some point in a Catholic visitation, a priest holds a wake service, including readings from the Scripture and prayers. Occasionally a rosary is still said. During informal visitations, food is often served.

### E. WHO GETS TO "LIE IN STATE?"

"Lying in state" means that a dead body is ceremoniously exposed to public view with great pomp and solemnity. Riches and fame alone do not give the deceased the prerogative of lying in state. To lie in state is an honor permitted only to deceased rulers and to the few others, such as extraordinary generals or statesmen, who have given service of historic proportion to their nations. Lying in state is not unusual, though, as there are many national leaders, and they all die. What is unusual is how this rite has occasionally been carried out.

The body of Roman Emperor Constantine not only lay in state, but presided over the Empire after his death. When he died of natural causes at "the mature age of sixty-four" his body was transported to the palace at Constantinople where it was placed on a special golden bed. "Every day, at the appointed hours, the principal officers of the state, the army, and the household, approach[ed] the person of their sovereign with bended knees and a composed countenance, offer[ing] their respectful homage as seriously as if he had been still alive."[24] This lasted until his potential successors finished their skulduggery and bloodletting, and the next emperor was crowned.

The Romanov czars of Russia took lying in state to an extreme. Their bodies were laid out for weeks in open coffins at Saint Peter and Paul Cathedral in St. Petersburg. Thousands of subjects passed the corpses and kissed the icons clasped in their hands.[25] The Soviets extended this just a bit farther with the body of Lenin, keeping him (or a wax-enhanced double) on public exhibit for decades after his death.

On occasion, notables have lain in state because no money could be raised for their funerals. That was the situation with Queen Anne of Denmark, the wife of King James I of England. Although she died on March 2, 1610, and the King wanted a quick burial, she lay in state for ten weeks until enough money could be raised to provide a properly elaborate royal burial. As was the norm, her widower the King did not attend the funeral, since it was not royal protocol for him to attend a funeral of his inferiors, even that of his own queen.[26]

Some years later when Oliver Cromwell, the Lord Protector of Great Britain, died on September 3, 1658, he had a ritual lying in state. His coffin lay on a catafalque from October 18 to November 10, covered with a life-size wax effigy of him. His body, however, was thought to have already been secretly interred in Westminster Abbey. Rumors at the time said that embalmers had botched the job, necessitating a quick burial. It is also possible, however, that the government was worried that rebel monarchists would steal his body.[27]

In the late twentieth century, the most famous lying in state was that of President John F. Kennedy. While his body lay in state in the Capitol rotunda, thousands of ordinary citizens filed by in a public expression of grief and shock. He was interred after a nationally televised funeral procession.

## F. WHO GETS A PARADE?

Funeral processions allow and encourage the public to acknowledge and honor the dead. Most people get the type of attention provided by parades only at their weddings and funerals. Today, anyone can have a funeral cortege who has enough friends with cars to participate. These automobile processions exemplify the notion that "For many, the 'famous for fifteen minutes' part comes at the end."[28] They do not come close, however, to the grand funeral parades that are normally reserved for the rich and famous (or infamous).

Funeral parades are nothing new. Ancient Scythians, in what is now part of Russia, had funeral processions that lasted forty days, and stopped at each of the villages of clans related to the deceased. At the same time, Greek and Roman funeral processions were announced by heralds and included stops for orations on the way to the public funeral. In their funeral processions, Julius Caesar's body was borne by the Roman magistrates, and Augustus Caesar's by the senators of Rome.

In Samoa, interment of chiefs was often delayed for many days so that the corpse could be carried to the various places he normally visited in life and the people could pay their respects.[29]

One of the longest funeral processions in history was that of Nero Claudius Drusus Germanicus, a consul of Rome and the father of Emperor Claudius. After he died in Germany while commanding Roman forces, authorities carried his body back to Rome, a trip of over 600 miles requiring them to cross the Alps. The body was first borne by tribunes and centurions and then by the chief men of the cities along the route.[30]

Somewhat shorter, but more common, were Scottish funeral processions to bury the deceased near their forefathers. Mourners sometimes carried bodies 70 miles or more over "coffin roads," using multiple companies of bearers who rotated the load among them. One such solemn procession bore the body of the beloved Lady Mackenzie of Gairloch, who died in childbirth in the late nineteenth century. Five hundred volunteers, divided into four companies, silently carried her coffin on its week-long journey.[31] Scottish funeral processions were not always solemn, however, as attested to by Flora MacDonald's 16-mile journey to the grave in Skye, during which participants consumed at least three-hundred gallons of liquor.[32]

Between the thirteenth and eighteenth centuries, solemn European religious funeral processions were composed of priests, monks, candle bearers and paupers. In the Middle Ages, many people left wills specifying who would be in their funeral cortege. The presence of priests and the poor in a funeral procession lent honor to the dead. One will dated 1202 specified that 101 poor priests should be in the funeral procession.[33]

Beginning in the eighteenth century, Paris was the scene of enormous funeral processions, and the populace "was awakened every morning at four o'clock by a bell announcing the cart which carried the dead from the Hôtel-Dieu [a large hospital] to the cemetery at Camart."[34] When a French King was to be interred, the formalities of L'Ancien Régime, which ended with the funeral of Louis XVIII in October 1824, demanded that transporting the body "to Saint-Denis was carried out by the *banouards* [salt carriers] who, after having had the privilege of salting and boiling the dead kings, inherited that of bearing the sovereign's coffin."[35]

Some funeral processions have been unhealthy for observers.

Anyone who met the funeral procession of a Mongol prince was immediately slain and then "ordered" to accompany the prince as an escort. Similar practices were also followed in the Kimbunda area of Africa.[36] In the Solomon Islands, members of the funeral cortege themselves felt threatened. They routinely took a different route back to their village than they took going to the grave, lest the deceased's ghost follow them.[37] In the Philippines, Tagologs try to avoid meeting funeral processions, since they are considered bad luck. If they meet one while going to gamble or collect a debt, they postpone that activity until a more auspicious time.[38]

Most large funeral processions have been for very famous people.

Napoleon, for example, eventually had a funeral parade worthy of his fame, although it only occurred during his second interment. When he died on St. Helena in 1821, his body was buried simply by a few companions and his guard of British Grenadiers. With a change in French politics, though, his body was returned to France for more formal ceremonies in December 1840. Although the weather was bitterly cold, more than 600,000 people, including King Louis Philippe, lined the streets for his cortege.

Similarly, people crowded the streets and all other vantage points to see the Duke of Wellington's funeral parade in 1852, the grandest of the nineteenth century. The funeral procession of this general, who defeated Napoleon at Waterloo, took almost three months to plan and was a spectacular military event. Large bodies of troops, including one captain, one subaltern, one sergeant, one corporal and five privates from *every* British Army regiment participated; thousands of additional military men lined the route or followed in the procession. The giant funeral car carrying his body was so heavy that sixteen horses could barely move it. An enormous parade in his honor (but without the body) was also held in Austria, where the Austro-Hungarian Emperor and his entire army, one of the largest in the world, participated.

All British royalty normally had public funeral parades until the nineteenth century, and London's poor looked forward to these events. At each funeral, poor people from London's churches were chosen to walk in the procession. If the dead royal was male, men were selected; if female, women. Each participant was given a suit of warm black clothing he could then keep. Competition for these positions was fierce.[39] Yet not everyone approved of these elaborate events. In 1832, during discussions concerning the Anatomy Act in England, Henry Hunt proposed what he thought was a better idea for some of those famous corpses: "I would recommend, in the first place that the bodies of all our kings be dissected, instead of expending seven or eight hundred thousand pounds of the public money for their interment. Next, I would dissect all our hereditary legislators. After that, the bishops, with a host of those priests and vicars who feed themselves, and not their flocks."[40]

During the Victorian period in England, any notable, or anyone with sufficient funds, could have an elegant funeral procession. Mimes and other attendants carrying the trappings of mourning preceded an elaborately decorated hearse. The hearse was usually trimmed in silver and gold and was pulled by six black horses decorated with ostrich feather plumes. The hearse's sides were usually glass, exposing the elaborate coffin to public view.[41] These funeral processions demonstrated the deceased's wealth and power. They also indicated the regard the family had for the deceased, and even more than weddings, helped to establish a family's social position.[42] Queen Victoria herself had an elaborate funeral parade, the most impressive part of it being a short trip across the Solent River aboard the Royal Yacht *Alberta*. The yacht was accompanied by thirty-eight Royal Navy battleships, cruisers and destroyers, five German ships, and one ship each from Portugal, France and Japan. They formed a double line, and the yacht passed between them as their Minute guns fired and their bands played the *Dead Marches* of Chopin and Beethoven.[43]

The Victorian period also saw a different type of postmortem parade. After hangings in Britain, bodies, after being cut down, were "placed in a handcart and drawn through the streets in full public view—possibly as a warning to evil-doers—with the City Marshal in full ceremonial uniform leading the way and the hangman and his assistant riding in the cart. Arrived at the surgeon's hall, which was in the neighbourhood...the body was taken inside, stripped and laid on a table while a surgeon made an incision in the presence of the City Marshal."[44]

The United States has also had its share of impressive funeral processions. Abraham Lincoln's funeral caravan in 1865, for example, was on a train that, over fourteen days, traveled the 1,700 miles from Washington, D.C. to Springfield, Illinois. The train, drawn by thirteen locomotives, was decorated with portraits of Lincoln wreathed in evergreen and black draperies. Over seven million people saw it. At every major stop, the coffin was removed and opened so that the public could see Lincoln's face.

During the funeral parades of presidents and other famous heroes, a saddled horse is led behind the casket. In John F. Kennedy's cortege, the horse was quite skittish. Perhaps it knew the origin of this custom; important persons' mounts were once killed at the graveside and buried with them. As late as 1781, this custom was used in a formal ceremony when a calvary general, Count Friedrich Kasimir Boos von Waldeck, was buried with his sacrificed horse in Treves, Germany.[45] In accordance with this tradition, former president and general Ulysses S. Grant also had his horse buried with him.

In some locales, commoners also get elaborate funeral parades.

A traditional funeral procession in northern China can be immense, involving men scattering spirit-money, displaying written testimonials to the deceased, and carrying plaques with his titles or official posts, enormous testimonial banners, and items for graveside sacrifice. Trailing behind are musicians, monks, priests, a chief mourner, other male relatives, the coffin with pallbearers, women and children, and other guests. These giant processions usually move very slowly, stopping at each roadside altar to make an offering.[46]

Elaborate funeral parades are also a New Orleans tradition. Their best-known elements are the jazz bands that play as they lead the funeral cortege down the street. Much quieter is the traditional Amish funeral that can, however, include a long funeral procession, especially when an elder with many relatives dies. One man had 274 direct descendants when he died. His funeral procession included 125 horse-drawn carriages.[47]

## G. WHAT HAPPENS TO CORPSES OF FAMOUS RELIGIOUS FIGURES?

Being too famous has often been detrimental to a simple (and lasting) interment. Saints have been routinely dismembered so that their parts could be used as religious icons. T.S. Eliot noted that the "Saint and Martyr rule from the tomb."[48] Many of their parts, however, are not in the tomb.

The bones and bodies of Christian saints have long been on the move, in some instances being exhumed multiple times. Parts of saints' bodies have often been distributed widely for use as religious relics. Some of these have been kept in reliquaries for centuries. These containers are often rings enclosing small finger bones, crystals covering chips of bone, or gold cases surrounding limbs.

Reliquaries exist in churches throughout Europe. One example of such a reliquary contains Saint Camillo de Lellis' finger, gouty foot, and the half of his heart preserved in the church of Santa Maria Magdelena in Rome. The rest of his heart was divided among other brotherhoods of his order. Many baroque German and Austrian churches contain the skeletons of saints in glass-fronted cases, often dressed in Roman armour and velvet tunics. The well-preserved body of St. Catherine of Bologna, who died in 1463, can be seen through glass in the convent of Poor Clares at Bologna, where she was once the prioress. Reliquaries in Spanish churches often contain more gold decoration than bone; those in Portugal generally have more bone than gold.

St. Cuthbert's bones are renowned for having travelled widely and frequently throughout England and Scotland. During the several centuries after he died in A.D. 687 on the Farne Islands off Northeast England, his remains were repeatedly moved. His relics even played a part in motivating William the Conqueror in battle during the eleventh century.[49] William's corpse did not fare well either. While his body was buried in St. Etienne at Caen, his heart was left to Rouen Cathedral and his entrails to the Church of Chalus. Even his body gave its caretakers problems. When attendants tried to stuff his ample body (King Philip of France said he looked like a "pregnant woman") into a stone sarcophagus, it burst and filled the church with a horrid stench.[50]

The hearts of St. Ignatius (d. A.D. 107), St. George (d. A.D. 303), St. Benoit (d. A.D. 547) and St. Catherine of Sienna (d. A.D. 1590), among others, have all been preserved as holy relics.[51] In some cases the saint's heart was removed at death, in others it was removed many years or even centuries later. What was actually recovered, however, may be open to question.

In an example of crass commercialism, the remains of St. Amandus, who died about A.D. 684, were surreptitiously moved, in 1762, from Rome to Oberammergau, Austria, as a tourist attraction.[52] Only later did the city's passion play draw more tourists.

This behavior with Saint's remains, however, contrasted violently with popular Christian belief which paralleled the pagan fear of death without burial. Many people were convinced that unless their body was buried, and the grave remained unviolated, they would not be able to arise on the Last Day. A common Christian saying went "He who goes unburied shall not rise from the dead."[53]

The Catholic Church has rigid customs for some of its potential saints. When a Pope dies, the *cardinal camerlingo*, in purple vestments, inspects the corpse, calling out the Pope's name three times. If there is no answer and no sign of life, he is pronounced dead. When death does not occur in the Vatican, the body is shaved, washed and immediately embalmed. Attendants then dress the body in its pontifical vestments, including mitre and chalice, and carry it in a large open litter to St. Peter's Church. If death occurs in the Vatican, the body is immediately carried, by the back stairs, into Sixtus V's Chapel. After laying there for twenty-four hours, it is embalmed. The body is then carried to the chapel of the Blessed Trinity, where it lays for three days, in an open coffin so that mourners can kiss the corpse's feet. After three days, the body is again embalmed and laid in a lead coffin within a cypress coffin. The body must then lay in St. Peter's Basilica for at least a year. After that time, if the deceased Pope had indicated a wish to be buried elsewhere, another church can have the body—if it pays a large enough sum to St. Peter's for the privilege. It is said that the cost goes up with the odds that the Pope will be canonized in the future.[54]

Buddhist reliquaries have also met unusual fates. In late 1993, for example, Nepalese officials reported that international gangs had stolen Buddha's *asthi dhatu*, believed to be Buddha's mortal remains. They are thought to have been smuggled out of Nepal for sale to foreigners.[55]

## H.  WHAT HAPPENS TO CORPSES OF MONARCHS AND PRESIDENTS?

The corpses of secular leaders were also often distributed widely. A common practice for monarchs and warriors, especially from the twelfth to the eighteenth centuries, was to bury their hearts separately from their bodies. Many knights of the Middle Ages, to prove their loyalty, directed that their hearts should be removed, after death, and buried at the feet of the noblemen they served.

A corpse's heart, as the traditional seat of emotions, was often buried at a favorite spot to which the body could not be removed. This tradition may have restarted in historical times with the enshrinement of the heart of D'Arbrissel, founder of the Order of Fontevrault in 1117.[56]

When Richard I died in 1199, his "lion-heart" was removed and his body was buried at Fontevaud and some internal organs were interred at Chaluz. In 1838, 700 years after his death, investigators discovered the lead-encased heart in Rouen. The heart of King Philip of Navarre was also removed at death, but was kept by his queen until she also died and had his heart buried with her. In 1514 Anne of Brittany's heart was buried at the Carthusian Church at Nantes, and in 1621 the Cardinal de Guise's heart was buried at Notre Dame Cathedral in Paris.[57] Topping them all, Charles V's high constable, Bernard Du Guesclin, had four tombs, one for his flesh, one for his heart, one for his intestines, and one for his bones. Only the bones were buried at the exalted St. Denis cemetery.[58]

The hearts of the post-restoration Stuarts were encased in silver and covered with purple velvet. Robert Bruce, the hero of Scotland, asked that his heart be buried in the Church of the Holy Sepulchre in Jerusalem. Unfortunately, the gentleman transporting this relic was killed en route. The heart, however, was recovered and eventually brought to Scotland's Melrose Abbey.[59]

Dismembering and honoring parts of dead leaders was not only a Western tradition. Among the Ovimbundu of Angola, for example, the king's jawbone was traditionally removed from the corpse five months after death and cleaned by putting it on an anthill. It was then wrapped into a large bundle and placed with his umbilical cord in a temple.[60] And among the Tanala of Madagascar, the king's eye teeth were traditionally preserved as sacred relics along with crocodile teeth.[61]

Though not quite a queen, Eva Perón attracted a huge following after her death in 1952, and the public's memory of her continued to hold Argentina's Peronist Party together. She remained such a potent symbol that, three years after her death, political enemies stole her corpse and hid it in Italy for 16 years. Subsequently, different Argentine regimes, for their own political motives, had the body moved to different sites, until it was finally interred in the family crypt in Argentina. In a like manner, the return of Ferdinand Marcos' body to the Philippines was thought to have served as a rallying point for right-wing political activity. His family stored the body in a refrigerated crypt outside of Honolulu from his death in 1989 until it was allowed into the Philippines for burial in late 1993. Emperor Haile Selassie, who ruled Ethiopia for several generations and died mysteriously in 1975 was found buried under the floor of the office of the man who overthrew him, Megnistu Haile Mariam. According to Ethiopian radio, "The reason why Mengistu chose this site was to see that the body did not rise from the dead."[62]

Some famous people, even when they have specifically requested simplicity, have often had elaborate funerals. Queen Mary II of England, who died in 1694 had a very costly and elaborate funeral, even though she had expressed in writing that she wished no expense to be incurred at her funeral.

One might reasonably wonder what happened to the bodies of former U.S. presidents. Most have simple markers on their graves. Those who died in office, however, normally have much more elaborate gravesites, as do Andrew Johnson, Ulysses S. Grant, and Dwight D. Eisenhower. Some graves are nearly hidden away, such as that of James Madison, whose grave in Montpelier, Virginia, is reached by a one-lane dirt road.[63] Abraham Lincoln's body, however, took an interesting course after burial. Over the next 36 years people repeatedly tried to kidnap the casket for ransom. The body was hidden in cellars and secretly buried elsewhere and the public unknowingly paid homage to an empty sarcophagus. In 1901, it finally came to rest, within tons of concrete, in Springfield, Illinois' Lincoln Tomb.[64]

## I. WHAT HAPPENS TO CORPSES OF OTHER FAMOUS PEOPLE?

The corpses of many famous people who were neither religious nor secular leaders have also come to strange ends. A few examples suffice to demonstrate just how strange some dispositions can be.

After the poet Percy Bysshe Shelley died in a boating accident, his heart was snatched from the funeral pyre and returned to England. In 1723, when the Duke of Orléans died, his body was opened so his heart could be placed in a special box. Before the Duke's Great Dane could be stopped, however, it gobbled up a quarter of the heart, greatly disturbing the embalmers.[65]

In modern times, Robert Livingstone's heart (as in "Mr. Livingstone, I presume") was buried in Africa after he died; his body was returned to Westminster Abbey.[66] Although Frédéric Chopin's heart is in the church of the Holy Cross in Warsaw, his body is at Père-Lachaise, Paris, France. (His French tomb is often used as a mailbox for lovers.)[67] Likewise, when noted physicist Albert Einstein died in 1955, most of his body was cremated and the ashes scattered. His brain, however, was preserved by a Princeton Hospital pathologist for analysis, since Einstein's was purportedly the most brilliant mind of the twentieth century. (At two and two-thirds pounds, it was hardly of extraordinary size, as the average weight of a male human's brain is three pounds.)

The most famous body existing as a secular icon is that of Jeremy Bentham, a philosopher who helped found Utilitarianism. He requested that upon his death, his skeleton be placed on display at University College, London. Before he died in 1832, he willed his body to his physician friend, Southwood Smith, with instructions for a public dissection (invitation only, please) and "the skeleton he will cause to be put together in such manner as that the whole figure may be seated in a chair usually occupied by me when living, in the attitude in which I am sitting when engaged in thought in the course of the time employed in writing." His body was to be an "Auto-Icon," set within a box and clothed in his own clothes, hat and walking stick, adding, "said Box or case with the contents there to be stationed in such part of the room as to the assembled company shall seem meet...".[68] His body still sits in its case, being opened periodically. His head, alas, has been replaced by a wax copy topped by a panama hat; his desiccated head rests between his feet. His request was designed to help pass the English Anatomy Act of 1832 and to dispel public concern about dissection.

The modern author, Thomas Hardy, left a request that he be buried in his local churchyard. He was so famous, however, that a compromise was reached. His ashes were buried in the poet's corner of Westminster Abbey, and his heart was buried near his home.[69] Similarly, the great Italian composer, Giuseppe Verdi, gave his friends strict instructions to bury him without public fanfare or display. Yet more than 100,000 people lined the way to his funeral and he is interred in an ornate marble tomb.

## J. HOW HAVE CORPSES SERVED AS POLITICAL SYMBOLS?

Corpses have also been used as political and secular symbols. While the Roman Emperor Constantine ruled after death, at least one corpse was reportedly made queen *after* she died. In 1355, Inez de Castro was beheaded by the King of Portugal for not abandoning his son, the prince, as he commanded. Prince Pedro did not take this well, later deposing his father and assuming the throne in 1357. After killing his lover's executioners and trying to eat their hearts (he couldn't), Pedro had Inez disinterred and moved the body to a beautiful masoleum in the abbey at Alcobaça. Supposedly, Pedro had her corpse enthroned beside him in April 1361 as Queen of Portugal. All of his courtiers were required to show obeisance by kissing her hand.[70]

To exercise social control, dead Inca luminaries were mummified and, on great occasions, taken to preside over major feasts. A large collection of Inca mummies was used in this fashion as late as 1559. A traditional practice in the New Hebrides was to bake the skeletons of former chiefs into idols.[71] Among the Khasis of Assam, bodies of dead chiefs were made into mummies and buried in hollowed-out tree trunks so they could be visited periodically.

Until 1824, French royal funerals were considered entertainment, the *menus plaisirs du roi*. They eventually went on so long that embalming the body became necessary. As soon as the king had died, his body was washed, embalmed, and enclosed in three nested coffins—soft wood, lead, and oak, covered by embroidered black velvet. At one time, a wax death mask, wearing the crown and draped with the royal cloak, was kept on the death bed for ten days. During that time, servants laid out the king's clothes, and served meals to the corpse, while the princes, princesses, prelates, and officers continued normal court activities.[72]

## K. REFERENCES

1. Fraser J: *The Aborigines of New South Wales.* Sydney, Australia: Commissioners for the World's Columbian Exposition, 1892, p 80.
2. *I Samuel* 28.
3. Kastenbaum RK, Kastenbaum B, eds: *Encyclopedia of Death.* Phoenix, AZ: Oryx Press, 1989, p 196.
4. Ibid., p 197.
5. Tegg W: *The Last Act: Being the Funeral Rites of Nations and Individuals.* London: William Tegg & Co, 1876, p 48.
6. Edgeworth M: Quoted in: O'Súilleabháin S: *Irish Wake Amusements.* Cork, Ireland: Mercier, 1967, p 18.
7. Puckle BS: *Funeral Customs—Their Origin and Development.* London: T Werner Laurie, 1926, pp 62-63.
8. Gordon A: *Death is For the Living.* Edinburgh: Paul Harris, 1984, p 36.
9. O Súilleabháin S: *Irish Wake Amusements.* Cork, Ireland: Mercier, 1967, p 18.
10. Gittings C: *Death, Burial and the Individual in Early Modern England.* London: Croom & Helm, 1984, p 106-107.
11. Hagberg: Hwbch. des d. Abergl. 5, pp 239-246. Cited in: O'Súilleabháin, *Irish Wake Amusements,* p 160.
12. McNeil JT, Gamer HM: *Medieval Handbooks of Penance.* New York: Columbia Univ Press, 1938, pp 318-19.
13. Hunt T: *Wedding Days of Former Times.* 1845. As quoted in: Coffin MM: *Death In Early America.* Nashville: Thomas Nelson, 1979, p 87.
14. Coffin MM: *Death In Early America.* Nashville: Thomas Nelson, 1979, p 85.
15. Hannah Fisher, RN, MLS: Interview. Tucson, AZ: May 1993.
16. Habenstein RW, Lamers WM: *Funeral Customs the World Over.* Milwaukee: National Funeral Directors Association, 1963, p 621.

17. Anima N: *Childbirth & Burial Practices Among Philippine Tribes.* Quezon City, Philippines: Omar Pub, 1978, pp 84-85, 100.
18. Ibid., p 44.
19. Kalish RA, Reynolds DK: *Death and Ethnicity—A Psychocultural Study.* Los Angeles: Ethel Percy Andrus Gerentology Center, Univ of Southern CA, 1976, p 47.
20. Dolan C: Burying tradition, more people opt for 'fun' funerals. *Wall Street J.* May 20, 1993, p A1+.
21. Twain M: Pudd'nhead Wilson's Calendar. From: *Pudd'nhead Wilson.* 1894. Quoted in: DeVoto B, ed: *The Portable Mark Twain.* New York: Viking Press, 1946, p 558.
22. Kliman A. Cited in: Editors of Consumer Reports: *Funerals—Consumers Last Rights.* New York: WW Norton, 1977, p 104.
23. Draznin, Y: *The Business of Dying.* New York: Hawthorn Books, 1976.
24. Gibbon E: *The Decline and Fall of the Roman Empire.* vol 1, chapter 18. In: *Great Books of the Western World.* vol 40. Chicago: Encyclopaedia Britannica, 1952, p 263.
25. Bland O: *The Royal Way of Death.* London: Constable, 1986, p 15.
26. Ibid., pp 44-45.
27. Ibid., p 57.
28. Hanzon L, Koepsel T, Harnett J: *Passages.* San Francisco, CA: Lonnie Hanzon, 1990, p 6.
29. Bendann E: *Death Customs: An Analytical Study of Burial Rites.* New York: Alfred A Knopf, 1930, p 202.
30. Tegg, *The Last Act,* p 49.
31. Gordon, *Death is For the Living,* p 61.
32. Ibid., p 38.
33. Ariès P: *The Hour of Our Death.* New York: Oxford Univ Press, 1981, pp 166-68.
34. Ragon M: Sheridan A, trans: *The Space of Death: A Study of Funerary Architecture, Decoration, and Urbanism.* Charlottesville, VA: Univ Press of Virginia, 1983. Originally published as *L'espace de la mort: Essai sur l'architecture, la décoration et l'urbanisme funéraires,* Albin Michel, 1981, pp 140-41.
35. Ibid., p 151.
36. Basevi WHF: *The Burial of the Dead.* London: Geo. Rutledge & Sons, 1920, p 129.
37. Bendann, *Death Customs,* p 61.
38. Anima, *Philippine Tribes,* p 42-43.
39. Bland, *Royal Way of Death,* p 59.
40. Richardson R: *Death, Dissection and the Destitute.* London: Routledge & Kegan Paul, 1987, p 100.
41. Curl JS: *The Victorian Celebration of Death.* Detroit: Partridge Press, 1972, p 2.
42. Ibid., p 20.
43. Bland, *Royal Way of Death,* pp 194-95.
44. Haestier R: *Dead Men Tell Tales: A Survey of Exhumations, From Earliest Antiquity to the Present Day.* London: John Long, 1934, p 124.
45. Basevi, *Burial of the Dead,* p 34.
46. Watson JL, Rawski ES, eds: *Death Ritual in Late Imperial and Modern China.* Berkeley, CA: Univ of California Press, 1988, p 43.
47. Smith EL: *The Amish.* Lebanon, PA: The Amish, 1966, p 33.
48. Eliot TS: *Murder in the Cathedral.* 1935.
49. Tegg, *The Last Act,* p 219.
50. Fraser A: *The Lives of the Kings and Queens of England.* New York: Alfred A Knopf, 1975, p 30.
51. Habenstein RW, Lamers WM: *The History of American Funeral Directing.* Milwaukee, WI: National Funeral Directors Association, 1985, p 83.
52. Haestier, *Dead Men Tell Tales,* p 59.
53. Ariès, *Hour of Our Death,* p 31.
54. Tegg, *The Last Act,* p 82-87.
55. Robinson G: Stolen remains. *World Press Review.* 1993;40(10):30.
56. Habenstein, Lamers, *History of American Funeral Directing,* p 83.

57. Ibid., p 84.
58. Ariès, *Hour of Our Death,* p 262.
59. Haestier, *Dead Men Tell Tales,* p 65.
60. Habenstein, Lamers, *Funeral Customs the World Over,* p 268.
61. Ibid., p 302.
62. Capital line: And in Ethiopia. *USA Today.* February 18, 1992, p 4A.
63. O'Donnell J: *The Paths of Glory: A Guide to the Gravesites of Our Deceased Presidents.* West Bethesda, MD: Huntington Pub, 1991.
64. The surprising story of Lincoln's Casket. *Parade Magazine.* Dec 13, 1992, p 22.
65. Ariès, *Hour of Our Death,* p 388.
66. Hastier, *Dead Men Tell Tales,* p 67-68.
67. Ragon, *Space of Death,* p 101.
68. Bentham J: His will. As quoted in: Tegg, *The Last Act,* p 258.
69. Haestier, *Dead Men Tell Tales,* p 67-68.
70. Castro, Inez de. In: *The New Encyclopaedia Britannica.* vol 2. (micropaedia). Chicago: Encyclopaedia Britannica, 1987, p 941.
71. Habenstein, Lamer, *Funeral Customs the World Over,* p 389.
72. Ragon, *Space of Death,* p 150-51.

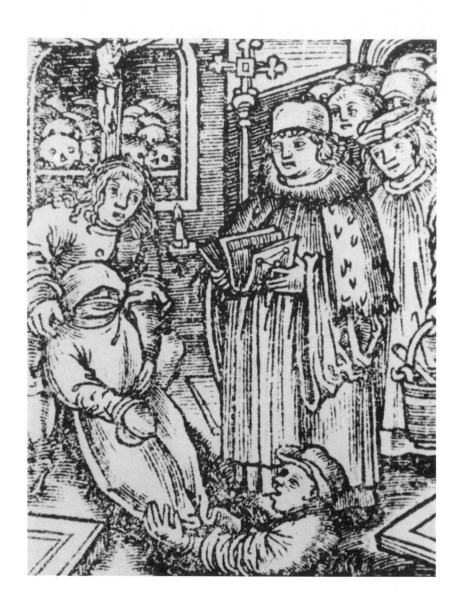

Medieval funeral. Originally published by Renward Cysat: *Nutzlicher und kurtzer Bericht, Regiment und Ordnung,* in *pestilentzischen Zeiten zu gebrauchen.* Munich, 1611. (Reproduced with permission. National Library of Medicine.)

# 11: BLACK TIE AFFAIRS

*What is a funeral, and what unusual aspects sometimes surround it? What U.S. government regulations govern the industry, and how can one customize funeral rituals, make casket choices, perform memorial services, and determine costs? How are these rites altered in times of crisis and on the battlefield?*

## A. WHY HAVE A FUNERAL?

People have funerals as a response to death and to honor the dead. While customs differ, formal rites marking the passage from life to death have been present in every region of the world throughout history. Some anthropologists argue that humans have burials to re-establish and reaffirm relationships among the living, with the most elaborate funerary rites in societies with a strong kinship system. As one funeral historian said, "A funeral is the knot on the bow of life."[1] Not everyone, however, believes funerals are valuable.

Mourners use funerals to remember the deceased and to honor them by showing respect to the body that housed the person during life. Unless we can, as one minister suggested, "abolish death," most people feel that they should acknowledge it through an appropriate rite of passage—the funeral. Nearly all Judeo-Christian clergy also believe that the funeral is important both for its psychological and religious value.[2] In most societies, an individual has two deaths—a biological death and a social death. Physicians denote the biological death; funerals denote the social death and the deceased's separation from the community.[3]

In some societies a person may be biologically dead for quite a while before social death occurs. In the Malay Archipelago, for example, a person's corpse is buried in a temporary grave while the body decomposes. The family must serve the corpse meals at the grave twice a day until the final burial occurs months or years later. Until this final burial, the community does not feel that the deceased has completely departed the living community.[4] In the United States, we do not wait as long for the funeral, but normally hold it on the third day after death.

The funeral industry sees "a funeral service as a social function at which the deceased is the guest of honor and the center of attraction."[5] In Western countries, funeral homes market, advertise and sell funerals; without the funeral, the funeral industry has no business. Therefore, it promotes and protects the concept of funerals with all of the force it can muster. As a National Funeral Directors Association (NFDA) president said, "Without the funeral, we need not be concerned with the issue of advertising as we will have no product to advertise."[6]

The funeral industry recognizes that "People tend to buy products they need. People also buy products to enhance their image."[7] Accordingly, the industry builds the perception of need and image enhancement into traditional funeral industry services by emphasizing the services they provide, including:

1. Care and maintainance of the deceased's remains while options are considered.
2. Help in meeting health, sanitation and other legal requirements after death.
3. Providing information on and procuring a variety of disposition and interment products.
4. Preparation of the body according to the family's wishes for viewing and final disposition.
5. Overseeing the post-death ceremonies and rituals.
6. Providing post-death support and counselors for the bereaved survivors.
7. Arrange for the ultimate disposition of the remains.

Some people feel, as did Ambrose Bierce, that the funeral is "a pageant whereby we attest our respect for the dead by enriching the undertaker, and strengthen our grief by an expenditure that deepens our groans and doubles our tears."[8] Byron agreed, saying of George III's funeral,

> The fools who flocked to swell or see the show,
> Who cared about the corpse? The funeral
> Made the attraction, and the black the woe,
> There throbbed not there a thought which pierced the pall;
> And when the gorgeous coffin was laid low,
> It seemed the mockery of hell to fold
> The rottenness of eighty years in gold.[9]

Voicing the negative view of modern funerals, Ernest Morgan, writing for the Continental Association of Funeral and Memorial Societies, said:

An elaborate funeral, centered around a corpse, gives major emphasis to negative aspects of death, both physical and financial. This remains true no matter how thoughtful the sermon, how impressive the surroundings, or how gracious the funeral director. Furthermore, the competitive social display implicit in a "fine" funeral ("expected of the family because of their position in the community") is in itself a negative and unworthy manner in which to signalize death.[10]

The nineteenth-century poet and social critic, Matthew Arnold, said it even more clearly:

> Spare me the whispering, crowded room,
> The friends who come, and gape, and go;

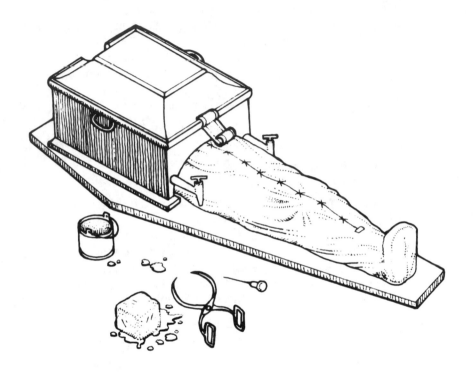

Corpse cooler

> The ceremonious air of gloom —
> All which makes death a hideous show[11]

Despite the critics, funerals continue to be a part of the social fabric and the punctuation ending most lives.

## B. HOW DO VARIOUS RELIGIONS' FUNERALS DIFFER?

Charles Berg, in *The Confessions of an Undertaker,* wrote that "In the domain of religion it is custom which has largely influenced ritual...it is custom that is the chief factor in the evolution of observances in connection with death and burial."[12] Exactly. Most groups have enfolded their secular funerary customs within their religion resulting in remarkably different funeral customs through the ages.

Predating the more modern wake, the Trausi people of ancient Thrace, in southern Europe, laughed and rejoiced at funerals, saying, "now he is free from a host of sufferings, and enjoys the completest happiness." With remarkable consistency, relatives of a Trausi newborn sat around the child and wept for the woes that would befall it.[13]

More somber were pre-Christian Roman and Greek burials, which were often held at night, lest they pollute the sunlight.[14] Their formalities, similar in many ways to modern customs, began when relatives closed the dead person's eyes and mouth. Before *rigor mortis* set in, they laid out the body, washed and anointed it, and wrapped it in a suitable garment. They placed a coin in the corpse's mouth as Charon's fare to carry the departed soul over the River Styx and hung a lock of the corpse's hair on the door to signify that the family was in mourning.[15]

*Protestant* funerals vary more than those of any other U.S. religious group, due to the diversity of sects. The only common denominator among Protestants is to have a funeral followed by a committal service. A visitation period often precedes the funeral. Protestants traditionally hold funerals in churches, and their clergy will often allow non-parishoners to have funerals in their church.[16] One exception is Christian Scientists, who hold the services in funeral homes or at the grave sites.

A denomination's book of worship determines the ritual — a balance of Bible readings, prayers, a sermon, meditation, and a eulogy, usually interspersed with organ music and hymns. The casket normally resides at the front of the church, where congregants file by at the end of open-casket funerals. The Presbyterian Church suggests closing the casket and covering it with a pall during funerals so that "attention in the service be directed to God."[17] After the funeral a hearse leads a motorcade to the grave site where there is a short committal service.

*Roman Catholic* funeral rites are usually more formal than those of Protestants. They usually include a wake, a funeral Mass (once called a "Requiem Mass" and now referred to as a "Mass of the Resurrection") and the burial. In general, Roman Catholic and Orthodox Christian clergy prefer to hold services only for their own parish members.[18]

The family, parish priest and funeral director normally plan the funeral service. Depending upon the priest, there can be considerable variation in the service. It generally begins with a procession to the church from the funeral home. The casket is met at the church door by a white-robed priest (to symbolize the joy of faith that overcomes sadness and death[19]) and brought down the aisle. The funeral itself, accompanied by music, consists of a set of prayers within the Mass, including opening prayers, Bible readings, a homily, the liturgy of the Eucharist, communion, and the closing rite of commendation. Ambrose Bierce, not a lover of these events, said that the Requiem was "a mass for the dead which the minor poets assure us the winds sing o'er the graves of their favorites."[20]

In 1989, the Roman Catholic Church revised its ritual for funerals. In the new rite, *The Order of Christian Funerals,* the family takes a more active role in the funeral prayers and liturgy. A funeral procession to the cemetery is followed by a brief committal rite. The family does not usually stay for the burial, but is invited to leave once the rites are completed.

An *Eastern Orthodox* funeral begins with close family and friends reciting the *Trisagion*, a series of three short prayers, over an open casket. They then close the casket and move the body to the church. The body enters the church feet first and remains with feet toward the altar while the priest leads the funeral service, the *Parastas* ("standing service"). At the end of the service the casket is opened, whenever possible, and the mourners file past. The graveside committal service consists of readings and a short prayer.[21]

Traditional *Jewish* funeral and burial practices have changed little since the rabbinic reforms in the fourth century A.D.. They emphasize speed, simplicity and confronting the fact of death. Ideally, a corpse, dressed in white, is buried before nightfall or at least within 24 hours of death. They base this on *Deuteronomy 21:23,* "But thou shalt surely bury him on the same day." This rule, however, is now often broken to allow out-of-town relatives time to arrive.

Prior to burial, Jews treat the corpse with the same respect they show a Torah that can no longer be used and so must be buried. Traditionally, they watch the body, and ritually cleanse and purify it before burial. Attendants may not perform any religious observance near the corpse, since doing so would mock the unfortunate dead person who cannot himself perform these acts. During the period between death and burial, relatives are absolved from performing all positive commandments except arranging the funeral.

In many communities, the fraternal society, *Chevrah Kaddisha*, normally makes these arrangements.

The Jewish funeral service is generally similar for individuals of all social strata. The rabbi conducts the service in the funeral home, not the synagogue or temple. The service normally consists of prayers, the *Twenty-third Psalm,* and a eulogy for the dead. Flowers are not customary. The body, in a plain wood, closed casket must be present, since the funeral is considered primarily a rite of separation.

A motorcade to the cemetery ends with a brief committal service. In Israel, the only service is at the graveside and the body is buried within hours, in only a shroud.[22] Mourners, including family, customarily shovel dirt into the grave, acknowledging that death has actually occurred. A separate "unveiling" of the gravestone with a short service is held within a year after death.

*Buddhists* in the United States usually hold open-casket funerals at funeral homes. A monk, surrounded by burning incense, leads the family in a series of chants punctuated by ringing a gong. A meal of rice, peas and carrots is prepared at the funeral home and taken to the crematorium. When possible, the family walks to the crematorium. A monk leads a thirty-minute committal service at the crematorium.[23]

Traditionally, *Hindu* families prepare the body for the funeral. In Western countries, however, especially the United States and Canada, this is now the responsibility of the mortician. Many Hindu customs regarding visitation and the funeral depend upon the person's original nationality and cultural background. In the United States, the funeral is generally held in a funeral home. A priest leads prayers and chants amidst candles and incense. Some families still insist that they carry the body to the cremation chamber (retort) and light the fire.[24]

Most *Moslem* funerals are held with open caskets at the cemetery. The body is buried as quickly after death as possible. As a Jordanian woman said,

> Three things are urgent. The marrying of a ripe virgin. — And the meal for the guest. And burying of the dead. His honour demands it. He must be buried quickly, so that he shall not smell. On the day he dies, he must be put into his grave. Only if he dies in the evening may he be buried on the following morning. There are certain things that must be avoided or not done after sunset, and burying is one of them. But it is horrifying to have a dead person above earth, especially in the darkness of night.[25]

The casket, carried to the cemetery by male family members, is buried with the head oriented toward the south and the face pointed east. Relatives hold the funeral service within 50 feet of the grave. Over a period of about 20 minutes, the men in the party chant the funeral prayer, the *Janaazah*

447

*Namaaz*, and then lower the coffin into a grave lined with concrete or surrounded by wood.[26]

The typical *non-religious*, or *Humanist* funeral service is usually divided into opening words of welcome and explanation to the mourners, thoughts on life and death including selected poetry or prose readings, tributes to the person by those who knew him or her well, the committal or removing of the casket from view, and closing words of strength and gratitude to the mourners.[27] After these services, the body is most often cremated. Since no specific rules govern this type of funeral, there is wide variation depending upon the wishes of the family, the deceased and community custom.

Modern American funerals typically follow the pattern of the Protestant majority. Given the cultural diversity in the United States, however, much variation exists.

Recently, memorial services without the body present have replaced traditional funerals for some Protestant denominations, such as Friends United Meeting, Unitarian-Universalist Association, Mennonite Church, Church of the Brethren, United Presbyterian Church, United Church of Christ, Disciples of Christ, and the American Baptist Churches. Such services are also favored by Protestant clergy on the West Coast of the United States, while the clergy in other Judeo-Christian groups promote traditional public services with the body present.[28]

In the past, there was less variation. Ariès describes American funerary practices through the mid-nineteenth century as follows: "The carpenter made the coffin (not yet the "casket"); the family and friends saw to its transport and to the procession itself; and the pastor and gravedigger carried out the service."[29] A more complete description was supplied by Farrell, a funeral historian:

> Before the 1880s in the U.S., when a person died, the body was usually placed on a sheet-draped board placed between two chairs, and washed by women of the household. They held the mouth closed with a forked stick wedged between the breast bone and the chin, fastened with a string around the neck. They used a coin to keep the eyelids closed. A winding sheet or shroud was used to clothe the body. In summer months, they placed a large block of ice in a tub beneath the body, with smaller pieces on the board. The local cabinet or furniture maker supplied the six-sided simple coffin, which after 1850, was sometimes lined with cloth. After a simple home funeral, mourners viewed the body and closed the coffin. They took the body to the graveyard and placed the coffin in the grave dug by the sexton or friends. The mourners then filled the grave and the ritual was over.[30]

## C. CAN SOMEONE HAVE A CUSTOM FUNERAL?

Most funerals in the United States follow a standard pattern. According to Alex Ghia, partner in a San Francisco alternative funerary service, "If you've been to one funeral in the United States, you've been to them all."[31] As LeRoy Bowman said, "The American funeral appears to be an anachronism, an elaboration of early customs rather than the adaptation to modern needs that it should be."[32]

Funerals do not have to be routine, however. A spokesman for the California Funeral Directors Association estimates that in the San Francisco Bay and Los Angeles areas as many as twenty percent of funerals are nontraditional, but "less than a half percent are unconventional elsewhere in the state."[33]

Attending one's own funeral while still alive is the ultimate custom funeral. Many people feel as Maria Edgeworth (in *Castle Rackrent*) did when she had one of her characters say, "I've a great fancy to see my own funeral afore I die."[34]

One person who did see his own funeral was one "Sir Giles" a nineteenth-century English aristocrat, who, after supposedly dying abroad, actually participated in his own interment. After his trusted servant suggested that "this stranger" act as an official funeral attendant, Giles helped, while in disguise, to bury another body in his place. While this deception has been used to hide murders or to bilk insurance companies, such was not Sir Giles' intent. Rather, he wanted to rid himself of his social burden and property, preferring to live a humbler life. He was never heard from again. His servant related the story on his deathbed.[35]

More macabre were the daily funerals held by King Charles V of Germany and Spain after he abdicated his thrones in 1555/56 and entered a monastery in Yuste. For the last three weeks of his life he demanded that he have a funeral service every day and be carried around in the coffin which was ultimately used for his burial.[36,37]

Most people seem to gravitate toward their religion's and community's "traditional" funeral services, either from a fear of criticism from friends and relatives or to have the touchstone of a familiar ritual during times of grief. Castigating the funeral industry for moving toward customized funerals, one funeral historian wrote that

> The biggest mistake within the trade during the last ten years has been, in my opinion, the 'customizing' of funerals as a result of the corporate image promoted by some of the conglomerate holding companies. Funerals are not commodities; rather they are highly important and emotional social events forming the final ritual in the calendar of life. They should not be marketed as though they were package holidays—even though there is an element of

journeying into the unknown—and the offer of fringe benefits and insurance policies somehow cheapens the service further.[38]

With changes in culture and customs, however, increasing numbers of Americans cannot relate to traditional religious rites and want to customize their own funerals. One woman, whose hobby was vegetable gardening, left instructions that her casket be covered with vegetables. It was.[39] At the January 1991 funeral of Inka Dink, the clown, he was dressed in his costume—a blue hat atop a yellow wig, an immense red bow tie, red-checkered suit, yellow- and red-striped stockings, and enormous bright yellow shoes. His friends applied the complicated clown makeup and the open casket was canopied by a 40-foot balloon arch. Many attendees were in full clown regalia, and the Clown's Prayer was read at the ceremony.[40]

Some custom funerals simply involve friends and loved ones in a more direct way, such as moving the casket; others extend to having raucous parties with rock 'n' roll music, food, and spirits. At "farewell party" services, recalling the Irish wakes of the past, participants are feted with balloons, wild music, colorful attire, champagne and videotaped farewells.[41] However, audio or video tapes of the deceased played during the ceremony can be rather unnerving.

Mike Sullivan of Oceanside, California takes the unusual one step farther. He videotapes funerals and cremations. According to him, people want the tapes so they can "hear all the good things that family and friends have to say" about the deceased. Occasionally relatives may also use the tapes to bolster the deceased's reputation, a kind of postmortem "spin control." One woman ordered forty copies of her husband's funeral tape to distribute to friends and relatives for this purpose.[42]

While some funeral directors accommodate unusual requests, not all will. To fill this need, firms specializing in custom funerals have arisen. One of the best known, San Francisco's Neptune Society, offers stylish, creative and individualized funeral services. Death boutiques have developed in California and France. San Francisco's Ghia Gallery offers, among other items, designer burial robes and customized urns and coffins. The French store offers off-the-rack burial equipment at cut-rate prices. (French funeral directors are furious.)

In Pensacola, Florida, the Junior Funeral Home offers a drive-by viewing window to pay last respects to the deceased (According to the owner, they did it as a promotional ploy.) Only about a half dozen drive-by viewing windows exist in the United States.[43] In Memphis, Tennessee, the Family Heritage Casket Gallery sells unusual caskets, including a golfer's special which is lined with green velvet with a small flag under the lid denoting the 18th hole.[44]

Some Californians use a burial pall to customize funerals. An ancient device, the pall covers the coffin during a funeral. In a modern twist, funeral attendees pin something to the pall that reminds them of the deceased. The family keeps the pall as a reminder of their loved one. Commonly funeral attendees attach photographs, letters, ribbons, and personal messages. In one case, a young deceased woman's friend pinned diamond earrings on the pall with the message, "You always borrowed them, anyway." The family put them inside the coffin. In some instances, as at weddings in some cultures, attendees pin money to the pall to help the family pay funeral and other necessary expenses.[45]

One family found an eight-page letter and a set of keys attached to their daughter's pall. She had died in a motorcycle accident when in her early twenties. The letter was from a young man, a successful lawyer who had met their daughter while he was a foreign exchange student from Italy. Although her family disapproved of him, they had continued to exchange letters over the years. Not long before her death she had joined him on a European vacation. They travelled together around the continent and got engaged at a *pension* in France. The keys were to the room they shared. He offered them to her parents as a gift.[46]

## D. WHAT DO CORPSES WEAR?

Corpses can wear anything (or nothing). Except as demanded by religion or tradition, there is no dress code for the dead.

As a sign of respect, survivors have usually tried to clothe corpses for burial. Western societies first buried their dead in everyday clothes, later switched to shrouds (and occasionally nudity), and reverted to clothes in modern times.

Prehistoric people buried their dead in everyday clothing, occasionally with an extra robe or covering.[47] Ancient Romans enhanced this practice by dressing their dead in their best robes. Under the robes, Romans clothed the bodies of ordinary citizens in white togas, and those of magistrates and other officials in their *praetextae*, long white robes with purple edging. If the deceased had been awarded a crown for bravery in life, he wore it in death.

Early Christians, however, questioned the need to sumptuously dress the dead. "Why," said St. Jerome (in *Vitâ Pauli*), "does a desire for appearance exist amid mourning and tears? Why should the dead be clothed in sumptuous vestments? Cannot the rich rot away unless in the same gorgeous apparel that decorated them when alive?" Early Christians adopted the practice of burying their dead in a shroud, essentially a cloth sack. (See illustration, p 453.)

Shrouds were usually made of plain cloth. In England before the seventeenth century, bodies of the poor, if not naked, entered their graves wrapped in linen shrouds. During the same period, children who died within a month of baptism were buried in shrouds made of their "chrisoms," or baptismal robes. These robes were bound to the body by "swaddling" bands.

"Swaddling" now refers to all infant clothing. Relatives often loosened the shroud at the corpse's hands and feet so the dead could speedily escape on Resurrection Day. For similar reasons, Cypriots, who traditionally bury their dead in a full set of outdoor clothing, complete with hat, shoes and gloves, still burn a hole in the surrounding shroud through which the corpse's head emerges.[48]

One of the most elaborate and famous depictions of a shroud is on the marble statue of John Donne, the famous English poet. Located in London's St. Paul's Cathedral, this sculpture depicts Donne, who died in 1631, in a full-flowing shroud surrounding his life-like face. No wonder it was life-like. Donne, several years *before* his death, had posed naked, except for the shroud, for a picture from which the bust was done. He kept the picture on a wall by his bed.[49]

A variant of the shroud was the simple winding sheet, a cloth wound around the corpse until it looked like a mummy. When bodies were buried in only a winding sheet, they often had a "mortcloth" laid over them during the funeral and while being carried to the grave. Mortcloths, always black, often made of velvet, and lined with satin, were usually the property of guilds, burghs, trade corporations and some privately run charities. A variant is still used in modern Britain, where the "shroud" is simply laid over the body and tucked in.

In 1686 the Scottish Parliament, to boost its linen trade, passed the *Act anent Burying in Scots Linen,* prohibiting anyone from clothing a corpse in "rich materials." The law required winding sheets and grave clothes to be made of plain linen, coarse flax, or hemp cloth without any decoration, and to be spun in Scotland. Despite heavy fines for violations, the law was ineffective.

In 1707, the Scots passed another law to promote the wool industry. It made clothing the dead in anything but woolen cloth a crime.[50] Alexander Pope, who did not think much of a similar English law (1666) wrote in his *Moral Essays*:

> 'Odious! in woolen! 'twould a saint provoke,'
> (Were the last words that poor Narcissa spoke)
> 'No, let a charming chintz and Brussels lace
> Wrap my cold limbs, and shade my lifeless face'[51]

The English law, however, supposedly kept at least 200,000 pounds of rag linen which was needed for a budding paper industry from rotting in graves.[52]

Eventually, the concept of resurrection demanded that communities bury important people in fine clothes. Over the centuries, authorities enacted many laws permitting only corpses of the rich to be clothed for burial. Shrouds for the rich, sometimes embroidered in black, were referred

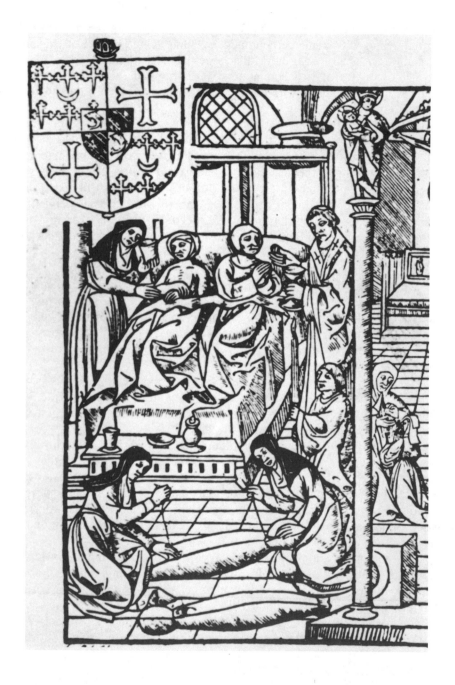

Nuns shrouding corpses before burial in the 16th-century Hôtel Dieu, Paris. (Reproduced with permission. National Library of Medicine.)

to as "sable" by poets, although they weren't. However, a fancy bull's hide shroud was used by some early nobles, including King Henry I of England, his son Prince Henry, King John, and James III of Scotland.[53] In the Middle Ages, the corpses of rich commoners were wrapped in cerecloth, a fine fabric soaked or painted with an adhesive, such as wax, to hold the cloth closely to the body and exclude air.

Several groups have continued to maintain traditional burial dress. Gypsies still bury corpses in their best suit of clothes—turned inside out. The Chinese customarily clothe their dead in very costly and elaborate clothing, according to the dead person's status and profession. In the past, a ruler not only wore elaborate clothes, but also had up to fifty extra suits placed in his tomb; a student's corpse was buried with a rich assortment of black silk robes. At the other end of the spectrum, dead children in China were often wrapped by their parents in matting and laid at street corners where they were collected for burial by a man in a black cart drawn by a black cow.[54]

Jews continue to bury their dead in shrouds, (the *Tachrichim*), and the Greek Orthodox bury their clergy in only a hair cloth. The corpses of Church officials in other Christian denominations often wear the distinctive dress of their office, such as their robes or priest's collars. Mormons who have had temple ordinances (special instruction) are normally dressed in white with a green apron.

The Amish, who traditionally wear black during life, dress their dead in white for burial. The only other occasion on which they wear white is at their wedding. This pattern derives from a scriptural passage, "and they shall walk with me in white; for they are worthy."[55]

Eventually authorities and the funeral industry coerced most groups in Western societies to bury their dead in grave clothes. These clothes can either be purchased specifically for burial, or can be those the person wore in life. The clothing must also cover the entire corpse, because despite rumors to the contrary, morticians do clothe the entire body, even when the casket remains closed or when just the top half of the body is exposed to view.

In the United States, specific burial clothing is made in a few styles for men and hundreds of styles for women. This clothing, unlike normal apparel, opens in the back so it can easily be put on a supine corpse. Modern American corpse clothes are often chiffon, crepe, or lace-over-taffeta, pastel-colored dresses for women, supplemented as necessary by stockings, undergarments, and matching shoes. Men are fitted with dark suits.

Charles Berg noted in 1920 that

Burial garments, while their sale is a source of profit to the undertaker, seldom afford satisfaction to the purchaser, unless it

454

be men's garments, which are priced at a figure considerably less than that of a new suit of clothes, and for the purpose, compare very favorably in appearance. Procuring ladies' garments from the undertaker should only be resorted to in emergency, for such garments do not add to the 'natural' appearance of the one who is so unfortunate as to have to be clothed in them. The styles in ladies wear change from season to season, and the undertaker is yet to be found who can keep up with the change of styles and still work off his old stock.[56]

Most people, however, are now buried in their own clothes. Contrary to the old saw that you can't take it with you—if it fits, you can wear it. This, however, can lead to complications. One woman selected, before her death, the clothing in which she wished to be buried and carefully put it away in a drawer. When she died, however, her daughter refused to allow her mother to be buried in those clothes, saying they were "definitely out of fashion."

People sometimes choose unusual attire in which to be buried. Corpses have been buried in jumpsuits, pajamas, house coats, graduation caps and gowns, golf clothes, wedding dresses, and clown suits. Bella Lugosi, the star of 1930s and 1940s horror films, was buried in a Dracula cape in 1956. The Gypsy Mortuary in Los Angeles has buried a number of cross-dressers. "There are some guys wearing ladies wear," said funeral director Louis Baez. "There are also girls wearing men's suits."[57]

Howard Belkoff, a New Jersey funeral director relates that in 1975, when a 19-year-old boy died of an overdose of drugs and alcohol, his parents had his body dressed in jeans and a T-shirt for burial. True to his lifestyle, they also slipped two marijuana joints into the coffin.[58] Even six feet down, a corpse can make a fashion statement.

If a mortician stymies a corpse's fashion desires, however, it can be costly. At his 1989 funeral in Washington state, his wife fitted Dick Hughes out in his prized black Stetson cowboy hat. She was shocked to hear that a relative was wearing the hat several months later, presumably given to him by the funeral director, the deceased's son-in-law. The widow sued and won $101,000 from the funeral home for breach of contract, negligence, violating a state code, and outrageous conduct.[59]

A recurring urban legend is that the clothes a corpse wears can often have dire effects on the living. As Brunvand describes it:

A girl who was going [to an important banquet] decided it was important enough to have a new dress. She bought one at a local department store, a simple but exquisite gown. At the dance after the dinner, her escort noticed a peculiar odor while they were dancing. She had been feeling faint, and she believed it was the odor. She thought the dye in the dress had faded; so she went to the washroom and took off the dress. There was nothing wrong; so she went back to the dance again. However, she felt more faint, and the odor still remained. She thought she had better sit down, and on the way back to their table, she fainted. Her escort took her home, and called a doctor. She died before he got there. The boy explained about the odor, and the doctor investigated the dress and found that the dress had a familiar odor. He ordered an autopsy, and they discovered that the girl had formaldehyde in her veins. The drug had coagulated her blood, and had stopped the flow. They investigated the department store where she had bought the dress and learned that the dress had been sold for a corpse and had been returned and sold to the girl. When she perspired and her pores opened, she took in the formaldehyde which killed her.[60]

While this macabre story continues to make the rounds, funeral homes do not reuse corpses' clothing. Even if the clothes were recycled, the amount of formaldehyde in a dress, even if it was saturated, would not kill anyone. Just ask any (older) physician who was exposed to much higher concentrations of formaldehyde when he, without gloves, survived months of dissecting a formaldehyde-soaked cadaver.

## E. WHAT IS FUNERAL MUSIC?

Funeral music can range from a toneless chant to the traditional poetic songs of the Ashanti, and from simple religious hymns to modern popular tunes. It consists, in short, of anything the planners wish and their own culture permits.

Christian funerals traditionally included a dirge. The dirge is a slow, mournful musical composition or poem. Shakespeare had Cymbeline's two sons sing such a composition at their half-brother's funeral.

> Guiderius: Fear no more the heat o' the sun,
> Nor the furious winter's rages;
> Thou thy worldly task hast done,
> Home art gone, and ta'en thy wages.
> Golden lads and girls all must,
> As chimney-sweepers, come to dust.
>
> Arviragus: Fear no more the frown o' the great;
> Thou art past the tyrant's stroke;
> Care no more to clothe and eat;
> To thee the reed is as the oak.
> The sceptre, learning, physic, must
> All follow this, and come to dust.

456

Guiderius: Fear no more the lightning-flash,
Arviragus: Nor the all-dreaded thunder-stone;
Guiderius: Fear not slander, censure rash;
Arviragus: Thou hast finish'd joy and moan.

Both: All lovers young, all lovers must
  Consign to thee, and come to dust.[61]

At one time, hymns played on organs were the most common funeral music for Christian services in the United States. Today, however, most funerals use piped-in, pre-recorded music. One U.S. minister would like to "ban 90% of present vocal music now being used at funerals."[62] They believe that such (Christian) hymns as "In the Garden," "Beyond the Sunset," and "I Believe" are "prime examples of 'tear-drawing' music which counteracts the message of joy and hope the minister is trying to convey through the spoken word."[63]

Concurring with that idea, many families now choose music that reflects the deceased person's tastes. The selections range from religious or classical music to modern country-western or pop-rock. On occasion, families even bring in their own musicians and instruments.

Recently, the music industry began requiring funeral homes (as well as bars, stores, and others using their copyrighted music) to pay royalties for each use. ASCAP and BMI, the two major music-licensing enforcement agencies, now get an average of $3.77 for the music played at each funeral. While this may not seem like much, if the fee is collected for only two-thirds of the U.S. deaths each year, it generates $4.5 million!

Other cultures are also experiencing changes in their funeral music. Traditional Chinese funeral music was designed to accompany the corpse and settle the spirit. It came in two forms, a high-pitched piping from an oboe-like instrument usually played by a paid musician, and percussion from cymbals, gongs or drums played by the priest. Both sets of instruments were played during key sections of the funeral.[64] Since the 1930s, Western-style marching brass bands, wearing white uniforms and military-style caps also often accompany the traditional musicians—and they may play at the same time.[65]

## F. WHAT ARE FUNERALS LIKE IN TIMES OF CRISIS?

As might be expected, funerals are, at best, perfunctory when the population faces the crises of epidemics, war or disaster. They also sometimes permanently change a society's funeral practices.

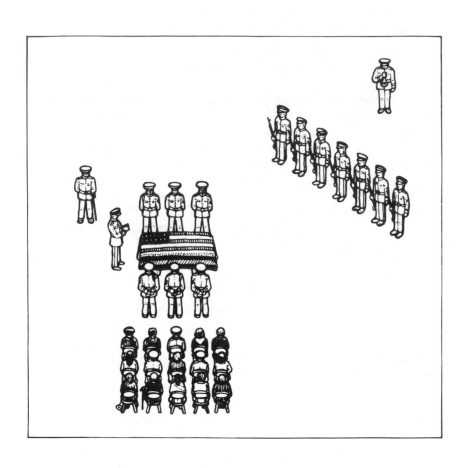

Military funeral and honor guard

458

In Italy during the plague of 1348, the masses of dead began to stink and the populace became concerned that the odor and "vapors" would add to the disease. In Venice, they ceased their normal practice of exhibiting unburied bodies in front of their houses "to invoke compassion of their neighbors," and quickly buried the bodies. As Marchionne di Coppo Stefani, a contemporary commentator said:

> All the citizens did little else except to carry dead bodies to be buried...At every church they dug deep pits down to the water level; and thus those who were poor who died during the night were bundled up quickly and thrown into the pit. In the morning when a large number of bodies were found in the pit, they took some earth and shovelled it down on top of them; and later others were placed on top of them and then another layer of earth, just as one makes lasagne with layers of pasta and cheese.[66]

Bubonic plague struck London in 1665, giving rise to some of the first regulations to protect the living from the dead. Laws banned friends and children from accompanying the body to the grave or visiting the deceased's house, barred the corpse from the church when many people would be present, required the grave to be at least six-feet deep, and mandated that corpses only be buried at night. To warn others of the danger, authorities marked the deceased's house with a large red cross and the words, "Lord have mercy on us."[67] (see illustrations, pp 574 & 606.)

During some epidemics or famines so many people died at once, as in 1690s Scotland, that reportedly "the living were so much wearied with burying the dead that they ceased at last to do so." During epidemics, Scots transported bodies in reusable iron or wood coffins so that infection would not be spread from an uncontained body to the living. In times of epidemic or famine the reusable coffins were extremely economical, since up to fifteen people could be buried in one day using a single coffin.

In *The Plague,* Camus describes the stage in an epidemic when coffins become scarce and begin to be reused for the mass burials of corpses:

> For then coffins became scarcer; also there was a shortage of winding-sheets, and of space in the cemetery...At one moment the stock of coffins...was reduced to five. Once filled, all five were loaded together in the ambulance. At the cemetery they were emptied out and the iron-gray corpses put on stretchers and deposited in a shed reserved for that purpose, to wait their turn. Meanwhile the empty coffins, after being sprayed with antiseptic fluid, were rushed back to the hospital, and the process was repeated as often as necessary...At the far end of the cemetery two big pits had been dug. One was reserved for the men, the other for the women...At the bottom of each pit a deep layer of quicklime

459

steamed and seethed...The naked, somewhat contorted bodies were slid off into the pit almost side by side, then covered with a layer of quicklime and another of earth, the latter only a few inches deep, so as to leave space for subsequent consignments...The corpses were tipped pell-mell into the pits and had hardly settled into place when spadefuls of quicklime began to sear their faces and the earth covered them indistinctively.[68]

In some cases, coffins were used to ensure that the "dead" stayed dead. The husband-wife team responsible for burials during a cholera epidemic in Gloucester in 1849, testified that as soon as someone was declared dead they put them into a coffin and screwed the lid down. Sometimes the victims revived before burial and violently kicked and pounded on the sides of their coffin for release, but they were never removed from their coffin since, as the pair said "they had got to die anyway."[69]

Coffins also sometimes became scarce during crises in the United States. During the influenza epidemic of 1918, so many people were dying that undertakers thought themselves lucky even to have rough boxes to use as coffins. In Washington, D.C., while soldiers hastily dug graves in preparation for the masses who would soon die, the health commissioner commandeered two railroad cars full of coffins for their use.[70] And after the famous Johnstown, Pennsylvania flood, survivors retrieved material floating down the Conemaugh River to fashion crude coffins for the large number of dead.[71]

In modern European Russia burials have been disrupted due to an economic and social, rather than a medical, crisis. In a society that reveres the dead much more than in other Western countries, abandoned bodies numbered fewer than ten per year in Moscow before the collapse of communism and its economy. Yet families now routinely abandon their dead, preferring that the state pay for disposition. This is not surprising, given that the cost of the simplest funeral can be 6,000 rubles, or about half of a year's salary.[72]

## G. WHAT HAPPENS TO BODIES ON THE BATTLEFIELD?

During battle, corpses are of secondary concern. Once the fighting ceases, however, survivors usually want a proper disposition for their dead comrades. Ancient civilizations greatly respected their battlefield dead. The Athenians, for example, often failed to pursue defeated foes so they could take time to honor their dead. They even dismissed excellent generals who had failed to sufficiently honor their battlefield dead. Occasionally some of the ancients were so embarrassed that they had no dead after a large battle, that they erected tombs for "their dead" anyway, so they could "obtain credit with those who should come after them."[73]

The horror and confusion of war often disrupts orderly corpse disposal. After the Turks savagely suppressed a revolt in 1876, for example, Bulgarian bodies so littered the countryside that proper burial was impossible. An American reporter described the horror he witnessed:

> Some weeks after the massacre, orders were sent to bury the dead. But the stench at that time had become so deadly that it was impossible to execute the order, or even to remain in the neighbourhood of the village. The men sent to perform the work contented themselves with burying a few bodies, throwing a little earth over others as they lay, and here in the churchyard they had tried to cover this immense heap of festering humanity by throwing in stones and rubbish over the walls, without daring to enter. They had only partially succeeded. The dogs had been at work there since, and now could be seen projecting from this monster grave, heads, arms, legs, feet, and hands, in horrid confusion. We were told there were three thousand people lying here in this little chuchyard alone, and we could well believe it. It was a fearful sight — a sight to haunt one through life.[74]

In May 1871, the French Communards revolted in Paris and a visiting Englishman described what happened to their bodies after the final battle:

> The hollow was now filled up by dead. One could measure the dead by the rod. There they lay, tier above tier, each successive tier powdered over with a coating of chloride of lime — two hundred of them patent to the eye, besides those underneath hidden by the earth covering layer after layer. Among the dead were many women...The ghastly effect of the dusty white powder on the dulled eyes, the gnashed teeth, and the jagged beards cannot be described.[75]

During World War I, British soldiers suffered massive casualties at Gallipoli in southeastern Europe. Hastily burying their dead, one soldier wrote, "We pushed them into the sides of the trench but bits of them kept getting uncovered and sticking out, like people in a badly made bed. Hands were the worst; they would escape from the sand, pointing, begging — even waving!"[76]

Near the close of World War II as the Japanese Imperial Army straggled out of Burma, "the army's route was marked by heaps of corpses, gruesome mile markers for a campaign of 'monumental folly and death.' "[77] In battle, these same Japanese soldiers would often cut off the penis of an enemy corpse and stuff it in the dead soldier's mouth.[78]

The bodies of civilians caught in the midst of modern warfare often get worse treatment than those of soldiers. One witness of the atomic bomb attack on Hiroshima in World War II wrote, "Under the bridge countless corpses were floating. Only scraps of clothing were left on them."[79] Weeks went by until many of these corpses were buried.

While Americans now go to great lengths to retrieve and inter all of their war dead, that has not always been the case. During the American Revolution, the battlefields "strewn with unidentified and unclaimed dead soldiers gave some anatomists a wealth of material with which to work."[80] Dr. John Collins Warren wrote of "his virtually unlimited supply of corpses from the New York-New Jersey campaign."[81]

The Civil War, the first "modern war," demonstrated what happens to bodies on the battlefield. Although visitors to the Gettsyburg National Park now see row upon row of marble tombstones, it was quite different in the days following the battle. Observers said

> ...it would be a long time before all the misshapen cadavers could be buried. They were everywhere—behind stones and rocky crags, in fields, in woods, upon the hills...everywhere. Burial details swung out and managed to get most of the things which had once been men into hasty graves. But without any system it was rather slapdash and perfunctory. Inverted muskets, their bayonets rammed into the earth, or pieces of board penciled with brief information, or just stones, marked the sites of superficial graves. And in a short time the woods and fields at Gettysburg became a hodgepodge burial ground."[82]

Unfortunately many of these hasty graves reopened with each rainfall, revealing their grisly contents. Authorities quickly had to rearrange the graves into the permanent and suitable cemetery dedicated by Lincoln. The U.S. government established the first Graves Registration Unit in 1864. Its task was to make positive identification of Federal soldiers killed in battle, so their bodies could be reinterred in national cemeteries. The last bodies, however, were not located and reburied until 1914.[83]

While some U.S. military dead were returned home from the Mexican and Indian Wars, no bodies were embalmed before shipment until the Civil War.[84] During the Civil War, embalming and corpse shipment was at first unregulated. The only corpses embalmed were those whose families could pay for the service.

In 1898, with the outbreak of the Spanish-American War, the relatively new National Funeral Directors Association (NFDA) offered to form a company of embalmers to accompany the troops; the War Department declined the offer. As in the Civil War, families of dead U.S. soldiers hired their own embalmers to go to Cuba or Puerto Rico, to find and disinter the bodies, embalm them as best they could, and return the remains the the United States. At the end of the war, the War Department began prohibiting this practice, allocating $200,000 for the newly formed Army Burial Corps to return all U.S. dead to the United States at government expense. The Corps was staffed by civilian employees of the War Department. In 1899, during the Philippine Insurrection, U.S. dead were embalmed in Manila and then sent back to the United States. Although the transport took 40 to 60 days, the bodies reportedly arrived in viewable condition.[85]

During World War I, the United States buried most dead soldiers in newly established European cemeteries after General Pershing declined another offer from the NFDA to send embalmers. He believed there was little interest in repatriating fallen soldiers' bodies.[86] These cemeteries are still maintained by the American Battle Monument Commission.

One World War II American combat surgeon graphically described feelings toward dead comrades:

> They expected us somehow to whisk the torn bodies off into decent invisibility like undertakers, but in our world a dead man simply had to lie there, naked to the snow or the rain, dying over again anytime anybody looked at him or came into the range of his staring eyes. Our dead had to be dumped like rubbish and ignored.
>
> A corpse is like a newborn infant in its terrible need for protection; it cries out for care. We always performed some small ritual; we pulled a field jacket over torn viscera, we covered a face, sometimes by turning a man on his abdomen (covering people's faces seemed important), and we often stuck his weapon in the ground by the muzzle or the bayonet and put his helmet on it.[87]

In recent wars, the U.S. military has been very careful with its dead soldiers. After confusion at the start of the Korean War, a daily airlift carried U.S. dead to an embalming facility in Kakura, Japan. The bodies were then shipped home by boat. In the early days of the Vietnam War, cadavers were packed in ice inside a rubber pouch and shipped to Clark Field, Philippines, about 700 miles away. There, workers with the Air Force Mortuary embalmed the body and flew it to the United States. (Some U.S. soldiers' body bags were reportedly also used to ship heroin back to the United States.) Later, when the number of casualties increased, the Air Force began embalming bodies at its mortuary at Ton Son Nhut Airport, near Saigon. In July 1966, the Army took over mortuary duties and added a second mortuary at Da Nang. All embalming continued to be performed by civilians, under military supervision.[88] Yet many bodies were lost, and for many years Vietnam continued to use some remains as political hostages.

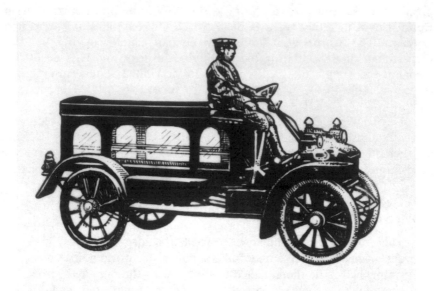

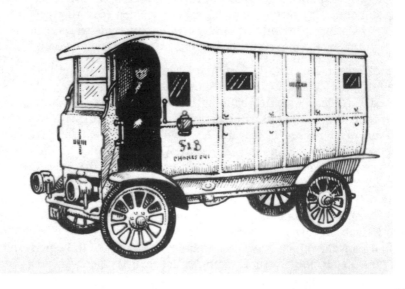

Early motorized hearse and hearse-ambulance

464

In the Grenada, Panama, and Desert Storm operations, the military recovered all bodies (or pieces of every body) allowing definite identification. (See Chapter 4, *How can a person be identified from partial or decomposed remains?*)

## H. WHAT ARE COFFINS?

"Coffin" is the general term for all types of boxes in which corpses are buried. Most commonly, however, the term "coffin" refers to the centuries-old design of an eight-sided burial box tapered to fit the human body. This traditional coffin widens from the head to the shoulder area, and then narrows toward the feet. In some cases, such as with the coffins of English royalty in the past, the box was rounded to closely fit the head and shoulders. These "anthropoid" coffins, mimicking Egyptian sarcophagi, were popular in England from the fifteenth to the seventeenth centuries.[89]

Over the millennia, people have fashioned coffins in many styles and from a variety of materials. In Iron Age Palestine, simple wooden or clay boxes served as coffins for a secondary burial of bones, rather than for the initial interment.[90] Later, the Greeks used wood, stone and baked clay coffins at different periods in their history.[98] The Chinese, who have used coffins to bury at least some of their dead since the Neolithic Period (30,000 to 6,000 B.C.), have in the last few centuries sealed corpses in (what they hoped were) airtight coffins. To accomplish this, they secured the coffin lids not only with nails, but also with caulking compounds.[92] In some instances precautions were so elaborate that the coffin was indeed airtight. (See the Chinese Princess, page 185.)

In an attempt to thwart body snatchers, Edward Lillie Bridgman patented a wrought-iron coffin in 1818. With no screws, hinges, or movable parts, it could not be opened from the outside. As with today's caskets, the iron coffin was relatively imperishable and limited the recycling of graves (the common practice). For this reason, many graveyards refused to bury iron-encased bodies until the courts ruled in Bridgman's favor. His iron coffin, however, did not prevent bodies from being snatched, since resurrectionists could break open the lids with sledgehammers.[93]

In the United States until the late nineteenth century, relatives often brought bodies to carpenter's shops where coffins were custom-made. Making coffins in advance of death was considered an abhorrent idea. As Charles Berg noted, "The idea that one could be so audacious as to make preparation in advance of death and to profit by the transaction was not readily accepted."[94] When one legendary "Aunt Jerushy" died, her body was dutifully brought to the carpenter. After her coffin was made, however, she began to regain color in her cheeks, indicating that she was still alive. Reportedly, the carpenter who had made the coffin ranted that "Color or no color, she's goin' in this box right now. The funeral's all set for four o'clock and I don't calc'late t' lose my five dollars."[95] The funeral, however, was delayed—for several years.

Later, furniture dealers began to both sell coffins and act as morticians. Until the mid-twentieth century, some funeral directors still operated out of furniture stores in the American Midwest. Gradually though, American society accepted the transition from cabinet maker/coffin seller, to furniture dealers who carried a stock of ready-made coffins, and finally to funeral director/coffin retailers.

Coffins have long taken the brunt of burial reform. Joseph II, the Holy Roman Emperor from 1765 to 1790, for example, decreed that coffins could only be made with flat tops. His subjects ignored the edict, calling these coffins "nose squeezers" because of their effect on the corpse's proboscis. He then ordered that no coffins be used, and that too was ignored. Fed up with the whole thing, the palace finally announced that "His Majesty no longer cares how they bury themselves in the future."[96]

In Western societies, being buried in a box of any type was once a mark of social standing. "The coffin was—and, to some extent, still is—a status symbol, its finish and furniture indicative of the social standing of the deceased. No fifteenth-century peasant or artisan expected to be buried in a coffin; by contrast no noble would have been subjected to shroud burial in the churchyard."[97] In sixteenth-century Sussex, England, for example, except for the mayor, his wife, or councilmen, only those licensed by the mayor could be buried in coffins. They referred to this as being "chested" or "boxed." If a carpenter "boxed" an unlicensed body, he could be fined.[98]

Traditional coffin-shaped burial boxes are now rarely used in the United States. Beginning in the 1970's, however, "old-fashioned" pine coffins were once again available at a number of non-industry outlets. San Francisco's Ghia Gallery, for example, currently stocks a traditional pine coffin called "Mr. Coffin," which they make themselves and sell for $325 (1992). While some people do use these coffins for burial, many are made into wine racks, hope chests, bars, coffee tables, grandfather clocks, bookshelves and closets. The funeral industry is not amused.[99]

## I. WHAT ARE CASKETS?

Technically, *casket* is merely the American euphemism for *coffin*. Some people, however, use the terms *coffin* or *casket* to indicate the shape of a burial box. Yet the terms coffin and casket are still used interchangeably. The *New York Times,* for example, does not differentiate between the terms in its stories.

The nineteenth century saw the introduction of rectangular coffins, termed "burial chests" or "burial cases," which later became known as caskets. Justifying his 1849 patent application for a casket, C. Barstow said, "the burial cases formerly used were adapted in shape nearly to the form of the human body, that is they tapered from the shoulders to the head, and from the shoulders to the feet. Presently, in order to obviate in some degree the disagreeable sensations produced by a coffin on many minds, the casket, or square form has been adopted."[100] By 1927, one writer noted that "the old wedge-shaped coffin is obsolete. A great variety of styles and grades of caskets is available in the trade, ranging from a cheap, cloth-covered pine box to the expensive cast-bronze 'sarcophagus.' "[101]

Over the past two centuries, designers have made many strange and elaborate caskets. They obtained U.S. patents for caskets made of cement, pottery and glass, although none of these gained public acceptance.[102] Wood predominated until the mid-twentieth century, when steel caskets became common.[103]

Today, caskets made of cloth-covered softwood or particle board constitute about 10% of total casket production in the United States. The most expensive caskets, about 3% of all caskets made, are those constructed of polished copper, bronze or stainless steel. Fewer than 1% of all U.S. caskets are made of plastic, fiberglass, zinc, aluminum or cultured marble.[104] A common industry statement (and the title of an article in *Mortuary Management*) is that "If God meant us to have fiberglass caskets he would have planted fiberglass trees."

Nearly three-fourths of all caskets now made in the United States are steel. Barbara Jones, in her book *Design for Death*, has one of the best descriptions of the modern casket: "Not rectangular, because hardly any angles are visible at all, the thing is the oxidized metal offspring of a cumulus cloud and a half-sucked lozenge, and it is called a casket. All the forms are vulgar and coarse; debased classical, gothic, jazz, baroque, or nondescript. The finish is superb."[105] Metal caskets, however, are declining in popularity, and wood is once again gaining favor with consumers.

United States funeral directors now sell more hardwood caskets than they did in the past. While the casket industry no longer considers the old pine box part of its line, hardwood caskets, such as oak, poplar, cherry, maple, walnut and mahogany, constitute about 15% of the U.S. casket market. One-seventh of these sales are for Jewish funerals which traditionally require wooden caskets without any metal in their constructions.[106]

In some funeral homes hardwood caskets constitute up to 40% of their casket sales.[107] Wood casket advocates believe that the rise in sales is due to wood caskets fitting relatives' sensibilities better than steel.[108]

Wooden casket makers disdain any distinction between "protective" and "non-protective" caskets, a common method funeral directors use to categorize their caskets. Wood, of course, decomposes, rendering it "non-protective." They point out that, rather than protecting the corpse, "80 to 90 percent of a casket's function is provided before burial," by providing a sentimental "memory picture."[109]

Conservationists question how much valuable wood is used in the form of caskets each year (unknown) and how much metal is wasted. Decomposing wood is seen as more environmentally sound than the steel. Industry figures say that more than 200 million pounds of steel is used each year in caskets.[110]

Modern caskets come in "full-couch" and "half-couch" styles. The full couch allows a body to be laid with the head at either end for viewing of either the right or left side. While showing the right side of the face is customary, a full-couch casket allows showing the left side if an injury or illness has affected the right side. This can also be accomplished in half-couch caskets, but requires special equipment.

Modern caskets can be quite elaborate. Most casket interiors are lined with velvet, crepe or taffeta in many colors and designs. Some even come with built-in interior lighting.[111] Some death boutiques, such as San Francisco's Ghia Gallery, offer brightly colored, biodegradable caskets ($500), leopard print caskets ($700), and light-weight Egyptian sarcophagi ($7,600). Elaborate burial containers, however, are not confined to Western countries. One casket maker near Accra, Ghana makes caskets that commemorate the deceased's occupation. For a devoted mother, he makes her coffin in the shape of Mother Goose, for the fisherman who first used an outboard motor, he makes a motor-shaped coffin, and for those who can afford it (in life as well as death), he makes the popular Mercedes-Benz-shaped coffin.[112]

Some customs, however, ban elaborate burial boxes. Traditional Jewish law specifies that bodies be buried in plain wooden coffins with no adornment or metal parts. These boxes, known as *Aron*, use wooden pegs as fasteners. Going one step farther, traditional Irish custom was to remove nails from a coffin immediately before lowering it into the grave. This supposedly allowed the dead to have no difficulty in freeing themselves on Resurrection Day.

## J. HOW DO YOU PURCHASE A CASKET?

Caskets are usually unconsidered purchases. Except for those who have bought caskets under a preneed plan, individuals purchasing caskets are quite susceptible to being swayed into expensive selections. Comparison shopping by grieving relatives is not considered acceptable funeral behavior. As Mark Twain wrote, "There's one thing in this world which a person don't say—'I'll look around a little and if I can't do better I'll come back and take it.' That's a coffin. And take your poor man, and if you work him right he'll bust himself on a single layout. Or especially a woman."[113]

Twain must have had negative experiences with the nineteenth-century funeral industry, since in *Life on the Mississippi* he wrote that when the child of a poor man died, the boy's plain wooden coffin cost $26. (The father had never made more than $400 per year in his life.) Twain commented, "It would have cost less than four [dollars] if it had been built to put something useful into."[114] Ernest Morgan, a writer who advocates simpler body disposition agreed, saying "Things like metal burial vaults, and caskets with innerspring mattresses make about as much sense as a fur-lined bathtub, but they help wonderfully in running up the bill!"[115] An anonymous traditional riddle perhaps best describes the situation:

> The man who made it didn't want it.
> The man who bought it had no use for it.
> The man who used it didn't know it.

Currently, nearly 96% of U.S. families not opting for cremation purchase caskets. According to the Federal Trade Commission's survey, the retail price of caskets has just kept pace with inflation, although the wholesale price has increased more rapidly. They interpret this to mean that while funeral directors once derived their primary income from the sale of caskets, they now (perhaps because of the FTC Funeral Rule) must take a greater percentage of their profit from other goods and services.[116]

Yet caskets still generate big profits for funeral homes. In 1990, the average metal casket's wholesale price was $482 and a wooden casket's was $722. With a minimum markup 2.5 times the wholesale price, this netted the funeral home a profit of $723 on the average metal casket, and $1,083 on a wooden casket.[117] Sentiment doesn't come cheap.

Some funeral homes reportedly charge their customers up to 20-times more than the price they paid for a casket. According to Alex Ghia, a woman who had just buried her sister in a $3,700 casket, recently came into his San Francisco gallery and was aghast when she saw the same casket priced at $750 (which was double his wholesale price).[118] Howard Belkoff, a New Jersey funeral director, says that an unwritten rule among his state's funeral industry is that a "conscionable mark-up" on caskets is two to three times wholesale cost.[119]

Other funeral homes promote the sale of elaborate and oversized caskets for an additional cost, even when they are not really necessary. The industry puts considerable thought into developing new and better display areas for caskets, since funeral directors have found that the arrangement of the caskets materially affects the amount of sale. According to Jessica Mitford, the purpose of the numerous texts, symposia and study courses on this topic reflect the goal of "selling consistently in a bracket that is above average."[120] She says that casket makers, using the same technique as furniture makers from whom they are descended, construct the inexpensive caskets so hideously that only those who cannot afford more expensive selections will by the cheaper models.[121] A funeral sociologist observed:

In some large funeral homes, caskets priced either extremely high or extremely low are placed in annexes off the main room. The main room itself contains caskets of varying prices. Explaining why high-priced caskets should be in an annex, funeral home workers "explained that those people wishing to select an especially expensive casket deserved to be treated exclusively and to be taken to a room in which only the best were shown. Conversely, anyone wanting the cheapest casket possible also deserved to be so segregated." The room for the inexpensive caskets was "small and crowded because it is not profitable to display inexpensive merchandise to the exclusion of moderate to more expensive merchandise."[122]

According to Alex Ghia, an industry rebel, "the casket industry in the United States is controlled by a few large companies, such as the Batesville Casket Company, that require approval of a funeral home's showroom and require the home to carry a minimum of 70% of their caskets."[123] According to Mr. Ghia, a videotape about caskets made by one company and shown to clients has a tag line saying that "with each casket we will plant a tree." The U.S. Forest Service told him this meant that for each casket sale they received 18 cents to plant seedlings![124]

To recoup any lost income, some funeral homes charge customers a handling fee of several hundred dollars if the family wants to use a casket purchased from a low-price retailer. The Federal Trade Commission is considering banning this practice as anti-competitive.[125]

One sales technique relies on a consumer's inclination to buy a medium-priced casket. Funeral directors show their most expensive caskets first, leaving the least expensive until the end. They feel that purchasers will calculate a considerably different price if they cut the most expensive casket price (say, $5,000) in half, rather than doubling the least expensive price ($600).[126] The difference between these two "averages" ($2,500 v. $1,200) is $1,300! If they first showed the most expensive commercial caskets, costing over $15,000, the price difference would be much higher.[127]

Caskets come in several sizes, as seen in Table 11.1. Funeral directors rarely stock larger-sized caskets, so their profit decreases if they must specially order these caskets. Therefore, they employ several methods to make larger corpses fit in standard caskets in order to avoid using the costly larger caskets. For obese bodies, they position the elbows as far forward as possible or turn the body slightly in the casket. And with very tall bodies, they flex the legs and omit using shoes.[128]

Casket purchasers are sometimes surprised when the casket fails to work as it should. Funeral homes have been taken to court when caskets have fallen apart while being carried, when they have not completely closed, when "air- and water-tight" caskets have allowed water in or gasses from the decomposing body to leak out, and when the handles fell off, injuring pall bearers.[129] Nineteenth-century Scottish carpenters were fined £1 for making defective coffins. Today, most large casket companies cover wholesale buyers, normally funeral homes, with multimillion-dollar liability insurance policies for claims against the performance of their caskets.

### K. DO CASKETS PREVENT BODY DECAY?

Certainly not those currently in use. Despite claims to the contrary, sealed caskets do not prevent a body's decomposition. In 1975, a $500,000 lawsuit was filed in Puerto Rico alleging that a casket failed to prevent decomposition of a corpse after a 3-week interment, despite a written guarantee. The manufacturer stated that no casket can protect a body from decay "indefinitely."[130]

Funeral directors emphasize excellent sealing qualities to sell their most expensive caskets. However, Dr. Jesse Carr, former Chief of Pathology at San Francisco General Hospital, stated that an embalmed corpse fares far worse in a hermetically-sealed metal casket than otherwise. "If you seal up a casket so it is more or less airtight, you seal in the anaerobic bacteria—the kind that thrive in an airless atmosphere...These are putrefactive bacteria, and the results of their growth are pretty horrible...In fact, you're really better off with a shroud, and no casket at all."[131]

With the intent of assisting bodies to decompose *more rapidly*, Francis Haden, a British surgeon, patented his "necropolis earth-to-earth" coffin in 1875. The corpse was placed in a wooden box with holes bored into it,

---

## TABLE 11.1: Standard Casket Sizes

| METAL | *Standard* | 6 ft 7 in X 24 in |
|---|---|---|
|  | *Oversized* | 6 ft 9 in X 26 in<br>X 28 in<br>X 31 in |
| WOOD | *Standard* | 6 ft 3 in X 22 in |
|  | *Oversized* | 6 ft 6 in X 24 in<br>X 26 in<br>X 28 in |

---

similar to the practice of Orthodox Jews. The box was then packed with moss and put into a wire mesh basket. His coffin worked, but only the London Necropolis Company adopted it. Haden estimated that if all of England used his method, only 2,000 acres would be needed to bury their dead *forever*.[132,133]

He further suggested that the bodies of great men who were to be interred in Westminster Abbey should first lie imbedded in a charcoal air-circulating crypt for a year, thereby assuring that little would remain of their corpses.[134] In 1881, the French architect J. Courtois-Suffit proposed using Haden's concept so Paris would need only a single fifty-acre cemetery. He commented that with this technique "the human remains are respected, the nonvolatilized residues are preserved intact...Nothing is changed from the present practice of burial."[135] Authorities rejected his proposal.

## L. CAN COFFINS BE REUSED?

Reusing a coffin is not as unusual as it might seem. Coffins have long been reused in two ways: the same coffin was used for more than one body, and the same person has used one coffin in multiple ways.

At one time coffins were used only to transport bodies of the poor to their graves, where they were removed from the box and buried in shrouds or winding sheets. The coffins were then returned to the church for another funeral. In 1563, the Scottish General Assembly required every county parish to have a reusable coffin so that the poor would not be transported to their graves unboxed. In the Scottish Highlands they used a *sgulan ruhairbh* or "death hamper," carried to the grave using a bar passed through three pairs of loop handles. After pall-bearers lowered the hamper with its body into the grave, they dumped the body out and retrieved the hamper for future use. In parts of Scotland, the poor continued to be buried without permanent coffins until the mid-nineteenth century.

Elsewhere, parish churches used other types of reusable coffins. Reusable iron or wood coffins, called "slip coffins," had hinged openings on the bottom, so they could be lowered halfway into the grave and then opened, dropping the bodies. While expedient, these coffins often cost four times more than disposable boxes. Parishes, therefore, kept close track of their slip coffins.

Coffins have also been used by the living prior to their use for burial. One eighteenth-century Scot bought a lead coffin and kept it filled with bottles of wine in his bedroom. A Mrs. Delaney wrote about a similar use in 1750: "Sir William Pendarvis's house was the rendezvous of a very immoral set of men. One of his strange exploits among other frolics, was having a coffin made of copper, and placed in a great hall...it was filled with punch, and he and his comrades soon made themselves incapable of any sort of reflection; this was often repeated, and hurried him on to that awful moment he had so much reason to dread."[136]

In England, Colonel Luttrell turned up at a large London masquerade party dressed *as* a coffin in 1771. According to another party goer, Luttrell's coffin disguise cast such a "pall of gloom" over the proceedings that he was asked to leave soon after his arrival.[137]

Civil War troops at Gettysburg used rubber interment sacks, meant to replace standard coffins, as sleeping bags, stretchers and inflatable boats. The sacks, weighing 8 lb. 6 oz., looked like long, flat socks with lacing at the open end. They never caught on with civilians after undertakers launched a campaign against this "rubber sack abomination."[138]

Others have been a bit more restrained in their use of coffins. Chinese sons, as a sign of respect, once gave their parents coffins that were kept on display in their houses.[139] To foster humility and an awareness of man's mortality, some orders of monks have traditionally slept in the coffins in which they were ultimately buried. The celebrated actress, Sarah Bernhardt, was photographed lying in a casket she kept in her bedroom. Using a coffin during life is not unknown in modern America, as was shown by a recent letter to Ann Landers' column. A woman wrote that her husband was aghast at her wanting to use her coffin as a bench in the family room; Ann said to go ahead and do it.[140]

Reusable caskets are also part of the modern funeral industry. Renting a casket for a funeral prior to cremation is much cheaper than buying the same item. After the funeral, the body is cremated in a sturdy cardboard box, rather than in the expensive casket. Rental caskets can also be used for funerals held before whole-body burials at sea. The body enters the water in only a shroud or winding sheet. Clergy accept the concept of rental caskets in approximately the same proportion as they accept cremation. Eastern Orthodox and Jewish clergy are opposed, and Roman Catholics and Protestants mostly approve or are neutral. Black clergy favor this concept less than most other Protestant clergy.[141]

## M. IN WHAT OTHER TYPES OF CONTAINERS ARE BODIES BURIED?

Coffins have not been the only containers used for burials. In Iron Age Palestine, it was not uncommon to bury infants, children and sometimes adults in storage jars. When a tall child or adult was buried in a jar, part of the body was placed in each of two jars and the rims of the jars were sealed together.[142] Ancient Greeks living on the Isle of Rhodes also buried infants and small children in jars. These jars, often quite large, were laid on their sides, either on the ground or, occasionally, in trenches cut out of the rock. They then blocked the mouths of the jars with a stone and covered them with dirt.[143]

Among the most elaborate burial containers in history were those of the ancient Ethiopians who, after mummifying their dead, covered the bodies in gypsum and painted them in a lifelike manner. They then placed the bodies in hollowed crystal pillars, thereby allowing them to be viewed from all sides. They kept these pillars at home for a year and then were put on public display.[144]

Approximations of coffins have sometimes been used. In Brittany, people once buried corpses in rough crates made with only a top and bottom plank and held together by blocks of wood at the neck, under each arm, and near the ankles.[145] French children once had even cruder burial containers. Before the French Revolution, the French often buried their children bound in bark stripped from Chestnut trees. This caused so much damage to the trees, however, that the practice was banned.[146] In a similar fashion, some Philippine tribes once made coffins (*tarimban*) from split bamboo held together by bamboo strings.[147]

While normally used for cremations, "alternative containers" can also be used to bury bodies. Alternative containers (the official government term) are the corrugated fiber boxes sold by funeral homes or packing equipment companies. A South African firm, Timbalyte International, now franchises distributors of its cardboard coffins. The company expects its franchisees to finish the coffins at home and sell them to funeral homes at a 300 percent markup.[148]

Inexpensive, homemade plywood boxes can also be used as coffins. For morbid workmen, Ernest Morgan's book, *Dealing Creatively with Death,* describes how to construct such a homemade coffin.[149] An Alameda, California undertaker and former Baptist minister, appropriately named Al Carpenter, sells build-it-yourself pine coffin/bookcase instructions for $9.95 through his company, Direct Funeral Services. He says of this, "I think grandpa would look a heck of a lot better in a box made by the grandchildren than in one from a factory in Ohio."[150] He urges people to "shop before they drop." His own casket sits in a corner of his office. "It only took me two hours [to build]," he said. "It was a lot of fun."[151] For a classier alternative, some people now have themselves buried in cabinet-quality furniture which they first use during life as settees, linen chests or cabinets.

Examples of other unusual burial containers include those with the logo from major universities (made by a Tennessee company),[152] those made in the shape of boats by the Ilongos of the Philippines,[153] and one in the shape of a Cadillac Seville purchased by the family of a Chicago gambler for over $7,000.[154] The Ghia Gallery also sells replicas of Egyptian sarcophagi modeled on King Tut's. These elaborate burial containers are made by a Nevada artist and sell for about $7,600. While several have been sold, few buyers actually use them for burials.[155]

## N.  SHOULD I HAVE AN OPEN- OR CLOSED-CASKET FUNERAL?

Whether one has an open- or closed-casket funeral depends mainly on religious tradition and social custom.

Belief in the psychological benefit to mourners of open-casket funerals and viewings varies with one's religious orientation. Fully 99% of Eastern Orthodox clergy, 84% of Roman Catholic priests, and 76% of Protestant ministers believe viewing is helpful to families. Yet ninety-three percent of Jewish rabbis think viewing is not of any value. The few rabbis who do think viewing is of value restrict it to the immediate family.[156] These findings correspond to a Christian tradition that allows or encourages viewing the body and a Jewish tradition that prohibits it. Non-religious individuals normally opt for a closed-casket, which they see as being a more person-centered rite than the open-casket or body-centered funeral.[167]

Even if a casket is open for viewing before the funeral, both clergy and funeral directors dislike reopening it in the church. Nevertheless, the custom of open-casket funerals tenaciously persists, with 65% of U.S. funerals preceding burial having open caskets.[158,159] Most clergy prefer that the casket be sealed permanently before the beginning of the funeral service and not be reopened. As one minister said, "opening the casket after the service has an adverse psychological effect on the family and takes away from the message of hope in the service."[160] The only exception is among the Eastern Orthodox, who normally want the casket to remain open throughout most of their funeral service.[161]

In some cultures an open-casket funeral has played a role in healing the ill or preventing disease. Rudyard Kipling cites this belief in *Our Fathers of Old,*

> If it be certain as Galen says—
> And sage Hippocrates holds as much—
> "That those afflicted by doubts and dismays
> Are mightily healed by a dead man's touch."[162]

Ulcers and cancerous growths were long believed healed by the touch of a dead man's hand. In Scotland, those who took part in a funeral believed they not only had to see the body before it was shrouded, but also touch the body if they were to avoid being haunted. If the deceased had been murdered, the body had to be touched for it to decompose. In England, Cornish children kissed the dead to ensure themselves a long life and physical strength. (See also Chapter 8, *Wayward Bodies.*)

## O.  WHAT IS PROPER FUNERAL ETIQUETTE?

People often feel uncomfortable at funerals because they do not know how to behave. In general, mourners need only follow the instructions given by the funeral director and minister. They are aware of mourners' discomfort and try to alleviate it as much as possible.

At a viewing, although friends and family mingle and socialize freely, proper etiquette demands that a visitor first approach the casket and afterwards comment on how good the deceased looks.

At the funeral itself, unless one is tapped to be part of the ceremony (usually only immediate family and very close friends), one need only sit in the pew. Mourners make their condolences to the family either before the service or after the burial. Many mourners wear black. According to Ariès, this alleviates some strain because "the wearing of black expresses mourning and dispenses with more personal or dramatic demonstrations."[163]

Is it proper for children to attend funerals? Modern child-development experts now believe that children as young as five-years old should be allowed to attend funeral or memorial services, especially if the deceased was someone close to them, such as a member of the family, a neighbor, a family friend, or an important person in their school. The reality of the funeral is often far less frightening than the fantasies a child may have about it. It may also, as with adults, help to confirm that the person no longer will be part of their life, and allow the grieving process to begin. As with adults, however, not all children are ready to confront death, and they should never be forced or embarrassed into attending.[164]

In most Western societies, mourners are expected to spend an appropriate amount on such accoutrements as flowers. The amount varies according to how close they were to the deceased, with many considering it tactless for those not close to the deceased to send too large a wreath.[165] Some individuals and groups shun flowers, preferring that the money be given to charity or spent to help the family meet expenses. Many people send food to the family so they will not be burdened with everyday chores during their mourning period.

Feasting after funerals has a long tradition. In Georgia, the former Soviet republic, the funeral feast, held on the grave, includes hot *khachapuri* cheese cake, *lobio* bean soup, *satsivi* chicken, and *tamada* wine.[166] In the United States, many cultures traditionally serve food at home for mourners, sometimes for several days after the funeral. A growing custom, however, is to invite those attending the funeral to a restaurant for lunch. As one New Jersey restaurant owner said, "In the beginning, some people thought it was a little strange, but now it's commonplace."[167]

Disrupting or preventing a funeral is far removed from proper etiquette. One must wonder, therefore, what prompted the canons of the Church of England to explicitly prohibit clergymen from refusing to bury or delaying the burial of a corpse. Likewise, English secular law prohibits anyone from obstructing a clergyman from reading a burial service in a parish church or conspiring to prevent a burial.[168] The United States has recently seen examples of extremely offensive funeral behavior. In an act of extraordinarily bad taste, one radical Topeka, Kansas church group picketed the funerals of people they suspected died of AIDS. Not only is picketing a funeral tacky, the Kansas legislature also made it illegal in 1992.[169]

## P. CAN I HAVE A FUNERAL IF I WILL BE CREMATED OR FROZEN OR MY BODY WAS LOST?

Yes and no. This is because technically, a funeral refers to a service held with the body present. If the body is not present, the service is called a memorial service. (See below.)

If a body is to be cremated, there is no reason why a funeral cannot be held before the cremation. Ornate caskets are often rented for use during these services; afterwards the body is placed in a less-expensive, combustible casket or shroud.

If the body is to be cryonically frozen however, the time constraints of the freezing process make a funeral impractical. Similarly, if the body has been destroyed or lost in an accident, there can be no "funeral." In these cases, however, mourners often hold one or more memorial services for the deceased.

## Q. WHAT IS A MEMORIAL SERVICE?

A memorial service is a ceremony used to remember the deceased. The corpse is not present at a memorial service, which often is held after cremation, burial, or the loss of a body, as in a death at sea.

No strict format exists for memorial services; there is great variation in their timing, location and leadership. The service may be held from a few days to weeks, or even months after death. Many mourners hold memorial services in places of worship, although they are also held in homes, funeral homes, or at other sites which hold special meaning for the family. Clergy run some memorial services; others are run by friends and relatives of the deceased who offer remembrances of the individual.

Memorial services commonly have at least one of three purposes: they "rehabilitate" the image of the deceased by recollecting past memories from better days; they bond survivors together with the identity of a deceased person who was important to them; or they allow survivors to console each other and then to resume their normal lives.[170] As one minister said, "reminiscence of the past life is more uplifting than dwelling upon the throes of death."[171]

Catholic memorial services most commonly occur after loss of the body or when the body is donated to medical science and center on the Funeral Mass. Modern Protestants frequently use memorial, rather than traditional funeral, services for any death. Other religious groups have standard memorial services that can be used as is, or modified to the family's circumstances. One of the most austere is the Quaker memorial meeting, conducted in candlelight with a background of recorded music. The service consists only of mourners' testimony about the deceased. Standard secular and humanist memorial ceremonies are also available. One of the best sources for these services is Ernest Morgan's *Dealing Creatively with Death.*

Yet the funeral industry has repeatedly disparaged memorial services, especially when chosen over an open-casket service. They refer to these rites as "disposal services," suggesting that they are cold, unfeeling affairs in which the deceased is treated like garbage.

When a body has been lost, is buried elsewhere, or has been cremated, a memorial monument or *cenotaph*, can still be erected. Some people erect these monuments in cemeteries, others near religious buildings, or in places that have special meaning to the deceased, family, or friends. Examples of well-known cenotaphs are the Washington Monument and Jefferson and Lincoln Memorials in Washington, D.C.

## R. WHAT IS DIRECT BURIAL OR CREMATION?

"Direct burial" or "direct cremation" is going directly from death to burial or ashes, without detouring for embalming, or a funeral, viewing, wake, or other ritual. The funeral industry pejoratively describes it as a "minimum service request." Funeral directors view such requests with alarm, even disdain.

In a November 1991 article in *The Director,* the official publication of the National Funeral Director's Association, Michael Kubasak, a Burbank, California funeral director said "There is no simple formula to turn direct disposal requests into full service 'traditional' funerals."[172] The article describes how a funeral director's receptive attitude and flexibility can often propel the family into accepting some of the additional services the funeral home offers. As Kubasak said,

> Nothing works all the time, but my success rates are high, and family satisfaction even higher...Every funeral director and counselor probably sees value in cremating the deceased in a hardwood casket following viewing and a ceremony. Inurnment of the remains in a solid bronze urn would be icing on the cake...it can be a more frequent occurrence if you reflect on your attitude and study ways to improve your communication skills...During the (family) conference, highlight legal requirements and procedures that must be satisfied.[173]

## S. WHAT DO FUNERALS COST?

Families in most Western societies believe it is important to spend the "correct" amount on funerary expenses.[174] The "correct" amount can be exorbitant, with Americans alone spending over $7 billion annually on funerals. Beginning in the 1960s, the federal government took steps to help control these costs.

Yet Americans have complained of high funeral costs since at least 1651, when the Province of Massachusetts General Assembly passed a measure critical of these charges.[175] Rarely, though, would a modern funeral bill look like that for a Hartford, Connecticut man who drowned in 1678:[176]

| | |
|---|---|
| A pint of liquor for those who dived for him | 1s |
| A quart of liquor for those who brot him home | 2s |
| Two quarts of wine and one gallon of cyder to jury of inquest | 5s |
| 8 gallons and 3 quarts wine for funeral | £1-15s |
| Barrel cyder for funeral | 16s |
| 1 coffin | 12s |
| Windeing sheet | 18s |

After the 1963 publication of Jessica Mitford's *The American Way of Death,* the federal government demanded that the funeral industry discuss prices with its (living) customers. The effort had little success. In 1984, the Federal Trade Commission established rules requiring, among other things, itemized bills (Appendix I). But as one funeral director noted, "The FTC gave us a license to steal. In the past, funeral homes never charged separately for benches, register books, candles, etc. Now everything must be itemized. It seems like we are nickel and diming the family."[177]

Funerary costs consist of four types of expenses:

1. The professional and staff charges for funeral directors, use of facilities and equipment, and caskets and vaults;
2. Expenses paid either through the funeral director or separately, such as minister fees, flowers, obituaries, limousines, burial clothing, and special transportation of the body;
3. Cemetery costs: grave and interment (opening and closing grave) or cremation charge, urn and any formal disposition site.
4. Memorial monument or marker for a grave or niche.

This section discusses only the first two items. The others are discussed in Chapters 12 and 13. (Note that some funeral directors may lump charges somewhat differently, into: (1) Professional services; (2) Facility charges—including storage of the body and use of the chapel; (3) Transportation; (4) Merchandise—including the casket; and (5) Cash disbursements—money paid to cemetery, gratuities, ministers, etc.)[178]

The professional services component of these charges varied by region, with New England's funeral directors being the most expensive and those in the South Atlantic states the least expensive. New England's funeral directors charged about $80 more and those in the South Atlantic states about $57 less than the national average in 1991.[179]

In the early 1990s, the average funeral home had an income of more than $546,000 and the average funeral (with all accoutrements) cost $4,610.[180] In 1991, one out of four U.S. families paid more than $4,000 for funerals (services plus casket), although in 1986 fewer than one in twenty families paid this much, and in 1981 only one in two hundred families.[181] The money they spent on funerals, however, was not evenly distributed. More money has routinely been spent on funerals for older people than for younger people, and more for natural or accidental deaths than for suicides.[182] By 2002, an average American funeral will cost about $5,701.[183]

Even faced with this large expense, little comparison shopping for funeral homes occurs, with 85% of people selecting a funeral home before contacting a home to discuss arrangements. Ninety-five percent only contact one funeral home, 65% of the time by phone.[184] And, although the FTC has made it easy to shop for services by phone, only about 4% of those arranging funerals take advantage of this opportunity.[185]

Estate attorneys point out that "the funeral director enjoys a preferred status among the estate's creditors; his bill must be paid by the estate before any other debts except administrative expenses (court costs, attorney fees, and Personal Representative fees) are paid, even though his charges may deplete the estate entirely."[186] Yet some funeral directors go to extraordinary lengths to collect on their bill.

One Flint, Michigan, funeral director held the body of an 80-year-old man for more than three years while he sued the family over a $3,605.59 funeral bill. A spokesman for the Michigan funeral Directors Association said that while it is "very unusual...there are no state laws requiring funeral home directors to continue with burials or funerals if satisfactory financial arrangements have not been made."[187]

In Japan, the average Japanese funeral costs more than $10,000, although cremation is inexpensive or free, displaying the body is rare, corpses are preserved with dry ice rather than embalming, and the funeral director normally makes the coffin from a kit. Why are they so expensive? The funeral is still elaborate. The funeral director converts the family's home into a chapel with a lavish portable altar, wall and ceiling coverings, chairs or floor mats, garden and waterfall displays, and a catering service. The family also purchases gifts for mourners and elaborate wreaths for a public display of their mourning.[188]

With funerals so expensive, one may wonder whether a person might refuse to die rather than pay the cost. One epitaph noted this by saying:

> Here lies one who for med'cines would not give
> A little gold, and so his life he lost;
> I fancy now he'd wish again to live,
> Could he but guess how much his funeral cost.[189]

## T. WHAT REGULATIONS GOVERN FUNERAL OPERATIONS AND COSTS?

There are many rules! Not only does the U.S. Federal Trade Commission (FTC) have rules governing the funeral industry (Appendix I), but each individual state has its own regulations. Some groups within the funeral industry also have their own guidelines (Appendix J). The FTC's "Funeral Rule," 16 C.F.R. §453, became effective in April 1984. Its proponents sought to "increase consumer access to accurate information about prices and legal requirements prior to and at the time of purchase of a funeral."[190] With the Rule in effect, purchasers are supposed to learn the actual funeral costs in advance and buy only those goods and services they really want.[191] The Rule requires funeral directors to supply the family with price information over the telephone, a complete price list of merchandise and services at the beginning of the "arrangement conference," and an itemized statement of costs at the end of that meeting.

Unfortunately, the Funeral Rule has had little effect on consumers. Not only did the amount of money spent on a funeral increase by more than 9% after the Rule went into effect (even after an inflation adjustment), but also only one-third of funeral directors provided purchasers with both the required general price list and the final itemized statement during the initial arrangements meeting.[192] Even when a price list was provided, it often came late in the meeting, after consumers had already agreed on their purchases. Customers who got the information early spent significantly less on the funeral than those who got it late or not at all.[193]

Arizona obtained a partial exemption from the Funeral Rule because its law complied with or exceeded the Rule's requirements. Arizona's law provides some significant consumer protections that the federal government did not mandate, such as requiring funeral homes to provide price lists by mail, to display their least expensive caskets, to release remains promptly upon request, to refrain from disparaging remarks about alternative goods or services, to put prices on the displayed caskets, and to distribute consumer information pamphlets.[194] Unfortunately, even with enhanced regulations, the Arizona Auditor General found "consumers may still lack adequate information about services and costs prior to making funeral arrangements."[195]

The NFDA says that the Funeral Rule would have included extra consumer protections if they had not strenuously lobbied against them. They convinced the FTC to drop requirements for funeral directors to: (1)

display their three least expensive adult caskets and to have these items available in all colors within 12 hours; (2) explain that outer burial enclosures are also for sale at some cemeteries; (3) provide, upon request, written explanations of any legal requirement which necessitates any service or merchandise; (4) pass along any rebates, commissions or trade volume discounts; and (5) include the following statement on all advertising: "funeral prices vary considerably. For information on prices for funeral merchandise and services, call ..."[196]

The FTC is actively investigating and prosecuting funeral homes throughout the country which violate the Funeral Rule. Financial penalties can be substantial, although in only a few cases do the benefits reach the consumers who were treated shabbily or defrauded.

Every state except Colorado requires licensing of funeral directors and embalmers, although the need for this has been questioned.[197] Colorado disbanded its Board in 1982 and has suffered no ill effects. Many states, especially in the West where "sunset" laws exist, have repeatedly tried to disband their funeral boards, mainly composed of funeral directors.[198]

## U. HOW DO YOU PAY FOR FUNERALS?

Paying for funeral expenses with something other than a life's savings involves advance planning. People normally pay for funerary expenses using personal savings, insurance, or trusts.

Many people fear a pauper's burial and will scrimp in life to assure themselves that they will receive a "decent burial." Others arrange to pay for their funeral through life or funeral insurance, governmental allowances (social security, veterans administration, workman's compensation, welfare, etc.), or union or fraternal organization benefits. Some people use the prepayment plans offered by funeral homes. Most often, however, families of the deceased end up paying for the funeral and burial out of their savings or inheritance.

Arranging to prepay some funeral and burial costs, however, is not the same as pre-planning. Pre-planning and prepaying are different concepts, although they are frequently linked by the funeral industry into *preneed* and *prearrangement* planning.

Prepaying began in the southern United States with "burial insurance" during the 1930's depression.[199] Pre-planning involves telling family, friends, and funeral homes exactly what you want done (or have already arranged to have done) when you die. For most people this is much harder than simply paying for funerary services, since it involves talking about what is often regarded as a taboo subject. The instructions can, however, also be left in written form (see Chapter 13, *A Hand From the Grave*). Individuals have three ways to prepay U.S. funeral costs: individual plans, state-regulated trusts, and life insurance. Each has its own benefits and problems, so will be discussed separately.

In *individual plans* (sometimes called Totten Trusts), the individual sets aside the money and manages his own funeral expense account. The account must contain, after inflation, sufficient funds to guarantee the type of funeral and burial desired. In 1992 people needed $3,500 to fund such an account at the basic level. This was the average cost of an adult funeral, not including limousines, flowers, newspaper notices, or the clergyman's honoraria. It also did not include the burial plot, grave marker, mausoleum, or the cost of opening and closing the grave.[200] By 2002, an individual plan will need to contain $5,701, the anticipated average U.S. funeral cost.[201]

When funding an individual plan, one should factor in any potential death benefits. In the United States, survivors of those covered by Social Security receive a lump sum payment of $255 by filing Form SSA8 within two years of the person's death. The payment can also be made directly to the funeral director or included as part of a prepayment package. Others who may be entitled to death benefits include survivors of U.S. veterans, employees or retirees of some governmental agencies or private businesses, and members of some fraternal orders or unions. In Canada, the Last Post Fund pays for "an honourable burial" for those who have served in Canada's wartime military and lack the resources to provide for their own funeral and burial.

Individual plans can be set up in several ways. The key to a successful plan is to avoid probate, which can delay post-death distribution of monies for more than a year—a long time to wait for a funeral. Without using a lawyer, individuals may establish a savings account with the appropriate amount of money designated as "payable on death" to the funeral home. Alternatively, individuals can start a joint account with a family member (thereby avoiding probate), from which that person can pay funeral expenses. An attorney can also set up a *Totten Trust* with a funeral home as the beneficiary on the person's death.

The benefits of individual plans are that the person maintains control of the money, the money is transferrable to another location or funeral home if necessary, cash can be used anywhere, and any excess income accrues to the individual or the estate. The main problem with such plans is that there is no way to lock in a guaranteed price for funeral services as there may be with funeral industry-sponsored plans. After reviewing all of the options, however, the American Association of Retired Persons (AARP) urges people to consider establishing individual plans.[202]

The funeral industry offers two other common methods of prepaying funeral and burial costs: trusts and insurance.

*State-regulated* trusts are available in 48 states (not Vermont, Alabama, and the District of Columbia). After a person signs a prearrangement (pre-planning) agreement for specific funeral services and pays the full cost, the funeral director places a portion of that money (*trusting* amount) into a commercial funeral trust overseen by state regulators. The amount placed in the account varies by state law, with more than half the states requiring that all of the money be put in the account. Some states, such as Mississippi (50%) and Florida (70%), require much lower deposits. The funeral home keeps any money not put into the account.[203]

The benefits of using a state-regulated, funeral home-run trust are the ease of setting it up and the price guarantee for funeral services. Most, but not all, such plans guarantee that the trust funds will cover the agreed-upon funeral services. The main problem with these plans is that many states have no provisions for payment if the trust cannot pay benefits at the time of need, due to losses or fraud. Also, these plans are usually not transferrable out of state and are often not transferrable between funeral homes.

Another funding mechanism is *insurance*. With an insurance plan, the individual buys a life insurance policy through the funeral home with a value equal to the cost of the agreed upon funeral services. The funeral home is named as the beneficiary. This is the fastest-growing funding mechanism used for funerals, possibly because unlike the other methods, not only does the funeral home lock in a customer, but it also usually gets a 10 to 20 percent commission on the sale of the policy.

Again, the benefits are in the simplicity and the price guarantee, when they exist. Another benefit of buying insurance is that most states have a "cooling off" period during which the buyer can cancel the policy without penalty. As with other insurance, these plans' provisions vary with the company underwriting the policy. While state insurance commissions regulate insurance companies, they are not all financially stable. State insurance commissions can answer any questions about them. As with state-regulated trusts, these plans cannot usually be transferred out of state or between funeral homes. Six states (Georgia, Maryland, Montana, New York, South Carolina, Wyoming) have banned insurance-funded preneed plans.[204]

While most people pay for their preneed contracts in one payment, most funeral homes and cemeteries also offer installment plans, believing that "most Americans feel they can afford anything they want given the opportunity to make payments over time."[205] More than 80% of the funeral industry uses trusts to hold these large sums of money. New Jersey's prepaid funeral fund trust alone is worth more than $60 million. It is managed by the state's Funeral Directors Association.[206] One conglomerate, Service Corporation International, sold over 29,000 preneed funeral contracts in 1992. This represents more than $100 million in contract face value.[207]

Funeral home preneed plans do not usually cover cemetery expenses. (They can, however, easily be included in individual plans.) Cemetery preneed plans are often poorly regulated (or not regulated in some states) and subject to much more variation than funeral plans. Since cemetery costs (grave site, grave marker, vault, mausoleum) are mostly for goods, rather than services, they involve a sale of property. This property, however, cannot be used until death, and so must stay in the possession of the cemetery. Where the value of the merchandise is put into a trust account, cemetery managers deposit only the wholesale cost of the items (much less than is paid). In other cases, nothing is deposited and the items are simply warehoused until needed.

Virtually all funeral homes and cemeteries offer preneed arrangements if state laws allow them. In 1990 alone, more than 1.2 million preneed funeral contracts were sold in the United States by funeral homes, and industry experts estimate that by the year 2000, 5 million preneed contracts will be sold each year.[208] At the time of death, about 23% of Americans have some type of pre-arrangement with a funeral home,[209] and about 28% of adult Americans have made cemetery arrangements.[210]

## V. HOW ARE PRENEED FUNERALS MARKETED?

Preneed sales are slick, high-powered assaults on the public. The purpose of preneed selling is for the funeral home to secure a customer in advance of need, and in the case of cemeteries, to eliminate the funeral director from interference in their (sometimes dubious) sales practices. The aggressive sales techniques that preneed vendors favor cannot be used for selling merchandise and services "at-need," that is, at the time of death, because high-pressure sales alienate most customers who are in mourning.

Preneed salesmen pitch their products through direct mail, cable television advertising, "grief seminars" or "grief counseling," open-house events, senior citizen fairs, and mall shows.[211,212] They are motivated by large potential profits. Preneed sales organizations receive approximately 50% commission on their sales, with 20% to 40% of the sales price going to the salesman. Cemeteries with preneed plans spend four to ten times more for preneed selling than for the planning, development and landscaping of the cemetery.[213]

As early as 1937, Jackson described memorial park preneed sales crews of 50 to 500 promoting burial lots as investments. In southern California alone, he estimated that aggressive preneed campaigns had induced the public to invest $20 million for graves, $15 million of which were difficult or impossible to resell if not needed.[214]

Some jurisdictions feel that preneed selling has gotten out of hand. The state of Virginia, for example, bars these plans from being sold by phone, and even in person the salesman must be both a licensed funeral director and an insurance agent. These restrictions, hotly contested by the funeral industry, were upheld by the U.S. Supreme Court.[215]

## W. HOW COULD PRENEED PLANS BE IMPROVED?

Preneed plans clearly need improvement, being one of the most frequent subjects of complaint to regulatory agencies. Because of this, at least eleven states, including California, Florida and Illinois have enacted stricter laws to control abuses in the sale of preneed funeral plans.[216]

Investigating preneed plans, the Arizona Auditor General found that although these plans do allow the consumer to shop around, purchase the type of funeral he desires, and minimize distress for loved ones at the time of death, "consumers who purchase preneed funeral plans do not always receive merchandise or services purchased."[217] He found that while, on the average, preneed plans save consumers about $400 in funeral expenses, the plans are vulnerable to abuse, especially since the untutored purchasers and the often lengthy and complex contracts "offer great opportunity for misrepresentation."[218] Part of the problem may stem from the two ways individuals can pay for preneed plans. The first is to make one payment for all specified services. The second method involves paying a specified amount, but the funerary services at death depend on the amount of money and interest accrued in the account. This leads to many misunderstandings.

Consumers would be better protected in preneed funeral purchases if any preneed contract clearly included: (1) a list of the specific funeral services and merchandise included, (2) any provisions for substitution of goods and services, (3) the disposition of the funds paid and the treatment of accrued interest, and (4) a mandatory "cooling off" period during which the purchaser can void the contract without penalty. No current statute has all of these provisions.[219]

The preneed acquisition of funeral services and cemetery lots avoids pressuring survivors into making a quick purchase at the time of need. Preneed cemetery lot purchase may be useful for families who are settled in one location. Yet, as Ernest Morgan suggested, "the moral is look around, investigate all possibilities, do your own buying, and don't let a smooth salesman push you about."[220]

## X. HOW DOES THE BODY GET TO THE BURIAL SITE?

Ever since man stopped burying his dead where they fell, he has had to transport them to their burial sites. Over time there have been many methods, routine to exotic, for getting the corpse to its final resting place.

The first step is usually to get the corpse out of the home. Even this can present a problem. Fear of dead spirits encourages people to do unusual things. In Scotland, suicides had to be removed not by the door, but through a window or a hole knocked in the wall. This practice has been very common throughout the world.

In the Fiji Islands, it was once the custom to break down the side of the house to carry out a dead body, even though the door was wide enough. Some Indian Hindus remove a corpse who died on an inauspicious day through a temporary hole in the wall. In Siberia, the Koryak customarily carried their dead out under the corner of their tent and the Chukchee lifted their dead out through their tents' roofs. Among Native Americans, the Algonquins carried their dead out through holes made opposite the door, and the Tlingit removed theirs through temporary holes in the rear corner of the houses. Not quite as dramatic, but symbolizing the same process, a common custom in France, Germany and Switzerland until at least the early twentieth century was to remove a tile from the roof where a dead body lay.[221]

In modern Western society, workers sometimes must enlarge available entryways to get corpses out of the home. Not unusual is the story related by one medical examiner who had to call the fire department to cut an opening in the wall of a trailer so a 400-pound corpse could be removed.[222] Nearly every fire department in the United States has had to do this on occasion.

The next step is to transport the body to the grave site. At the end of the nineteenth century, full of whiskey from a lively wake, the members of one funeral procession in Shetland stopped to brawl among themselves. When the fighting was over, they went home. Only the next day did they remember that they had neglected to bury the body. A small group then went to the site of the brawl, retrieved the body and buried it. A similar funeral procession, in the same state of inebriation, is said to have come upon a crossroads, with both roads leading to a church cemetery. The drunken arguments over which graveyard they were to proceed to got nowhere, so they buried the body at the crossroads and dispersed.

A common belief in England was that a creditor could have the body of a deceased person "arrested" and held until the debt was paid. In truth, although this occasionally occurred, this behavior constituted a criminal act.[223] Likewise, it was believed that permitting a funeral procession to transit private land would from then on make that path a public right-of-way. While this was false, English and Scottish funeral processions are still exempted by law from paying tolls.[224]

While motorized hearses now carry most Western corpses, the hearse has evolved over time. Even today, though, alternatives are sometimes still used. (See illustrations, pp 464 & 496.)

An early method of transporting bodies to the grave was on a bier. The bier is a low wooden stand used to support a shrouded body, or more commonly today, a coffin or casket. It often has shoulder rests for the pall bearers. When it was used as transportation, it often doubled as a catafalque for the coffin during the funeral service.[225]

The next improvement in funerary transportation was the hand-drawn hearse. One example of this death cart still exists in Allonby, England, although it is no longer used. This hand-drawn hearse has four wood wheels, iron tires, open sides and is topped with a fancy canopy. It closely fit Ambrose Bierce's description of a hearse as "Death's baby-carriage."[226]

In the late nineteenth century, the hallmark of a U.S. undertaker was his elaborate horse-drawn hearse. The hearse was driven by coachmen in top hat and tails, and for each funeral it was decorated with a variable number of plumes, the number indicating the deceased's importance.[227] Even more elaborate was the one-hundred-foot-high white cardboard elephant used for a royal funeral in Mandalay in 1909. It was one of the largest hearses ever built. As late as 1971, one Brooklyn funeral home used a horse-drawn hearse when a woman demanded, and got, the same horse-propelled hearse for her funeral that had carried the bodies of both her husband and her father.

As the twentieth century dawned, motorized hearses appeared. Los Angeles had four funeral trolley cars, two of which, the *Descanso* (Resting Place) and the *Pariaiso* (Paradise) made two to three trips each day. The cars carried both the casket and mourners from the mortuary to one of the local cemeteries. The price for this service ranged from $15 to $25. When the *Descanso* was finally taken out of funeral service, it was renamed and used as a regular trolley. Its mahogany fixtures and stained-glass windows, however, informed potential riders of its former use—they stayed away. It usually travelled empty until sometime later when its owners completely renovated it.[228] About the same time, elaborately decorated trolley cars were also used as hearses in Burma.

In 1910 in Cleveland, Ohio, a funeral car was built to accommodate thirty-six people plus a casket. It could even travel to the graveside and act as a chapel in inclement weather. In 1916, Packard built a funeral bus that carried the casket and flowers just behind the driver, with up to twenty mourners in the rear. This vehicle now resides at the American Funeral Service Museum in Houston, Texas.[229] In Israel, corpses are still frequently transported on funeral buses. A team from the *Chevrah Kaddisha*, usually three men, travels to the site of a Jewish death by bus, cleans the body, shrouds it, places it in the bus with the family, and then goes directly to the cemetery.[230]

Gondolas long provided transportation for dead Venetians. They were used from the early nineteenth century when Napoleon banned using local churchyards as cemeteries, requiring the city to create the San Michele cemetery from two small islands. Only after World War II did motorboats mostly replace them. The black-draped funeral gondolas are now only seen in funeral processions for luminaries, such as the famous musician, Igor Stravinsky, who was buried in Venice. In that procession, the first gondola carried Venice's Greek Orthodox Archimandrite, the second carried the flower-laden casket, and others followed carrying family and friends.[231]

Until the 1970s, many U.S. funeral homes also operated ambulance services, transporting both the living and the dead. In many smaller communities, one vehicle served as both ambulance and hearse. The joke (not so funny if you were the patient) was that if the drivers were slow enough, they would only have to make one trip—to the morgue. Through the 1960s, funeral homes in many regions tried to save their ambulance services as stiffer state and federal regulations and better-trained municipal and volunteer services emerged. Some funeral home-run ambulances, such as those in Danville, Virginia, survived (most only temporarily) by appealing to a populace fearful of change and increased costs.[232]

In remote Sitka, Alaska, the Prewitt Funeral Home reports that it is still "not unusual to fly 100 miles in a float plane to pick up a case, or spend four days accomplishing a funeral [such as when] I put a funeral coach on a car ferry for a one-and-one-half-day trip to Juneau, and flew there the next day with the remains. On the third day, I went to the grave site and held the service before putting the funeral coach on the ferry for the return trip home. On the fourth day, I finally flew home."[233]

Modern hearses are quite expensive, costing $30,000 or more. U.S. funeral directors feel that their customers demand relatively new hearses, and so usually trade them in for new vehicles every two to three years. Unfortunately, there is little market for old hearses, so the trade-in value is low. The difference, of course, is made up by the consumer.[234]

In 1991, the average cost of transporting a body from the place of death to the funeral home was $87.74. Using the hearse to transport the body to a local cemetery averaged $117.49. One should note, however, that in most states not only a licensed funeral director, but also a family member or another person who has been given authority to arrange a funeral can transport a body within the state. This often requires a permit, for a very small fee, from the county health department.[235] Very few families take advantage of being able to use personal vehicles to transport a relative's corpse.

## Y. HOW CAN I OBTAIN ADDITIONAL INFORMATION ABOUT FUNERALS?

If this book and the references are not sufficient, there are several other sources of information. For costly answers from an unknown source, one can always call the 1-900 telephone services advertised in magazines aimed at the older population. For $1.25 or more per minute, they will answer commonly asked questions about funerals and funeral planning. But additional information can be obtained more cheaply and directly.

Local funeral directors, national funeral agencies, the federal government (e.g., Federal Trade Commission, Veteran's Administration, Social Security Agency), and the American Association of Retired Persons are all pleased to furnish information about funerals, pre-planning, costs and other aspects of burial and cremation. Public libraries are another valuable source of this information.

## Z. REFERENCES

1. Litten, Julian: In: Palmer G, exec. producer: *Death: The Trip of a Lifetime.* Seattle, WA: KCTS-TV Public Broadcasting Station, 1993. (video production)
2. Minton F: Clergy views of funeral practices. *National Reporter.* April, May, & June 1981. Reprinted in: Fruehling JA, ed: *Sourcebook on Death and Dying.* Chicago: Marquis Prof Pub, 1982, pp 159-169.
3. Hertz R: *Death and the Right Hand.* London: Cohen & West, 1960, pp 27-86.
4. Helman CG: *Culture, Health and Illness: An Introduction for Health Professionals.* 2nd ed. London: Wright, 1990, p 202.
5. Strub CG, Frederick LG: *The Principles and Practice of Embalming.* 4th ed. Dallas, TX: Frederick, 1967, p 136.
6. Raether HC: *Funeral Service: A Historical Perspective.* Evanston, IL: NFDA, 1990, p 27.
7. Kubasak MW: *Cremation and the Funeral Director—Successfully Meeting the Challenge.* Malibu, CA: Avalon Press, 1990, p 101.
8. Bierce A: *Devil's Dictionary.* New York: Dover Pub, 1958, p 46.
9. Lord Byron (Gordon G): The Vision of Judgment. In: Bostetter EE: *George Gordon, Lord Byron—Selected Works.* New York: Holt, Rinehart & Winston, 1972, p 310.
10. Morgan E: *A Manual of Simple Burial.* Burnsville, NC: Celo Press, 1966, p 3.
11. Arnold M: "A Wish." In: Tinker CB, Lowry HF, eds: *The Poetical Works of Matthew Arnold.* London: Oxford Univ Press, 1950, pp 249-51.
12. Berg CW: *The Confessions of an Undertaker.* Wichita, KS: McCormick-Armstrong Press, 1920, p 13.
13. Herodotus: *History.* Book 5, verse 4. In: *Great Books of the Western World.* vol 6. 1952, p 160.
14. Berg, *The Confessions of an Undertaker,* p 16.
15. Tegg W: *The Last Act: Being the Funeral Rites of Nations and Individuals.* London: William Tegg & Co, 1876, p 31.
16. Minton, *National Reporter,* April 1981. Reprinted in: Fruehling, *Sourcebook on Death and Dying,* pp 159-162.
17. Office of the General Assembly: *The Constitution of the Presbyterian Church (USA) Part II, Book of Order.* Louisville, KY: Presbyterian Church, 1990, p W4.
18. Minton, *National Reporter,* April 1981.Reprinted in: Fruehling, *Sourcebook on Death and Dying,* pp 159-62.
19. Grollman EA, ed: *Concerning Death: A Practical Guide for the Living.* Boston: Beacon Press, 1974, p 106.
20. Bierce, *Devil's Dictionary,* p 111.
21. *Funeral Rites and Customs.* Dallas, TX: Professional Training Schools, 1991, pp 38-40.
22. Koosman S: *Cultural Variations in Funeral Practice.* (lecture.) National Funeral Directors Association Annual Convention. Baltimore, MD: 1989. (audiotape)
23. *Funeral Rites and Customs,* pp 6-8.
24. Ibid., pp 18-20.
25. Granqvist H: *Muslim Death and Burial—Arab Customs and Traditions Studied in a Village in Jordan.* Helsinke-Helsingfors: Societas Scientiarum Fennica, vol 34, 1965, p 55.
26. *Funeral Rites and Customs,* pp 36-37.
27. Willson JW: *Funerals Without God.* Buffalo, NY: Prometheus Books, 1990, pp 16-19.
28. Minton, *National Reporter,* April 1981. Reprinted in: Fruehling, *Sourcebook on Death and Dying,* pp 159-62.

29. Ariès P: *Western Attitudes Toward Death From the Middle Ages to the Present.* Baltimore, MD: Johns Hopkins Univ Press, 1974, p 96.
30. Farrell JJ: *Inventing the American Way of Death, 1830-1920.* Philadelphia, PA: Temple Univ Press, 1980, p 147-48.
31. Alex Ghia: Interview. San Francisco, CA: January 23, 1992.
32. Bowman L: *The American Funeral: A Study in Guilt, Extravagance, and Sublimity.* Washington, DC: Public Affairs Press, 1959, p vii.
33. Dolan C: Burying tradition, more people opt for 'fun' funerals. *Wall Street J.* May 20, 1993, p A1+.
34. Edgeworth M: *Castle Rackrent.* "Continuation of Memoirs." New York: Oxford Univ Press, 1964.
35. Tegg, *The Last Act,* pp 272-73.
36. Copperthwaite DR: *A Guide to the Ripley's Believe It or Not Collection of Oddities and Curiosities.* (pamphlet). Canada: Ripley International, 1978.
37. Ragon M: *The Space of Death: A Study of Funerary Architecture, Decoration, and Urbanism.* (Sheridan A, trans.) Charlottesville, VA: Univ Press of Virginia, 1983. Originally published as *L'espace de la mort: Essai sur l'architecture, la décoration et l'urbanisme funéraires.* Albin Michel, 1981, p 170.
38. Litten, *English Way of Death,* p 4.
39. Just Conversation. *Mortuary Management.* 1992;79(5):8.
40. Send in the clowns. *The Director.* 1991;62(11):34-38.
41. Snead E: Death is becoming less of a grave subject. *USA Today.* January 7, 1992, p 4D.
42. Connor M: "Videographers" record life's milestones. *Wall Street J.* June 30, 1992, p B1.
43. Woods A: Mourners will please pay respects at speeds not exceeding 15 mph. *Wall Street J.* September 23, 1993, p B1.
44. Solomon J, Roberts E: So many ways to say goodbye. *Newsweek.* September 7, 1992, p 51.
45. Alex Ghia, Interview, January 23, 1992.
46. Ibid.
47. Grinsell LV: *Barrow, Pyramid and Tomb.* London: Thames & Hudson, 1975, pp 30-38.
48. Adams J: Time to bury the past. *Nursing Times.* June 25, 1986, p 46-47.
49. Litten, *English Way of Death,* pp 65-66.
50. *32 Car. 2, c. 1.* Repealed by *54 Geo.* 3, c. 108.
51. Pope A: *Moral Essays.* Epistle 1. 1733.
52. Puckle BS: *Funeral Customs—Their Origin and Development* London: T. Werner Laurie, 1926, p 38.
53. Haestier R: *Dead Men Tell Tales: A Survey of Exhumations, From Earliest Antiquity to the Present Day.* London: John Long, 1934, p 23.
54. Puckle, *Funeral Customs,* p 37.
55. *Revelation* 3:4-5.
56. Berg, *Confessions of an Undertaker,* pp 61-62.
57. Burial garb. *Tucson (AZ) Citizen.* March 12, 1993, p 4C.
58. Howard Belkoff: Interview. May 5, 1993.
59. Cerio G, O'Donnell P: Hat spats. *Newsweek.* July 19, 1993, p 8.
60. Brunvand JH: *The Choking Doberman and Other "New" Urban Legends.* New York: WW Norton, 1984, pp 112-13.
64. Shakespeare W: *Cymbeline.* Act 4, scene 2, lines 258-76.
62. Minton, *National Reporter,* June 1981.Reprinted in: Fruehling, *Sourcebook on Death and Dying,* pp 166-69.
63. Ibid.
64. Watson JL, Rawski ES, eds: *Death Ritual in Late Imperial and Modern China.* Berkeley, CA: Univ of California Press, 1988, pp 14, 123-24.
66. As quoted in: Bassett S: *Death in Towns: Urban Responses to the Dying and the Dead, 100-1600.* Leicester, UK: Leicester Univ Press, 1992, p 145.
67. Curl JS: *The Victorian Celebration of Death.* Detroit: Partridge Press, 1972, p 34.
68. Camus A: *The Plague.* New York: Vintage Books, 1972, pp 164-67.
69. Hadwen WR: *Premature Burial.* London: Swan Sonnenschein, 1905, p 118.
70. Gordon R: *Great Medical Disasters.* New York: Dorset Press, 1983, p 88.
71. Coffin MM: *Death In Early America.* Nashville: Thomas Nelson, 1976, p 108.

72. Hamilton M: Some desperate Muscovites resort to abandoning their dead. *Arizona Daily Star.* Tucson, AZ: June 7, 1992, p F3.
73. Herodotus: *History.* Book 9, verse 85. In: *Great Books,* vol 6. 1952, p 306.
74. MacGahan J: The Turkish atrocities in Bulgaria. *NY Daily News.* August 2, 1876.
75. Forbes A: 'The Paris Commune: The Finale, 29 May 1871.' In: *Memorials of War and Peace.* 1894.
76. Thompson L: A Suffolk Farmhand at Gallipoli. In: Blythe R: *Akenfield.* David Higham Associates, 1969.
77. Ienaga S: *The Pacific War, 1931-1945.* New York: Pantheon, 1978, p 147.
78. Fussell P: *Thank God for the Atom Bomb and Other Essays.* New York: Summit Books, 1988, p 25.
79. Ienaga, *The Pacific War,* p 201.
80. Schultz SM: *Body Snatching: The Robbing of Graves for the Education of Physicians.* Jefferson, NC: McFarland, 1992, p 26.
81. Ibid.
82. McLaughlin J: *Gettysburg—The Long Encampment.* New York: Bonanza Books, 1963, p 182.
83. McLaughlin, *Gettysburg,* p 187.
84. Johnson EC: A brief history of U.S. military embalming. *The Director.* 1971;41:8-9.
85. Ibid.
86. Ibid.
87. Phibbs B: *The Other Side of Time.* New York: Pocket Books, 1987, pp 5-6.
88. Johnson, *The Director,* 1971.
89. Litten, *English Way of Death,* pp 90-92.
90. Abercrombie JR: *Palestinian Burial Practices From 1200 to 600 B.C.E.* (Ph.D. Thesis, Univ of Pennsylvania) Ann Arbor, MI: Univ Microfilms International, 1979, p 25.
91. Habenstein RW, Lamers WM: *The History of American Funeral Directing.* 2nd ed. Milwaukee, WI: National Funeral Directors Assn, 1981, p 20.
92. Watson, Rawski, *Death Ritual,* p 15.
93. Schultz, *Body Snatching,* p 45.
94 Berg, *Confessions of an Undertaker,* p 28.
95. Coffin, *Death In Early America,* p 100.
96. Joseph's caskets were too flat. *The American Funeral Director.* 1992;115(4):6.
97. Litten, *English Way of Death,* p 86.
98. Curl, *Victorian Celebration of Death,* p 29.
99. Alex Ghia, Interview, January 23, 1992.
100. Farrell, *Inventing the American Way of Death,* p 171.
101. Gebhart JC: *The Reasons for Present-Day Funeral Costs.* New York: self-published, 1927, p 8.
102. Habenstein, Lamers, *History of American Funeral Directing,* pp 175-79.
103. Holman JM: The undertaker's lot in America. *Casket and Sunnyside.* 1972;101(13):14-15.
104. Casket Manufacturers Association of America (CMAA): *Facts and Figures on the Burial Casket Industry.* Evanston, IL: (no date).
105. Jones B: *Design for Death.* Indianapolis: Bobbs-Merrill, 1967, p 74.
106. Marsellus J: *Highlights About Wood Caskets.* (lecture.) National Funeral Dirctors Association Annual Convention. Louisville, KY: 1990. (audiotape)
107. Ibid.
108. Wood caskets, children are topics of talks. *The American Funeral Director.* 1992;115(9):30.
109. Marsellus, *Highlights About Wood Caskets,* 1990. (audiotape)
110. CMAA: *Facts and Figures on the Burial Casket Industry.*
111. Ibid.
112. Palmer G, exec. producer: *Death: The Trip of a Lifetime.* Seattle, WA: KCTS-TV Public Broadcasting Station, 1993.
113. Twain M. As quoted in: Morgan, *A Manual of Simple Burial,* p 13..
114. Twain M: *Life on the Mississippi.* As quoted in: Harmer, *High Cost of Dying,* p 158.
115. Morgan, *Manual of Simple Burial,* p 13.

116. Daniel TP: *An Analysis of the Funeral Rule Using Consumer Survey Data on the Purchase of Funeral Goods and Services.* Washington, DC: Federal Trade Commission, February 1989, pp 12-13.
117. Marsellus, *Highlights About Wood Caskets,* 1990. (audiotape)
118. Ghia, Interview, January 23, 1992.
119. Howard Belkoff: Interview. May 5, 1993.
120. Mitford J: *The American Way of Death.* New York: Simon & Schuster, 1963, p 24.
121. Ibid., p 97.
122. Pine VR: *Caretaker of the Dead: The American Funeral Director.* New York: Irvington Pub, 1975, p 93.
123. Alex Ghia, Interview, January 23, 1992.
124. Ibid.
125. Rules may change in funeral industry. *Wall Street J.* May 19, 1992, p B1.
126. American Association of Retired Persons (AARP): *Pre-Paying Your Funeral.* Washington, DC: AARP, August 1992, p 13. (AARP Product Report D13188)
127. Anderson P: *Affairs In Order.* New York: MacMillan, 1991, p 44.
128. Mayer RG: *Embalming—History, Theory, and Practice.* Norwalk, CT: Appleton & Lange, 1990, p 208.
129. Troutman R, Crichton C: Funeral firm liability in defective caskets. *The American Funeral Director.* 1992;115(:)0+.
130. arsellus, *Highlights About Wood Caskets,* 1990. (audiotape)
131. Carr J: As quoted in: Mitford, *1merican Way of Death,* pp84-85.
132. Curl JS: A *Celebration of Death: An Introduction to some of the Buildings, Monuments, and Settings of Funerary Architecture in the Western European Tradition.* London: Constable, 1990, pp 299-300.
133. Tegg, *The Last Act,* p 370.
134. Ibid.
135. Courtois-Suffit J: Project de cimetière perpetuel par la crémation lente des gaz. *Moniteur des Architectes.* 1881:3.
136. Mrs. Delany: *Autobiography.* ca. 1720. Quoted in: Litten, *English Way of Death,* p 104.
137. Litten, *English Way of Death,* pp 104-105.
138. Habenstein, Lamers, *History of American Funeral Directing,* p 228-229.
139. Puckle, *Funeral Customs,* pp 47-48.
140. Ann Landers Column, *Tucson Citizen,* 1993.
141. Minton, *National Reporter,* May 1981. Reprinted in: Fruehling, *Sourcebook on Death and Dying,* pp 163-65.
142. Abercrombie, *Palestinian Burial Practices,* p 23.
143. Gates C: *From Cremation to Inhumation: Burial Practices at Ialysos and Kameiros During the Mid-Archaic Period, ca. 625-525 B.C.* Los Angeles: Institute of Archaeology, UCLA, 1983, p 28.
144. Herodotus: *History.* Book 3, verse 24. In: *Great Books,* vol 6, 1952, p 94.
145. Puckle, *Funeral Customs,* pp 47-48.
146. Puckle, *Funeral Customs,* p 41.
147. Anima N: *Childbirth & Burial Practices Among Philippine Tribes.* Quezon City, Philippines: Omar Pub, 1978, p 52.
148. Tannenbaum JA: For every niche, there's a franchiser wanting to fill it. *Wall Street J.* April 26, 1993, p B2.
149. Morgan E: *Dealing Creatively with Death.* 12th ed. Bayside, NY: Barclay House, 1990, pp 111-14.
150. Overheard. *Newsweek.* 1993;121:19.
151. Mortician urges: shop before you drop. *Tucson (AZ) Citizen.* March 23, 1993, p A2.
152. Dolan, *Wall Street J,* May 20, 1993.
153. Anima, *Burial Practices,* p 44.
154. Anderson, *Affairs in Order,* p 42.
155. Alex Ghia, Interview, January 23, 1992.
156. Minton, *National Reporter,* April 1981. Reprinted in: Fruehling, *Sourcebook on Death and Dying,* pp 159-62.
157. Hughes TE, Klein D: *A Family Guide to Wills, Funerals & Probate.* New York: Charles

493

Scribner's Sons, 1987, pp 138-39.
158. Holman, *Casket and Sunnyside,* 1972.
159. Daniel, *Analysis of the Funeral Rule,* p 6.
160. Minton, *National Reporter,* April 1981. Reprinted in: Fruehling, *Sourcebook on Death and Dying,* pp 159-62.
161. Minton, *National Reporter,* May 1981. Reprinted in: Fruehling, *Sourcebook on Death and Dying,* pp 163-65.
162. Kipling R: "Our Fathers of Old." In: *Rudyard Kipling's Verse,* Garden City, NJ: Doubleday Page, 1919, p 632.
163. Ariès P: *Hour of Our Death.* New York: Oxford Univ Press, 1981, p 164.
164. Segal J, Segal Z: Should children go to funerals? *Parents' Magazine.* 1992;67:236+.
165. Metcalf P, Huntington R: *Celebrations of Death.* 2nd ed. New York: Cambridge Univ Press, 1991, p 199.
166. Montefiore SS: Curious Georgia. *The New Republic.* June 29, 1992, p 17.
167. de Lisser E: House wines for these brunches, of course, will be from graves. *Wall Street J.* March 8, 1993, p B1.
168. Tegg, *The Last Act,* p 15.
169. Nationline: Funeral pickets. *USA Today.* April 28, 1992, p 3A.
170. Morgan, *Manual of Simple Burial,* p 9.
171. Minton, *National Reporter,* April 1981. Reprinted in: Fruehling, *Sourcebook on Death and Dying,* pp 159-62.
172. Kubasak M: Responding to minimum service requests. *The Director.* 1991;62(11):9.
173. Ibid.
174. Metcalf, Huntington, *Celebrations of Death,* p 199.
175. Raether, *Funeral Service: A Historical Perspective,* p 17.
176. Habenstein, Lamers, *History of American Funeral Directing,* p 128.
177. Howard Belkoff: Interview. May 5, 1993.
178. Ibid.
179. 1991 Federated Funeral Directors of America Report: Another decline in profitability. *The American Funeral Director.* 1992;115(7):26-28+.
180. Ibid.
181. Ibid.
182. Lester D, Ferguson M: An exploratory study of funeral cost for suicides (abst). *Psychological Reports.* 1992;70:938.
183. AARP, *Pre-Paying Your Funeral,* 1992, p 6..
184. Market Facts: *Report on the Survey of Recent Funeral Arrangers.* Washington, DC: Federal Trade Commission, 1988, p II-3-4.
185. Daniel, *Analysis of the Funeral Rule,* p 14-17.
186. Hughes, Klein, *Family Guide,* p 133.
187. Held for ransom. *Mortuary Management.* 1992;79(2):21.
188. Hast R: (editorial) *Mortuary Management.* 1992;79(7):4.
189. Anonymous epitaph. Quoted in: Strauss MB, ed: *Familiar Medical Quotations.* Boston: Little, Brown, 1968, p 150a.
190. Letter from Carol J. Jennings. Federal Trade Commission, November 1, 1991.
191. Daniel, *Analysis of the Funeral Rule,* p iv.
192. Ibid., p iv-vii.
193. Ibid., p vi.
194. *Federal Register.* October 21, 1987, p 39378.
195. State of Arizona, Office of the Auditor General: *A Performance Audit of the Board of Funeral Directors and Embalmers.* August 1983. Report 83-13.
196. You think it's bad now? *The Director.* 1992;63(3):52-53.
197. State of Arizona, *A Performance Audit,* August 1983.
198. Rostad CD: "Sunsetting" of state boards is a looming threat. *The American Funeral Director.* 1992;115(1):19+.
199. Fruehling JA, ed: *Sourcebook on Death and Dying.* Chicago, IL: Marquis Prof Pub, 1982, pp 143-44.
200. AARP, *Pre-Paying Your Funeral,* 1992, p 2.
201. Ibid., p6.

202. Ibid., p 14.
203. Ibid., multiple pages.
204. Ibid., p 10.
205. Gould GH: Using preneed to build volume. *The American Funeral Director.* 1992;115(9):22+.
206. New Jersey executive discusses regulation. *The American Funeral Director.* 1992;115(9):42.
207. Service Corporation International: *1992 Annual Report.* p 20.
208. Gould, *The American Funeral Director,* 1992.
209. Daniel, *Analysis of the Funeral Rule,* p 14.
210. Riley JW: Death and Bereavement. In: Sills DL: *International Encyclopedia of the Social Sciences.* vol 3. New York: Macmillan, 1968, pp 19-26.
211. Gould, *The American Funeral Director,* 1992.
212. Troutman R: *Cremation Liability.* (lecture.) Natrional Funeral Directors Association Annual Convention. Baltimore, MD: 1989. (audiotape)
213. Mitford, *American Way of Death,* p 133.
214. Jackson PE: *The Law of Cadavers and of Burial and Burial Places.* New York: Prentice-Hall, 1937, p 300-301.
215. Troutman, *Cremation Liability,* 1989. (audiotape)
216. State of Arizona, *A Performance Audit,* August 1983.
217. Ibid.
218. Ibid.
219. Ibid.
220. Morgan, *Manual of Simple Burial,* p 8.
221. Bendann E: *Death Customs: An Analytical Study of Burial Rites.* New York: Alfred A Knopf, 1930, p 59.
222. Wooters RC: A medical examiner recalls an array of experiences. *American Medical News.* June 2, 1992, p 27.
223. Tegg, *The Last Act,* p 15.
224. Ibid.
225. Litten, *English Way of Death,* p 128.
226. Bierce, *Devil's Dictionary,* p 55.
227. Holman, *Casket and Sunnyside,* 1972.
228. Kelly D, Fulton J: Long train running. *Mortuary Management.* 1992;79(2):16-17.
229. Solomon C: Ghouls, no, but they've dug up some macabre secrets of the grave. *Wall Street J.* October 30, 1992, p C1.
230. Koosman, *Cultural Variations,* 1989. (audiotape)
231. Bruning LD: Funerals in Venice...as unique as the city itself. *The American Funeral Director.* 1975;98(8):22-25.
232. Public opinion survey favored funeral home ambulance service. *The American Funeral Director.* 1969;92:46+.
233. Kendzie-Hodaway D: Miles from nowhere. *The Director.* 1992;64:10+.
234. Bleckman IA: *Death and Dying.* Queens Village, NY: Croner Pub, 1980, p 213.
235. Ghia Gallery: *General Information on Burials.* (pamphlet). San Francisco: Ghia Gallery, no date. (distributed in 1992)

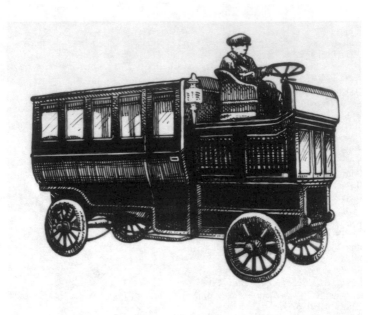

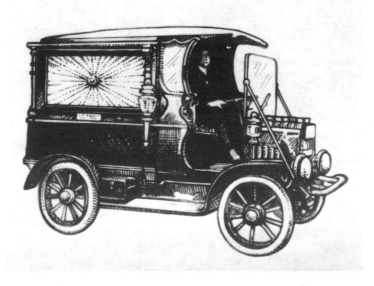

Early motorized hearses

496

# 12: FROM EARTH TO EARTH

*The final disposition for most bodies in the U.S. and Canada is burial. How does burial and "unburial" (exhumation) occur? What are mausoleums, catacombs, crypts, sarcophagi, vaults, grave liners, memorial parks, and memorial societies? How permanent are cemeteries and graves? Finally, who does the burial and how much does all of this cost?*

## A. WHY BURY A BODY?

People use earth burials to show respect for their dead, for health reasons, and to fulfill religious prescriptions.

The dead have been formally buried for at least 200,000 years. Neanderthals, with a sedentary population and a constant production of dead bodies, seem to have begun the custom. "Obviously, the smell of decaying flesh might alone be impetus to bury the body," said one anthropologist. But "when Neanderthals first started to bury their dead, they began by placing the body in the grave in either of two formalized ways: the flexed, or 'foetal' position; or the extended, or recumbent position. Neanderthals did not just cram the bodies into holes and cover them over."[1] Grave goods were often placed with these bodies in graves that were frequently laid out in an East-West axis or so that the face pointed East. Remains from these graves have been discovered at La Chapelle and Moustier, France, and in central Asia.[2-4]

As William Tegg said in 1876, burial is

> ...the prevalent method among civilised nations of disposing of the dead, by hiding them in the earth. As there is almost nothing else so deeply interesting to the living as the disposal of those whom they have loved and lost, so there is perhaps nothing else so distinctive of the condition and character of a people as the method in which they treat their dead.[5]

The word "burial" is from the Anglo-Saxon word, *birgan*, meaning to conceal. Verstegan said of the ancient Saxons:

> ...that the dead bodies of such as were slaine in the field were left lying upon the ground and covered over with turfes, clods, or sods of earth; And the more in reputation the persons had beene, the greater and higher were the turfes raised over their bodies, and this some used to call Byringing, some Beorging, and some Buriging of the dead, which wee now call berying, or burying of the dead, which properly is a shrowding or an hiding of the dead bodie in the earth.[6]

He goes on to relate burial to the establishment of cities, by saying that these earthen funeral monuments are called:

Beries, Baroes, and some Burrowes, which accordeth with the same sence of Byrighs, Beorghs or Burghs. From whence the names of diverse Townes and Cities are originally derived; Places first so called having beene with walls of turfe or clods of earth, fenced about for men to bee shrowded in, as in forts or castles.[7]

The ancient Romans, before cremation became more common, believed that the unburied were not admitted to the land of the dead, or at least had to wander the river Styx for a hundred years before entering. They customarily threw dirt on any unburied (dead) body they saw. Failure to do so required the person to sacrifice a hog to the god Ceres.[8] If any family member's body was known to be unburied, an empty tomb was raised to his memory and his heir annually sacrificed a victim, *Porca Praecidanea*, to Tellus and Ceres, to free himself and his kinsmen from pollution.[9]

Similarly, the Greeks believed that burial was one of their main responsibilities, since souls could not enter the Elysian Fields until the body was buried. They believed that their gods began the practice of burial, and it was, therefore, such a sacred duty that Greek soldiers returned the bodies of dead enemies to their kin for proper burial. When this wasn't possible, as with the Persians at Marathon, they buried the bodies themselves.

In China, Confucius equated immediate disposal of the dead with the great virtue of submission and love for superiors. The Chinese could perform no more righteous act than burying stray bones and covering exposed coffins.

A fundamental Judeo-Christian reason for burial stems from *Deuteronomy 32:43,* "And he makes atonement for the land of his people," suggesting that burial both honors the dead and is penance for the living. Biblical sources supporting earth burial include God's pronouncement to Adam in the Garden of Eden that he may enjoy life "till thou return unto the ground" (*Genesis 3:19*), and Abraham's statement at the interment of his wife, Sarah, to "give me a possession of a burying-place with you, that I may bury my dead out of my sight."(*Genesis 23:4*). Abraham bought a cave, Machpelah (Cave of Pairs), where Sarah, and eventually he and other patriarchs, were buried.[10]

Jews consider burial the only acceptable means of corpse disposal, since tradition requires that a body must decompose in a natural way and in contact with the earth to overcome its polluting influence. In Judaism, a "bad death" connotes an unburied corpse, the source of ritual uncleanliness (*tumah*). Being left unburied, either from scorn or neglect, has long been considered a horrible fate. Jeremiah leveled this dire biblical prophecy on Jehaiakim, saying "He shall be buried with the burial of an ass, drawn and cast forth beyond the gates of Jerusalem." He further laid the horror of non-burial on the invaders of Jerusalem, "They shall die of grievous deaths; they shall not be lamented; neither shall they be buried; but they shall be as dung upon the face of the earth: and they shall be consumed by the sword, and by famine; and their carcasses shall be meat for the fowls of heaven, and for the beasts of the earth."(*Jeremiah 16:4*) While Jewish tradition leans toward earth burial, Biblical evidence suggests that above-ground burial, such as in a mausoleum, may also conform with Jewish law.[11]

Thomas Aquinas felt that burial most benefits the living, "lest their eyes be revolted by the disfigurement of the corpse, and their bodies be infected by the stench..."[12] St. Augustine said, "Wherefore all these last offices and ceremonies that concern the dead, the careful funeral arrangements, and the equipment of the tomb, and the pomp of obsequies, are rather the solace of the living than the comfort of the dead." Disparaging costly funerary arrangements, he wrote that "in the sight of God that was a more sumptuous funeral which the ulcerous pauper received at the hands of the angels..."[13]

In Britain, funerary rites began changing from cremation to inhumation at the end of the second century A.D. The trend began in large towns, then spread to small towns and finally to rural areas. By the beginning of the fourth century A.D., inhumation was the dominant funerary rite in Britain. By the end of that century, burials in Roman Britain were east-west oriented, with the body coffined, extended, and supine—"the nearest the island ever got to a normative burial rite."[14]

Burial eventually became the dominant method of corpse disposal throughout Europe. It wasn't until the mid-eighteenth century, however, that Europeans raised concerns over the public health threat from the foul odors arising from common public graves.

Burial may hide a body from sight, but putrefaction continues. Bodies buried 1-foot deep or less still allow carrion insects or carnivorous mammals access to the corpse. On occasion, this aids investigators in finding hastily buried bodies.[15] To eliminate intrusions by carnivorous animals, burials must be *deep*; the traditional six feet seems to work fine.

## B. WHAT CHOICES ARE THERE FOR BURIAL?

Over the millennia, people in different cultures have been quite innovative in the way they have buried their corpses. They have been buried in pieces and intact, in different positions, at various locations, and with varying rites.

Interring an intact body is a *primary* or *articulate* burial. The body may either be stretched out *(extended burial)* or bent at the knees *(flexed* or *crouched burial)*. The body can also be tightly folded over and tied into a "fetal" position, or placed in a sitting, reclining, or standing position.

A body buried in pieces, after having first been cut up or exposed to be eaten by birds or other animals, is a "secondary," "disarticulate" or "fragmentary" burial. The pieces or bones are then usually buried in a haphazard manner, although occasionally, the bones or pieces are buried in a way that simulates their normal arrangement in life. This is a "false-extended" burial. In some cases, survivors may paint the bones before burial.

Bodies can also be initially buried, only to have all of them, or only the skulls, exhumed for reburial or placement in ossuaries. Skull reverence and burial has been common in many cultures.

In ancient Palestine, burial practices gradually changed over the centuries. In the fourteenth century B.C., primary burials, sometimes in jars or primitive coffins, predominated. This progressed to secondary burials, where exhumed bones were piled in caves. Around the tenth century B.C., some groups replaced this practice with cremation.[16] In biblical times, notables such as Abraham's wife Sarah were usually buried in caves. Many bodies were placed in natural cave niches sealed by large stones. The modern Jewish term for cemeteries, *beth hakvaroth*, means "the chamber of graves," reflecting the idea of cave burials. Originally, bodies were buried without coffins, but later were interred in coffins of cedar wood, earthenware, or in stone sarcophagi. Subsequently, elaborate labyrinthine complexes were hollowed out for burials, such as the catacombs at Beth She'arim near Haifa in Israel.[17]

Historically, bodies have been placed one, two, or many to a grave. When two bodies are placed in a single grave ("double" or "twin" burial), they are sometimes arranged in an embracing position, and paired burials of men and women are commonly found in graves from ancient Palestine.[18] In India, this is known as a Sati-type burial (not to be confused with the practice of *Sati*, or immolating the widow). From antiquity, small children have been buried with adults. Many were buried with their mothers who died during or shortly after childbirth. Until recently, very young or unchristened English children were often buried in the coffins of unrelated adult women, in the belief that their ghostly cries would then not torment their parents. In modern times, due to a lack of burial space, most Bermudians are buried eight to a grave. In New York's Potters Field, the cemetery for indigents and unidentified bodies, adults in pine boxes are stacked three deep in graves, infants seven deep.

In Western countries today, with rare exceptions, bodies may only be buried in authorized cemeteries. However, in the past this was far from the case. Basques, until 1787, buried their family members under the floors of village churches. In remembrance of this, the head woman in a Basque family still prays on a *tumba,* the spot in the church beneath which generations of her or her husband's family are entombed. In Scotland, burials within churches continued until the nineteenth century. The graves were often so shallow that bones stuck out of the ground, got in the way of worshippers feet, and were gnawed by dogs. One Highland church's records give this grisly report: "The floor of the church was oppressive with dead bodies, and unripe bodies had of late been raised out of their graves to give place to others for want of room, which frequently occasions an unwholesome smell in the congregation, and may have very bade effects on the people while attending divine service."[19]

Family burial plots were common on farms and estates. Condemning churchyard burials, a leader of the Brownists, forerunners of the English Congregationalists, said in 1590's Scotland, "Where learned you to burie in hallowed churches and churchyards, as though you had no fields to burie in? Methinks the churchyards, of all other places, should not be the convenientest for burial; it was a thing never used till Popery began; and it is neither comely nor wholesome."[20] In a bizarre twist to the idea of a family plot, Richard Wagner, the famous composer, prepared his own grave and took dinner guests into his garden to see his last resting place.

Rather than in a formal burial ground, Gypsies traditionally buried their dead at crossroads or under hedges. This suggests their attitude toward society, since from ancient times, crossroads were the place not only of executions, but where suicides and felons were buried. People used these sites because the traffic was thought to "keep the corpses down" and the roads going in different directions were supposed to confuse the spirits and prevent them from finding their way home. The last known example of this practice in England was the burial of John Mortland, who in 1823 murdered Sir Warwick Bampfylde. After his suicide, he was buried at a crossroad with a stake through his heart. Eighteenth-century New Englanders buried the bodies of suicides in common graves along the highway. This practice differs in purpose from that of burying victims of motor vehicle accidents by the side of the road where they died, still common in many parts of the world. The modern roadside burials stem from memorializing the place, as well as the person. They also serve as a graphic warning to motorists.

Many cultures once thought that the most proper site for a soldier's burial was where he fell in battle. After ancient battles, the dead were usually buried on the spot, and were commemorated by mounds on which they erected stone markers (*stelae*). During America's Revolutionary War, dead Continental Army soldiers who did not die in battle were buried in front of their camps.

Until the twentieth century, unbaptized Scottish babies and stillborns could not be buried in hallowed ground. Rather, they were buried at night in any available area. The nocturnal burial was based on *Psalm 58:8,* "As a snail which melteth, let every one of them pass away; like the untimely birth of a woman, that they might not see the sun." Stillborn children in Scotland are still rarely buried; hospitals or health authorities generally dispose of the bodies with other medical specimens.

In the past, some cultures have chosen to bury their dead in unusual

502

places. In India, the treatment of a dead body and the construction or placement of a grave was based on how the person lived his or her life. Among the Lo Dagga tribes of Africa, "sinners of suicide, murder, sexual intercourse outside human habitation" and the like were not buried in the village cemetery but far away, near water-courses or in trenches. The Bontocs of the Philippines inter most dead within their towns, but inter beheaded (murdered) men at the community's outskirts, facing the enemy, and reminding everyone of the need to avenge their deaths. And to help with the deceased's final outcome, some tribes in the Philippines bury their dead in the kitchen, beneath the water spout. The cool water is thought to prevent them from going to hell.[21]

Just as there are custom funerals, there have also been custom burials. The following are some unusual examples.

One of the most famous requests for a custom burial was made by Diogenes, the ancient philosopher and searcher for an honest man. He asked to be buried in a prone position "because in a little while everything will be turned upside down." It's unclear whether he ever got his wish. A more modern request was no less bizarre. Reuben John Smith, who died in Buffalo, New York on January 23, 1899, prearranged to be buried sitting in an oak recliner, beautifully upholstered in russet leather. He had also arranged to have his mausoleum equipped with his favorite checkerboard, a tin box with clippings about his burial, a table, candle and matches, and of course, a key to the mausoleum door.[22] Rather than a checkerboard, one woman was buried with a portable TV—tuned to her favorite soap opera.[23]

One special type of burial is available only to honorably discharged veterans of the armed services (or those on active duty)—a U.S. military burial. This formal ceremony, which can accompany any religious ritual, involves an honor guard, firing party, and a flag-draped casket. (See illustration, p 458.) Survivors can arrange these honors by contacting the military base nearest to the cemetery. U.S. veterans' families lately have had a more difficult time finding military honor guards for funerals, since the military is down-sizing and only half of American Legion Posts that once used to supply honor guards now have these units. Active duty base commanders can, at their discretion, charge families for the honor guard if the funeral is "too far" from the base.[24]

## C. WHEN ARE BODIES BURIED IN MASS GRAVES?

Mass burials have been used for, among others, paupers, victims of disasters, enemy soldiers, and wartime civilians.

Mass burial was once common for paupers. The Romans once buried their poor in mass graves outside the city walls—at a time when cremation was the "proper" method of corpse disposition. Eventually, Maecenas transformed one such graveyard into an elegant pleasure garden. Into the nineteenth century, the paupers' grave at Paris' *Cimetière des SS. Innocents* was thirty feet deep, twenty feet square, and contained up to fifteen hundred bodies. These graves stayed open, with their bodies or poorly constructed coffins exposed, until they were filled—approximately three years.[25] Not quite as formal, St. Pancras Guardians, a large British workhouse for the poor, saved money in the mid-nineteenth century by holding burials only twice a week. Each Tuesday and Friday they interred all of their dead in the same grave.[26]

Major disasters also sometimes warrant mass burials to protect the public health. In northern China, however, even when the frequent large-scale disasters warrant mass burials in shallow pits, they always are careful to place the corpses of men and women in separate graves.[27]

The disaster of war not infrequently results in mass burials. Only a few examples are mentioned.

One infamous mass burial was that of the 146 victims in the Black Hole of Calcutta who, during an anti-British uprising in 1756, were "thrown promiscuously into the ditch of an unfinished ravelin [a fortification ditch], which was afterwards filled with earth."[28]

During America's Civil War, the largest and most notorious Confederate military prison was at Andersonville, Georgia. More than 13,000 prisoners died there from lack of sanitation, water, food and medical care. John Ransom wrote in his diary:

> ...not less than 160 die each twenty-four hours...All day and up to 4 o'clock p.m., the dead are being gathered up and carried to the south gate and placed in a row inside the dead line. As the bodies are stripped of their clothing...the row of dead presents a sickening appearance. Legs drawn up and in all shapes. They are black from pitch-pine smoke and laying in the sun. Some of them lay there for twenty hours or more, and by that time are in a horrible condition.
>
> At 4 o'clock, a four- or six-mule wagon comes up to the gate, and twenty or thirty bodies are loaded onto the wagon and they are carted off to be put in trenches, one hundred in each trench, in the cemetery, which is eighty or a hundred rods away. There must necessarily be a great many whose names are not taken. It is the orders to attach the name, company, and regiment to each body, but it is not always done.[29]

Mass burials occurred worldwide during World War II. For example, after Japanese soldiers massacred all Chinese in Peking who looked like they might be soldiers, an eyewitness said, "The area was filled with crumpled, twisted corpses piled on top of each other in bloody mounds. Coolie laborers were set to work throwing bodies into the river...An officer

[said], 'There are about 20,000 dead Chinese there.' "[30]

As the war ended, desperation led to horrible behavior in Asia, too. At the end of World War II, as Soviet troops approached a secret Japanese unit that had performed bacteriological warfare experiments on prisoners of war, the Japanese killed the prisoners and "the bodies were thrown into a pit in a huge courtyard at the unit, doused with gasoline, and set on fire. Because of the great number of corpses, they did not burn thoroughly. The charred bodies were then put into a pulverizer."[31]

In the European theatre, Russians executed more than 4,000 Polish officers in the Katyn Forest near Smolensk and buried the bodies in a mass grave.[32]

Some of the largest mass graves, however, were those necessitated by the tens of thousands of unburied corpses that Allied troops found when they liberated German concentration camps at the end of the war. In one camp alone, troops (and former camp guards) quickly buried more than 30,000 bodies of those who hadn't survived the final weeks of confinement.

Modern America still has mass graves. Potters Field in New York City, for example, has one stone marker for each 150 bodies.[33] How many bodies have actually been buried there, however, is unknown.

## D. WHY ARE CORPSES ORIENTED WITH THE EARTH FOR BURIAL?

Burying the dead with a specific orientation to the earth has a long history. Many cultures believe that *geomancy* or harnessing the geographical forces of nature, which may stem from early sun-worship, benefits both the living and the dead. One early example is found in an Iron Age cemetery at Charvaise, France, where all but two of seventy bodies were buried with their heads pointing west and feet to the east, presumably to honor the sun. Many Christian cemeteries adopted this practice, explaining that the Lord's Second Coming would be from the east. In Wales, an east wind is still called "the wind of dead men's feet."

In ancient Egypt, the people lived on the east bank of the Nile (where the sun arose and "was born" each morning) and were buried on the west bank, where the sun died. Their form of geomancy also related to specific colors, with red being the male color, white and yellow the female colors. Thus, ancient Egyptians laid men's corpses on their right sides with their feet pointed toward the "red north" and their faces towards the "golden east." They placed women's bodies on their left sides facing the east with their feet towards the "white" or "yellow south."[34]

Geomancy also stemmed from a belief that the dead wanted to travel to their ancestral home. In the siting of the graves of some Pacific Island groups, for example, graves point toward the lands from which they believe their forebears came.[35] So important is orienting Chinese graves that geomancers often assume the role of religious figures in the funerary rites.

505

Other forms of corpse orientation stemmed from pagan customs which continued long after Christianity had a firm grip on Western societies. Burying bodies face down, for example, was not uncommon. Supposedly it prevented a witch or vampire from causing further trouble after death, because they could not find their way to the surface.[36] But according to folk legend, an infant buried face down, especially if first-born, prevented any other children from being born into that family. In Ireland and Britain, until well into the twentieth century, the "black north" side of a churchyard was reserved for suicides and murderers, who were refused Christian rites of burial and "were interred according to traditional pagan customs. The east was reserved chiefly for ecclesiastics, the south for the upper classes, and the west for the poorer classes. Funeral processions still enter the older churchyards from the east, and proceed in the direction of the sun towards the open graves. Suicides and murderers were carried in the opposite direction."[37]

The occasional body is buried vertically. Hindu ascetics, for example, are normally buried rather than burnt, usually in an upright posture with the body surrounded with salt.[38] The Muslim Maranaws of the Philippines once buried their dead in a standing position, although they now adhere to traditional Islamic burial practices.[39] While vertical bodies are more common in the East, some famous Westerners have been similarly interred. The noted dramatist Ben Jonson, perhaps to economize on space, was vertically interred in Westminster Abbey in 1637. Clement Spelman of Narborough, Norfolk, England, who died in 1672 insisted that he be buried upright so he would "not be trodden on." When his tomb was opened in 1865, the coffin was indeed, standing on end.[40] In the 1970s, members of a club for "Vertically Buried Loved Ones" placed bodies in upright plastic tubes deposited in deep holes.[41]

Most unusual of all was the burial position of Richard Hull, an eccentric buried beneath a stone tower on Leith Hill, England. He was buried sitting astride his horse—both being upside down. His rationale for requesting this placement was that they would be in the appropriate position on Judgment Day, when according to tradition, the world would be inverted.[42]

## E.  CAN I BE BURIED IF I WAS CREMATED?

Yes. At least a container with your cremated remains can be buried. Burial may be in a regular grave or, occasionally, in a special (and less expensive) section of the cemetery set aside for urn burials.

Since the disposal of cremated remains involves almost no restrictions, because under the law the corpse has already had its final disposition, they may also be buried at home or in a favorite place (see also Chapter 6, *The Eternal Flame*). How commonly this occurs, however, is not known.

## F. CAN ONLY PART OF ME BE BURIED?

Burying or reburying parts of bodies is an ancient custom that still persists. In Iron Age Palestine, people commonly first buried bodies and later exhumed the remains, only to reinter them with other remains, often in caves.[43] This practice, still common in many parts of the world, is termed "secondary burial."

Burying amputated limbs or other parts from the living in graves is more common. The Scots, who believed that the body must be as whole as possible for Resurrection Day, have long buried limbs in family graves to await arrival of the body. In early America, some grave markers even commemorate burying body parts. A Washington Village, New Hampshire, cemetery, for example, contains a marker with the inscription, "Here lies the leg of Captain Samuel Jones which was amputated July, 1807." Poor Sam caught his leg between some heavy timbers while building the town hall. Similarly, the Newport, Rhode Island cemetery has a marker placed by Mr. Tripp to "His Wife's Arm, Amputated February 20th, 1786."[44]

Even today, New York's public cemetery on Riker's Island has thousands of graves containing only amputated limbs. Through the 1970s, 20% of the burials in Potters Field were for severed parts from live people, rather than whole bodies of the dead.

Body parts from Popes are not buried, but get unique treatment. For example, John Paul II had pieces of his intestines removed in surgery after he was shot in May 1981. Rather than being cremated as are other discarded surgical specimens, his gut was taken to the *sacra praecordia* in the Church of Santi Vincenzo ed Anastasio. Since August 1590, when Pope Sixtus V died, the parts of Popes that embalmers (and now surgeons) remove have resided in large terra cotta jars in this very private repository. According to Catholic theology, the Popes' parts and bodies will be reunited on Resurrection Day.[45]

Not all body parts get such exalted treatment. John Moyle, a surgeon for the British Royal Navy described as part of the preparations for battle in 1686, putting a container near the operating table "to throw amputated limbs into till you have the opportunity to heave them overboard."[46]

In a sad aftermath to the Nazi atrocities of World War II, the Max Planck Institute for Brain Research finally agreed in 1989 to cremate 10,000 glass slides containing sections of brains from children killed at the Brandenburg-Görden euthanasia center. While the Institute received the brains of 697 of the more than 5,000 children killed at the center, the Institute's directors supposedly only learned of the connection between the specimens and the death camps in 1983 when historian Götz Aly tried to gain access to the collection.[47] One neuropathologist, Dr. Hallervorden, who received these brains via the unusually named *Charitable Transport Company for the Sick*, said of the batches of 150 to 250 brains he received at a time: "There was wonderful material among these brains...I accepted those brains of course. Where they came from and how they came to me was really none of my business."[48]

## G. HOW MUCH DO BURIALS COST?

A lot. Yet at one time Canon Law declared that there could be no charge for burial. Lyndwood's *Provinciale* states, "Let the right of burial and the sacraments of the Church be denied to none for lack of money, neither be anything demanded for Christening, let him that demandeth it be anathema."[49] English courts and Parliament later affirmed the right for a parishioner to be buried without fee in his parish graveyard.[50-52] This right moved with an individual to his new parish.[53]

Burial is no longer free though, and can often be very expensive. In part, this stems from the United States' cemetery costs and the cemetery industry never having been strictly regulated by the federal government, except as a minimal afterthought to the regulation of the funeral industry.

All cemeteries have what they term an "opening charge" for the labor involved in opening and closing a grave and any other services related to the actual interment. This charge is not generally included in any preneed payments and must usually be paid directly to the cemetery. Occasionally the cemetery directly bills the funeral director who then passes the costs on to the family. In the United States, cemetery charges for opening and closing graves run between $225 and $1,525. One New Jersey cemetery, for example, charges $1,395 for opening a grave on Sunday. This work takes a few minutes and is done with a backhoe.[54] They charge additional fees of $125 to $1,300 for installing grave markers.[55]

Some differences among cemeteries change the cost of interment. Questions to determine what the actual costs will be include:

1. If vaults or liners are required, does the cemetery provide them? How much do they cost, including installations?
2. Are chairs for the immediate family provided for the ceremony?
3. Are canopies or tents routinely provided for the ceremony, or is there an additional cost?
4. Does the cemetery charge for reseeding and resodding the grave?
5. Will cemetery employee be present to assure that everything goes smoothly?

Some cemeteries have levied some strange charges. For example, the Borough Council in Monmouth, England, developed a policy in May 1990 to double the burial fees (from £60 to £120) for those dying of AIDS. The Council justified these charges because of the extra costs for protective clothing for gravediggers and additional liming of graves to prevent the spread of infection. Persons dying of infections other than AIDS did not

508

have to pay extra fees. The Council finally admitted that they were woefully ignorant about the situation and rescinded the fees in September, 1991. No known AIDS deaths occurred in Monmouth during this interval.[56]

## H. WHY NOT BURY A BODY?

Throughout history, authorities have prevented the burials of certain bodies as a means of postmortem punishment, to serve as an example to others, to exercise political power, or for religious purposes, such as with saint's reliquaries.

Postmortem punishments were first recorded in *Joshua X* (26-27). Joshua found five Amorite kings, with whom he was at war, hiding in a cave. He killed them and then hung them, presumably as an example to potential enemies. He did, however, eventually bury their bodies rather unceremoniously. Later, the Romans retaliated against criminals who died during punishment by depriving them of burial. Their bodies were dragged to an infamous overlook, the *Scalae Gemoniae*, and hurled off.

The Greek Historian, Diodorus Siculus, described how some ancient Egyptians were refused burial. When friends and close relatives met with judges at the funeral, if "any accuser appears and makes good his accusation, that [the deceased] lived an ill life, then the judges give sentence, and the body is barred from being buried after the usual manner."[57]

Similarly, the medieval Catholic Church, as an ultimate reprisal and warning to others, refused to bury sinners and other excommunicants. Instead of interring these bodies, they exposed them to the elements or put them in the trunks of trees (*in concavo trunco repositum*). Monks described this as "the burial of an ass" or more clearly, "a dunghill." (*Sepultura asins sepeliantur, et in sterquinlinium super faciem terrae sint.*)[58]

In thirteenth-century England secular and ecclesiastical courts battled for control of the people, including their rites of burial. As described by a modern court, "From the year 1207-1213, the Interdict of Innocent the Third, kept out of their lawful graves all the dead, from the Channel to the Tweed. No funeral bell in the kingdom was permitted to toll; the corpses were thrown into ditches, without prayer or hallowed observance."[59] Eventually, the Church relented and they buried the backlog of corpses.

In thirteenth-century Hungary, Christian clergy required payment of one silver mark before they would allow those "murdered by sword, poison, or other similar means" to be buried. In 1279, only a Church Council was able to stop them from extending the practice to victims of fires, falls, collapsing buildings, and similar accidents. The practice, however, continued into the seventeenth century.[60]

At the end of the eighteenth century, the Bavarian government refused burial to the victims of duels, when duels were a major problem among the upper classes. Even nobles' bodies were turned over to anatomists for dissection. It is unclear, however, if this had much effect on the prevalence of duels.

There have been some unusual reasons for keeping bodies unburied. Diodorus Siculus said of ancient Greece, that among those in financial need, "It is a custom likewise among them to give the bodies of their parents in pawn to their creditors, and they that do not presently redeem them, fall under the greatest disgrace imaginable, and are denied burial after their deaths."[61]

In a celebrated nineteenth-century case, Martin Van Butchel kept his wife unburied for his own financial gain. An annuity had been bequeathed to her "so long as she should be above ground." Mr. Van Butchel was not inclined to give up this annuity following his wife's natural death, and had her pickled with the assistance of Dr. John Hunter. He kept her at home, and continued to receive her annual income. To earn additional revenue, he also put her on public display "Any day between Nine and One, Sundays excepted." When he remarried, his new wife would not tolerate her predecessor in the house, so he bequeathed the body to the Royal College of Surgeons in London, where it remained for 150 years until bombs destroyed it during World War II.[62,63]

The Catholic Church kept one of the world's greatest violin maestros unburied, at least in sacred ground, because of rumors that he had sold his soul to the devil in exchange for his world-renowned virtuosity. Niccolo Paganini (1782-1840), whose name means "little devil," was thought to have made a Faustian pact to attain his greatness. He did not help matters by professing agnosticism during life. In 1843, the Church finally gave permission to bury his body in consecrated ground, but officials in his home town of Genoa refused to bury him there until 1896. Routinely, the Church has kept its saints' bodies or parts of the bodies unburied to serve as religious icons (see Chapter 10, *What happens if you are too famous?*).

In modern times, U.S. courts have held that bodies may not be exposed to the elements because of our standards of decency. Yet burial at sea has been seen as permissible when necessary.

## I. WHY "UNBURY" A BODY?

Removing an already-buried body from a grave is called *disinterment* or *exhumation*. Forensic scientists now generally perform exhumations to examine or reexamine corpses for medicolegal or scientific purposes. Cemeteries also sometimes exhume bodies to rebury the remains elsewhere (see also Chapter 4, *What is an exhumation?*). In the past, however, corpses have often been disinterred to seek delayed vengeance or for personal reasons. (See illustration, p 513.)

At one time the Catholic Church commonly tried the dead for heresy and other offenses. If convicted, their remains were exhumed, and if the punishment for the offense during life would have warranted a death penalty, their remains were burned. Otherwise, the remains were usually reburied in unhallowed ground. Pope Formosus' (816-896) body was disinterred twice for his crimes. Pope Stephen VII, spurred by political motives, had the dead Pope's body exhumed, dragged through the street and, after trying the corpse in what is popularly called the "Cadaver Synod," cut off his fingers of consecration. His remains were again buried, but Pope Sergius III repeated the trial, disinterment and punishment.[64]

Although St. Ivo of Chartres stated in 1100 that the dead could neither be tried nor denied burial, several bodies were subsequently tried, exhumed and "punished," including Gherardo of Florence (d. 1250) who was tried for heresy in 1313 and John Wyclif (d. 1384) who was tried for heresy in 1425. Not to be outdone, adherents of the Church of England, during a period of anti-Catholic sentiment, convicted Thomas Becket, the Archbishop of Canterbury and Chancellor to Henry II (d. 1170), of high treason around 1540. They exhumed his remains and publicly burned his bones.[65]

More spontaneous public exhumations have also occurred. During a serious cholera epidemic in a Hungarian village during the Middle Ages, probably from fright as much as anything, the town's people decided that the disease had been caused by a dead witch. Her body was exhumed and reburied face downwards to stop the plague. Although this had stopped previous plagues, it failed this time. They again exhumed the body, turned her grave clothes inside-out and reburied the body. Still, the disease raged on. They exhumed the body once more, removed the heart and cut it into four pieces, burning each piece at a corner of the village. It is unknown whether this helped.

In a similar, but prolonged episode, eighteenth-century Serbians began exhuming bodies and "killing" them, believing them to be vampires. A well-documented case was that of Peter Plogojowitz, whose body was exhumed in 1725, ten weeks after death. Blood at his mouth (actually a part of decomposition) supposedly indicated that he was a vampire.[66] They stabbed the corpse through the heart with a stake, and cremated it. Throughout the eighteenth and nineteenth centuries, New Englanders also unearthed corpses, within a few years of their burials, to mutilate or disrupt the remains in vampire-killing rituals. Rather than strangers, it was the surviving family members who often performed these rituals, most often on those who died of tuberculosis.[67]

Héloïse and Abelard, the famous unrequited lovers, were originally buried together. In 1630, however, an abbess got the notion that the burial of a monk and a nun in the same grave was indecent. (They went into the religious orders after they were forcibly separated during life.) She had the skeletons disinterred and reburied separately. During the French Revolution, their skeletons were disinterred again and purchased by a physician; later the remains were given to the museum of national antiquities where they joined the bones of the French writer, Molière, also on display. Héloïse's and Abelard's skeletons were eventually reinterred together in a special tomb. Molière's skeleton was reburied in the cemetery of Père-Lachaise.[68]

On January 30, 1661, the anniversary of the beheading of Charles I, for both political and religious motives, the British House of Commons unanimously voted to exhume the bodies of Oliver Cromwell (d. 1658) and his two compatriots, Ireton (d. 1651) and Bradshaw (d. 1659). The remains were removed from their exalted resting places in Westminster Abbey, and were then "in their shrouds, hanged by the neck until the going down of the sun." At sunset, their bodies were taken down, the heads were removed and placed on pikes outside Westminster for public exhibition. Their torsos were then thrown into a pit under the gallows at Tyburn prison. Cromwell's skull remained rotting on a spike for about eighteen years, until it was blown down in a storm and found by a passing soldier.[69] In 1781 the soldier's daughter sold the skull to a private citizen for £118, and it was later used as an exhibit in a peep show.[70] It now resides at Sidney Sussex College, Cambridge, the school Cromwell attended as a youth.

Also for political motives, in 1793 France, the body of Cardinal Richelieu was removed from its tomb in the Church of the Sorbonne and decapitated. (It was not uncommon during the French Revolution to decapitate the dead for crimes.) In 1866, a Richeliu descendant who had obtained the head returned it to the government who immured it in a mausoleum.[71]

Bodies have also been exhumed for personal reasons. Abraham Lincoln, for example, in an expression of unassuaged grief, reportedly had the body of his favorite child, Willy, disinterred twice so he could gaze upon the boy's face.

A romantic, albeit just as macabre, exhumation occurred at Highgate Cemetery, London. The well-known nineteenth-century poet, Dante Gabriel Rossetti, buried the only manuscript of several poems with the body of his wife, Elizabeth Siddall, who died from an overdose of laudanum, an opium compound. Seven years later, in 1869, he decided to retrieve the poems. One autumn night by the light of a great bonfire the lady's body was disinterred. Onlookers reported that the corpse's very long flaming red hair covered the manuscript and some strands were removed with the book. Only after the manuscript was dried and disinfected, however, was it returned to its author.[72]

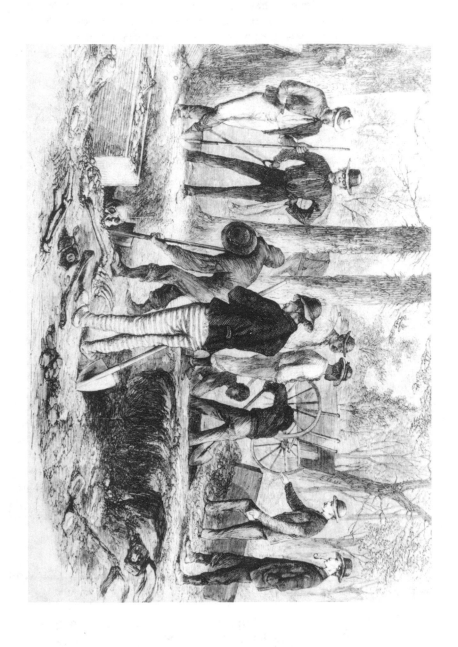

Exhumation of Union Civil War dead from the Battles of Fair Oaks and Seven Pines.
(Reproduced with permission. Library of Congress.)

513

Some ghost stories may have had their beginnings with exhumations. Tales of ghosts that "glow in the dark" may stem from seeing exhumed bodies containing luminous bacteria. These bacteria occasionally cover unembalmed cadavers, especially those buried in forests and other sites where dampness encourages the growth of wood fungi.

In recent times, authorities have permitted exhumations only for serious purposes and in "circumstances of extreme exigency."[73] English secular law, for example, once strictly forbade disinterments. This was overcome, in the public interest, by vesting exhumation authority in a religious officer, known as an "ordinary." This official could authorize the exhumation under church law. Statutes now permit exhumations if they are in the public interest. Disinterment is now usually allowed if it is designed to determine, among other things, a cause of death, or to move a body to another burial site, or establish a corpse's identity. Permission to exhume bodies has generally been denied if the request is simply to gather information for a civil suit or to establish inheritance rights.[74-76]

One example of an exhumation to establish identity was the tabloid-type fiasco at Highgate Cemetery, London, in 1907. When a Mrs. Druce claimed that her supposedly dead husband was alive and really the Duke of Portland, authorities exhumed the body in her husband's grave. Mr. Druce's coffin did indeed contain his remains.[77]

In modern times, a person's remains may be exhumed and transferred from one burial site to another for several reasons. Not uncommonly, a family or friends may wish to move a person's remains so they can "rest" near those of relatives. If all interested parties, such as next-of-kin and owner of the cemetery (not including the estate's executor) agree, this is normally approved. When cemeteries are abandoned the remains may also be removed to another site. Occasionally, especially with deaths in foreign countries, a body will be buried temporarily with the clear intent of subsequently moving it to its "final" resting spot. This usually causes no problems as long as death was not from a serious, easily transmitted disease, such as diphtheria, typhus, or plague. In those cases, the bodies normally can be exhumed only if they are in hermetically sealed container.

## J. WHEN ARE FAMOUS CORPSES EXHUMED?

Many corpses of famous people have not been allowed to "rest in peace." Tombs of the famous are often reopened for historical, scientific or other reasons.

The tomb of King Edward I of England, for example, was reopened in 1774 merely to document his burial clothes and accoutrements (a robe of gold and silver tissue and another of crimson velvet, a scepter in each hand and bejewelled crown). St. Dunstan's remains were secretly exhumed in 1508 more than 500 years after his death to retrieve part of his crown as a holy relic.

Those exhumed are not always treated kindly. The body of King John (of Robin Hood fame) was accidentally exposed during repairs to the Worcestershire Cathedral in 1797. One worker took this opportunity to use a piece of the tyrant's body as fish bait—with which he actually caught a fish.[78] During the French Revolution, the body of King Henry IV was exhumed and torn to pieces by a mob, and when the Bolsheviks took control of Russia in 1918, they entered the Kremlin to open the tombs and mock the bodies of the dead Czars. It is claimed, however, that when they opened the tomb of Ivan Groznyi (the Terrible), his body was so well preserved and his visage so fierce that they quickly closed the tomb and left.

The tomb of the boy princes, Edward V and Richard, Duke of York, both killed by King Richard III, was opened first in 1674 and again in 1932. The skeletal remains of the brothers who had been first imprisoned and then murdered in the Tower of London, were examined both times to ascertain that the remains were indeed theirs, to determine a cause of death, and to try to determine who really murdered them. The first exhumation was actually accidental, since their bodies had been hidden by Richard III. The second was done for scientific and historical reasons. Their identities and that of their killer were confirmed, although after this length of time, no cause of death could be verified.[79]

To test an old conspiracy theory, forensic scientists exhumed the body of Zachary Taylor, twelfth President of the United States, in the early 1990's. They tested the remains for poisons using modern scientific methods (none were found). (Permission to exhume and reautopsy John F. Kennedy has, however, been repeatedly denied.[80])

Similarly, the body of Dr. Carl Weiss, alleged assassin of Senator Huey Long of Louisiana, was exhumed to find missing bullets (none found). Lee Harvey Oswald, President John F. Kennedy's assassin was exhumed (to test one of the many conspiracy theories) to be sure that he and not a Soviet agent was buried in his grave—it contained his remains.[81] In 1985 the purported remains of the notorious war criminal, Dr. Josef Mengele, the German mass murderer at the Auschwitz death camp were exhumed from a small cemetery near Sao Paulo, Brazil. All types of available analysis, including video superimposition of facial photographs were used to ascertain the corpse's identity. It was he.[82] In 1992, the Russians released a report that in 1945 they had found the charred bodies of Adolph Hitler and Eva Braun. The bodies were stuffed in a munitions box and taken to a Soviet field hospital where they underwent autopsy and were buried. Later the Soviets exhumed the bodies at least twice for identification and reautopsy.[83] The bodies *were* those of Hitler and Braun.

Today, instead of immediately exhuming the bodies of the famous dead, some investigators "explore" the remains using ground-penetrating radar. The Tennessee grave of Meriwether Lewis, the noted American explorer, was investigated using this method in August 1992 on what would have been Lewis' 218th birthday. Scientists and historians tried to find out if there was evidence indicating whether the explorer had killed himself or he had been murdered.[84] Other researchers have tried to get permission to exhume the skulls of Lizzie Borden's parents in Fall River, Massachusetts in an attempt to better reconstruct the gruesome axe murder. Lizzie, who supposedly "took an axe and gave her father 40 whacks, and when that job was neatly done, gave her mother 41," (actually, it was 11 and 18 axe blows, respectively) was never convicted and the skulls then disappeared. They are now believed to be buried in the same grave as the rest of her parents' bodies.

## K. WHAT IS A CEMETERY?

Ambrose Bierce claimed that a cemetery is "an isolated suburban spot where mourners match lies, poets write at a target and stone-cutters spell for a wager."[85] True or not, a cemetery does contain the remains of human bodies. A church lawyer once said, "Churchyards are dormitories for human bodies."[86] Societies' notion of where the cemetery should be situated, how the land should be used, and what threat the cemetery holds for the populace have all changed over time.

The word cemetery derives from the Greek (*koimeterion*) and Latin (*coemeterium*) words for a sleeping chamber. These words may have been chosen because some ancient societies designed their burial chambers to imitate dwellings for the living. Other ancients, such as Bronze Age Gauls and Britons, however, merely cut bottle-shaped shafts in their chalky ground and used them as common graves for slaves (as well as other refuse). When a shaft was full, they planted a tree to seal the hole. Some Scots used a variation of this crypt burial until the end of the eighteenth century.

The cemetery's location has long concerned societies. Many cultures considered it illegal to bring the dead within their cities. In pre-Christian Rome, only Vestal Virgins, certain priests, and honored generals were allowed to be buried within the city's walls. Yet in ancient Greece, before cremation became common, families buried bodies within their homes. This may, in part, have stemmed from the ninth-century B.C. ruler, Lycurgus, the originator of Spartan laws, who decreed that the dead should be buried within cities so that the "youth might be accustomed to such spectacles, and not be afraid to see a dead body, or imagine that to touch a corpse or tread upon a grave would defile a man."[87]

The Thebans had a law that no person could build a house without providing a burial site for his dead. Kings and great men, however, were buried either in, or at the foot of, mountains—a custom that later spawned the building of large monuments over the graves of the high and mighty.

Plato, however, in his *Laws*, disallowed burial in any field fit for agriculture, reserving only dry and sandy ground for burials, since "no man, living or dead, shall deprive the living of the sustenance which the earth, their foster-parent, is naturally inclined to provide for them."[88] In early Christendom, burial was always outside the city walls. Only in A.D. 752 did St. Cuthbert get Papal permission to place burial grounds (churchyards) adjacent to churches.

While Romans believed that the grave or monument: *tumulus, sepulcrum, monumentum* or *loculus,* was more important than the surrounding grounds, Christian Europe completely reversed this, making the sacred burial ground their focus of attention. In medieval Europe, Christians buried their dead in the church, against its walls, in the surrounding area, or under its rain spouts. *Cemetery* originally designated the outer part or atrium of the church. An alternative name for this area appropriately translates as charnel house, since the medieval rectangular churchyard was formed by the church along with arcades or charnel houses piled with dead bodies.

Some cemeteries were once located inside churches. This became so prevalent that in the seventh century the Council of Nantes prohibited burials in the church proper, but allowed burials in the atrium or porticus in special cases, mainly for illustrious personages. Their pronouncement, however, did not slow in-church burials. Eventually more than twenty church councils up through the eighteenth century condemned in-church burials, but they had little effect.

Cemeteries have enjoyed a variety of uses over time—and some still do. Originally, cemetery land was generally flat and open, since very few occupants could afford tombstones. Medieval cemeteries, as part of church property, were places of asylum and refuge. People built houses and lived in the cemeteries, first because of their role as refuge and later because of the privileges (such as no taxes) enjoyed by those residing there. (In Egypt, due to the shortage of housing, millions of people still live in cemeteries.)[89]

The authorities also saw cemeteries as having multiple uses. In 1457, for example, the Scottish Parliament mandated that weekly archery practice and quarterly weapons demonstrations be held in the churchyard, and in 1593 ordered that prisons, stocks and irons for the punishment of idle, begging vagabonds should be placed there.

Open land was scarce inside towns, and what there was of it was used fully. So cemeteries functioned as central meeting places in which to conduct business; shops were established alongside the charnel houses. Cemeteries were also the sites of Sunday fairs and markets. Activity was not limited to business, since dancing and gambling were also common cemetery activities. Eventually, this behavior caused enough furor that church councils had to specifically forbid, under threat of excommunication, dancing or the presence of mummers, jugglers, theatrical troops and musicians within cemeteries. Even so, a 1657 text still notes "five hundred sorts of sports which can be seen within these galleries...In the midst of this throng of public writers, seamstresses, booksellers and second-hand clothes dealers people had to go about conducting a burial."[90]

They didn't ban farming, however. So, while still under Dutch governance, the ruling council of New York City noted in its court minutes of June 17, 1665, that "the Churchyard of this City lies very open and unfenced, so that the hogs root in the same." A commentator in 1861 wrote of American cemeteries, "...the curate's cow grazes in the village churchyard and feeds his children from his parishioner's remains."[91]

When Paris' *Cimetière des SS. Innocents* was to be closed in the eighteenth century, the main objection was that it was the one place where families of every social strata met and mingled. (Unfortunately, locals also used the cemetery as a garbage dump.)[92] By the mid-eighteenth century, French cemeteries ceased to be "places of public intercourse, meetings, and festivities. Innumerable edicts forbade people to dry their clothes there or to thresh wheat, to hold fairs or markets, to graze cattle, to play tennis or bowl, to dump refuse, to open taverns, to organize dancing and assemblies."[93]

During the same period, especially in France and Italy, cemeteries and the graves of loved ones became the center of much individual religious activity. The public would no longer tolerate the centuries-old practice of dishonoring the remains of the dead. Cemeteries began to rapidly increase in size, some being designed to serve both as parks which families could visit and as shrines for famous people. As William Tegg said of English cemeteries of the late nineteenth century, "the new cemeteries are in many instances cheerful open places of recreation, and in them the place of rest for the dead has rather tended to improve than to undermine the health of the living."[94] A modern U.S. example of just such a design is Arlington National Cemetery, where the garden of the Custis-Lee mansion preserves the appearance of a private estate. As the famous U.S. sculptor, Augustus Saint-Gaudens, wrote in 1901, "Nothing could be more impressive than the rank after rank of white stones, inconspicuous in themselves, covering the gentle wooded slopes and producing the desired effect of a vast army in its last resting place."[95]

Even today, some cemetery owners in "high rent" districts, especially owners of memorial parks with flat markers instead of tombstones, allow public jogging, skiing, and snowshoeing in an effort to forestall developers from acquiring their cemeteries. A suburban Pittsburgh cemetery, for example, once allowed cross-country racing, and Boston's fifty cemeteries are still favorite places for bird watching. Leonard Knott, in his book, *Before You Die*, suggests that cemetery owners at least draw the line at allowing picnics, especially when memorials might be used as barbecues. As one cemetery manager said, "Would you want to find somebody with a lunch spread out on your mother's grave?"[96]

Cemetery managers have been permitted to establish related activities, such as mortuaries, crematoria, plant and flower nurseries on their grounds. But there are limits. When a Louisiana cemetery allowed drilling for oil on the property, a court said that cemetery land, once committed to that purpose, could not be used for inconsistent purposes—and descendents of those buried were due compensation for mental anguish.[97]

Modern Jewish and Catholic cemeteries do not allow these activities. Catholics base this on modern Canon Law, which requires "appropriate norms on the discipline to be observed in cemeteries, especially regarding the protecting and fostering of their sacred character."[98] Yet in Mexico, some cemeteries periodically become tourist attractions. Traditional cemetery-based ceremonies during the Days (and Nights) of the Dead have been changed from simple religious ceremonies to tourist attractions. While elsewhere people celebrate a sanitized holiday of Halloween, rural Mexicans visit cemeteries to light candles, decorate the graves, and commune with the dead. At the most popular sites, such as in Patzcuaro and Oaxaca, thousands of tourists often outnumber the celebrants.[99]

Cemeteries eventually became recognized among some cultures as the source of contagion, especially during the plagues in the Middle Ages. As this feeling grew, steps were again taken (as in ancient times) to separate the final resting places of the dead from those of the living. One writer said of a church cemetery in 1775:

> Here nauseous weeds each pile surround
> And things obscene bestrew the ground;
> Skulls, bones in mouldering fragments lie,
> All dreadful emblems of mortality.[100]

The French National Assembly, for sanitation reasons, passed a law in 1804 requiring that cemeteries be situated on high ground and that every corpse be buried at least five feet deep. Britain and the United States also passed laws regulating cemeteries in the late nineteenth century. Yet in London, an article in a local magazine as late as 1843 noted that London "stores and piles up 50,000 of its dead, to putrefy, to rot, to give out exhalations, to darken the air with vapours...50,000 desecrated corpses each year stacked in some 150 limited pits of churchyards."[101]

## L. WHAT IS A MEMORIAL PARK?

Cemeteries with grave markers that are flush with the ground are termed memorial parks. They appear to be vast lawns with strategically placed shrubbery and sculptures. As a 1928 observer said of these facilities, "We have been to cemeteries where we have received the impression of a waffle-iron imprint pattern with some monuments dropped around here and there and a few trees thrown in for good measure."[102] In the United States, memorial parks began to appear in large numbers in the late 1920s and 1930s. By 1937, about 600 memorial parks existed in the United States. As Jackson said, "A memorial park is frankly designed for profit-making; it treats the practice of burial as an industry."[103]

To the owners, the major benefit of memorial parks over traditional cemeteries is their lower maintenance costs. Groundskeeping, a major expense for cemeteries, can be accomplished primarily with large mowing equipment, rather than the hand mowers (and increased labor costs) needed to trim around upright gravestones and tombs. Memorial parks may be free-standing or exist as parts of cemeteries which also offer monument sections, mausoleum entombment, and columbaria.

## M.  WHO MAY USE VETERANS CEMETERIES?

Civil War dead were the first to be interred in U.S. veterans cemeteries. These cemeteries were established as an emergency measure to deal with the problem of thousands of unexpected corpses, many of whom were unidentified and so could not be returned for family burials. In 1872 Congress formalized national cemeteries, extending burial rights in them to "honorably discharged soldiers in a destitute condition." A second system of national cemeteries was also established for those who had lived in the National Homes for Disabled Volunteer Soldiers. Gradually, both systems merged and liberalized their entry requirements. The requirement for destitution was ignored and starting in 1890 spouses, and subsequently all unmarried minor children, and with special approval, unmarried disabled adult children of veterans, could be interred in national cemeteries.[104] These rules continue today.

By 1990 there were 113 cemeteries managed by the Veterans Administration, Arlington National Cemetery managed by the Army, and 24 overseas military cemeteries managed by the American Battle Monuments Commission. Today the system would be even larger if veterans' groups and the Veterans Administration's efforts to increase the number and size of these cemeteries had not been repeatedly stymied by professional cemetery associations. Cemetery professionals have successfully lobbied for a burial allowance to subsidize private burials, rather than for funds to maintain and enlarge the national cemetery system. Private cemeteries still receive over 85% of veteran burials, as is attested by the more than 250,000 grave markers the government shipped to private, religious and municipal cemeteries for veteran burials in 1987. The most common reason cited for private burial is because a veteran's home is more than 100 miles from a national cemetery.

In the 1970s, state and federal governments joined in establishing state owned and managed national cemeteries. This was to alleviate overcrowding in current national cemeteries. Still, it is estimated that most existing national cemeteries will be full (except for the inurnment of cremains in columbaria) by 2020.

## N.  HOW ARE CEMETERIES PLANNED?

While U.S. cemeteries were once part of the community structure, they now exist as separate entities far removed from daily life.

American cemeteries were once adjacent to places of worship or close to the community. So entwined were early American cemeteries with their communities that colonists camouflaged their cemeteries to confuse the Indians about the number of their dead. Puritans used their churchyard cemeteries as places to stroll between church services or to have picnics, and many people set up family cemeteries on their own properties. Eventually, because of urbanization and a change in mortuary architecture, cemeteries were moved to the periphery of the cities.

Cemeteries today are usually separate from their communities, and are for the most part very profitable enterprises. This profit stems from their tax-free status, cheap land, and the ability to reinvest preneed and perpetual care funds. Jessica Mitford, in 1963, provided an example of a cemetery's intense land use by citing one Los Angeles "lawn type" facility:

| | |
|---|---|
| Adult graves | 1,815 per acre |
| Additional graves; made available by reserving one-half of each acre for double-depth interments | 907 |
| Babyland (three in the space occupied by one adult) | 120 |
| *Total number of graves* | *2,842   per acre* |

She adds that another such facility projects 3,177 "plantings" per acre of land used for ground burial.[105] Cemeteries certainly produce a better income for land use than the plantings of traditional farmers.

Older cemeteries, with their pleasant walkways and open spaces, often have their plots farther apart than modern ones. Some cemetery architects have suggested closing some roads (which would increase the distance from the road to a grave to more than six hundred feet—the length of two football fields) to provide more burial space, or transforming unused open areas to "estate gardens that are highly desirable and that command a good price." As they say, "No opportunity should be lost to reclaim unused land in the older cemetery. A land reclamation program..[will]..renew business for a number of years at today's prices."[106]

The physical isolation of cemeteries from the living has also decreased their cultural importance over the past century. Nevertheless, at least one industry writer implausibly speaks of the cemetery as "serving many of the cultural and social needs of living people...The cemetery is assuming its rightful position as a source of spiritual inspiration and discipline, as a custodian of our social and cultural heritage, and as an important, and perhaps indispensable guardian of all our freedoms so far won."[107]

Under modern U.S. law, a cemetery is established if the land has been set aside and marked for the purpose of burying human remains.[108] Under some state statutes, any site containing six or more buried bodies also constitutes a cemetery.

One of the world's best known cemeteries is Forest Lawn Memorial Park in Los Angeles. Evelyn Waugh described it in *The Loved One*, a book and later a (bad) movie which the funeral industry detested and condemned. Forest Lawn, ever eager to find new sources of income, contains concert halls, wedding chapels, movie theaters, museums, and gift shops. It has been variously described as the 'Côte d'Azure of burying grounds,' 'a Disneyland for the dead,' or 'God's own million-dollar acre.' One of the largest pieces in its considerable art collection that includes more than 700 statues, is the *Crucifixion* by Jan Styka, housed in an 850-seat air conditioned auditorium. More than 2 million visitors tour the grounds each year.

## O. HOW DO I BUY A CEMETERY LOT?

Cemetery lots are easy to buy; the trick is buying what you really want and need, and not falling prey to a societal aberration described by a funeral sociologist: "The culture of capitalism eventually...promoted competition among individuals...[and, in cemeteries] competition for the choice lots that established social status, and to some social mobility, even after death"[109]

Modern cemeteries must sell lots to survive financially. They have, therefore, developed very slick sales techniques, public relations, and advertising programs. Direct mail solicitations now target specific ethnic, socioeconomic and religious groups. Television advertising has recently been added to radio and newspaper advertising campaigns and telephone marketing. Sales staffs adopt modern hard-sell methods and they couch their pitch within the more socially acceptable topics of estate planning and will preparation. They must be doing a good sales job—Americans spend about  Cemetery plots generally cost $100 to $3,500. However, the exclusive Westwood Village Memorial Park in Los Angeles (where Marilyn Monroe and many other stars are buried) requires a minimum $15,000 entry fee.[110]

One key objective for cemetery sales is to eliminate the middlemen, such as funeral directors, between themselves and the buyer. Then they have an opportunity to push their whole line of products, including not only burial lots, but also grave markers, grave vaults and liners, tombs, mausoleums, and the like. They can also more easily sell their services, such as opening and closing graves, setting grave markers, and "perpetual" care. Eliminating the middlemen also increases their profit margin.

Buyers often wonder how many lots they should buy. This depends upon each individual's situation. In our mobile society, the need for multi-generational plots has dwindled. Yet buyers should consider the fact that if several adjacent burial sites are desired, they many not be available if they are not purchased simultaneously. One answer may be to investigate lot-exchange plans whereby owners may exchange lots in participating cemeteries all over the United States. The key, however, is to not make a decision either in haste or in the midst of emotional turmoil.

Cemeteries sometimes offer price discounts for new sections that they plan to develop. Buyers should be certain to investigate what alternatives will be available if the section is not ready by the time it is needed. No matter what type of lot is being purchased at a private cemetery, it is wise to at least consider not only the cemetery's local reputation, but also its standing with the National Association of Cemeteries, the American Cemetery Association, or the Pre-Arrangement Interment Association of America.

The families of some preneed buyers find that when it comes time to use the plot, the cemetery staff seems to find ways to add costs and generally make life difficult. Rather than valued customers, family members are now treated only as potential dupes who can possibly be soaked for a little more cash.

To avoid problems, potential purchasers should ask some questions before buying cemetery lots, including:

o  Who owns the cemetery?
o  Who manages the cemetery?
o  Is there a fund for perpetual care?
o  Who administers the care fund?
o  Does the cemetery meet my religious needs?
o  Does the cemetery meet my (and my family's) esthetic needs (location, neatness, landscaping)?
o  Will the cemetery accommodate any other specific needs I have (specific type of marker, tomb, interment of cremains, etc)?
o  Are there restrictions on the size of grave markers?
o  Will someone always be available to help visitors?
o  Are rules for placing flowers and visiting the grave reasonable?
o  Will the cemetery buy back the lots? If so, what are the conditions?
o  Can I sell my lot to another person? What are the rules?
o  Does the cemetery participate in trading lots with cemeteries in other parts of the country? If so, are there any restrictions?

Some cemeteries sell (and people buy) graves at extraordinary prices. Ultra-Orthodox Jews believe that the Mount of Olives, in Israel, will be the first place people will be resurrected on Judgement Day, and that those sites near noted religious scholars will be given priority. Therefore, grave sites in the cemetery on the sacred Mount can cost $20,000 if positioned near a noted rabbi.[111] Another expensive lot is rather unusual. The Hearpia Project Company, a Tokyo funeral home, is accepting applications for a cemetery they plan to build on the moon. Japan's National Space Development Agency will transport the bodies beginning about 2020. Right now, however, they are still trying to determine whether the sales are legal.[112]

## P. WHAT IS A GRAVEDIGGER'S JOB?

A gravedigger, of course, digs graves. While at one time the deceased's family and friends dug the grave, eventually the position became formalized.

In 1576, for example, the Scottish Assembly required that every parish have a gravedigger, or "grave-maker," who also acted as the registrar of deaths. The gravedigger was required to put some order in the graveyard, fill up and level graves as they settled, collect all human bones into one place, and keep the graveyard clean. He also received payment for supplying turf to cover new graves, ringing the "dead bell" and other incidentals. Payment for individual graveyard services was generally determined by the size and depth of the grave.

In the areas of early America populated by the Dutch, the schoolmaster was given the task (and the extra money that went with it) of digging graves when they were within the church itself. Perhaps the schoolmaster was chosen because the job had to be done meticulously if the church interior was to be kept neat and tidy.[113] The job paid well (and was even considered something of a racket by the authorities), so was a highly desirable and prestigious position. There was occasionally even some joy in the job, as described by Douglas Jerrold in *Ugly Trades*, "The ugliest of trades have their moments of pleasure. Now, if I were a grave-digger, or even a hangman, there are some people I could work for with a great deal of enjoyment."

While gravediggers now both dig the grave and close it, into the late nineteenth century closing the grave was still the pall bearers' job. In many cases this process became a contest of strength to see who could throw the most dirt in the least amount of time.[114] Into the 1940s, despite the old law requiring gravediggers, mourners dug the graves for many burials in Scotland. The lack of official gravediggers was as much due to the remoteness of some villages as it was to the cost of the gravedigger's services. The body often lay on the ground in the cemetery while the grave was dug.

Manually digging a grave takes between three and eight hours, depending upon the ground conditions. One trick gravediggers used in rocky cemeteries was to leisurely pre-dig a grave and then fill it in with sand. Then, when a grave was needed quickly, only the sand needed to be removed. Therefore, one of the most important technological advances in the cemetery industry was the backhoe, a mechanical gravedigger, developed in the 1950s. By the 1980s, every medium to large cemetery owned at least one backhoe. Mechanically digging a grave now takes about fifteen minutes. The inflated cost, of course, belies this fact.

Gravediggers remain a very important part of the burial process. Quoted in *USA Today*, one funeral director said, "You can't just take any person coming off the street and say, 'Here's a shovel, dig a grave.' "[115] Unionized gravediggers in Cook County, Illinois recently emphasized their importance when they went on strike. Bodies began to pile up, since there was no one available to bury them. The situation was especially "grave" for Jewish families, since Jewish law requires that bodies be buried as soon as possible after death. A judge ruled that Jewish bodies could be buried in plots already owned by the families, and that cemeteries had to provide shovels, wheelbarrows, plywood and lowering devices. Rabbis even started a hotline to help families in need. But since most area cemeteries required concrete grave liners, weighing 2,000 to 3,000 pounds, it was unclear to many in the funeral business whether laymen had the ability to prepare graves for burial.[116] When striking New York-area gravediggers began throwing rocks at hearses arriving at the cemeteries, many funeral directors put bodies into receiving vaults or refrigerated them in their funeral homes, rather than be accosted.[117] Yet gravedigging is not really that complicated. New York's Potters Field cemetery for indigents has successfully used Riker Island prisoners as gravediggers for many years.

## Q. HOW PERMANENT ARE INDIVIDUAL GRAVES?

One clown asks another in Shakespeare's *Hamlet*, "What is he that builds stronger than either the mason, the shipwright, or the carpenter?" Gravedigger is the riddle's answer, because the "houses that he makes last till doomsday."[118] Shakespeare's characters, however, knew little of the truth. Graves are often far from permanent. In fact, one of the clowns was present a short while later when he and Hamlet discover the skull of Yorick (as in "Alas, poor Yorick!") who had been buried 23 years before.

Archaeologists, builders and nature continually disinter significant quantities of human remains.

Archaeologists, or at least amateur historians, have, since the beginning of history, retrieved the remains of those from previous civilizations for display, inspection and occasionally, reverential treatment. They generally have shown little regard for the skeletal fragments of people who could no longer be individually identified, or who had no descendants to guarantee respectful treatment.

United States law now allows Native Americans to request the return of pilfered tribal remains and sacred and ceremonial objects from museums. Museums, however, have up to five years to catalogue the items before returning them for disposition. Some states have similar laws.[119] But it is often difficult to determine to which tribe the remains belong. Such was the case with a 1,250-year old skeleton unearthed by ditch diggers in Mesa Verde National Park. Eight different tribes, each with its own funerary rites, inhabit the area and claimed the body.[120] In another case, archaeologists and representatives from the Hopi, Zuni, and White Mountain Apache tribes met in June 1993 at Grasshopper, on the Fort Apache Indian Reservation in east-central Arizona, to decide the fate of 696 sets of human remains of Mogollon Indians (who no longer exist as a distinct group) dating from around A.D. 1300, and unearthed during a 30-year-long archaeological dig. The Apaches claim the remains since they now own the land, although the tribe did not live in the area when the Mogollons disappeared around 1400. The Hopi and Zuni claim the remains based on biological or cultural affinity. The Acoma and Laguna tribes can also claim that the remains are those of their ancestors, according to archaeologists.[121]

These remains are only a small part of the more than 3,000 sets of human remains at the Arizona State Museum in Tucson, unearthed from various archaeological sites over the past century and secreted behind a metal grating in a dark corner of the building. Most are prehistoric, primarily Mogollon and Hohokam, with some Anasazi.[122]

Most European graves have long been considered merely temporarily occupied. In medieval Europe, for example, the poor were buried in vast common graves, the *fosses aux pauvres*. When one pit was full, it was covered with earth and an old pit was reopened. The bones from the latter were then taken to the charnel house. Even the wealthy, originally buried under flagstones inside the church, were eventually disinterred and sent to the charnel house, in a process termed *secondary* burial. Most people accepted this practice as long as the bones remained near the church. Occasionally, the charnel houses were even decorated. In 1423, artists painted the celebrated *Danse Macabre* on the rear wall of the charnel house of the *Cimetière des SS. Innocents* along the Rue de la Ferronnerie. (See illustration p xviii.) The mural, in which thirty fleshless dead conversed with thirty living people was destroyed in 1660 to widen the street.[123] Although the practice of reusing graves was banned elsewhere in Europe during the eighteenth century, it continued in Brittany, Naples, and Rome. Through the nineteenth century in Breton, France, the gravediggers continued to remove the bones of the buried after five years in the grave. During an average lifetime, a gravedigger "worked over the whole length of the cemetery six times," meaning that he had reused the cemetery for six generations of corpses. Disinterred bones went to the charnel house.[124]

These removals, however, were not always appreciated. One late eighteenth-century physician at the University of Montpelier, France complained of "the scandalous, and at the same time dangerous custom of carrying the remains of unburied bodies, bones, often surrounded with flesh, partially decomposed, to places called reservoirs, to make room for new bodies, and thus to render graves the source of perpetual gain."[125] More graphically, the 1838 London's *Weekly Dispatch* wrote of typical churchyard removals:

> What a horrid place is Saint Giles's church yard! It is full of coffins, up to the surface. Coffins are broken up before they are decayed, and bodies are removed to the "bone house" before they are sufficiently decayed to make their removal decent...Here, in this place of "Christian burial," you may see human heads, covered with hair; and here, in this "consecrated ground," are human bones with flesh still adhering to them.[126]

In a similar ritual that still occurs in southern China, bodies are buried for seven to ten years, after which a bone specialist exhumes the bones. The specialist sorts the bones, reconstructs the skeleton, and dabs the larger bones with red dye (a blood substitute). He then wraps the smaller bones in red paper and places them in a large pot with the skeleton that has been bent into a fetal position. The bones are eventually reburied in a permanent tomb.[127]

Commenting on their reuse of graves, a Jordanian woman said, "If someone has recently been buried in the grave it must not be opened. No bad smell should be allowed to escape. When the deceased is laid in an old grave, the bones of those who have died before him are pushed aside to make room for him. Many people say: I should like to be with this one or that one."[128]

English common law states that a grave is only held temporarily (not owned), and its use terminates "with the dissolution of the body."[129] It bestows the "right of appropriation of the soil to the body interred therein until its remains shall have so mingled with the earth as to have destroyed its identity."[130] This was one argument against using iron caskets which would not disintegrate within a reasonable time. As one court said, "the period of decay and dissolution does not arrive fast enough in the accustomed mode of depositing bodies in the earth, to evacuate the ground for the use of succeeding claimants."[131] It went on to say that if graves are not reused, "A comparatively small portion of the dead will shoulder out the living and their posterity. The whole environs of this metropolis must be surrounded by a circumvallation of churchyards, perpetually enlarging."[132] In New

Orleans the law still allows people to reuse a grave after a year and a day. Some graves (actually the tombs) have ten or more names listed as occupants. [133]

Camus describes in *The Plague* what measures were taken to increase available burial space during an epidemic, " It became necessary to find new space and to strike out in a new direction. By a special urgency measure the denizens of grants in perpetuity were evicted from their graves and the exhumed remains dispatched to the crematorium."[134]

Modern cemeteries in many countries routinely "rent" a grave for two to thirty years. At the end of that period, they disinter and rebury the bones in accordance with that country's cemetery laws. Vancouver, British Columbia, a neighbor of Seattle, successfully uses a 30-year renewable lease for graves. In London, England, the wealthy have for many years obtained 99-year leases on their graves at prestigious cemeteries; graves for purchase, though, are scarce. In some places, a few "perpetual" graves may be available at exhorbitant prices.

Taiwanese provide "perpetual" cemetery care in an interesting way. They hold an annual tomb-sweeping festival, *Ching Ming*, when families pay honor to their ancestors by restoring and beautifying family burial sites while offering prayers to the spirits. In a similar ceremony, some Southern U.S. families "scrape" the growth off their forebears' graves. It is unknown whether this practice is done out of a belief that grass on the grave is disrespectful to the dead, or whether it is merely a custom persisting from Western Africa.

Hugh Bernard, in *The Law of Death*, suggests that there are three legal principles in the United States regarding moving graves or entire cemeteries:

1. As between the interests of the dead in silent and undisturbed repose and the interests of the living in material growth and progress of the country—its cities, its defense, and its public works—the interests of the living prevail. No cemetery is immune to the laws of eminent domain, although in the case of national cemeteries, there is little practical likelihood of displacement.
2. The law does not lightly sanction or order the disinterment and reinterment of the dead, but will endeavor to resolve the interests of the different parties (the deceased, the survivors, and the public) as equitably as possible.
3. Few cases in this area are susceptible of neat and pat solutions; most involve an *ad hoc* approach with a careful weighing of the specific relationships, personalities, degrees of kindred and affinity, etc., and to some extent at least the customs and practices of groups, religions, races, etc., involved.[135]

## R. HOW PERMANENT ARE CEMETERIES?

European and United States cemeteries have been routinely deconsecrated and razed. The poet John Donne well knew this when he wrote:

> When my grave is broke up again
> Some second guest to entertain,
> (For graves have learnt that woman-head
> To be to more than one a bed)
> And he that digs it spies
> A bracelet of bright hair about the bone,
> Will he not let us alone?[136]

At the end of Louis XVI's reign, in 1785, the 600-year (or more) old *Cimetière des SS. Innocents* was razed, plowed, dug up, and built over. This 1.5-acre cemetery in the middle of Paris may have existed since Roman times, and had been walled off with a special drainage system since 1186. In the years before it was closed to burials in 1780, the cemetery saw more than 3,000 burials a year. Yet over six winter months between December 1785 and October 1787, the remains were disinterred and moved to catacombs (except those that went to museums or laboratories). Grave markers were removed (some were preserved for historical reasons), the accompanying church and charnel house were destroyed, and the entire area was disinfected and covered in cement. This was all done without any noticeable public concern and with the approval of religious, medical and judicial authorities.[137]

During the French Revolution, cemeteries were stripped of their lead coffins which were melted down for bullets; the bodies were consigned to the city ditch. During this period, authorities also sold *La Tombe Isoire*, a well-known burial site, and the new owner erected a dance hall on the property. Proprietors of the very chic "Hall of Victims" would allow only those who had lost close friends or relatives in the Revolution to be admitted. Reportedly their slogan was "We dance midst tombs."[138]

The search for the remains of American Revolutionary War naval hero, John Paul Jones, testifies to the impermanence of cemeteries. The admiral had been buried in Paris in 1792. However, in 1905 when the U.S. ambassador to France, Horace Porter, tried to find the remains, he was slowed by the fact that the cemetery had been successively used as a garden, a dumping area, the site of a laundry, and the site of several dilapidated buildings.[139] (The remains were eventually located, identified by a team of forensic experts and now reside at the U.S. Naval Academy in Annapolis, Maryland.)

Some communities were overly concerned with their cemeteries, and this could be used against them. In 1670, for example, Leopold of Vienna extorted four thousand florins from the city's Jewish population to prevent desecration of their cemetery. By the mid-eighteenth century in Europe, graves were individualized and grave sites were sold in perpetuity. By the second half of the nineteenth century when Napoleon III attempted to deconsecrate the Parisian cemeteries that had been encroached upon by urban sprawl, a massive public outcry halted his efforts.

In the early United States, some graveyards were also reused. After the Methodist Church graveyard in Lancaster, Pennsylvania was filled to capacity, they simply added three more feet of soil above the existing graves and resold all of the sites. The town authorities eventually stopped this dubious practice.[140] During the Middle Ages in Europe, however, Jewish cemeteries did the same thing out of necessity, since authorities allotted them only small amounts of land for their burial grounds.[141]

The lack of cemetery permanence is seen in New York City, where at one time forty cemeteries flourished south of Fourteenth Street; few still exist. The City's Potters Field, used for indigent burials, was established at Madison Square (as in the Gardens) in 1794. As New York City expanded, it was soon moved to Washington Square, then Bryant Square, then Third Avenue and 50th Street, then Ward's Island and finally, in 1870, to Harts Island. The city built up over the old cemeteries and remains were rarely moved.

The early twentieth century also saw marked urban development in Singapore which required moving multiple Chinese cemeteries to acquire valuable building space. Not all remains were treated equally, however. As one writer said:

> The remains of a bygone merchant were carried [to a new cemetery] under a canopy and covered with fine silk and accompanied by relatives and friends and bands of Chinese musicians while the next procession would consist of three coolies, two of whom carried the remains done up in an old "gunny" bag slung on a carrying pole, and the third coolie preceded the procession, holding in one hand a few sprigs of bamboo with a red flag fastened to one of them and piping away on [an] old tin-whistle.[142]

After banning cemeteries from the city in the 1930s, San Francisco disinterred all the remains in the many cemeteries surrounding what is now the Neptune Society's Crematorium. The process of relocating 90,000 remains took 9 1/2 years. The remains went to four cemeteries in Colma, which became known as "Cemetery City."[143,144] The stone markers, however, were widely dispersed. Some were buried at the beach in Ocean Park, while others went to Aquatic Park to build sea walls. The public bought many for use as stepping stones and to build retaining walls.[145] The land is now the site of a large residential community and part of the University of California.

One recent example of the impermanence of cemeteries in the face of urban progress was the 1989 displacement of an old Dutch Reformed Church cemetery in Wynberg, Cape Town, South Africa. The cemetery had graves dating from 1848 to 1984 (and reburials with dates as early as 1811). The land was needed, however, for an urban development project. Of the 479 people supposedly buried in the cemetery, only 219 remains were disinterred for reburial, and not all of those with great care. The remains of the other 260 corpses presumably became part of the foundation for the new urban environment.[146]

In what the National Funeral Directors Association called the worst cemetery disaster in U.S. history, about half of the 1,400 graves in Hardin, Missouri's cemetery washed away when the Missouri River flooded in the summer of 1993. Citizens of Hardin spent nearly $500,000 to retrieve and identify corpses that flood waters had disinterred and floated downstream. Yet they were unable to locate 127 bodies and had to reinter the 476 that remained unidentified in a mass grave.[147,148]

In the United States, the purchaser of a cemetery lot does not acquire absolute ownership (a freehold or fee simple right, in legal jargon), but rather a right to use the land (easement) in accordance with the contract with the cemetery and conforming to cemetery and civil regulations. Cemetery lots are tax exempt. Some cemeteries have state-supervised endowment-care trusts for maintaining the grounds "in perpetuity." The payment for this trust can either be part of the cost for a cemetery plot or a separate fee. Some cemeteries do not have such arrangements. Many states have passed legislation mandating that municipalities assume responsibility for the maintenance of old graveyards.

Family graveyards or plots are often lost, abandoned, or in need of major upkeep. The funeral industry has taken note of that. Some caskets, such as those from Batesville Casket Company, now come with a "memorial record tube" that is attached to the casket and provides identification of the remains "should it be necessary to move a casket at a future date."

In U.S. law, there is a difference between halting further burial in a cemetery and discontinuing its use and maintenance as a cemetery. Even if no further burials occur, even if there is no more land for graves, the land remains a cemetery dedicated to the bodies already interred. If, however, its use as a cemetery is to be abandoned, the bodies usually must be disinterred and reburied elsewhere. Once this is done, the land can revert to other uses.[149] Occasionally relatives have refused to have bodies moved. In Chicago, for example, the bodies in an old cemetery in Lincoln Park were disinterred and reburied to make the land public space. One family refused. Their relative remains in a mausoleum in the park, with shrubbery discreetly hiding it from the park's many visitors.

Some cemetery industry experts have suggested that future societies may wish to recycle cemeteries simply to reclaim metals and reuse valuable land. In some cases this already occurs, as when a cemetery is no longer kept up, the graves become unrecognizable, and the public begins using the land for another purpose. The law considers this to be abandonment, and allows new uses for the land.[150]

## S.  WHAT ARE BURIAL VAULTS AND GRAVE LINERS?

A burial vault or grave liner is a rigid structure within the grave, surrounding the casket. Originally, these devices (mortsafes) were designed to keep grave robbers from disturbing the grave. As the public grew less concerned about grave robbing in early twentieth-century America, the industry had to market this product in other ways.

Grave liners are box-like structures most often made of concrete, steel, fiberglass, or copper, with a loose-fitting slab cover to support the earth that will be filled in over it. The industry claims that these devices prevent the ground from caving in and protect the casket from the elements. Wooden coffins or caskets often collapse and the ground settles over them, leaving a depression. In these cases, using a liner spares the cemetery the added expense of filling in "unsightly depressions" and allows them to maintain their lawns more economically. But if the caskets are sold to be perpetually intact, where are these sunken areas coming from? Or is the concern expressed simply another way to generate income?

Grave vault makers claim that their products also retard the deterioration of the body by protecting the casket from the elements and by providing another sealed layer around the body. Vaults may also double as grave-liners. Their actual purpose may best be illustrated by this insightful French commentary:

> The corpse is whisked away, shut up as soon as possible in the coffin which, itself, is shut up in a vault. The vault, acquired by the bourgeoisie in the nineteenth century, became widespread in the twentieth. This 'super-coffin,' this 'coffin of coffins,' is an index of the 'fever of the preservation...it is no longer enough to protect the corpse, we now have to protect what protects the corpse.'[151]

Vaults are often made of steel and vary in thickness and in the coating that is applied. One manufacturer recommends that funeral directors sell vaults by saying, "You don't need a vault. However, if you're concerned about the protection of your loved one's remains from the elements in the earth, you would want to have a vault that protects that casket from outside moisture and the elements that are in the earth. If you're not concerned about that, then don't worry about a burial vault."[152] No one, however, has actually shown that burial vaults have any significant effect on corpse preservation.

Most U.S. cemeteries now require grave vaults or liners for interments. Courts have upheld the right of a cemetery to require a vault or some type of enclosure to surround the casket or coffin.

Liners cost $130 to $395, while vaults cost $195 to $8,000.[153]

## T. WHAT WERE EARLY GRAVE MARKERS?

Since antiquity, people have used grave markers as memorials to their dead. But as General Lew Wallace, author of *Ben Hur*, wrote, "The monuments of the nations are all protests against nothingness after death; so are statues and inscriptions; so is history."[154] These "protests" from most ancient grave markers have dissolved with time, since they were made of wood or soft stone. Those of hard stone, such as the millennia-old obelisks of Egypt, still exist.

Massive stone tombs marking grave sites first appeared in France before 4,000 B.C., and were later erected in Spain, the British Isles, Scandinavia, Germany and Holland. Many predate the pyramids of Egypt. In China, it wasn't until the Sung dynasty (A.D. 960-1279), that people other than rulers and the gentleman/official class could erect shrines to their ancestors. Commoners were denied this right, since it prevented access to their gods thereby denying them political power.[155] Many of them undoubtedly erected simple stone cairns over graves, as is still done in some cultures.

In northern Europe after the Black Death, the horrible realities of decay and corruption began appearing on the tombs of the nobility. At Tewkesbury, for example, the corpse of John Wakeman is shown being devoured by a mouse, serpents, worms, and snails. These *memento mori* monuments are called the *gisant*-type of sepulchral art, intended to have an admonitory effect on the living. Contemporary poets vividly described this, as in this verse:

> *Et dans ces grands tombeaux,*
> *où leurs âmes hautaines*
> *Font encore les vaines*
> *Ils sont mangés des vers.*
>
> [And in these great tombs,
> where their haughty souls
> Still act in their conceited ways
> They are eaten by worms.][156]

Until the eighteenth century, it was rare for most Europeans to visit graves. Instead, they placed 12- to 16-inch-wide memorial plaques on church walls. Despite the notations suggesting that they were grave markers, these plaques simply denoted that the person's body had been consigned to the church. They usually contained simple inscriptions such as "Here lies John Green, who died 24 November 1492. Merchant." Some slightly larger plaques depicted the deceased person in a religious scene. Others commemorated donations to the churches. These donations usually stipulated that the church would periodically hold religious services for the salvation of the deceaseds' souls forever.

Grave stones began to depict the dead in seventeenth-century Europe. These depictions included representations of skeletons or bones, rather than the decomposing bodies previously seen. In some cases, such as with French King Louis XII and his queen, Anne of Brittany, even the embalmer's stitching can be seen on the bellies of their effigies, which lie in the abbey church of St. Denis.

During epidemics and famines, few grave markers were raised. The populations were so busy burying the dead that raising markers wasted too much time and energy. While many died, for example, during Scotland's Seven Years' Famine (1695-1703), few gravestones exist for that period.

Until World War I, most Western cemeteries were identical. Markers were either the horizontal flat tombstones or vertical stones attached to walls. In the United States, beginning in colonial times, only vertical markers (steles) were normally used. They contained biographical information and, often, short verses. Small vertical foot markers were common. More elaborate markers were usually reserved for the famous, or later, for the wealthy. Families, however, sometimes used large "wolf stones" over a common family grave. These large flat stones not only marked the graves, but also discouraged others from disturbing the bodies.

Stonecutters in the early United States often signed their names or initials at the bottom of the stone. Many of these identifications have disappeared as the stones have settled into the earth. One enterprising stonecutter actually advertised on his wife's grave marker in the Springdale, Ohio cemetery: "Here lies Jane Smith, wife of Thomas Smith, Marble cutter, Monuments of the same style, $350."[157]

Many historical grave markers have disappeared. They have been taken by souvenir hunters for personal collections and for museums. One such recipient was the renowned Old Sturbridge Village in Sturbridge, Massachusetts. They recently had to return eleven historic headstones taken from a cemetery in nearby Gilmanton, New Hampshire.[158]

## U. WHAT CHOICES ARE THERE FOR GRAVE MARKERS TODAY?

As the twentieth century dawned, both the United States and Scandinavia moved toward simple markers, while the rest of Europe turned to the more extravagant and baroque.

United States grave markers were once made of marble, slate or sandstone. These materials weathered so badly, though, they were replaced almost exclusively by granite and bronze. Bronze is generally less expensive than granite.

Granite, an igneous and uniquely durable rock, comes in black, gray, pink, soft reds and white. Granite lasts; quality granite in Egyptian carvings shows little wear after 5,000 years. Quality stones have a uniform grain texture and color, without discoloration, cracks, seams or discernible patterns. Granite is also very heavy, weighing about 180 pounds per cubic foot. A marker of 3' X 8" X 2' with a base measuring 4' X 1'2" X 8" (7.15 cubic feet) weighs approximately 1,287 pounds.

Markers are normally made by professionals who sell their wares through dealers. The industry proudly refers to their markers, statues and icons as "items of dignity, strength and lasting beauty."[159] The best manufacturers of granite markers often complete the entire production process themselves, from quarrying the stone to cutting the design and lettering. Most will guarantee their memorials unconditionally and without time limitations to be free from any defects in material and workmanship. The best guarantee, sometimes called the "double protection" guarantee, is one in which either the purchaser or the cemetery can make a claim for repair or replacement. The catch, however, is that these guarantees must be backed by either a solid reputation or a parallel guarantee by a manufacturers' association. A sandblasted manufacturer's seal must be on the marker for any guarantee to be honored. No manufacturer offers a guarantee against vandalism, natural disasters, acts of war or cemetery negligence.

Just recently, a small movement toward more elaborate grave markers has surfaced in the United States. Some specialized manufacturers say that up to 10% of their business now deals with such personalized markers as busts of the deceased, playing cards and dice (for a gambler), electric guitars (hobby), or even a life-size Mercedes Benz statue.[160] In some other parts of the world, such as in the Philippines, traditional grave stones (*sundok*) have always been unique, being formed as totem poles, flying boats, horses, or other figures.[161]

Sandblasting inscriptions and designs and polishing the granite are intricate processes. Poor stones can be detected even after the marker has been carved, since only the best stone readily accepts fine carving and sandblasting. Inferior stones can be spotted when the edges of the lettering are crumbled, or if the carving appears rounded or rough. Poor carving can be detected when lines are of unequal width or depth, when the curves have flat spots, or when details are poorly shaped or proportions are faulty.

Polishing stones does not add to their durability. This fact is attested to in the cemeteries around Barre, Vermont, where some of the finest gray granite is quarried and those whose lives were guided by the stone are buried. These graves are marked mostly with matte finished (unpolished) stones.

Dealers will also sometimes cut the deceased's name and inscription on the marker, but their chief function is to sell the merchandise and properly set it in place at the gravesite. They are usually members of either the Monument Builders of America or the American Monument Association. Membership, however, does not guarantee that a dealer is reputable. If the dealer says a monument has a guarantee, be certain to get papers stating this.

Although the practice is uncommon, grave markers have been repossessed for non-payment. *USA Today* reported in 1991 that the Gate of Heaven cemetery, owned by the Roman Catholic Church, repossessed a woman's tombstone when her husband could not continue payments on it. The church official's comment was "I think we're being compassionate, but we're in business, too."[162]

## V. WHAT ARE EPITAPHS?

A grave marker's uniqueness often relates to its inscription, the epitaph. One of the best descriptions of this form of doggerel was penned by an Englishman, Richard Puttenham, who wrote, "An epitaph is an inscription such as a man may commodiously write or engrave upon a tombe in few verses, pithie, quicke, and sententious, for the passerby to judge upon without any long tariaunce."[163] The shortest epitaph on record has been said to be "Thorp's Corpse,"[164] although "Bismarck" is the sole epitaph on the gravestone of the famous German statesman. Much longer epitaphs abound. Yet, as Laurence Peter slyly wrote, "Many a tombstone inscription is a grave error."[165]

Epitaphs on grave markers have ranged from the sublime to the absurd. One classic epitaph from the ancient Epicureans reads, "I was not. I have been. I am not. I do not mind." Nicholas Ferrar, a seventeenth-century English writer, wrote an elegant epitaph for a relative, John Wodenote:

> John Wodenote's bones interred here do ly
> Could but his worth by words expressed by,
> Reader should'st weepe as fast as I,
> In Tearedrop'd rythmes, to his blest Memorie.[166]

At one time epitaphs became so bizarre in the U.S. that an old cemetery had a restriction against "advertising on tombstones." One wonders how this law would have applied to the gravestone of Frances G. Fear in Buena Vista, Colorado, whose epitaph reads "Before I knew the best part of my life had come, it had gone."[167] To use this saying, her husband had to agree to put the author's name (Ashleigh Brilliant) and a copyright symbol on the marker.[168] The courts have determined that the wording of epitaphs on monuments or markers may be regulated, to exclude offensive or vindictive language. This issue was tested in one New York court case when a family wanted the inscription: "Beneath This Stone Lies a Woman Who Loved Life But Was Murdered By A Doctor Whose Name Is Not Worthy To Appear Here."[169]

With an unusual sense of humor, one woman's epitaph in Bangor, England reads:

> Poor Martha Snell, hers gone away.
> Her would, if her could, but her couldn't stay.
> Her'd two bad legs, and a badish cough,
> But her legs it was as carried her off.[170]

The marker over the grave of a man who was buried with his two wives on either side of him is engraved with hands labeled "Mine" pointing to each of the two wives' graves. Each of their markers has a hand labeled "Ours" pointing at his.[171] Another gravestone in a Ruidoso, New Mexico, graveyard was clearly written by a Mr. Peas, who said, "Peas is not here, only the pod; Peas shelled out, went home to God." The last line of Casey Stengel, former New Yorks Mets manager's epitaph reads, "There comes a time in every man's life, and I've had plenty of them."[172]

Additional epitaphs, witty, pithy and sad can be found in Chapter 14, *Say It Gently: Words, Sayings and Poetry About the Dead.*

## W.  DO U.S. VETERANS GET FREE GRAVE MARKERS?

The Veterans Administration will supply an upright headstone, flat stone marker, flat bronze marker, or a niche marker, or will contribute the average cost for these markers toward the private purchase of a commercially-sold monument.

Those eligible for this benefit include veterans of wartime and peacetime U.S. military service who were discharged from active duty "under conditions other than dishonorable," persons whose deaths occurred under honorable conditions while serving in the U.S. Armed Forces, and veterans' dependents who are buried in national, military post, base, or state veterans' cemeteries. The VA-supplied grave markers must include the name, branch of service and birth/death years. They may also include (without cost) a religious emblem, military grade/rank, war service, and birth/death month and day. Limited additional information can be inscribed at private expense. Markers are usually shipped within 60-90 days of receipt of VA Form 40-1330. Shipping is at government expense, but placing the marker in private cemeteries is not covered by the VA. Additional information and forms can be requested from Monument Service (42),

Department of Veterans Affairs, 810 Vermont Avenue, NW, Washington, DC, 20420.

## X. WHAT ARE CATACOMBS?

Catacombs are a series of below ground chambers and passages used to house the dead. The word itself has uncertain origins, being used in its Latin form, *catacumbas*, as early as the fifth century A.D. to designate the subterranean cemetery under the Basilica of St. Sebastian on the Apian Way, near Rome. The term was later extended to the network of burial chambers in other parts of Rome. Most catacombs were probably first quarries, which were only later converted to burial chambers. Many of the structures were first used by non-Christians, and were subsequently appropriated by Christian sects.

Rome has the most famous catacombs, a labyrinth of graves, placed one above the other like bunks. The galleries, resembling mines, are long and narrow, usually about eight-feet high and five-feet wide, twisting and turning in all directions, with niches for bodies hollowed into their sides. At irregular intervals, the galleries expand into wide, lofty chambers, often covered with frescoes. In times of trouble, early Christians sometimes used the catacombs as places of refuge or worship.

Although the structure is contained in only a small area, it has been estimated that if the tunnels were stretched into a straight line, they would extend the entire length of Italy. Many of the tunnels, however, have been destroyed over the centuries. As early as the eighth century A.D., catacombs were razed by the Lombards besieging Rome. To avoid their desecration, many saints' remains were subsequently removed from the catacombs and placed in churches. Most of this extensive labyrinth was covered up and forgotten until 1578, when it was fortuitously rediscovered. Catacombs also exist in Naples, Palermo, and Syracuse, Italy; and in Israel, Greece, Syria, Peru, Iran, Cyprus and Paris.[173,174]

The catacombs of Paris were originally immense stone quarries which supplied the city with building material. On April 7, 1786, officials began to disinter bones and bodies from several Parisian church cemeteries, moving the remains to the catacombs. The *Cimetière des SS. Innocents* and the cemeteries at St. Eustache and St. Etienne des Grès supplied most of the bodies. These processions of the dead took place only during winter nights (to decrease the odor and the number of onlookers), and were accompanied by chanting church officials. In the catacombs, the remains were decorously arranged—arm bones piled with other arm bones, leg bones with other leg bones, and all intersected with rows of skulls. Smaller bones were tossed in the back. By the time they were done, these catacombs contained the reinterred remains of between three and six million Parisians.

## Y. WHAT IS A MAUSOLEUM?

Mausoleums are buildings in which bodies can be entombed above ground in a process called *immurement*. Mausoleums have been used throughout the world, continuing to be some of the best-known buildings. They have become increasingly popular in the United States.

Entombing the dead, rather than burying them, has a long history. Elaborate stone entombment structures predate by many centuries the famed pyramids of Egypt, with tombs being some of the grandest buildings in the world. The first structure termed a "mausoleum" was one of the Seven Wonders of the World. Built about 350 B.C. in Halicarnassus, in Asia Minor, this 140-foot-high pyramid, with a complex interior, served as the tomb for Artemisia, the wife of Mausolus, king of Caria. It was destroyed, probably by an earthquake, during the thirteenth or fourteenth centuries. Only its steps remained when the Crusaders took Jerusalem in 1404. Relics excavated from this mausoleum still exist in the British Museum.

The earliest tombs for Egyptian Pharaohs were simple mausoleums, but they gradually evolved into the elaborate pyramids known to the world today. One of the word's greatest tombs is the Great Pyramid of Cheops. Composed of more than 5 million tons of stone, it stands 481-feet high, is 755-feet square, and covers over 13 acres. The pyramids were furnished to meet the needs of the dead, and sometimes even included toilet facilities. Yet only the *very* wealthy can afford to employ between 100,000 and 400,000 men for more than the twenty years to build their mausoleums.

Like the Pharaohs, Chinese emperors selected their own burial sites and often began building their tombs within mausoleums while they still lived. However, since the location of the tomb was supposed to affect the fortunes of the dynasty, wrangling over its exact positioning was often prolonged and rancorous. Even after death, the Chinese maintained their hierarchy through their tombs. During the seventeenth-century Ming Dynasty, for example, a person's rank determined the size and complexity of his tomb. Princes had tombs measuring 100 paces in circumference and nearly 20-feet high, surrounded by ten-foot-high walls, and decorated with four human statues and two statues each of horses, tigers and sheep. Noblemen of the ninth rank, however, were allowed tombs only 20 paces in circumference, less than six-feet high, and with no surrounding wall or statues.[175]

Ancient Roman nobles often built giant mausoleums which held up to 700 bodies for themselves and their extended family and servants.[176] If they suddenly died (there was a rash of assassinations), their friends and heirs were obligated to complete the construction.[177] Later, European nobility vied with one another to have larger and grander mausoleums than those of their competitors. This led to one of the world's most magnificent cemeteries, the twelfth-century Campo Santo in Pisa, Italy, which is filled with garish monuments, vaults and mausoleums. Other ornate and world-renowned tombs include the castle of St. Angelo, the tomb of Caecilia Metella, and the Taj Majal.

Perhaps the world's most beautiful building is a mausoleum, India's famed Taj Majal. Built in 1631, it commemorates the love Mogul Shah Jahan had for his queen, Mumtaz Mahal, who died during the birth of their fourteenth child. The building's design epitomized the Persian view of the world, with the dome symbolizing the vault of heaven over a square building, representing the world below. The building is replete with inlaid marble and decorated with precious stones. The queen's crypt is one of the most elaborate parts of the building. Ironically, Shah Jahan, imprisoned in 1657, spent the last nine years of his life staring from his cell at the Taj Majal, where he also was eventually entombed.[178]

Mao Tse-tung's remains lie within an imposing memorial building called Mao's Chi-nien t'ang (Memorial Hall). Situated in T'in-an men Square between the Revolutionary History Museum and the Great Hall of the People, this 112-foot-high building, completed in 1977, involved the labor of more than 700,000 people. The building was designed not for visitors, but for "homagers." Homagers must walk up imposing sets of steps to reach the entrance. Mao's 10-foot-high statue greets visitors in an anteroom, in a design supposedly inspired by the Lincoln Memorial. The body itself lies on a black granite catafalque in an inner room, under a trapezoidal crystal. The body appears sallow, the face wrinkled. Ironically, Mao's monument does not conform with his view of how the state was to dispose of the bodies of dead revolutionary Chinese (through cremation). Indeed, a joke common among Peking intellectuals just after the monument was built went: "A *t'u-pao-tzu* (bumpkin) from the countryside visits his city cousin, who takes him to see Mao's tomb. 'Ai-ya,' the bumpkin says. 'It's so big! Chairman Mao always wanted to be just like one of us. He never wanted to distance himself from the masses. How could you build him such a big and imposing *ling-mu* (mausoleum)?' 'Oh,' answers the city cousin, 'just to prove that he's really dead.' "[179]

In Europe and South America, tradition dictates that many of the wealthy still be entombed in mausoleums, rather than being cremated or buried.

Ambrose Bierce commented on mausoleums, saying:

Worms'-meat ... The contents of the Taj Mahal, the Tombeau Napoleon and the Granatarium. Worms-meat is usually outlasted by the structure that houses it, but "this too must pass away." Probably the silliest work in which a human being can engage is construction of a tomb for himself. The solemn purpose cannot dignify, but only accentuates by contrast the foreknown futility.[180]

540

He goes on to say:

> Ambitious fool! so mad to be a show!
> How profitless the labor you bestow
>     Upon a dwelling whose magnificence
> The tenant neither can admire nor know.
>
> Build deep, build high, build massive as you can,
> The wanton grass-roots will defeat the plan
>     By shouldering asunder all the stones
> In what to you would be a moment's span.[181]

Over the past two centuries, mausoleums have been particularly popular in non-Protestant U.S. cemeteries, especially those catering to the wealthy. Huge cathedral-like structures, designed by world-famous architects and incorporating Tiffany stained-glass windows, were built for families such as the Rockefellers and the Vanderbilts. Even Jewish cemeteries, such as Bayside and Salem Fields in Brooklyn, had mausoleums for above ground burial, in contrast to modern Jewish teachings on earth burial (although they more closely adhered to the biblical tradition of cave burial).[182]

In the United States, New Orleans is the only site where above ground entombment is the most common form of body disposal. That is due to geography as much as culture. Since New Orleans is barely kept dry by its levees, and the water table lies close to the ground's surface, underground interment of bodies there would lead to many unfortunate and unexpected surfacings. In 1788, after a flood, a fire and an epidemic devastated the city, authorities established the St. Louis cemetery, containing the first of the famous above-ground, oven-like tombs, designed so that the flood-waters could not reach the bodies and endanger health. "These tombs contained *loculi*, or oven-like recesses, into which coffins were placed. After the bodies had decayed, the coffins were removed and burned. The bones were then swept through a hole to fall into a recess or *caveau* below that contained family bones...Costs of stone were high, however, and so stucco-faced brick, wood, and iron were the cheapest materials for tombs, although they did not survive long in a pristine state in the swampy cemeteries."[183]

In the 1870s, an increasing public demand for entombment led to the establishment of community mausoleums. Marketed to the middle class, these structures offered entombment within a larger mausoleum, albeit at a substantial cost. The prices charged were based on location. Hallway entombments were a base price, while niches in small private vault rooms off the corridor were priced considerably higher. A classic mausoleum from the early twentieth century, the Cathedral of Memories in Hartsdale, New York, contains 8,800 crypts, 250 private family rooms, and an 80-seat chapel. A similar structure is Forest Lawn's Great Mausoleum.

As mausoleums became more common, the odor from corpses became a problem. So that the living would not be offended by the smell of unburied, unembalmed corpses, special provisions were taken to seal the caskets entombed above ground. Frequently, bodies were placed in coffins which were then sealed in one or more leaden caskets.

Mausoleums vary in size, from those made for only one casket to those housing many caskets from an extended family. Mausoleums that contain more than one family crypt are usually two to three stories high. One mausoleum in Nashville, Tennessee, the Woodlawn Mausoleum, however, stands twenty stories high and will accommodate 129,000 bodies. Nashville natives have dubbed it "Death Hilton."[184] Nashville is not alone in high-rise mausoleums, though. Rio de Janeiro, Brazil, boasts a $14,000,000, 39-story mausoleum known as "the big condominium in the sky."[185]

Most mausoleums are enclosed structures. Some sun belt states, however, also have unroofed garden mausoleums with honeycomb-like crypts. And other areas of the country have developed more open, unheated mausoleums, often surrounding centrally-heated chapels. These are much less costly to maintain than traditional indoor, heated mausoleums and are thus favored by the funeral industry.

Mausoleums are still being built in the United States, especially outside of the midwestern states. Once reserved for the rich and famous, mausoleum interment is becoming attractive for its physical appearance and visible memorialization, even though it costs $1,500 to $25,000 plus the cost of opening and closing the crypt. Some cost even more. Irving Thalberg's tomb in Forest Lawn cost $800,000 at the time of his death.[186] The mausoleum for the Helmsleys (of tax-evasion infamy) has a stained-glass representation of the New York City skyline and reportedly cost hundreds of thousands of dollars.[187] Why people want above-ground interment is unclear, but the cemetery owners' motives are obvious. Interest in mausoleums seems to be directly related to an increase in disposable income and a growing acceptance of displays of social and economic distinctions (conspicuous consumption).

Cemetery owners' interest in mausoleums result from their large profits on garden and other open mausoleums (due to the economical use of space compared to earth burials), their low maintenance costs, and the package, including use of the cemetery chapel and marker, they can sell (and be paid for) on a "preneed" basis. Cemeteries can charge much more for a mausoleum than a standard grave, there can be 10,000 bodies per acre (versus at most about 3,000 per acre at a crowded standard cemetery), and it guarantees room for future customers since there are generally about 14 crypts in each mausoleum. As one mausoleum builder graphically put it, "A mausoleum can take a ten-acre cemetery and change it into a 100-acre cemetery by going up."[188]

## Z. WHAT ARE THE DIFFERENCES AMONG TOMBS, SEPULCHERS, CRYPTS & SARCOPHAGI?

All of these terms denote structures that house corpses, and since any of them can hold one or more bodies, it may sometimes be difficult to differentiate among them. As Ariès points out, "Washington, D.C. is a city filled with commemorative monuments, such as those to Washington, Jefferson, and Lincoln—which are 'tombs' without sepulchers..."[189] By this he means, without bodies.

The *tomb* or *sepulcher* is the basic burial structure. Although it can simply indicate a hole in the ground for the burial of a corpse, it more commonly indicates a structure or vault for interment, either below or above ground. As Barbara Jones describes it, the tomb is "the final word, the lasting praise, the *durable* memento, the paperweight to pin down the poor soul for ever."[190]

A subterranean burial vault or chamber, often beneath the floor of a church is called a crypt. Modern terminology also uses this term for the space in a *mausoleum*, an above-ground structure, usually of stone, in which one or more bodies are entombed. (See also *What is a mausoleum?*) The body itself can reside in a regular coffin or in a sarcophagus, a stone coffin which is usually inscribed and adorned with sculptured figures. A few very expensive modern sarcophagi are made of copper.[191] Sarcophagi can also function as above-ground, one-body mausoleums.

The earliest existing tombs in North America are the great burial mounds built by Native American cultures flourishing in the Ohio Valley from 1000 to 300 B.C. These conical dirt heaps contain the bodies of the tribes' important members and those others who were slain to serve them in death as well as burial objects.[192]

In ancient Rome, everyone, including slaves, had burial places or *loculi* marked with that person's name and often his portrait. Around the fifth century A.D. identification on tombs became rare. Personal identification of tombs did not reappear again in Europe until the thirteenth century, and then only for very important personages. In mid-eighteenth century Europe, tombs began to once again commonly commemorate people after their deaths.

United States cemeteries that permit erection of crypts, tombs, sarcophagi & mausoleums normally require the purchase of multiple grave sites (lots). The number of lots that must be purchased depend upon the size of the monument and the peculiarities of the individual cemetery.

# KENNETH V. ISERSON

## AA. WHAT LAWS & RELIGIOUS RESTRICTIONS GOVERN BURIAL AND CEMETERIES?

Multiple laws and religious rules have always governed burials. Many of these are covered in Chapter 11, *What differences exist between funerals in different religions & cultures?*. The different perception of funerary customs is well illustrated by the story told by Puckle, an early twentieth-century writer in 1926:

> A soldier going to place flowers on the grave of a fallen comrade met a native carrying a food offering to his ancestral tomb. Amused by this superstitious absurdity, the soldier asked him when his ancestors would emerge from their tomb to enjoy their meal. "About the same time as your friend comes up to smell your flowers," he answered.[193]

Whether it is religious or social custom, a common practice among many religions and societies is for a close relative to throw the first spadeful of earth on the coffin. According to the Scots, "it is regarded as a sacred duty and is not declined even by the most afflicted widow." Jews also still observe this custom, and in Israel, mourners completely refill the grave. Paradoxically, ancient Jewish graves in Iron Age Palestine sometimes contained offerings of pig bones. This has been explained as not violating Jewish dietary laws, since the dead were also considered "unclean."[194]

In ancient Rome, persons killed by lightning (a death from the gods) were buried on the spot where they died. The site was consecrated by sacrificing sheep, and was enclosed within a wall to prevent anyone committing the sacrilege of treading on the grave.[195]

Islamic bodies are often placed into niches cut into the side of the graves. After a body is placed in the niche, the grave is bricked up before the main grave is filled. The grave itself must be oriented so that the deceased's face is toward Mecca.

Although ecclesiastical law in Europe, especially England, normally controlled burial practices and cemeteries in the past, this was not true in the United States. As one court said, "The repudiation of the ecclesiastical law and of ecclesiastical courts by the American colonies left the temporal courts the sole protector of the dead."[196] Nevertheless, state statutes normally vest the trustees of various religious societies with the control of the graveyards they own. Public graveyards are controlled by the municipality in which they are located. In the United States, large private cemeteries with specific areas designated for particular faiths, and large nonsectarian sections are the rule. Individual Jewish and Catholic cemeteries, however, still prevail, with burial normally restricted to members of those faiths.

Common social proscriptions often break down in cemeteries,

544

sometimes demonstrating a measure of irony. Such is the case when enemies are buried side-by-side, as in the cemetery behind the Koshevo Hospital in Sarajevo, Bosnia-Herzegovina. In that crude cemetery, Serbs, Croats and Bosnian Muslims who killed each other in their brutal ethnic civil war now are interred in the same burial ground.

## AB. WHAT ARE MEMORIAL SOCIETIES?

Memorial or funeral societies are membership-fee organizations that assist families in making funeral arrangements. Burial societies have existed since ancient Rome, although they were occasionally used for shady purposes. Roman fraternal organizations, *collegia*, to which up to one-third of the population belonged, were not only burial societies, but heavily involved in violent political activity around the first century B.C. In their burial mode, they assessed an entry fee and a monthly contribution from members. Upon the death of a member, a lump sum was paid to the heir or whoever organized the funeral. Some fraternal organizations still follow this practice. The communal funds held by some *collegia* disappeared after plagues ravaged Rome, killing off most members.[197] In early England, it was "said that in the guise of 'benefit and burial societies,' [nonconformists] could obtain some protection for their communal property."[198]

The first memorial society in the United States was formed by a Seattle church in 1939, the People's Memorial Association. They sought simple, dignified funerals as "an alternative to the elaborate and costly services pushed by many undertakers." By 1952 they had 650 members and by 1979, 57,000. Between 1965 and 1974, services for 6,956 members cost $1.67 million (avg $240). If they had paid prevailing rates, these same services would have cost $10 million. Yet by 1950, the U.S. only had seven memorial societies. After that, they spread much more quickly, mainly among Protestant groups.[199]

Memorial societies are all non-profit, democratic, and cooperative. Most are members of the Continental Association of Funeral and Memorial Societies (formed 1963) or the Memorial Society Association of Canada (formed 1971). They stress simplicity, dignity, economy, education, and the right of individuals to arrange the disposition of their own bodies.

Society members own and control these organizations. Most require the individual or family to do some funeral pre-planning so that the pressure is taken off loved ones at the time of death. Upon joining a memorial society, a member will usually be asked to complete a prearrangement form that indicates preferences about the disposition of his or her body after death. This form is filed with the society and with a participating funeral home, and can be changed at any time. Many societies, especially those organized through labor unions, offer funerals and burials at lower-than-usual cost.

All legitimate Funeral Reform or memorial societies are nonprofit and membership-controlled. Membership is generally transferrable among societies within North America. While "pseudo-memorial societies" have occasionally been set up as 'fronts' for funeral directors, they are not non-profit organizations controlled by members, nor are they members of the national memorial society organizations. Non-profit memorial or funeral societies differ markedly from the "preneed" solicitations from for-profit cemeteries, funeral homes and crematoria. The former is a service, the latter merely a business arrangement.

More than two hundred memorial societies, primarily run by volunteers, exist throughout the United States and Canada. While the societies once emphasized cremations to the exclusion of burials, either can usually now be obtained. Individuals can cancel their membership at any time. Some societies are specifically organized to help families hold memorial services without the body present, instead of holding the routine open-casket funeral. They also smooth the process of planning, thus eliminating nearly all transactions with funeral directors.

Although there are a handful of funeral home cooperatives in the Midwest, most current memorial societies do not themselves perform funerals or sell funerary merchandise at a low cost. They simply help with preplanning and contract for lower costs through private funeral homes. The funeral industry still controls the prices and the activities. The basis of the memorial society's cost savings is simplicity, collective bargaining, and knowing where to go for the best price.

Two types of memorial societies exist: (1) contract; and (2) cooperating/advisory. *Contract* societies have formal agreements for funeral, cremation, burial and associated services at moderate costs for members. *Cooperating/advisory* societies maintain no formal contract with the funeral industry, but may have verbal agreements with funeral homes. They can steer members to these services. As one investigator noted, "On occasion, morticians who do agree to cooperate are subjected not only to pressure and ostracism from other morticians but also even to disciplinary measures from the state board of funeral directors. In some cases, state boards have prevented a special relationship between a memorial society and an undertaker."[200]

Eventually, more non-profit memorial societies may assume the responsibility for funerals, cremations and burials. They then will become a major threat to the funeral industry establishment.

## AC. REFERENCES

1. Pardi MM: *Death: An Anthropological Perspective.* Washington, DC: Univ Press of America, 1977, 11.
2. Turner AW: *Houses for the Dead.* New York: David McKay, 1976, p 3-4.
3. Gargett R: *Current Anthropology.* 1989;30:157-90.
4. Polson CJ, Brittain RP, Marshall TK: *The Disposal of the Dead.* 2nd ed. Springfield, IL: Charles C Thomas, 1962, p 16.
5. Tegg W: *The Last Act: Being the Funeral Rites of Nations and Individuals.* London: William Tegg & Co, 1876, p 9.
6. Weever J: *Ancient Funeral Monuments.* 1631, pp 6-7. Cited in: Jackson PE: *The Law of Cadavers and of Burial and Burial Places.* New York: Prentice-Hall, 1937, p 7.
7. Ibid.
8. Tegg, *The Last Act,* p 45.
9. Bendann E: *Death Customs: An Analytical Study of Burial Rites.* New York: Alfred A Knopf, 1930, p 48.
10. Cameron JM: The bible and legal medicine. *Med Sci Law.* 1970;10:7-13.
11. Jacob W: *Contemporary American Reform Responsa.* New York: Central Conference of American Rabbis, 1987, pp 163-64.
12. Aquinas T: *Summa Theologica.* Supplement to Third Part, Q. 71, Article 11.
13. St. Augustine: *The City of God I.* Chapter 12.
14. Bassett S: *Death in Towns: Urban Responses to the Dying and the Dead, 100-1600.* Leicester, UK: Leicester Univ Press, 1992, p 32-34.
15. Rodriguez WC, Bass WM: Decomposition of buried bodies and methods that may aid in their location. *J Forensic Sciences.* 1985;30(3):836-52.
16. Abercrombie JR: *Palestinian Burial Practices From 1200 to 600 B.C.E.* (Ph.D. Thesis, Univ of Pennsylvania) Ann Arbor, MI: Univ Microfilms International, 1979, p 170-79.
17. Kaganoff BC: From Machpelah...to Beth She'arim. *The American Cemetery.* 1973;46:32+.
18. Abercrombie, *Palestinian Burial Practices,* p 22.
19. Gordon A: *Death is For the Living.* Edinburgh: Paul Harris, 1984, p 91.
20. Ibid., p 81.
21. Anima N: *Childbirth and Burial Practices among Philippine Tribes.* Quezon City, Phillippines: Omar Pub, 1978, p 86, 93.
22. Coffin MM: *Death in Early America: The History and Folklore of Customs and Superstitions of Early Medicine, Funerals, Burials, and Mourning.* Nashville: Thomas Nelson, 1976, p 137-38.
23. Dolan C: Burying tradition, more people opt for 'fun' funerals. *Wall Street J.* May 20, 1993, p A1+.
24. Scharnberg K: The changing face of honor guards. *American Legion.* 1993;134(5):26-27.
25. Walker GA: *Gatherings From Grave Yards.* London: Longman, 1839. Reprinted by Arno Press, New York: 1977, p 123.
26. Crowther M: *The Workhouse System 1834-1929.* London: Batsford, 1981, p 242.
27. Watson JL, Rawski ES, eds: *Death Ritual in Late Imperial and Modern China.* Berkeley, CA: Univ of California Press, 1988, p 47.
28. Holwell JZ: "The Black Hole of Calcutta." From: *Annual Register.* 1857.
29. Ransom JL: *Andersonville Diary.* Auburn, NY: 1881, pp 87-88.
30. Ienaga S: *The Pacific War, 1931-1945.* New York: Pantheon, 1978, p 186.
31. Ibid., p 89.
32. Nagorski A: At last, a victory for truth. *Newsweek.* October 26, 1992, p 41.
33. Palmer G, exec. producer: *Death: The Trip of a Lifetime.* Seattle, WA: KCTS-TV Public Broadcasting Station, 1993.
34. Mackensie DA: *Ancient Man in Britain.* London: Blackie & Son, 1932, p 170.
35. Basevi WHF: *The Burial of the Dead.* London: Geo Rutledge & Sons, 1920, pp 37-41.

36. Barber P: *Vampires, Burial, and Death: Folklore and Reality.* New Haven, CT: Yale Univ Press, 1988, p 49.
37. Mackensie, *Ancient Man in Britain,* pp 171-72.
38. Pallis CA: Death. In: *The New Encyclopaedia Britannica.* vol 16. (Macropaedia). Chicago: Encyclopaedia Britannica, 1987, p 1039.
39. Anima, *Burial Practices,* p 88.
40. Litten J: *The English Way of Death: The Common Funeral Since 1450.* London: Robert Hale, 1991, p 167.
41. Anderson P: *Affairs In Order.* New York: MacMillan, 1991, p 42.
42. Puckle, *Funeral Customs,* pp 160-61.
43. Abercrombie, *Palestinian Burial Practices,* p 25.
44. Coffin, *Death in Early America,* p 184.
45. Gordon R: *Great Medical Disasters.* New York: Dorset Press, 1983, pp 203-04.
46. Roddis LH: *A Short History of Nautical Medicine.* New York: Paul B Hoeber, 1941, p 73.
47. Dickman S: Brain sections to be buried? *Nature.* 1989;339:498.
48. Alexander L: *Neuropathology and Neurophysiology, Including Electroencephalography in War-time Germany.* Combined Intelligence Objectives Subcommittee, Item No. 24, File No. XXVII-1. July 1945, pp 1-65. As quoted in: Horan DJ, Mall D, eds: *Death, Dying and Euthanasia.* Frederick, MD: Univ Pub of America, 1980, p 575.
49. Lib. v, tit. ii, *De Simonia.* As cited in: Jackson PE: *The Law of Cadavers and of Burial and Burial Places.* New York: Prentice-Hall, 1937, p 27.
50. *Topsall v. Ferrers,* Hob. 175, 80 Eng. Rep. 322.
51. *Fruin v. Dean and Chapter of York,* 2 Keb. 778, 84 Eng. Rep. 491.
52. *Andrews v. Cawthorne,* (1744) 125 Eng. Rep. 1308.
53. Jackson PE: *The Law of Cadavers and of Burial and Burial Places.* New York: Prentice-Hall, 1937, p 64.
54. Howard Belkoff, funeral director: Interview. May 15, 1993.
55. American Association of Retired Persons (AARP): *Cemetery Goods and Services.* (brochure). Washington, DC: AARP, no date, p 7.
56. The latest word: About face. *Hastings Center Report;* Nov/Dec 1991, p 47.
57. Jackson, *Law of Cadavers,* p 63, note 3.
58. Ibid., p 63, note 5.
59. *Matter of Widening Beekman Street.* 4 Bradf. (N.Y. Surr. Preps.) 503.
60. Ariès P: *The Hour of Our Death.* New York: Oxford Univ Press, 1981, p 12.
61. Jackson, *Law of Cadavers,* p 63, note 3.
62. Tegg, *The Last Act,* p 274.
63. Coffin, *Death in Early America,* p 140.
64. Jackson, *Law of Cadavers,* p 92, note 7.
65. Ibid., p 93.
66. Barber, *Vampires, Burial, and Death,* pp 5-7.
67. New Englanders 'killed' corpses, experts say. *Associated Press.* October 30, 1993.
68. Ragon M: *The Space of Death: A Study of Funerary Architecture, Decoration, and Urbanism.* (Sheridan A, trans) Charlottesville, VA: Univ Press of Virginia, 1983. Originally published as *L'espace de la mort: Essai sur l'architecture, la décoration et l'urbanisme funéraires,* Albin Michel, 1981, p 98.
69. Bland O: *The Royal Way of Death.* London: Constable, 1986, p 58.
70. Haestier R: *Dead Men Tell Tales: A Survey of Exhumations, From Earliest Antiquity to the Present Day.* London: John Long, 1934, p 52.
71. Ragon, *Space of Death,* p 96.
72. Curl JS: *The Victorian Celebration of Death.* Detroit: Partridge Press, 1972, p 100.
73. *Thompson v. Deeds,* 93 Iowa 228, 230, 61 N.W. 842.
74. *Danahy v. Kellogg,* 70 Misc. 25, 126 N.Y. Supp. 444.
75. *Perth Amboy Gas Light Co. v. Kilek,* 102 J.J. Eq. 588, 141 Atl. 745.
76. *State v. Clifford,* 81 Wash. 324; 142 P. 472.
77. Curl, *Victorian Celebration of Death,* p 100.

78. Haestier, *Dead Men Tell Tales*, p 46-47.
79. Ibid., pp 70-76.
80. Nationline: No Kennedy exhumation. *USA Today*. July 8, 1992, p 3A.
81. Norton LE, Cottone JA, Spher IM, DiMaio VJM: The exhumation and identification of Lee Harvey Oswald. *J Forensic Sciences*. 1984;29:19-38.
82. Helmer RP: Identification of the cadaver remains of Josef Mengele. *J Forensic Sciences*. 1987;32:1622-44.
83. The search for Adolf Hitler. *Prodigy News Service*. July 14, 1992.
84. Explorer's grave to be examined. *St. Louis Post-Dispatch*. August 16, 1992, p 8D.
85. Bierce A: *Devil's Dictionary*. New York: Dover Pub, 1958, p 21.
86. Pardovan. 1709, pp 173-74. Quoted in: Jackson, *Law of Cadavers*, p 177.
87. Plutarch: *The Lives of Noble Grecians and Romans—Lycurgus*. In: *Great Books of the Western World*, vol 14, 1952, p 46.
88. Plato: *Laws XII*. In: *Great Books*, vol 7, 1952, p 793.
89. Man I: The rifts in Egypt's "village." *World Press Review*. 1993;40(7):32.
90. Berthold: La ville de Paris en vers burlosques. *Journal d'un voyage à Paris en 1657*. Quoted in: Dufour V: *Paris à travers les âges, (Paris 1857-82)*. vol 2.
91. Burial. *The North American Review*. 1861.
92. Sourkes TL: The origins of neurochemistry: the chemical study of the brain in France at the end of the eighteenth century. *J Hist Med*. 1992;47:322-39.
93. Ragon, *Space of Death*, p 145.
94. Tegg, *The Last Act*, p 17.
95. Jackson KT, Vergara CJ: *Silent Cities*. New York: Princeton Architectural Press, 1989, p 26.
96. Dempsey D: *The Way We Die*. New York: MacMillan, 1975, pp 194-95.
97. *Humphreys v. Bennett Oil Corp.*, 195 La. 531, 197 So. 222 (1940).
98. Curley TP: Catholic Funeral Ritual emphasizes burial service. *The American Funeral Director*. 1992;115(2):38-44.
99. Rice J: Days of the dead. *Arizona Daily Star*. Tucson, AZ: October 31, 1993, p A16.
100. Haestier, *Dead Men Tell Tales*, p 136.
101. *The Builder*. London: 1843, p 104. Quoted in: Curl, *Victorian Celebration of Death*, p 35.
102. Taylor AD: Landscape composition in modern cemetery design. *The American City*. March 1928.
103. Jackson, *Law of Cadavers*, p 300.
104. Grycznski, ES, Tolleson LJ, Audie EH: *Taps—A Guide to Military-Oriented Burial*. Alexandria, VA: Retired Officers' Assn, 1990, p 11.
105. Mitford J: *The American Way of Death*. New York: Simon & Schuster, 1963, pp 127-28.
106. Drewes DW: *Cemetery Land Planning*. Pittsburgh, PA: Matthews Memorial Bronze, 1964, p 85.
107. Ibid., p vii.
108. *Concordia Cemetery Assn v. Minnesota, etc., Ry.*, 121 Ill. 199, 211, 12 N.E. 536.
109. Farrell JJ: *Inventing the American Way of Death 1830-1920*. Philadelphia, PA: Temple Univ Press, 1980, p 10.
110. Anderson, *Affairs in Order*, p 44.
111. Koosman S: *Cultural Variations in Funeral Practice*. (lecture). National Funeral Directors Association Annual Convention, Baltimore, MD: 1989. (audiotape)
112. Reaching for the moon. *The American Funeral Director*. 1992;115(1):6.
113. Coffin, *Death in Early America*, p 127.
114. Holman JM: The undertaker's lot in America. *Casket and Sunnyside*. 1972;101(13):14-15.
115. Johnson K: Ruling OKs burials despite strike. *USA Today*. January 10, 1992, p 3A.
116. Ibid.
117. Belkoff, Interview, May 22, 1993.
118. Shakespeare W: *Hamlet*. Act V, scene I, lines 45-46, 66.
119. *U.S. Public Law* 101-601.

120. Ditch digger finds prehistoric Indian grave. *The American Funeral Director.* 1992;115(8):82.
121. Erickson J: Return of Indian remains, artifacts to tribes 'a long, drawn-out process'. *Arizona Daily Star.* Tucson, AZ: June 6, 1993, p B1+.
122. Ibid.
123. Ragon, *Space of Death,* p 51.
124. Ariès, *Hour of Our Death,* pp 59-60.
125. Dr. Haguenot. In: Walker, *Gatherings From Grave Yards,* p 95.
126. *Weekly Dispatch.* London: September 30, 1838.
127. Watson, Rawski, *Death Ritual,* pp 16, 103.
128. Granqvist H: *Muslim Death and Burial—Arab Customs and Traditions Studied in a Village in Jordan.* Helsinke-Helsingfors: Societas Scientiarum Fennica, 1965;34:56.
129. Jackson, *Law of Cadavers,* p 353.
130. Ibid., p 101.
131. *Gilbert v. Buzzard and Boyer,* 3 Phill. 335, 161 Eng. Rep. 1342.
132. Ibid.
133. Koosman, *Cultural Variations,* 1989. (audiotape)
134. Camus A: *The Plague.* New York: Vintage Books, 1948, p 167.
135. Bernard HY: *The Law of Death and Disposal of the Dead.* 2nd ed. Dobbs Ferry, NY: Oceana Pub, 1979, p 4.
136. Donne J: *Progress of the Soul.* 1601.
137. Sourkes, *J Hist Med,* 1992.
138. Haestier, *Dead Men Tell Tales,* p 87.
139. Hill RB, Anderson RE: *The Autopsy—Medical Practice and Public Policy.* Boston: Butterworths, 1988, p 119.
140. Coffin, *Death in Early America,* p 126.
141. Kaganoff, *The American Cemetery,* 1973.
142. *Singapore Free Press.* As quoted in: Song Ong Siang: *One Hundred Years' History of the Chinese in Singapore.* Singapore: Oxford Univ Press, 1984, p 421. (reprint of 1902 book.) Cited in: Yeoh BSA: The control of "sacred" space: conflicts over the Chinese burial grounds in colonial Singapore, 1880- 1930. *J Southeast Asian Studies.* 1991;22:282-311.
143. *Cemeteries as Open Space Reservations,* HUD Report, 1970.
144. Emmitt Watson (caretaker and historian): Interview. Neptune Society Columbarium. San Francisco, CA: May 18, 1993.
145. Ibid.
146. van Wyk CW, Theunissen F, Phillips VM: A grave matter—dental findings of people buried in the 19th and 20th centuries. *J Forensic Odonto-Stomatology.* 1990;8(2):15-30.
147. Graham B: Work to recover bodies from flooded cemetery may cost $200,000. *Arizona Daily Star.* Tucson, AZ: September 5, 1993, p A16.
148. Price R: Washed-away bodies in 'God's care.' *USA Today.* November 11, 1993, p A3.
149. Jackson, *Law of Cadavers,* p 395.
150. *Campbell v. Kansas City,* 102 Mo. 339, 348, 13 S. W. 897.
151. Urbain J-D: *La Societe di Conservation.* Paris: Payot, 1978.: and Ragon, *Space of Death,* p 82.
152. Santore R: Interview—Dave Beck. *AFD Today.* 1992;4(6):1, 12-14.
153. AARP, *Cemetery Goods and Services,* p 7.
154. Wallace L. As quoted in: Peter LJ: *Peter's Quotations.* New York: Bantam, 1977, p 498.
155. Watson, Rawski, *Death Ritual,* p 30.
156. Unknown. Quoted in: Curl JS: *A Celebration of Death: An introduction to some of the buildings, monuments, and settings of funerary architecture in the Western European tradition.* London: Constable, 1980, pp 95-96.
157. Coffin, *Death in Early America,* pp 145, 156.

158. New Hampshire gravestones finally rest in peace. *The American Funeral Director.* 1992;115(6):82-83.
159. Mitford, *American Way of Death,* p 106.
160. Schwartz N: It's highly personal; It's "cemetery art". *Wall Street J.* September 3, 1992, p A1.
161. Anima, *Burial Practices,* p 65.
162. Nationline: Tombstone Debt. *USA Today.* November 21, 1991, p 3A.
163. Puttenham R: *The Arte of English Poesie.* As quoted in: Coffin, *Death in Early America,* p 183.
164. Items of Interest: Shortest Epitaph. *The American Funeral Director.* 1992;115(6):4.
165. Peter LJ: *Peter's Quotations.* New York: Bantam Books, 1979, p 498.
166. Doelman J: An unnoted funeral epitaph by Nicholas Ferrar. *Notes and Queries.* 1992;39(4):446.
167. Copyrighted as Brilliant Thought No. 1041 by Ashleigh Brilliant.
168. Stevens A: Exactly how many Brilliant Thoughts are there? 5,632. *Wall Street J.* January 6, 1992, p A1+.
169. *Ez Achaim Society v. Cohen,* 15 Misc. 2d 540, 181 N.Y.S. 2d 717 (1958).
170. Cited in: Haestier, *Dead Men Tell Tales,* p 137.
171. Coffin, *Death in Early America,* pp 180-81.
172. Koosman, *Cultural Variations,* 1989. (audiotape)
173. Tegg, *The Last Act,* p 20.
174. Kaganoff, *The American Cemetery,* 1973.
175. Information on display at the Royal Ontario Museum. Toronto, Canada: 1992.
176. Bassett, *Death in Towns,* p 18.
177. Tegg, *The Last Act,* p 62.
178. Bragg R: The legacy of the "king of the world." *World Press Review.* October 1992, p 51.
179. Wakeman F: Mao's remains. In: Watson, Rawski, *Death Ritual,* pp 254-88.
180. Bierce A: *Devil's Dictionary.* New York: Dover Pub, 1958, p 142.
181. Huck J (probably fictitious): quoted in Bierce A: *Devil's Dictionary,* New York: Dover Pub, 1958, pp 142-43.
182. Belkoff, Interview, May 22, 1993.
183. Curl, *Celebration of Death,* (1980), pp 146-47.
184. Hemphill P: Room at the top. *The New York Times.* February 13, 1972, p 10.
185. Dempsey, *The Way We Die,* p 196.
186. Harmer RM: *The High Cost of Dying.* New York: Crowell-Collier Press, 1963, p 44.
187. Anderson, *Affairs In Order,* p 44.
188 An anonoymous mausoleum builder. Indianapolis, IN: 1982. In: Jackson, Vergara, *Silent Cities,* p 112.
189. Ariès, P: *Western Attitudes Toward Death from the Midde Ages to the Present.* Baltimore, MD: Johns Hopkins Press, 1979, p 78-79.
190. Jones B: *Design for Death.* Indianapolis, IN: Bobbs-Merrill Co, 1967, p 203.
191. Belkoff, Interview, May 22, 1993.
192. Stuart GE: Who were the "mound builders"? *National Geographic.* 1972;142(6):782-801.
193. Puckle, *Funeral Customs,* p 171.
194. Abercrombie, *Palestinian Burial Practices,* p 189.
195. Tegg, *The Last Act,* p 48.
196. *Wightman v. Wightman,* (N.Y.) 4 Johns., Ch. 343.
197. Bassett, *Death in Towns,* p 20-24.
198. Maitland: *History of English Law.* 2nd ed. p 2. As quoted in: Jackson, *Law of Cadavers,* p 281.
199. Fruehling JA, ed: *Sourcebook on Death and Dying.* Chicago, IL: Marquis Prof Pub, 1982, pp 147-48.
200. Ibid.

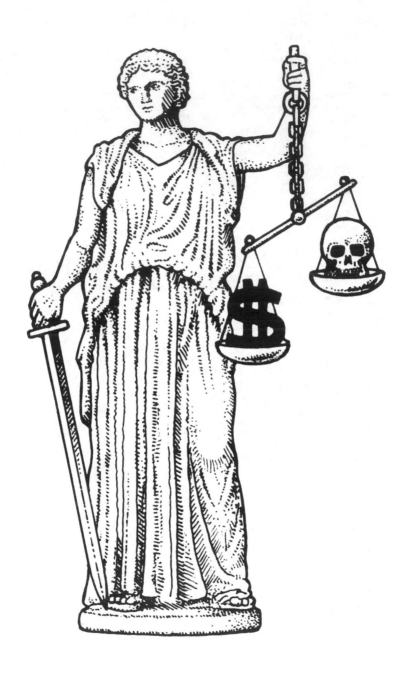

# 13: A HAND FROM THE GRAVE

*After burial or cremation the body may be gone, but some questions remain to be answered. What is the environmental impact of different corpse-disposal methods? What are the optimal methods for preserving a corpse? Who owns the body and what is the place of advance directives (living wills, etc.) in determining what will happen to the body?*

## A. WHAT WILL MY DISPOSAL DO TO THE ENVIRONMENT?

Environmentalists justifiably worry about what body disposal is doing to our soil and air. Ground water has been contaminated from decomposing bodies injected with chemical preservatives, including formaldehyde, which the Occupational Safety and Health Administration has classified as a hazardous chemical linked to cancer and birth defects. Many cemeteries require grave liners, but even when they are used it is not clear that they do much to stop the seepage.

Crematory emissions also pose environmental hazards. One funeral historian pointedly wrote of cremations, "Outside, as the mourners exchange greetings and inspect the wreaths, a plume of black acrid smoke rises from the ill-disguised chimney, bearing its load of burnt plastic and Terylene up, up and away to make its contribution to the 'greenhouse' effect. Cremation may be 'clean' but it's certainly not 'green.' "[1] Florida and California currently regulate their crematories, although few other states do. The Florida legislature, to reduce the output of potentially dangerous substances, recently required cremation temperature raised by 200°F, to 1,800°F (982°C). California may further regulate its cremation industry after studying the results of emission testing which indicated the presence of high levels of dioxins, trace metals or other pollutants from incinerated bodies and caskets. They may require crematories to relocate away from population centers, install scrubbers at about $150,000 each, or both. It is also possible that the Federal Clean Air Act implementation will mandate crematory monitoring, relocation or scrubbers across the country. This will invariably lead to an increased cost for cremations.[2]

Some environmentalists also worry about the effect of cremating people wearing plutonium-powered pacemakers. As one said, "there are all these people wandering around with little blobs of plutonium in their chests. When they're cremated, they release radioactivity into the environment."[3] In actuality, extremely few pacemakers have ever had plutonium batteries.

Somewhat facetiously, the executive director of the Crematory Association of America has been quoted as saying, "In the burial process there are problems with seepage. We have problems with incineration. So make it illegal to bury, illegal to burn, outlaw death and we'll be done with it."[4]

So what should the environmentally conscious do? "I think people were on to something 100 years ago," a staffer with the San Francisco's Natural Resources Defense Council said. "Stashing people in pine boxes and letting them decompose—ashes to ashes, you know."[5] Many people, however, seem to be anxious to hurry the process. In France during the fifteenth century, many people who could not be buried in Paris' *Cimetière des SS. Innocents* often requested that some earth from burial ground be placed in their grave, since the cemetery was known as "the flesh eater," reportedly decomposing bodies within twenty-four hours. At the time, prolonged preservation of the body was viewed by many as a curse.[6]

Richard Selzer has his fictionalized physician express the same sentiments:

> I want to be buried—unembalmed and unboxed—at the foot of a tree. Soon I melt and seep into the ground, to be drawn up by the roots. Straight to the top, strung in the crown, answering the air. There would be the singing of birds, the applause of wings.[7]

## B.  HOW CAN MY BODY BEST BE PRESERVED?

Historians have recorded many accounts of bodies, whether embalmed or not, that have survived years or even centuries in relatively good condition. How was this achieved? The essential ingredients appear to be initially disinfecting the body, as with embalming or soaking the body in alcohol, keeping it from carnivorous insects and animals, and preventing oxidation through use of an airtight casket. (A truly airtight casket, however, is nearly impossible to achieve according to scientists who still search for "pure ancient air" in sealed caskets.) Nevertheless, it is claimed that Napoleon's body, without embalming, survived intact for many years by being hermetically sealed in a casket. So too did the bodies of several kings of England, although some of those bodies may also have been embalmed.

If individuals desire to have their bodies preserved for centuries, a thorough embalming followed by impregnating the body in a block of plastic should work wonders. The danger, of course, is that it could work too well. Many specimens of human remains that are not as well preserved are currently on display in museums. Wouldn't these same museums pay top dollar in 100 years (or less) to display well-preserved remains? Perhaps this method should only be tried by the ultimate exhibitionist. No one is currently preserving human remains in this fashion, although modern mummification or plastination may work just as well. (See Chapter 5, *How does a mummy differ from an embalmed body?* and Chapter 3, *How are bodies prepared as dissection cadavers?*)

555

## C. WHO OWNS MY BODY AFTER DEATH?

In England, the deceased person's executor must dispose of the corpse. In the United States and Scotland, the next-of-kin has this responsibility. In no case does control of the body extend beyond that point.

A classic comment on the treatment of dead bodies was written by Justice Joseph Henry Lumpkin of the Georgia Supreme Court:

> Death is unique. It is unlike aught else in its certainty and its incidents. A corpse in some respects is the strangest thing on earth. A man who but yesterday breathed and thought and walked among us has passed away. Something has gone. The body is left still and cold, and is all that is visible to mortal eye of the man we knew...It must be laid away. And the law—that rule of action which touches all human things—must touch also this thing of death. It is not surprising that the law relating to this mystery of what death leaves behind cannot be precisely brought within the letter of all the rules regarding corn, lumber and pig iron. And yet the body must be buried or disposed of...And the law, in its all-sufficiency, must furnish some rule...in dealing with the dead and those sentiments connected with decently disposing of the remains of the departed which furnish one ground of difference between men and brutes.[8]

In England, from the eleventh-century Norman Conquest until the nineteenth century, the church controlled the body and its disposition after death. While the deceased's property, "heir-looms," were controlled by the secular courts and passed on to the rightful parties, heirs had no property rights to their ancestor's body.[9]

The position of English law is well stated by Judge Blackstone: "But, though the heir has a property right in the monuments and escutcheons of his ancestors, yet he has none in their bodies or ashes; nor can he bring any civil action against such as indecently, at least, if not impiously, violate and disturb their remains when dead and buried."[10] The traditional attitude toward corpses, passed down to modern law is that the corpse is *nullius in bonis*, no person's property.

In 1856, the New York Supreme Court commissioned a prominent jurist, Samuel B. Ruggles, to produce guidelines for dead-body cases, since they had such a case before them that they thought would be the first of many. As another court later quoted, the essence of his report was:

> 1. That neither a corpse, nor its burial, is legally subject, in any way, to ecclesiastical cognizance, nor to sacerdotal [priestly] power of any kind.
> 2. That the right to bury a corpse and to preserve its remains, is a

legal right, which the courts of law will recognize and protect.

3. That such right, in the absence of any testamentary disposition, belongs exclusively to the next-of-kin.
4. That the right to protect the remains includes the right to preserve them by separate burial, to select the place of sepulture, and to change it at pleasure.
5. That if the place of burial be taken for public use, the next-of-kin may claim to be indemnified for the expense of removing and suitably reinterring the remains.[11]

The phrase "next-of-kin" in paragraph (3) has normally given preference to the surviving spouse. The phrase, "to change it at pleasure," in paragraph (4) however, has been viewed with a jaundiced eye when there was no pressing reason for exhumation.

United States law now generally holds that the right to dispose of a person's remains rests, in order, with the surviving spouse, adult children, parents, and then siblings. The exact order is governed by each state's laws.[12]

Gradually, U.S. law accepted that next-of-kin had a general property right of "holding and protecting the body until it is processed for burial, cremation or other lawful disposition; selecting the place and manner of disposition, and carrying out the burial or other last rites; and the right to the undisturbed repose of the remains in grave, crypt, niche, urn, or elsewhere sanctioned by law."[13] Violations are actionable in courts of equity and law. The explicit nature of these rights has been summed up in the *Southern California Law Review*, as:

1. The right to a "Christian burial," using this phrase as the courts have done, not with reference to religious rites, but to a burial comporting with the prevailing sense of decency in the community.
2. The right (in the survivor) to select the place of burial. As to which of several survivors, in case of disagreement, the general rule provides the following order of precedence:
3. The wishes, testamentary or otherwise, of the deceased.
4. The wishes of the surviving spouse, if not estranged from the deceased, and unless these wishes are waived.
5. The next-of-kin, in order of relationship to the deceased: children of legal age, parents, brothers and sisters, and other more distant kin.
6. The executor or administrator of the estate, usually only to the extent of paying for the disposal.
7. The person under whose roof a death occurs, or the master of a vessel when a passenger or member of the ship's company dies.

These rights can be overridden when a preference might keep other sentimentally close persons from visiting the burial site, when the deceased's religious values would be violated, when a party has legally "dirty hands," (misconduct or wrong motives) or a specific law intervenes.[14]

The question of what rights relatives have over dead bodies through their obligation to bury the body has been mixed with the legal question of the body as (commercial) property. The right to possession of a corpse has repeatedly been termed a "quasi-property" right in the manner of a "sacred trust" that a court will uphold.[15] The exact nature of this right is still being worked out in the courts, and the courts are awarding damages against the funeral industry among others. Common causes of legal action include delaying interment, unjustified or improper mutilation of the body, performing an unauthorized autopsy or an autopsy that goes beyond what was authorized, unlawful disinterment, or interference at or with a grave.[16]

There is a difference between ownership and control. In medical examiner cases, the medical examiner has control of the body until he or she completes the examinations required by law. In many cases the medical examiner or the investigator releases the body immediately upon death, after notification by phone. But in a very complex case, he may need to hold a body for more than 36 hours to get the samples needed to complete his examination.

In the past, some U.S. crematories charged $25 for releasing ashes to survivors. The Federal Trade Commission (FTC) pointed out that the crematory did not acquire any property rights to the cremated remains simply by providing cremation services. They said of this practice, "the right to dispose of the remains vested in the deceased's wife or next-of-kin according to state law. The crematory is paid separately for the cremation services it renders. The consumer gets no goods or services for the $25 or more he must pay to obtain the remains. Such a charge is nothing more than a ransom..."[17]

Another "right" sometimes claimed for the deceased is that of privacy. In the modern climate of AIDS and other communicable diseases, does the deceased have a right to privacy after death? Legally, it appears that the right to privacy does not extend into the grave, although many states follow the American Medical Association's recommendation that they guard information about deaths from HIV infection more than other causes of death.[18] United States common law holds that the only rights a dead body has (except as noted in statute) exist for the purposes of burial.[19-22]

The responsibility to pay for burial extends from the responsibility to bury the corpse. This derives, in part, from the civil law of ancient Rome. The spouse or other "householders" have the primary responsibility for funeral expenses, followed by the estate or someone charged in life to care for the individual. Lastly, the state may have to intervene and pay for burial or other disposition.[23]

South African law, derived from Roman and Dutch law, is that a dead person has neither rights nor duties. Yet the wishes of the deceased as expressed in a will can direct what is done with the body. If no directions were left, the relatives, generally the heirs, may determine what is done. Failing this, the state decides on and pays for the disposition.[24]

## D. CAN A CORPSE BE HELD FOR NONPAYMENT OF DEBTS?

No. In pre-industrial England, creditors occasionally intervened to stop a burial, since it was generally thought to be legal until 1804 to use this technique to "torture the compassion of friends" into paying the deceased's debts.[25]

In 1598, according to the records of the Church courts in Essex, Thomas Bett "did go into the grave made for the body of Edward Godfrie and did there arrest the body with very unseemly, unrelevant and intemperate speech, whereby [the] minister would not bury him or read the burial service for him."[26] A similar incident in 1689 was recorded in the parish register of Sparsholt, Berkshire, "The corpse of John Matthews, of Fawley, was stopped on the church way for debt August 27. And having lain there four days was by justices warrant buried in the place to prevent annoyances—but about six weeks after it was by an Order of Sessions taken up and buried in the churchyard by the wife of the deceased."[27] Even the famous were not spared this indignity. In 1700 the body of the poet Dryden was seized to collect a debt, and as late as 1784 the body of Sir Bernard Taylor suffered the same misfortune. There is no record that creditors ever recovered their money, and in the early nineteenth century both statutes and courts clearly made such practices illegal.[28,29]

In the United States, detaining bodies to assure the payment of debts has never been condoned. Laws in Rhode Island and Massachusetts forbidding the practice, however, suggest that it was tried.[30,31] In addition, U.S. common law has long held that it is not larceny to steal a corpse,[32] although a corpse may not be held as security for funeral costs[33] and cannot be withheld by an express company or returned to the sender when shipped COD.[34,35] However, a Flint, Michigan funeral director is holding the corpse of James McDill, who died on February 26, 1989, until the family pays him $3605.29 in unpaid funeral expenses. Says J. Merril Spencer, owner of House of Spencer Mortuary, "The body is still in the basement of my parlor, and will stay there until they pay me." There are no Michigan state laws requiring burial if there has been no payment.[36]

559

## E. DO I HAVE A CHOICE ABOUT WHAT HAPPENS TO ME AFTER DEATH?

A person of sound mind may normally direct the disposal of property and disposal of his or her body in any reasonable manner. "Reasonable" is the operative word, however. Jackson points out, "as a practical matter unreasonable or eccentric testamentary (after-death) directions are avoided by the courts upon one ground or another."[37]

Sir Benjamin Richardson, an early proponent of cremation, wished to be cremated upon death, although his family was adamant that they would prevent that from happening. Since British law gave all rights of disposal to the next-of-kin, it seemed he had no options. However, he amended his will so that if he was not cremated his entire fortune (a considerable sum) would go to the cremation society. After his death his family and the clergy first refused to allow cremation, but after finding this codicil in his will, they relented and inherited the loot.[38]

Thomas Hardy had Michael Henchard, a character in his *The Mayor of Casterbridge*, detail in his will what he did *not* want done after his death:

> That Elizabeth-Jane Farfrae be not told of my death,
>     or made to grieve on account of me.
>     & that I be not buried in consecrated ground.
>     & that no sexton be asked to toll the bell.
>     & that nobody is wished to see my dead body.
>     & that no mourners walk behind me at my funeral.
>     & that no flours be planted on my grave.
>     & that no man remember me.
> To this I put my name.[39]

One may request an elaborate funeral and burial consistent with one's social status, but if there is no money available the wishes expressed may not be carried out. As a New York court said of a ne'er-do-well, "as he left nothing of account behind him, the surrogate ought not to take the [costly] way of living of the deceased into consideration...An extravagant mode of life adds nothing to the real position of a poor man, and, while the expense of the funeral is often determined by position in life, in this case the mode of life should not be taken into consideration."[40]

Charles Lindbergh, the first man to fly solo across the Atlantic Ocean, laid out exactly how he wanted to be buried, what the funeral was to be like, and what hymns he wanted sung, as he lay dying of leukemia. As soon as he died, his wishes were carried out: he was dressed in his normal clothes, and buried, without embalming, in a plain wooden coffin.

Winston Churchill, while he was still in fine health and reportedly downing a quart of whiskey a day, laid out every detail of his funeral. He planned the order in which the British regimental guard marched, the music they played, the route to St. Paul's Cathedral, the fly-over by the surviving RAF pilots who had fought in the Battle of Britain, and the path to Chartwell Cemetery. The funeral went exactly as planned. On the other hand, Churchill's friend, President Franklin D. Roosevelt, also left explicit instructions for his funeral in a four-page letter dated December 26, 1937. He wanted a very simple funeral with no hearse, lying-in-state or embalming, and burial in an unlined grave in a plain wooden casket. Unfortunately, these instructions were found in his safe three days after his burial. For instructions to be followed after death, someone has to know about them in advance!

In the Netherlands, as of 1991, persons over the age of 16 deemed mentally incompetent and unable to make decisions for themselves during life, still have the right to direct what will happen to their bodies after death.[41]

## F. WHAT ARE ADVANCE DIRECTIVES AND CAN THEY INCLUDE AFTER-DEATH INSTRUCTIONS?

It was not unusual for physicians, such as Sir William Osler, the famous Canadian physician (1849-1919), to use their wills to request an autopsy, hoping that the knowledge gained by it would assist all physicians, or at least the physicians who had treated them. They also often left detailed medical histories to aid the dissector. In 1772 an unknown London physician suffering from what we now know was *angina pectoris*, wrote in Medical Transactions in the *Critical Review*:

> If it please God to take me away suddenly, I have left directions on my will to send an account of my death to you, with a permission for you to order such an examination of my body, as will shew the cause of it; and, perhaps tend at the same time, to a discovery of the origin of this disorder, and be productive of means to counteract and remove it.[42]

Three weeks later when the doctor died, John Hunter, the noted surgeon and anatomist (and occasional consort of body snatchers) dissected his body, but unfortunately did not make the connection between the state of his coronary (heart) arteries and his symptoms.[43]

Today, if one wishes to donate organs, he should do so through the use of an organ donor card, and not a will, since by the time someone finds a will and takes it through probate, the organs or tissues will be unusable.

According to law, if a will causes defamatory statements to be printed about survivors, the estate can be sued.[44] In one case, a Pittsburgh man left a will directing that "two busts be executed ...as legacies to two of the most unprincipled scoundrels who ever appeared before a court of justice." Since the dead man's property was repeatedly subdivided and built up and now forms the core of the city, this clause has been read many hundreds of times as titles have been examined.[45]

Guidelines for expressing your wishes about the disposal of your body are included in the following section. This information will assist your family and friends greatly in feeling that they have done what you wanted. As lawyers who advise on individuals funeral pre-planning have said, "If your survivors have no idea as to your preferences, they are likely to put up little resistance to the arguments of a funeral director in favor of the most expensive funeral they can (or think they can) afford. These arguments center on three areas in which your survivors may be vulnerable: (1) social status and conspicuous display...(2) an appeal to grief and guilt...and (3) a denial of the reality of death."[46] This vulnerability is compounded by inexperience and time pressure to complete arrangements.

Optimally, you will complete information in the following section and discuss it with your relatives or whomever will make your funeral arrangements. Give them a copy of your wishes, and keep a copy in the records that will be opened immediately after your death. (Not in a safety deposit box.)

## G. BODY-DISPOSAL INSTRUCTIONS AND DISCUSSION GUIDE

Full Name: _____

Maiden/Other Name: _____

Usual Address: _____

Birth Date: _____ Birth Place: _____

Social Security Number: _____

Spouse's Full Name: _____

1. How you should dispose of my body:
    [ ] Interred (buried), not embalmed.
    [ ] Interred (buried), embalmed.
    [ ] Cremated, not embalmed.
    [ ] Cremated, after embalming.
    [ ] Do above *after* organ/tissue donation.
    [ ] Donate entire body. (Precludes organ donation)

2. I wish to donate:
    [ ] My entire body for research, study or transplant.
    [ ] Any organs or tissues that can be used for transplantation, research or study.
    [ ] The following specific organs or tissues:
        [ ] Corneas (eyes)
        [ ] Heart/lungs
        [ ] Liver
        [ ] Pancreas
        [ ] Skin
        [ ] Bone
        [ ] Other _____

    [ ] I have already made arrangements for this with:

    _____

3. I [ ] do; [ ] do not have funeral or burial insurance. The policy is with

    _____

    (company) and the policy number is _____

563

4. I prefer _____funeral home or funeral director.

    They [ ] have, or [ ] have not been previously contracted.


5. I prefer my hair and makeup be prepared by the following individuals:
    [ ] hair _____
    [ ] makeup _____
    [ ] funeral home
    [ ] no preference


6. I want to be dressed in _____
    [ ] Shroud only
    [ ] Shroud over clothing
    [ ] No preference


7. I would like to be buried with (jewelry, favorite possessions, etc):

_____

_____


8. I prefer a:
    [ ] funeral (with the body present)
      [ ] open casket
      [ ] closed casket
    [ ] memorial (without the body present)
    [ ] no formal service

9. I prefer a [ ] publicly announced; or [ ] family-only funeral or memorial
    service.

10. I prefer to have any service to be:
    [ ] in a church/ mosque/ synagogue
    [ ] at the funeral home/crematory
    [ ] at the graveside only
    [ ] at home, or
    [ ] somewhere else (specify) _____

11. I want a [ ] religious, [ ] fraternal order, [ ] military/veterans or [ ]
    secular ceremony. (These are not necessarily mutually exclusive )

12. I want the service run by a: (enter name if known)
    [ ] minister: _____
    [ ] priest: _____
    [ ] rabbi: _____
    [ ] other: _____

13. I have a preference for:
    [ ] music: _____
    [ ] readings: _____
    [ ] prayers: _____
    [ ] other: _____

14. I [ ] do; or [ ] do not want "calling hours," [ ] with, or [ ] without an open casket.

15. I want to be interred (buried) at _____ cemetery.

16. I own a [ ] plot, or a [ ] mausoleum.
    The deed for the plot is kept: _____

    It is in the name of _____

17. I [ ] do, or [ ] do not want to be buried with anyone else.

    If with someone, who? _____

18. I want a specific type of:
    [ ] Casket: _____

    [ ] Vault: _____

    [ ] Grave marker: _____

19. I want this written on my marker: _____

    _____

20. I want this symbol/ decoration on my marker: _____

    _____; None [ ]

21. I [ ] do,  or [ ] do not want a veteran's marker.

22. I was in the _____(branch of military) from
_____to _____(dates). I was discharged at
_____(place) on _____(date).

23. My discharge papers are located _____

24. If cremation, I want this done with my ashes:
    [ ] Inurned
    [ ] Buried
    [ ] Kept at home
    [ ] Scattered
    [ ] Other: _____

25. I want a specific type of:
    [ ] Urn: _____

    [ ] Columbarium: _____

26. I want my ashes scattered:
    [ ] At sea
    [ ] At another site: _____

27. The following people should be notified of my death:

    Name: _____
    Address: _____
    Phone: (     ) _____

    Name: _____
    Address: _____
    Phone: (     ) _____

    Name: _____
    Address: _____
    Phone: (     ) _____

    Name: _____
    Address: _____
    Phone: (     ) _____

28. I prefer to have or not to have the following people at my funeral, if
     possible:

Name: _____
Address: _____
Phone: (    ) _____
[ ] Come to funeral; [ ] Not come to funeral

Name: _____
Address: _____
Phone: (    ) _____
[ ] Come to funeral; [ ] Not come to funeral

Name: _____
Address: _____
Phone: (    ) _____
[ ] Come to funeral; [ ] Not come to funeral

Name: _____
Address: _____
Phone: (    ) _____
[ ] Come to funeral; [ ] Not come to funeral

Name: _____
Address: _____
Phone: (    ) _____
[ ] Come to funeral; [ ] Not come to funeral

Name: _____
Address: _____
Phone: (    ) _____
[ ] Come to funeral; [ ] Not come to funeral

29. Other family and friends are listed in my address book/rolodex/
     computer listing, which is located _____
     The computer listing is accessed by typing _____

_____

_____
_____

30. I want mourners to send:
    [ ] Flowers.
    [ ] Donations. To whom? _____

31. I want something special in my obituary: _____

_____

    Send copies of the obituary to the following periodicals:

_____

32. I have a cost limit on any of the services mentioned above:

_____

33. My lawyer is _____
        Phone:_____

34. My life insurance company/agent is _____
        Phone: _____

35. My will is located:

_____

36. The executor of my estate is:

_____
        Phone: _____

## H. COSTING IT OUT: A COST-COMPARISON CHART
## OF POSTMORTEM ACTIVITIES

The cost of postmortem activities varies widely. The following charts, however, give some average costs from which to get an idea of the relative expense of various items.

---

## Table 13.1: Average Expenditures on Various Types of Funerals, 1981 and 1987 (1981 Dollars)

|               | 1981      | 1987      |
|---------------|-----------|-----------|
| Open Casket   | $ 2,618.  | $ 2,818.  |
| Closed Casket | 2,339.    | 2,512.    |
| Cremations    | 990.      | 1,054.    |
| Other         | 2,029.    | 2,276.    |

Adapted from Daniel TP: *An Analysis of the Funeral Rule Using Consumer Survey Data on the Purchase of Funeral Goods and Services*. Washington, DC: Federal Trade Commission, February 1989.

---

# Table 13.2: The Cost of Funeral Services—1990 National Data

| | |
|---|---|
| Non-declinable professional service charges. | $ 668.33 |
| Embalming | 226.23 |
| Other body preparation (cosmetology, casketing, hair) | 90.71 |
| Use of viewing facilities | 189.04 |
| Use of facility for ceremony | 185.76 |
| Other use of facility | 193.93 |
| Transfer of remains to funeral home | 87.74 |
| Hearse (local) | 117.49 |
| Limousine (local) | 94.65 |
| Other auto | 66.99 |
| Acknowledgement cards | 19.32 |
| Forwarding remains to another funeral home | 794.58 |
| Receiving remains from another funeral home | 738.22 |
| Direct cremations (family provides container) | 824.03 |
| Immediate burial (family provides container) | 835.99 |
| Direct cremations (funeral home provides container) | 886.10 |
| Immediate burial (funeral home provides container) | 1,048.57 |

## Average Retail Selling Price for Caskets (1991)

| | |
|---|---|
| Minimum alternative container | $ 163.19 |
| Cloth covered wood | 490.87 |
| 20 gauge steel, non-sealer, crepe interior | 816.90 |
| 18 gauge steel, velvet interior | 1754.41 |
| Copper, sealer, velvet interior | 3255.40 |
| Select hardwood, crepe interior | 1919.89 |
| Other | 1848.89 |

## Average Retail Selling Price for Burial Vaults (1991)

| | |
|---|---|
| Two piece concrete box | $ 421.59 |
| 12-gauge non-galvanized steel vault | 827.73 |
| 10-gauge galvanized steel vault | 1207.17 |
| Asphalt coated concrete steel vault | 595.88 |
| Concrete vault with non-metallic liner | 720.14 |
| Other | 786.36 |

Adapted from the National Funeral Directors Association's 1991 Survey of Funeral Operations based on the general price lists required by the Federal Trade Commission.

## FUNERAL HOME COSTS AND PROFIT

This information is from the Federated Funeral Directors of America. These figures are based on 164,980 funerals conducted by nearly 1,400 firms in 30 states in 1989. According to their information, the retail cost of the average adult funeral has more than tripled since 1968, although the business costs have increased more than that. The typical profit margin had decreased 26% in inflation-adjusted dollars since 1968. In 1988, the profit margin on funerals had decreased to the lowest level in 30 years. Some of their representative figures:

**AVERAGE ADULT FUNERAL GROSS SALE**       **$4104.16**
      **(NOT INCLUDING CEMETERY)**

Of this amount, operating expenses are *costed out against each funeral*. Some of the more interesting (but not all) of these expenses are listed below:

| | |
|---|---:|
| Salaries, payroll taxes, and benefits | $ 999.13 |
| Rent/Depreciation/Utilities/Maintenance/Taxes | 501.46 |
| Insurance/Depreciation (Automobile) | 91.42 |
| Advertising | 62.65 |
| Telephone | 42.38 |
| Insurance (General) | 31.90 |
| Bad Debts | 31.18 |
| Business Promotion Meals/Entertainment | 24.41 |
| Preparation Room Supplies | 19.53 |
| Discounts | 17.88 |
| Conventions/Meetings | 12.72 |
| Leased Music | 3.77 |

They claim a pre-tax profit of $295.37 per funeral, or 9.87%. Omitted is their profit on burial vaults, which range in average price from $422 to $1,207.

A non-medicolegal autopsy costs on average $900-1,100. Medicolegal (forensic) autopsies are free. Organ and tissue donation does not cost the family or estate anything. Whole body donation (to a medical school) may involve transportation charges, although in some cases this is covered for in-state deaths.

# I. REFERENCES

1. Litten J: *The English Way of Death: The Common Funeral Since 1450.* London: Robert Hale, 1991, p 3.
2. Inman R: *Cremation Liability.* (lecture). National Funeral Directors Association Annual Convention. Louisville, KY: 1990. (audiotape)
3. Schulte B: Disposing of the deceased. *Arizona Daily Star.* Tucson, AZ: May 28, 1991, p 5A.
4. Ibid.
5. Ibid.
6. Ragon M: *The Space of Death: A Study of Funerary Architecture, Decoration, and Urbanism.* (Sheridan A: trans) Charlottesville, VA: Univ Press of Virginia, 1983. Originally published as *L'espace de la mort: Essai sur l'architecture, la décoration et l'urbanisme funéraires,* Albin Michel, 1981, p 360.
7. Selzer R: *Mortal Lessons: Notes on the Art of Surgery.* New York: Simon & Schuster, 1987, p 140.
8. *Louisville & N.R. Co. v. Wilson,* 123 Ga. 62, 51 S.E. 24, 25 (1905).
9. *Darcy v. Presbyterian Hospital,* 202 N.Y. 259, 95 N.E. 695.
10. *2 Bl. Comm. 429.*
11. *Bogert v. City of Indianapolis,* 13 Ind. 134, 140 (1859).
12. Inman, *Cremation Liability,* 1990. (audiotape)
13. Bernard HY: *The Law of Death and Disposal of the Dead.* 2nd ed. Dobbs Ferry, NY: Oceana Pub, 1979, p 13.
14. Ibid., pp 15-17.
15. Jackson PE: *The Law of Cadavers and of Burial and Burial Places.* New York: Prentice-Hall, 1937, p 124.
16. Ibid., pp 458-75.
17. FTC Planning Memorandum. Cited in: Editors of Consumer Reports: *Funerals—Consumers' Last Rights.* New York: WW Norton, 1977, p 171.
18. American Medical Association Council on Ethical and Judicial Affairs: *Confidentiality of HIV Status on Autopsy Reports.* Presented to the AMA House of Delegates. Chicago, IL: June 1992.
19. *American Express Co. v. Eppley,* 5 Ohio Dec. (Rep.) 337.
20. *Southern Life & Health Ins. Co. v. Morgan,* 21 Ala. App. 5, 105 So. 161.
21. *Matter of Beekman St.,* (N.Y.) 4 Bradf. Surr. 503.
22. *Long v. Chicago, etc.,* R. Co., 15 Okla. 512, 86 P. 289.
23. Jackson, *Law of Cadavers,,* pp 69-81.
24. Nathan C: Ethical and legal aspects to death: the burial. *Medicine and Law.* 1989;8:445-54.
25. Jackson, *Law of Cadavers,* p 119.
26. Gittings C: *Death, Burial and the Individual in Early Modern England.* London: Croom & Helm, 1984, p 66.
27. Ibid.
28. Jackson, *Law of Cadavers,* p 119.
29. *Reg. v. Scott,* (1841) 2 Q.B. 248, 114 Eng. Rep. 97.
30. *Act 1811,* Gen. Laws (1932), C 272, Sec. 70.
31. Rhode Island, Gen. Laws 1923, Sec. 5261.
32. *Toppin v. Moriarty,* 59 J.J. Eq. 115, 44 Atl. 469.
33. *Jefferson County Burial Soc. v. Scott,* 218 Ala. 354, 118 So. 644.
34. *American Express Co. v. Eppley.*
35. Jackson, *Law of Cadavers,* p 121.
36. Held for Ransom. *Mortuary Management.* February 1992, p 20.

37. Jackson, *Law of Cadavers*, pp 81-82.
38. Puckle BS: *Funeral Customs—Their Origin and Development.* London: T Werner Laurie, 1926, pp 222-23.
39. Hardy T: *The Mayor of Casterbridge.* 1894.
40. *Matter of Moran,* 75 Misc. 90, 134 N.Y. Supp. 968.
41. van der Woude J: De Wet op de lijkbezorging en de verpleegkundige. *TVZ.* 1991:12:402-404.
42. Hill RB, Anderson RE: *The Autopsy—Medical Practice and Public Policy.* Boston: Butterworths, 1988, p 45.
43 Ibid.
44. Jackson, *Law of Cadavers*, p. 431-32
45. Ibid.
46. Hughes TE, Klein D: *A Family Guide to Wills, Funerals & Probate.* New York: Charles Scribner's Sons, 1987, p 84.

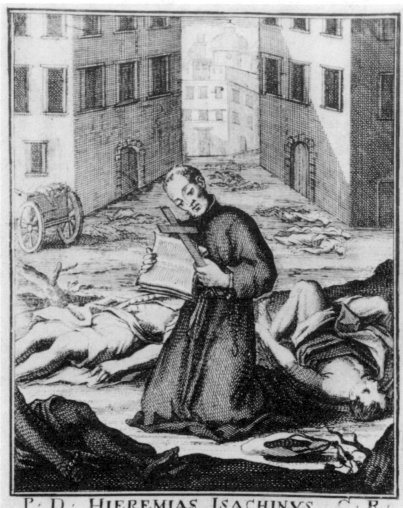

P · D · HIEREMIAS ISACHINVS C · R ·
*A' Secretis Pauli IV, et a' Cubiculo.*
*Veneto a' Senatu contentiose' Pio V: expetitus ac a D Carolo*
*Speculum Perfectionis a' Sixto V: publice Depredicatus,*
*Diuitiarum, Purpurq, ac Vitq contemptor;*
*Quam Patauina' in Luc. Spiritum sibi ipsi comendans,*
*Miraculorum uel Viuens Patrator, consumpsit.*

*The plague dead.* A memorial engraving for Italian priests who died while tending plague victims. Originally published in Padua, Italy. (Reproduced with permission. National Library of Medicine.)

574

# 14: SAY IT GENTLY: WORDS, SAYINGS AND POETRY ABOUT THE DEAD

*From the Bible onward, writers, including those who wrote on tombstones, have used death and the dead as a common theme. Sometimes their writing was humorous, sometimes it was insightful, and sometimes it was tragic. This chapter cites some representative examples.*

One is hard put to stop being dead.

MM Pardi.

Death has got something to be said for it;
There's no need to get out of bed for it;
Wherever you may be,
They bring it to you, free.

Kingsley Amis.

I went to Rosie's funeral,
I heard the preacher say,
"Here lies the shell,
The nut has passed away."

L. Morrison L, ed: *A Diller A Dollar.* New York: Thomas Y Crowell, 1955.

The three main fears Americans have: 1) public speaking; 2) speaking about death; 3) dying.

J DeMars, 1990.

575

KENNETH V. ISERSON

When you come past my grave
And I am dead and rotten,
Just hold your nose
And keep on trottin'.

L Morrison, ed: *A Diller A Dollar.*

For there is a sickening sense in which a corpse is a human being that has
been returned to its sheerest humanity; there is something truly universal
about a corpse.

L Wieseltier L: After memory. *The New Republic.* 1993;208(18):16-26.

I bequeath myself to the dirt to grow from
          the grass I love,
if you want me again look for me under
          your boot-soles.

Walt Whitman's *Song of Myself.*

Show me the manner in which a Nation or community cares for its dead and
I will measure with mathematical exactness the tender mercies of its people,
their respect for the law of the land, and their loyalty to high ideals.

William Ewart Gladstone.

So mix his body with the dust! It might
          Return to what it *must* far sooner, were
The natural compound left alone to fight
          Its way back into earth, and fire, and air;
But the unnatural balsams merely blight
          What Nature made him at his birth, as bare

As the mere million's base unmummied clay —
          Yet all his spices but prolong decay.

Lord Gordon G. Byron, speaking of George III's funeral.

Mummy, n. An ancient Egyptian, formerly in universal use among modern civilized nations as medicine, and now engaged in supplying art with an excellent pigment. He is handy, too, in museums in gratifying the vulgar curiosity that serves to distinguish man from the lower animals.

> By means of the Mummy, mankind, it is said,
> Attests to the gods its respect for the dead.
> We plunder his tomb, be he sinner or saint,
> Distil him for physic and grind him for paint,
> Exhibit for money his poor, shrunken frame,
> And with levity flock to the scene of the shame.
> O, tell me, ye gods, for the use of my rhyme:
> For respecting the dead what's the limit of time?

Scopas Brune, in Bierce A: *Devil's Dictionary.*

Embalm, v.t. To cheat vegetation by locking up the gases upon which it feeds.

Ambrose Bierce, *Devil's Dictionary.*

> Done with the work of breathin; done
> With all the world; the mad race run
> Through to the end; the golden goal
> Attained and found to be a hole!

Squatol Johnes, in Bierce A: *Devil's Dictionary.*

In the sweat of thy face shalt thou eat bread, till thou return unto the ground; for out of it wast thou taken; for dust thou art, and unto dust shalt thou return.

*Genesis* 3:19, God to Adam.

> Golden lads and girls all must,
> As chimney-sweepers, come to dust.

Shakespeare, *Cymbeline*,IV, ii.

_____ and who would lay
His body in the city burial-place,
To be thrown up again by some rude sexton,
And yield its narrow house another tenant,
Ere the moist flesh had mingled with the dust,
Ere the tenacious hair had left the scalp,
Exposed to insult lewd, and wantonness?
No, I will lay me in the village ground;
There are the dead respected.

H.K. White.

The burial of the cadaver is *caro data vermibus* [flesh given to worms].

Lord Coke, *Third Inst,* p 203.

The womb shall forget him; the worm shall feed sweetly on him; he shall be no more remembered.

*Job* 24:20.

But man dieth, and wasteth away: yea, man giveth up the ghost, and where *is* he?

*Job* 14:10.

We must all die; we are like water spilt on the ground, which cannot be gathered up again.

*2 Samuel* 14:14.

There are two ways of not thinking about death: the way of our technological civilization, which denies death and refuses to talk about it; and the way of traditional civilizations, which is not a denial but a recognition of the *impossibility of thinking about it directly or for very long* because death is too close and too much a part of daily life.

P Ariès, *The Hour of Our Death.* p 22

578

O carrion, who art no longer man,
Who will hence keep thee company?
Whatever issues from thy liquors,
Worms engendered by the stench
Of thy vile carrion flesh.

Pierre de Nesson (1383-1442). *Vigiles des morts: Paraphrase sur Job*.


Hamlet: Imperious Caesar, dead and turn'd to clay,
Might stop a hole to keep the wind away.
O, that that earth, which kept the world in awe,
Should patch a wall to expel the winter's flaw.

Shakespeare, *Hamlet, Prince of Denmark*, V,i.


Behowlde youre selves by us sutch once were we as you
And you in tyme be even duste as we are now.

Epitaph in St. Bartholomew the Great, London, 1558, in Jones B: *Design for Death*, p 148.


The Ilocano tribe in the Philippines say the *dung-aw* at death. A portion, translated into English says:

Oh, holy rose-colored cheeks,
And eyes that have been closed!
Let me kiss them, though hardened,
Ah my son, what shall I do
In the midst of what I suffer?

Anima N, *Childbirth & Burial Practices*, p 57.


Each conduit of the body
Constantly produces putrid matter
Out of the body.

Pierre de Nesson (1383-1442). *Vigiles des morts: Paraphrase sur Job*.


579

Nunc, vero inter saxum et locum durum sum.
(Now, I really am between a rock and a hard place.)

Henry Beard, *Latin for All Occasions.*


...ah bone, is the pit of a man after the cumbering flesh has been eaten away.

Selzer R, *Mortal Lessons,* p 51.


In memory of Jane and Ama Sweetman
1st and 2nd wives of
Rev. Joseph Sweetman
Strangers in life,
Our dust mingles in the grave.

(The two women died 20 years apart and did not know each other.)

Portion of an epitaph, in Coffin MM, *Death in Early America,* p 180.


This is the fruit of the earth taken, its flesh torn. This is it given over to standing, toward rot. It is the principle of corruption, the death of what is, the birth of what is to be. You are wine.

Selzer R, *Mortal Lessons,* p 130.


Soon ripe
Soon rotten
Soon gone
But not forgotten.

Epitaph on a Massachusetts tombstone, in Wallis CL, *Stories in Stone*, p 181.


Oh, would that I could lift the lid and peer
within the grave and watch the greedy worms
that eat away the dead.

Epitaph on a Massachusetts tombstone, in Wallis CL, *Stories in Stone*. p 185.

Dead, the body is somehow more solid, more massive...it is only what it is—a mass, declaring itself, an ugly emphasis.

Selzer R, *Mortal Lessons,* p 135.

Colder and colder grows the flesh, as the last bit of warmth disperses. Now you are meat, meat at room temperature.

Selzer R, *Mortal Lessons,* p 136.

> O what shall be done with our dead, old boy?
> We'll run out of ground very soon.
> Why, pack 'em in straw for a bed, old boys,
> And freight 'em straight to the moon.
>
> O what shall be done with our dead, old boy?
> It seems a shame to waste 'em.
> So after your tears are shed, old boys,
> Why, spit 'em and roast 'em and taste 'em.

Sung by a physician and his barroom cronies, in Selzer R, *Mortal Lessons,* p 140.

Death is nothing to us, since when we are, death has not come, and when death has come, we are not.

Epicurus, *Diogenes Laertius*, Book 10, sec 125.

As one dies, so dies the other. They all have the same breath, and man has no advantage over the beasts...all are from the dust, and all turn to dust again.

*Ecclesiasticus* 3:19-20.

Six feet of earth make all men of one size.

Old American proverb.

581

Under the wide and starry sky
Dig the grave and let me lie
Glad did I live and gladly die
        And I laid me down with a will.

This be the verse you grave for me
"Here he lies where he longed to be"
Home is the sailor, home from the sea
        And the hunter home from the hill.

Robert Louis Stevenson (epitaph) & *Requiem.*

Haul up the flag, you mourners,
Not half-mast but all the way;
The funeral is done and disbanded;
The devil's had the final say.

Karl Shapiro, *Elegy for Two Banjos*, st. 1 and 14.

And we all go with them, into the silent funeral,
Nobody's funeral, for there is no one to bury.

T.S. Eliot, *Four Quartets. East Coker*, II, 1940.

With one auspicious and one dropping eye,
With mirth in funeral and with dirge in marriage,
In equal scale weighing delight and dole.

Shakespeare, *Hamlet, Prince of Denmark* I, ii, 11.

Let no one pay me honor with tears, nor celebrate my funeral rites with weeping.

Quintus Ennius in Cicero, *De Senectute* XX.

Their bodies are buried in peace; but their name liveth for evermore.

*Ecclesiasticus* 44:14.

Marley was dead, to begin with. There is no doubt whatever about that. The register of his burial was signed by the clergyman, the clerk, the undertaker, and the chief mourner. Scrooge signed it. And Scrooge's name was good upon 'Change for anything he chose to put his hand to.

Old Marley was dead as a doornail.

Charles Dickens, A Christmas Carol, 1843.

The soil out of which such men as he are made is good to be born on, good to live on, good to die for and to be buried in.

James Russell Lowell, Garfield, 1881.

Snow was general all over Ireland. It was falling on every part of the dark central plain, on the treeless hills, falling softly upon the Bog of Allen and, farther westward, softly falling into the dark mutinous Shannon waves. It was falling, too, upon every part of the lonely churchyard on the hill where Michael Furey lay buried. It lay thickly drifted on the crooked crosses and headstones, on the spears of the little gate, on the barren thorns. His soul swooned slowly as he heard the snow falling faintly through the universe and faintly falling, like the decent of their last end, upon all the living and the dead.

James Joyce, Dubliners, The Dead, 1916.

The waters were his winding sheet,
    the sea was made for his tomb;
Yet for his fame the ocean sea,
    was not sufficient room.

Richard Barnfield, Epitaph on Hawkins, 1595.

Death is a debt we all must pay.

Euripides, Alcestis, 419.

It is a poor thing for anyone to fear what is inevitable.

> Tertullian, *The Soul's Testimony,* IV.


The Doctor said that Death was but
A scientific fact.

> Oscar Wilde, *The Ballad of Reading Gaol*, part III.


Let the experiment be made on a worthless body.

> Latin Proverb.


Nothing can be done
To keep at bay
Age and age's evils, hoar hair,
Ruck and wrinkle, drooping, dying,
        death's worst, winding sheets,
        tombs and worms and tumbling to
        decay.

> Gerard Manley Hopkins, *The Leaden Echo and the Golden Echo*.


I like that Saxon phrase, which calls
        The burial-ground God's-Acre!

> Henry Wadsworth Longfellow, *God's-Acre*.


The CEMETERY is an open space among the ruins, covered in winter with violets and daisies. It might make one in love with death, to think that one should be buried in so sweet a place.

> Percy Bysshe Shelley, *Adonais*, 1821.


O me, why have they not buried me deep enough?
Is it kind to have made me a grave so rough,
Me, that was never a quiet sleeper?

> Alfred, Lord Tennyson, *Maud*, 1855.

## Say It Gently

Upon my buried body lay
Lightly gently earth.

Francis Beaumont, *The Maid's Tragedy*, II.i.

We buried him darkly at dead of night,
The sods with our bayonets turning.

Charles Wolfe, *The Burial of Sir John Moore at Corunna*.

But there, everything has its drawbacks, as the man said when his mother-in-law died, and they came down on him for the funeral expenses.

Jerome K. Jerome, *Three Men in a Boat*, 1889.

And when they buried him the little port
Had seldom seen a costlier funeral.

Alfred, Lord Tennyson, *Enoch Arden*, 1864.

I will teach you my townspeople how to perform a funeral
for you have it over a troop of artists—
unless one should scour the world—
you have the ground sense necessary.

William Carlos Williams, *Tract*.

The men that worked for England
    They have their graves at home...
And they that rule in England,
    In stately conclave met,
Alas, alas for England
    They have no graves as yet.

G.K. Chesterton, *Elegy in a Country Churchyard*.

The wind doth blow to-day, my love,
    And a few small drops of rain;
I never had but one true love;
    In cold grave she was lain.

I'll do as much for my true-love
    As any young man may;
I'll sit and mourn all at her grave
    For a twelvemonth and a day.

*The Unquiet Grave*, English Traditional Ballad

Reader behold! and shed a tear
Think on the dust that slumbers here,
And when you read the fate of me,
Think on the glass that runs for thee.

Early American epitaph, in Coffin, *Death in Early America*, p 225.

What hopes lie buried here.

Early American epitaph, in Coffin MM, *Death in Early America*, p 228.

Sometime we'll understand.

Early American epitaph, in Coffin MM, *Death in Early America*, p 228.

Here lies a wife
Of two husbands bereft:
Robert on the right,
Richard on the left.

Early American epitaph, in Coffin MM, *Death in Early America*, p 179.

Promoted to higher service.

Epitaph, Major Hilda Freed, Salvation Army plot, Oak Ridge Lutheran Cemetery, Hillside,
IL, 1939, in Jackson KT, Vergara CJ: *Silent Cities*, p 68.

586

Mary Nichols is my name
Ireland is my nation
Catholic Church is my belief
Heaven is my expectation.

Epitaph, New Orleans cemetery, in Jackson KT, Vergara CJ, *Silent Cities,* p 54.

Let me live in a house
By the side of the road
Where the race of men go by
The men who are good
And the men who are bad
As good and as bad as I

Epitaph, Cypress Lawn Cemetery, Colma, CA, 1975., in Jackson, Vergara, *Silent Cities,* p 40.

On fame's eternal camping grounds
His silent tent is spread,
And glory guards with solemn rounds
The bivouac of the dead.

Epitaph for a Union officer, Alexander Hays, Allegheny Cemetery, Pittsburgh, 1864., in Jackson, Vergara, *Silent Cities,* p 24.

References to the realities of death, when bodies became compost and food for worms, were frequently found in the inscriptions on the *gisant-* (reclining) type of monument, such as:

*Nunc putredo terrae et cibus verminorum.*

[Now I give off a smell of the earth and am food for worms.]

Curl JS: *A Celebration of Death,* 1980.

Epitaph grimly punned on the death of the 'Fair Rosamund':
*Hic jacet in tumba Rosa mundi, non Rosa munda;*
*Non redolet, sed olet, quae redolere solet.*

[Here lies in the grave Rose of adornment, not an elegant Rose;
She doesn't stink, but she smells, which she is accustomed to do.]

Curl JS: *A Victorian Celebration of Death.*

587

Julian Skaggs, a retired West Virginia coal miner, was known as a practical joker. He liked, for example, "giving a hand to a stranger," when he would shake hands and leave them holding his artificial limb. When he died in 1974 and his body was cremated, he instructed his family to put a marker in the family plot with the epitaph:

> I made an ash of myself.

Meyer RE: *Cemeteries and Gravemarkers: Voices of American Culture.* Ann Arbor, MI: UMI Research Press, 1989, p 90.

The family of a friendly Philadelphia car salesman, Porter H. Waite, inscribed this epitaph epitomizing his personality,

> "Hi everyone! Have fun. See you later."

Meyer RE, *Cemeteries and Gravemarkers,* p 95.

The epitaph of Captain Jonathan Poole, Wakefield, Massachusetts, who died, age 44, December, 1678:

> Frinds sure would prove to far unkind
> If out of sight they leave him out of mind
> & now he lies transform'd to native dust
> In earths cold womb as other mortals must
> Its strange his matchless worth intomb-d should ly
> Of that his fame should in oblivion dy

Tashjian D, Tashjian A: *Memorials for Children of Change: The Art of Early New England Stonecarving.* Middletown, CT: Wesleyan University Press, 1974, p 237

The epitaph of Jedediah Aylesworth, Arlington, Vermont, died age 16 years, March 18, 1795:

> This youth tho Young was lov'd by all
> By old & young by great & small
> His generous soul his obliging way
> Amongst his acquaintance bore their sway
> But death that conquerer bow'd his head
> And now he lies among the dead
> Yet he shall rise & leave the ground

Tashjian D, Tashjian A, *Memorials for Children of Change,* pp 248-49.

The epitaph of Ebenezer Cole, Shaftsbury, Vermont, who died at age 82:

> You see the place where I am laid,
> Death is a debt that must be paid;
> And as by me you find it true,
> And time will prove it so by you.

Tashjian D, Tashjian A, *Memorials for Children of Change.* p 249.

The Park family stone, Burgess Cemetery, Grafton, Vermont, dated 1803:

> Youth behold and shed a teer,
> Se fourteen children slumber here
> Se their image how they shine,
> Like flowers of a fruitful vine.
>
> Behold and se as you pass by -
> My fourteen children with me lie,
> Old or young you soon must die,
> And turn to dust as well as I.

Tashjian D, Tashjian A, *Memorials for Children of Change,* p 257.

"The May Briant and children stone" Norwell, Massachusetts, 1724:

> Here lyes ye body
> Of Mrs Mary Briant
> Wife of Mr Thomas
> Briant who dyed
> November the 30th
> 1724 aged 39 yeares
> & in har arms doth
> Lye ye corps of two
> Lovely babes born
> Of har 8 days before
> Har death one a son
> Nathaniel dyed ye day
> Before har a daughtr
> Named Hannah dyed a few ours after har

Tashjian D, Tashjian A, *Memorials for Children of Change,* p 260.

Come come. Fate is rancorous, but not to that extent. Look at Mammy. What rid me of her, in the end? I sometimes wonder. Perhaps they buried her alive, it wouldn't surprise me.

Beckett S: *Molloy*. NY: Grove Press, 1955, p 109.

...he knew how the dead and buried tend, contrary to what one might expect, to rise to the surface, in which they resemble the drowned. And he had made allowance for this when digging the hole.

Beckett S: *Malone Dies*. NY: Grove Press, 1956, p 38.

Here lies Malone at last, with the dates to give a faint idea of the time he took to be excused and then to distinguish him from his namesakes, numerous in the island and beyond the grave.

Beckett S, *Malone Dies*, p 101.

Do not stand at my grave and weep,
I am not there, I do not sleep.
I am a thousand winds that blow;
I am the diamond glints on snow.
I am the sunlight on ripened grain;
I am the gentle autumn's rain.
When you awaken in the morning's hush,
I am the swift uplifting rush
Of quiet birds in circled flight,
I am the soft star that shines at night.
Do not stand at my grave and cry,
I am not there; I did not die.

Anon. Reprinted by Van Buren A: *Arizona Daily Star*. July 11, 1993, p 4D.

John Felt epitaph, Rockingham, Vermont, 1805, died age 23:

> Be bold and se as you pass by
> As you are now so once was I,
> As I am now so you must be
> Prepair for death & follow me.

Tashjian D, Tashjian A: *Memorials for Children of Change,* p 269.

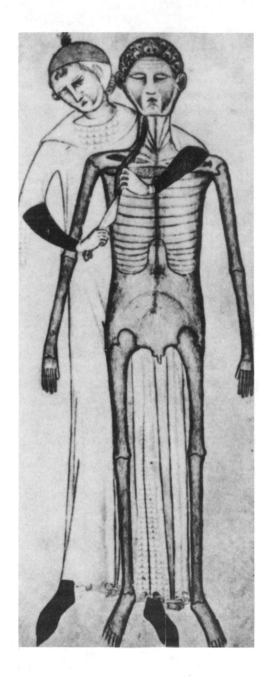

*Anatomical dissection.* Originally published by Guidonis de Vigevano, 1345. (Reproduced with permission. National Library of Medicine.)

# 15: GLOSSARY

ACCESSORY CHEMICALS: Hardening compounds, preservative powders, sealing agents, mold preventatives and other chemicals used in addition to routine arterial embalming fluids.

ADIPOCERE: A grayish-white cheesy substance, principally hydrolyzed fat, that a corpse's tissues may turn into if exposed to cool moist soil or water. Also known as grave wax.

ADVANCE DIRECTIVE: A class of legal documents, such as living wills, that allow individuals to specify in advance what medical care they desire. They only go into effect if the person lacks the capacity to make valid decisions at the time they are necessary.

AIRTRAY: An outer container covering a casket or body used for air shipment of corpses.

ALGOR MORTIS: The body's cooling after death.

ANATOMICAL GIFT: An organ, body part or the entire body from a deceased person which is donated for the use of others.

ANTEMORTEM: Before death.

ARON: The wooden casket with wooden pegs used by Jews.

ARRANGEMENT CONFERENCE: The initial meeting between the funeral director and those wanting to purchase his services.

ARTERIAL PRESERVATIVE: The usual chemicals injected into a body in the embalming process.

ASHES: Usually used to describe the remains after cremation, they are actually purified human skeletal remains or fragments. An average adult's weighs from 3-9 pounds.

AUTOLYSIS: The breakdown of the corpse's tissues by the body's own digestive enzymes.

AUTOPSY: The medical examination of a corpse, generally done to determine the cause of death.


BAR MINEN: Jewish term for a deceased person.

BARROW: A large mound of earth or stones placed over a burial site.

BELLY PUNCHERS: A derogatory term used for cavity embalmers by others in the industry. It derives from their method of "punching" holes through the abdominal wall with large trocars (needles).

BI-UNIT PRICING: A method of charging one fee for the casket and another for all other funeral services—now illegal in the U.S.

BIER: The stand on which a corpse, coffin or casket is placed prior to burial. It was once also used to transport the body to the grave, and in Scotland it also referred to the coffin.

BLEACHING AGENT: An agent often used to lighten skin stains on the corpse so these marks can be hidden with cosmetics It contains phenol or cavity embalming fluid.

BODY: Common term for a corpse.

BRAIN DEATH: A term used to indicate that a person is dead and lack of brain function was used to make that determination. An imprecise term, it is now being replaced by "death by brain criteria."

BURIAL CHEST: A nineteenth-century term for a casket.

BURIAL-TRANSIT PERMIT: A combined permit allowing cremation, burial or transportation of the body. These may be separate forms in some instances.

BURIAL VAULT: see VAULT.


CADAVER: A corpse. Generally used to indicate a body prepared for anatomical dissection.

CADAVER CARRIER: A specially designed stretcher used by hospital morticians to move bodies from patient care areas to the morgue.

CALCINATION: Reduction of a body to ash through the action of inert heat, rather than flames.

CALL: A funeral industry term for a funeral.

CANNIBALISM: Eating all or part of an individual from one's own species.

CANNULA: A hollow tube inserted into an artery through which embalming fluid is injected.

CANOPIC JARS: Vases used to hold vital organs of embalmed bodies, or occasionally, ashes of the dead.

CAPILLARY FLUSH: The rosy glow of the corpse's cheeks produced by the embalmer's cosmetic skills.

CASE: A funeral industry term for a funeral.

CASKET: Rectangular, rigid burial receptacle, usually made of wood or metal and lined with fabric. (Compare with COFFIN).

CASKET STANDARD: A catafalque.

CATACOMB: Underground cemetery with tunnels and recessed rooms dug out for tombs and coffins.

CATAFALQUE: Raised, flat structure on which corpse is laid or carried. Often very elaborate. In a crematory, it is used to pass the body into the oven.

CAVITY EMBALMING: Instilling embalming chemicals into the chest or abdomen to preserve these areas. The method is usually accompanied by draining gas and fluid from the internal organs through a needle.

CAVITY FLUID: The type of embalming fluid used to perform cavity embalming and other techniques. Very strong stuff.

CEMETERY: A site dedicated to the burial of human remains.

CENOTAPH: A monument which does not house a body, but which is erected to honor a dead person.

CERECLOTH: Historically, a fine fabric used to cover a corpse. It was soaked or painted with an adhesive, such as wax, to hold the cloth closely to the body.

CERTIFICATE OF DISPOSITION: A burial/cremation permit issued by a local government.

CHEVRAH KADDISHA: In Judaism, the "Holy Brotherhood" Society whose members devote themselves to burial and rites connected with it.

CHIN REST: A method of keeping a corpse's mouth closed.

CHRISTIAN BURIAL CERTIFICATE: A certificate from a Roman Catholic priest stating that the deceased is eligible for church rites. Also known as a Christian Burial Permit and Priestly Lines.

CHRISTIAN PRAYER SERVICE: A Roman Catholic service often used at wakes in place of reciting the Rosary.

CINERARIUM: A place for keeping the ashes of a cremated body.

CINERARY JAR: Another name for an ancient urn.

COFFIN: Eight-sided burial receptacle shaped to fit the human body. Rarely used in the U.S. (Compare with CASKET).

COLUMBARIUM: The structure containing recessed memorial niches for cremated remains. In modern structures, the niches are faced with protective glass, bronze, or marble.

COMMITTAL CHAMBER: Fancy term for the anteroom to a crematorium.

CONCURRENT DRAINAGE: Draining the blood from a cadaver while simultaneously infusing it with embalming fluid.

CORONER: An elected official, often without any special education, who supervises investigations of suspicious or unexplained deaths.

CORPSE: A dead body.

CORPSICLE: A cryonically preserved body (neologism).

CORTEGE: A funeral procession.

COSMETIC FLUID: Embalming fluid containing dyes to supply a more

COSMETIC FLUID: Embalming fluid containing dyes to supply a more normal appearance to the corpse.

CRANIAL EMBALMING: Passing a trocar through the nose and into the skull (through the cribiform plate) to remove tissue and fluid and inject embalming fluid.

CREMAINS: The bone-ash remaining after cremation.

CREMATION: The process of using heat and evaporation to reduce human remains to bone fragments.

CREMATION CHAMBER: The enclosed space within which cremation takes place.

CREMATION SOCIETY: A memorial or burial society which concentrates on cremations. Some are for-profit businesses.

CREMATORIUM: Also known as crematory; the building or portion of a building that houses the cremation chamber and facility to hold the body. It also refers to the surrounding facilities, including chapel, columbarium, garden, etc.

CRYOGENICS: The science which studies the effects of extreme low temperatures on physical systems and materials. Also, the technology which produces the above.

CRYONAUTS: A science fiction term to describe individuals who successfully return from cryonic suspension.

CRYONIC SUSPENSION: The freezing of a human who has died of a disease, at an extremely low temperature, in hopes that the body may be resuscitated after medical science improves. Also referred to, by its proponents, as cryonic preservation.

CRYONICS: The science and technology of cryonic suspension.

CRYOSTASIS: An alternative term for cryonic suspension.

CRYPT: Subterranean burial vault or chamber, often beneath the floor of a church, in which a body is placed. Modern cemeteries also refer to the space in above-ground mausoleums as crypts.


DEANIMATE: To die. A word used primarily by cryonics devotees.

DEATH CARE INDUSTRY: A term used by the funeral industry for itself.

DEATH CERTIFICATE: A legal form authenticating a death, and often includes the cause of death.

DEATH NOTICE: A paid advertisement announcing a death.

DECEDENT: A dead person.

DECOMPOSITION/DECOMPOSING: The process through which a corpse returns to dust.

DENTAL TIE: One method of keeping a corpse's mouth shut.

DEWAR: A multibody chamber constructed like a large vacuum thermos bottle and filled with liquid nitrogen, used to store cryogenically-preserved bodies and heads.

DIRECT BURIAL: Burial of a body without prior viewing, embalming, or cosmetic restoration. Usually followed by a memorial service.

DIRGE: A slow, mournful musical composition or poem traditionally used at funerals.

DISSECTION: As used in anatomy, the slicing of a body to identify and inspect its parts.

DRAINAGE: Removal of blood and other fluids through a large vein while arterial embalming is occurring.

DRAWING AND QUARTERING: A method of mutilating a corpse as postmortem punishment.

DURABLE POWER OF ATTORNEY FOR HEALTH CARE: A form of advance directive that empowers a person's agent to make health care decisions for him if he is unable to do so.

ELEGY: A melancholy poem or song written in elegiac couplets and performed as a lament for the dead.

EMBALMER: A technician who embalms corpses.

EMBALMING: In modern times, the replacment of a corpse's fluids with disinfecting and preserving chemicals.

EMBALMER'S GRAY: The gray look of the face and neck that results from blood from the heart draining into these areas after death. Proper body positioning avoids this.

EMBALMING POWDER: A dry chemical preservative used either inside or outside of the body for surface embalming.

EMBALMMENT: An old technique of removing the internal organs, soaking and packing the body cavities with chemicals, and allowing the body to dehydrate.

EN BLOC: A way of removing a cluster of organs together during an autopsy to maintain their anatomical relationship for examination.

EN SITU: The method of examining organs during an autopsy while they are still in the body in their natural position.

ENTOMBMENT: Placement of the casketed body in an above ground mausoleum.

EULOGY: A laudatory speech, oftern given at funerals.

EXCARNATE: To strip off the flesh.

EXHUMATION: Removing a corpse from a grave, usually for examination or reburial elsewhere.

EXPERIMENTATION: Testing scientific hypotheses in a methodical manner.

FLOATERS: Bodies submersed in water for a period of time, usually long enough to have developed enough gas in the abdomen to float to the surface.

FORENSIC: Dealing with the law, as with a forensic pathologist who is the link between law and medicine.

FORMALDEHYDE GRAY: A gray discoloration of the body caused by an interaction between formaldehyde, a common component of embalming chemicals, and the hemoglobin in blood.

FORMALIN: A common tissue preservative used by pathologists. It is made of 36-40% gaseous formaldehyde (HCHO) in water. Usually used as a 10% solution in water.

FUNCTIONAL PRICING: Pricing the costs of the parts of the funeral independently of one another, i.e., itemizing the bill.

FUNERAL: An organized, purposeful, time-limited, culturally-regulated, group- centered response to death in which the body of the deceased is present for all or part of the rite.

FUNERAL CHAPEL: A building or room built to conduct funerals. Often associated with a funeral home, cemetery or crematorium.

FUNERAL DIRECTOR: A person who serves the public in all aspects of funeral service.

FUNERAL HOME: A commercial establishment devoted to the preparation of dead bodies, viewing of remains, and funeral services.

FUNERAL LIGHTING: The illumination used for display of the body in the casket.


GHUSL: Islamic bathing of the dead.

GIBBET: A metal cage in which the copses of criminals were publically displayed until after they rotted or were eaten by scavengers.

GRAVE: An excavation for burial of a body.

GRAVE LINER: A term sometimes used interchangably with Vault, it is a concrete enclosure assembled at the gravesite for the coffin. It is supposed to prevent collapse of the ground above. See also VAULT.

GRAVE MARKER: A monument to the deceased at the grave site.

GRAVE WAX: A more graphic term for adipocere.

GRIEF THERAPIST: The funeral industry's preferred euphemism for a mortician.


HARDENING COMPOUND: Substance used to solidify tissues during embalming.

HEAD FREEZE: Injecting very strong arterial embalming fluid into both major neck arteries (carotids) under high pressure to embalm without causing much swelling.

HEAD REST: Used to keep the head in position during embalming.

HEALTH CARE POWER OF ATTORNEY: Another term for a Durable Power Of Attorney For Health Care.

HEALTH CARE DIRECTIVE: Another term for a Durable Power Of Attorney For Health Care.

HEART TAP: Injecting embalming fluid directly into the aorta or heart—usually used in children.

HERMETICALLY SEALED: Airtight. Athough virtually no casket is truly airtight, today's "hermetically-sealed" caskets prevent the release of noxious odors.

HESPED: Eulogy delivered by a rabbi for the deceased.

HUMECTANT: Chemical used in cases of dehydration that allows the body to retain moisture.

HYPODERMIC EMBALMING: Injecting areas, such as the buttocks, shoulders, back of the neck and trunk walls with preservative to help embalm them.

HYPOSTASIS: Settling of the blood in the vessels in the most dependent (lowest) parts of the body; livor mortis.


IMMEDIATE BURIAL: See DIRECT BURIAL.

IMMUREMENT: To entomb within walls, such as in a mausoleum.

INHUMATION: A fancy word for burial, or interment of a body in a crypt or tomb.

INSTANT TISSUE FIXATION: See HEAD FREEZE.

INTERMENT: Burial.

INTERMITTENT DRAINAGE: Draining the blood and fluid only intermittently during arterial embalming. This allows pressure to build and the fluid to pass into smaller vessels.

INURNMENT: Placing cremated remains in an urn.

ITAI: Japanese term for a person's remains, as differentiated from the corpse. The *itai* has its own hopes and requests from the living.


KADDISH: Jewish prayer for the dead.

KEVER: Jewish term for the grave.

K'VURA: Jewish burial ceremony.

KNEELER: A low stool on which mourners may kneel at the side of a casket.

LAST OFFICES: A British term for the care given by nurses to a corpse. They normally include washing and shrouding.

LEVAYA: Jewish funeral procession.

LIVING WILL: A limited and inflexible form of advance directive.

LIVOR MORTIS: Purple discoloration of the skin in the dependent (lowest) part of the corpse from the pooling of blood.

MACERATE: To soften by soaking in liquid.

MASS OF ANGELS: Catholic funeral service for children.

MASS OF THE RESURRECTION: A Catholic rite celebrated on the day of burial, formerly called a Requiem Mass.

MAUSOLEUM: An above ground structure, usually of stone, in which bodies are entombed, usually within areas called "crypts."

MEDICAL EXAMINER: A pathologist employed by the government, normally specializing in forensic pathology, who must examine suspicious or unexplained deaths.

MEDICOLEGAL: Relating to medicine and law.

MEMORIAL HOME: Another name for a funeral home.

MEMORIAL NICHE: The enclosed space in which an urn with the ashes of a cremated body resides.

MEMORIAL PARK: Cemetery where graves are marked with markers flush to the ground instead of with monuments or gravestones.

MEMORIAL SERVICE: A funeral without the body present.

MEMORIAL SOCIETY: Voluntary group dedicated to providing members with inexpensive, pre-arranged funerals.

MEMORY PICTURE: Euphemism for the embalmed body as it is presented in an open-casket funeral.

MODIFYING AGENT: Chemicals added to the embalming process for a specific purpose. They may include humectants, buffers and water softeners.

MONTH'S MIND MASS: A Catholic rite celebrated one month after a death and funeral liturgy. When celebrated at annual intervals, it is called an anniversary Mass.

MORGUE: A site where corpses are stored.

MORTCLOTH: A fine cloth used to drape the body or coffin. Used primarily in Scotland until the twentieth century, it was normally reusable.

MORTICIAN: funeral director.

MORTUARY: A funeral home.

MULTIPLE CREMATIONS: Cremating more than one body at a time.

MULTIPLE-SITE INJECTION: Arterial embalming performed at more than one site. This is the recommended embalming method.

MUSCULAR SUTURE: The method of keeping a corpse's mouth closed by passing a needle and thread through the inside of the nose and securing it to the muscle of the lower lip and chin.

MULTI-UNIT PRICING: The practice of pricing the costs of the various components of the funeral and burial independently of one another, i.e., itemizing. This is now required by the U.S. Federal Trade Commission.

MUMMY: A corpse whose skin has been preserved over a skeleton, either through natural or artifical processes.


NECROBIOSIS: The process of decay or death in tissues or an entire body.

NECROGENIC: Arising from or produced by contact with corpses.

NECROGENOUS: Growing on dead or dying tissues or organs.

NECROLATRY: Worshiping the dead; sometimes associated with idolatry or supernaturalism.

NECROMANCER: One who carries on conversations with the dead, often to try to determine the future.

*NECROPHAGAUS:* A family of Clavicorn beetles including those that feed on dead and decomposing flesh.

NECROPHAGIA: Scientific name for cannibalism.

NECROPHILOUS: A fungi or beetle living on dead substance or carrion.

NECROPOLIS: A city of the dead or large burial site.

NECROPSY: An autopsy.

NECROSIS: Tissue death.

NEOMORT: Cadavers that are brain dead, but whose heart and lungs still function, if only through the use of mechanical devices.

NEUROSUSPENSION: Cryonic preservation of a patient's brain after death. The brain is usually stored intact within the head.

NICHE: A compartment or cubicle for the memorialization or permanent placement of an urn containing cremated remains.


OBITUARY: A news item announcing a death.

ORGAN/TISSUE BANK: An institution that coordinates organ donation between donors and receiving institutions.

ORGAN DONATION: Providing one's organs to another person to prolong or improve his life.

ORGAN DONOR: An individual who donates organs, tissue, or his entire body for transplant or medical science.

OSSUARY: Depository for the bones of the dead.

OVERLAP: A method of keeping the corpse's eyes closed by placing the upper lid over the lower lid.

PALL: The covering over a casket during the funerary rites.

PASCHAL CANDLE: A single candle placed between the casket and altar during the Roman Catholic funeral Mass.

PATHOLOGICAL INCINERATORS: The US government's term for crematories.

PERPETUAL CARE: The promise to maintain a cemetery forever.

PLAGIUM: Man-stealing, or body-snatching.

PLASTINATION: A modern technique to preserve dissected anatomical specimens using curable polymers.

POSTMORTEM: After death.

POSTMORTEM EXAMINATION: Often referred to as a "post," it is an autopsy.

POSTMORTEM STAIN: Discoloration caused by blood cell coloring seeping into the skin.

PRENEED: Purchase of funeral, burial or cremation services by a person before death.

PREPARATION ROOM: Another term for the embalming room.

PRESUMED CONSENT: Legal authority to remove a corpse's organs or tissues for transplant if there is no specific objection from the family, nor written objections left by the deceased.

PRIMARY BURIAL: The initial interment of a corpse.

PROCESSING: Pulverization.

PROSPECT: The term the funeral industry uses for a member of the deceased's family who will purchase services from it.

PYRE: An open fire used to cremate bodies.

PULVERIZATION: Grinding the residual bone fragments to crystal-sized particles after cremation.

PUTREFACTION: Destruction of the corpse by the bacteria contained within the body at death.

RABBIT PAW: The forefoot of a rabbit, dried and with nails removed, that is used to apply dry rouge to the dead.

REANIMATION: Term used for the potential reawakening of cryonically preserved patients.

RELIQUARY: A container in which sacred mementos, such as bone fragments, are kept.

REMAINS: A corpse or its parts.

RESTORATIVE ART: The funeral industry's term for the craft of embalmers and cosmeticians who work to recreate the natural form and color of a corpse.

RIGOR MORTIS: Stiffening of the body after death.

RITE: Ceremony.


SARCOPHAGUS: Stone coffin, usually inscribed and adorned with sculptured figures.

SECONDARY BURIAL: The ritual reburial of remains after disinterment, often with additional preparation of bones, such as by painting them.

SEPULCHER: A burial vault.

SEPULTURE: Burial.

SHELL EMBALMING: Preserving only the body surface, rather than the deeper tissues.

SHITAI: Japanese term for the corpse.

SHOMRIM: Jewish sitters who remain with a body from casketing to burial.

SHROUD: A white garment, often resembling a long-sleeved nightgown, in which corpses are buried.

SINGLE-UNIT PRICING: An older and somewhat deceptive method for pricing funerals, in which the cost of the funeral is dependent upon the cost of the casket—now illegal in the U.S.

SKULL CAP: The portion of the skull removed during an autopsy so the brain can be examined.

SLIP COFFINS: Coffins or caskets with hinged floors that were lowered into the grave with the bodies, but were then removed and reused after the bodies had been unloaded.

STRIPPING THE FLESH: The Zoroastrian and Parsee method of corpse disposition by exposing it to birds of prey. See also, Excarnate.


TACHRICHIM: In Judaism, the shroud of white linen in which the dead are buried.

TAHARAH: In Judaism, the traditional final bathing of the body.

THANATOLOGIST: An academic who is designated as an expert on death.

THANATOMIMESIS: Pretending to be dead.

THROAT CUTTER: An old derogatory term for arterial embalmers by those using other means of embalming. It derives from the incisions the embalmers make in the neck to expose the major arteries.

TISSUE DONATION: Providing one's skin or other tissue after death to another person to prolong or improve his life.

TOMB: Excavation for burial of a corpse; a structure or vault, below or above ground, for interment.

TONING COMPOUND: A warm brown color, which, when applied with a fundamental compound, such as flesh-pink, supplies the missing element to the complexion and mutes the fundamental color of a corpse's skin.

TRANSPLANTATION: Transferring an organ or tissue from a donor to a patient. The donor is usually dead (cadaveric donor), but in some cases can be alive at the time of donation (as with kidney donors).

TRISAGION: Three short prayers the Eastern Orthodox say over the deceased before the funeral.

TRI-UNIT PRICING: A method of charging separately for the casket, the mortuary facilities, and the personal services, including embalming—now illegal in the U.S.

TROCAR: Long hollow needle which embalmers use to remove fluid from the body and infuse embalming chemicals.

TROCAR BUTTON: A large plastic screw used to close holes in embalmed bodies.

TROCAR GUIDE: Imaginary lines used to guide the embalmer inserting the trocar into body cavities.

TUMULUS: An ancient grave mound; a barrow.


UNDERTAKER: A mortician or funeral director.

UNOS: Acronym for the national agency for transplantable organ procurement, the United Network for Organ Sharing.

UNVEILING: In Judaism, the prayer service surrounding the delayed consecration of a tombstone.

URN: A receptacle designed to permanently encase cremated remains.


VAULT: Burial structure or chamber, often arched, usually made of stone. Also, a prefabricated receptacle into which a casket and its contents is put, which is generally made of steel, concrete, fiberglass, or copper. The claim is that it prevents the ground from caving in and protects the casket from the elements.

VIEWING: A common U.S. Christian funerary custom in which friends and relatives see the corpse and visit with the family.

WAKE: Period between death and burial when the body is tended. Also often refers to the celebration held during this period.

WHOLE-BODY SUSPENSION: Preservation of the entire body in cryonic suspension.

WILL: A legal document effective after death detailing disposition of one's worldly goods.

WINDING SHEET: A sheet in which the corpse was wrapped or wound until burial, normally with the face exposed. It was tied or sewn above the head and below the feet to resemble a double-ended sack.

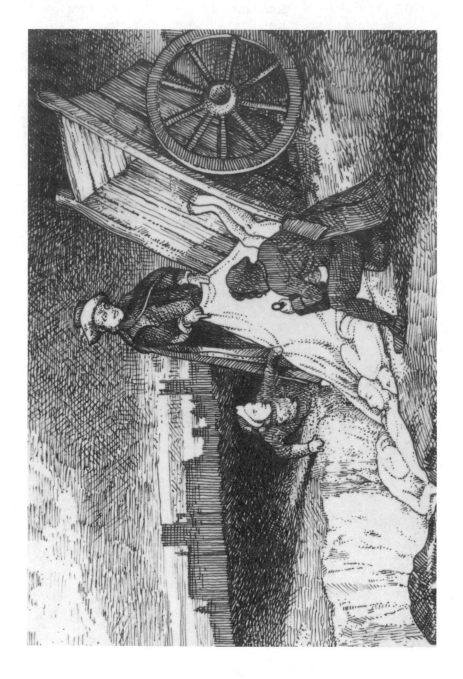

Mass burial in the plague pit.  Original print published by J. Franklin

# 16: APPENDICES

## A. TWENTY-SECOND WORLD MEDICAL ASSEMBLY,
Sydney, Australia, August 5-10, 1968.
(XXII World Medical Assembly. *World Medical J.* 1968:15(6):131-41.)

The determination of the time of death is in most countries the legal responsibility of the physician and should remain so. Usually he will be able without special assistance to decide that a person is dead, employing the classical criteria known to all physicians.

Two modern practices in medicine, however, have made it necessary to study the question of the time of death further: (1) the ability to maintain by artificial means the circulation of oxygenated blood through tissues of the body which may have been irreversibly injured and (2) the use of cadaver organs such as heart or kidneys for transplantation.

A complication is that death is a gradual process at the cellular level with tissues varying in their ability to withstand deprivation of oxygen. But clinical interest lies not in the state of preservation of isolated cells but in the fate of a person. Here the point of death of the different cells and organs is not so important as the certainty that the process has become irreversible by whatever techniques of resuscitation that may be employed.

This determination will be based on clinical judgement supplemented if necessary by a number of diagnostic aids, of which the electroencephalograph is currently the most helpful. However, no single technological criterion is entirely satisfactory in the present state of medicine nor can any one technological procedure be substituted for the overall judgment of the physician. If transplantation of an organ is involved the decision that death exists should be made by two or more physicians and the physician determining the moment of death should in no way be immediately concerned with the performance of the transplantation.

Determination of the point of death of the person makes it ethically permissible to cease attempts at resuscitation and in countries where the law permits, to remove organs from the cadaver provided that prevailing legal requirements of consent have been fulfilled.

## B. AD HOC COMMITTEE OF THE HARVARD MEDICAL SCHOOL TO EXAMINE THE DEFINITION OF BRAIN DEATH, 1968

An organ, brain or other, that no longer functions and has no possibility of functioning again is for all practical purposes dead. Our first problem is to determine the characteristics of a *permanently* nonfunctioning brain.

A patient in this state appears to be in deep coma. The condition can be satisfactorily diagnosed by points 1, 2, and 3 to follow. The electroencephalogram (point 4) provides confirmatory data, and when available it should be utilized. In situations where for one reason or another electroencephalographic monitoring is not available, the absence of cerebral function has to be determined by purely clinical signs, to be described, or by absence of circulation as judged by standstill blood in the retinal vessels, or by absence of cardiac activity.

1. *Unreceptivity and Unresponsivity*—There is a total unawareness to externally applied stimuli and inner need and complete unresponsiveness—our definition of irreversible coma. Even the most intensely painful stimuli evoke no vocal or other response, not even a groan, withdrawal of a limb, or quickening of respiration.

2. *No Movement or Breathing*—Observation covering a period of at least one hour by physicians is adequate to satisfy the criteria of no spontaneous muscular movements or spontaneous respiration or response to stimuli such as pain, touch, sound, or light. After the patient is on a mechanical respirator, the total absence of spontaneous breathing may be established by turning off the respirator for three minutes and observing whether there is any effort on the part of the subject to breathe spontaneously. (The respirator may be turned off for this time provided that at the start of the trial period the patient's carbon dioxide tension is within the normal range, and provided also that the patient has been for at least 10 minutes prior to the trial.)

3. *No Reflexes*—Irreversible coma with abolition of central nervous system activity is evidenced in part by the absence of elicitable reflexes. The pupil will be fixed and dilated and will not respond to a direct source of bright light. Since the establishment of a fixed, dilated pupil is clear-cut in clinical practice, there should be no uncertainty as to its presence. Ocular movement (to head turning and to irrigation of the ears with ice water) and blinking are absent. There is no evidence of postural activity (decerebrate or other). Swallowing, yawning, vocalization are in abeyance. Corneal and pharyngeal reflexes are absent.

As a rule the stretch of tendon reflexes cannot be elicited; i.e., tapping the tendons of the biceps, triceps, and pronator muscles, quadriceps and gastrocnemius muscles with the reflex hammer elicits no contraction of the respective muscles. Plantar or noxious stimulation gives no response.

4. *Flat Electroencephalogram* — Of great confirmatory value is the flat or isoelectric EEG. We must assume that the electrodes have been properly applied, that the apparatus is functioning normally, and that the personnel in charge is competent. We consider it prudent to have one channel of the apparatus used for an electrocardiogram. This channel will monitor the ECG so that, if it appears in the electroencephalographic leads because of high resistance, it can be readily identified. It also establishes the presence of the active heart in the absence of the EEG. We recommend that another channel be used for a noncephalic lead. This will pick up space-borne or vibration-borne artifacts and identify them. The simplest form of such a monitoring noncephalic electrode has two leads over the dorsum of the hand, preferably the right hand, so the ECG will be minimal or absent. Since one of the requirements of this state is that there be no muscle activity, these two dorsal hand electrodes will not be bothered by muscle artifact. The apparatus should be run at standard gains $10\mu v/mm$, $50\mu v/5mm$. Also it should be isoelectric at double this standard gain which is $5\mu v/mm$ or $25\mu v/5mm$. At least ten full minutes of recording are desirable, but twice that would be better.

It is also suggested that the gains at some point be opened to their full amplitude for a brief period (5 to 100 seconds) to see what is going on. Usually in an intensive care unit artifacts will dominate the picture, but these are readily identifiable. There shall be no electroencephalographic response to noise or to pinch.

All of the above tests shall be repeated at least 24 hours later with no change.

The validity of such data as indications of irreversible cerebral damage depends on the exclusion of two conditions: hypothermia (temperature below 90 F. [32.2 C]) or central nervous system depressants, such as barbiturates.

## C. UNIFORM DETERMINATION OF DEATH ACT
### 12 U.L.A. 271 (Supp 1985).

PREFATORY NOTE

This Act is silent on acceptable diagnostic tests and medical procedures. It sets the general legal standard for determining death, but not the medical criteria for doing so. The medical profession remains free to formulate acceptable medical practices and to utilize new biomedical knowledge, diagnostic tests, and equipment.

UNIFORM DETERMINATION OF DEATH ACT

1. An individual who has sustained either (1) irreversible cessation of circulatory and respiratory functions or (2) irreversible cessation of all functions of the entire brain, including the brainstem, is dead. A determination of death must be made in accordance with accepted medical standards.

2. This Act shall be applied and construed to effectuate its general purpose to make uniform the law with respect to the subject of this Act among states enacting it.

3. This Act may be cited as the Uniform Determination of Death Act.

[As of the end of 1992, this Act or a close modification, had been adopted in: AK, CA, CO, DE, DC, GA, ID, IN, KS, ME, MD, MI, MN, MS, MO, MT, NE, NV, NH, ND, OH, OK, OR, PA, RI, SC, SD, UT, VT, WV, WY.]

## D. UNIVERSAL DETERMINATION OF DEATH STATUTE (PROPOSED)

(Sass HM: Criteria for death: self-determination and public policy. *J of Med & Philosophy.* 1992;17:445-54.)

An individual who has sustained either (1) irreversible cessation of circulatory and respiratory functions, or (2) irreversibe cessation of all functions of the cntire brain, including the brain stem, or (3) irreversible cessation of higher-brain functions is dead. Competent adults, using advance directives may opt for any one of these criteria; proxy decisionmaking [sic] is not accepted, except in cases of parents deciding for their minor children. In the absence of advance directives, the irreversible cessation of all functions of the entire brain, including the brain stem, will signify death. Given global cultural diversity and different legal and religious traditions, states [involvement] in promoting their interest in protecting the life and dignity of their citizens in accordance with widely held values within their constituency may, as a matter of public policy, define different death criteria, such as those based on cessation of functions of the entire body or the heart, but should provide a conscience clause for individual choice. A determination of death must be made in accordance with accepted medical standards.

## E. UNIFORM ANATOMICAL GIFT ACT (U.S.)
(The template used by most state laws.)


PREFATORY NOTE

Human bodies and parts thereof are used in many aspects of medical science, including teaching, research, therapy and transplantation. It is a rapidly expanding branch of medical technology. Transplantation of parts may involve skin, bones, blood, corneas, kidneys, livers, arteries and even hearts. It is said that 6,000 to 10,000 lives could be saved each year by renal transplants if a sufficient supply of kidneys were available.

Transplantation may be effected within narrow limits from one living person to another living person. In such case, all that is required is an appropriate "informed consent" authorizing the surgical removal of the one and the implantation on the other. Tissues and organs from the dead can also be used to bring health and years of life to the living. From this source the potential supply is very great. But, if utilization of bodies and parts of bodies is to be effectuated, a number of competing interests in a dead body must be harmonized, and several troublesome legal questions must be answered.

The principal competing interests are: (1) the wishes of the deceased during his lifetime concerning the disposition of his body; (2) the desires of the surviving spouse or next-of-kin; (3) the interest of the state in determining by autopsy, the cause of death in cases involving crime or violence; (4) the need of autopsy to determine the cause of death when private legal rights are dependent upon such cause; and (5) the need of society for bodies, tissues, and organs for medical education, research, therapy, and transplantation. These interests compete with one another to a greater or lesser extent and this creates problems.

The principal legal questions arising from these various interests are: (1) who may during his lifetime make a legally effective gift of his body or a part thereof; (2) what is the right of the next-of-kin, either to set aside the decedent's expressed wishes, or themselves to make the anatomical gifts from the dead body; (3) who may legally become donees of anatomical gifts; (4) for what purposes may such gifts be made (5) how may gifts be made, can it be done by will, by writing, by a card carried on the person, or by telegraphic or recorded telephonic communication; (6) how may a gift be revoked by the donor during his lifetime; (7) what are the rights of survivors in the body after removal of donated parts; (8) what protection from legal liability should anatomical gifts have; (9) should such protection be afforded regardless of the state in which the document of gift is executed; (10) what should the effect of an anatomical gift be in case of conflict with laws concerning autopsies; (11) should the time of death be defined by law in any way; (12) should the interest in preserving life by the physician in charge of a decedent preclude him from participating in the transplant procedure by which donated tissues or organs are transferred to a new host. These are the principal legal questions that should be covered in an anatomical gift act. The Uniform Anatomical Gift Act covers them. The laws now on the statute books do not, in general, deal with these legal questions in a complete or adequate manner. The laws are a confusing mixture of old common law dating back to the seventeenth century and state statutes that have been enacted from time to time. Some 39 states and the District of Columbia have donation statutes that deal in a variety of ways with some, but by no means all, of the above listed legal questions. Four other states have statutes providing for the gift of eyes only.

These statutes differ from each other in a variety of respects, both as to content and coverage. They differ in their enumeration of permissible donees (some require that donees be specified, others permit gifts to be made to any hospital or physician in charge at death); they vary as to acceptable purposes for anatomical gifts (some, for example, do not include licensed tissue banks); they prescribe a variety of minimum ages for the donors; others differ as to the manner of execution of gifts and the manner of revocation. Some require delivery of the instrument of gift or filing in a public office, or both, as a condition of validity; others make no such provision. Since the statutes differ in important respects, a gift adequate in one state may or may not protect the surgeon in another state who relies upon the law in effect where the transplant takes place. In short, both the common law and the present statutory picture is one of confusion, diversity, and inadequacy. This tends to discourage anatomical gifts and create difficulties for physicians, especially for transplant surgeons.

In view of the foregoing, the need for a comprehensive act and an act applicable in all states is apparent. The Uniform Anatomical Gift Act herewith presented by the National Conference of Commissioners on Uniform State Laws carefully weighs the numerous conflicting interests and legal problems. Wherever adopted it will encourage the making of anatomical gifts, thus facilitating therapy involving such procedures. When generally adopted, even if the place of death, or the residence of the donor, or the place of use of the gift occurs in a state other than that of the execution of the gift, uncertainty as to the applicable law will be eliminated and all parties will be protected. At the same time the Act will serve the needs of the several conflicting interests in a manner consistent with prevailing customs and desires in this country respecting dignified disposition of dead bodies. It will provide a useful and uniform legal environment throughout the country for this new frontier of modern medicine.

## UNIFORM ANATOMICAL GIFT ACT

An Act authorizing the gift of all or part of a human body after death for specified purposes.

SECTION 1. [Definitions.]

    (a) "Bank or storage facility" means a facility licensed, accredited, or approved under the laws of any state for storage of human bodies or parts thereof.

    (b) "Decedent" means a deceased individual and includes a stillborn infant or fetus.

    (c) "Donor" means an individual who makes a gift of all or part of his body.

    (d) "Hospital" means a hospital licensed, accredited, or approved under the laws of any state; includes a hospital operated by the United States government, a state, or a subdivision thereof, although not required to be licensed under state laws.

    (e) "Part" means organs, tissues, eyes, bones, arteries, blood, other fluids and any other portions of a human body.

    (f) "Person" means an individual, corporation, government or governmental subdivision or agency, business trust, estate, trust, partnership or association, or any other legal entity.

    (g) "Physician" or "surgeon" means a physician or surgeon licensed or authorized to practice under the laws of any state.

    (h) "State" includes any state, district, commonwealth, territory, insular possession, and any other area subject to the legislative authority of the United States of America.

SECTION 2. [Persons Who May Execute an Anatomical Gift.]

    (a) Any individual of sound mind and 18 years of age or more may give all or any part of his body for any purpose specified in section 3, the gift to take effect upon death.

    (b) Any of the following persons, in order of priority stated, when persons in prior classes are not available at the time of death, and in the absence of actual notice of contrary indications by the decedent or actual notice of opposition by a member of the same or prior class, may give all or any part of the decedent's body for any purpose specified in section 3:

    (1) the spouse,

    (2) an adult son or daughter,

    (3) either parent,

    (4) an adult brother or sister,

    (5) a guardian of the person of the decedent at the time of his

death,

(6) any other person authorized or under obligation to dispose of the body.

(c) If the donee has actual notice of contrary indications by the decedent or that a gift by a member of a class is opposed by a member of the same or a prior class, the donee shall not accept the gift. The persons authorized by subsection (b) may make the gift after or immediately before death.

(d) A gift of all or part of a body authorizes any examination necessary to assure medical acceptability of the gift for the purposes intended.

(e) The rights of the donee created by the gift are paramount to the rights of others except as provided in Section 7 (d).

SECTION 3. [Persons Who May Become Donees; Purposes for Which Anatomical Gifts May be Made.] The following persons may become donees of gifts of bodies or parts thereof for the purposes stated:

(1) any hospital, surgeon, or physician, for medical or dental education, research, advancement of medical or dental science, therapy, or transplantation; or

(2) any accredited medical or dental school, college or university for education, research, advancement of medical or dental science, or therapy; or

(3) any bank or storage facility, for medical or dental education, research, advancement of medical or dental science, therapy, of transplantation; or

(4) any specified individual for therapy or transplantation needed by him.

SECTION 4. [Manner of Executing Anatomical Gifts.]

(a) A gift of all or part of the body under Section 2 (a) may be made by will. The gift becomes effective upon the death of the testator without waiting for probate. If the will is not probated, or if it is declared invalid for testamentary purposes, the gift, to the extent that it has been acted upon in good faith, is nevertheless valid and effective.

(b) A gift of all or part of the body under Section 2 (a) may also be made by document other than a will. The gift becomes effective upon the death of the donor. The document, which may be a card designed to be carried on the person, must be signed by the donor in the presence of 2 witnesses who must sign the document in his presence. If the donor cannot sign, the document may be signed for him at his direction and in his presence in the presence of 2 witnesses who must sign the document in his presence. Delivery of the document of gift during the donor's lifetime is not necessary to make the gift valid.

(c) The gift may be made to a specified donee or without specifying a donee. If the latter, the gift may be accepted by the attending physician as donee upon or following death. If the gift is made to a specified donee who is not available at the time and in the absence of any expressed indication that the donor desired otherwise, may accept the gift as donee. The physician who becomes a donee under this subsection shall not participate in the procedures for removing or transplanting a part.

(d) Notwithstanding Section 7 (c), the donor may designate in his will, card, or other document of gift the surgeon or physician to carry out the appropriate procedures. In the absence of a designation or if the designee is not available, the donee or other person authorized to accept the gift may employ or authorize any surgeon or physician for the purpose.

(e) Any gift by a person designated in Section 2 shall be made by a document signed by him or made by his telegraphic, recorded telephonic, or other recorded message.

SECTION 5. [Delivery of Document of Gift.] If the gift is made by the donor to a specified donee, the will, card, or other document, or an executed copy thereof, may be delivered to the donee to expedite the appropriate procedures immediately after death. Delivery is not necessary for the validity of the gift. The will, card, or other document, or an executed copy thereof, may be deposited in any hospital, bank or storage facility or registry office that accepts it for safekeeping or for facilitation of procedures after death. On request of any interested party upon or after the donor's death, the person in possession shall produce the document for examination.

SECTION 6. [Amendment or Revocation of the Gift.]

(a) If the will, card, or other document or executed copy thereof, has been delivered to a specified donee, the donor may amend or revoke the gift by:

(1) the execution and delivery to the donee of a signed statement, or

(2) an oral statement made in the presence of 2 persons and communicated to the donee, or

(3) a statement during a terminal illness or injury addressed to an attending physician and communicated to the donee, or

(4) a signed card or document found on his person or in his effects.

(b) Any document of gift which has not been delivered to the donee may be revoked by the donor in the manner set out in subsection (a), or by destruction, cancellation, or mutilation of the document and all executed copies thereof.

(c) Any gift made by a will may also be amended or revoked in the manner provided for amendment or revocation of wills, or as provided in subsection (a).

617

SECTION 7. [Rights and Duties at Death.]
(a) The donee may accept or reject the gift. If the donee accepts a gift of the entire body, he may, subject to the terms of the gift, authorize embalming and the use of the body in funeral services. If the gift is of a part of the body, the donee, upon the death of the donor and prior to embalming, shall cause the part to be removed without unnecessary mutilation. After removal of the part, custody of the remainder of the body vests in the surviving spouse, next-of-kin, or other persons under obligation to dispose of the body.
(b) The time of death shall be determined by a physician who tends the donor at his death, or, if none, the physician who certifies the death. The physician shall not participate in the procedures for removing or transplanting a part.
(c) A person who acts in good faith in accord with the terms of this Act or with the anatomical gift laws of another state [or foreign country] is not liable for damages in any civil action or subject to prosecution in any criminal proceeding for his act.
(d) The provisions of this Act are subject to the laws of this state prescribing powers and duties with respect to autopsies.

SECTION 8. [Uniformity of Interpretation.] This Act shall be so construed as to effectuate its general purpose to make uniform the law of those states which enact it.

SECTION 9. [Short Title.] This Act may be cited as the Uniform Anatomical Gift Act.

SECTION 10. [Repeal.] The following acts and parts of acts are repealed:
(1)
(2)
(3)

SECTION 11. [Time of Taking Effect.] This Act shall take effect.....

## F. THE HUMAN TISSUE GIFT ACT, 1971 (CANADA)

Her Majesty, by and with the advice and consent of the Legislative Assembly of the Province of Ontario, enacts as follows:

1. In this Act,
    (a) "consent" means a consent given under this Act;
    (b) "physician" means a person registered under The Medical Act;
    (c) "tissue" includes an organ, but does not include any skin, bone, blood, blood constituent or other tissue that is replaceable by natural processes of repair;
    (d) "transplant" as a noun means the removal of tissue from a human body, whether living or dead, and its implantation in a living human body, and in its other forms it has corresponding meanings;
    (e) "writing" for the purposes of Part II includes a will and any other testamentary instrument whether or not probate has been applied for or granted and whether or not the will or other testamentary instrument is valid.

## PART I INTER-VIVOS GIFTS FOR TRANSPLANTS

2. A transplant from one living human body to another living human body may be done in accordance with this Act, but not otherwise.

3.

    (1) Any person who has attained the age of majority, is mentally competent to consent, and is able to make a free and informed decision may in a writing signed by him consent to the removal forthwith from his body of the tissue specified in the consent and its implantation in the body of another living person.

    (2) Notwithstanding subsection 1, a consent given thereunder by a person who had not attained the age of majority, was not mentally competent to consent, or was not able to make a free and informed decision is valid for the purposes of this Act if the person who acted upon it had no reason to believe that the person who gave it had not attained the age of majority, was not mentally competent to consent, and was not able to make a free and informed decision, as the case may be.

    (3) A consent given under this section is full authority for any physician,
        (a) to make any examination necessary to assure medical

acceptability of the tissue specified therein; and

(b) to remove forthwith such tissue from the body of the person who gave the consent.

(4) If for any reason the tissue specified in the consent is not removed in the circumstances to which the consent relates, the consent is void.

## PART II POST MORTEM GIFTS FOR TRANSPLANTS AND OTHER USES
4.

(1) Any person who has attained the age of majority may consent,

(a) in a writing signed by him at any time; or

(b) orally in the presence of at least two witnesses during his last illness, that his body or the part or parts thereof specified in the consent be used after his death for therapeutic purposes, medical education or scientific research.

(2) Notwithstanding subsection 1, a consent given by a person who had not attained the age of majority is valid for the purposes of this Act if the person who acted upon it had no reason to believe that the person who gave it had not attained the age of majority.

(3) Upon the death of a person who has given a consent under this section, the consent is binding and is full authority for the use of the body or the removal and use of the specified part or parts for the purpose specified, except that no person shall act upon a consent given under this section if he has reason to believe that it was subsequently withdrawn.

5.

(1) Where a person of any age who has not given a consent under section 4 dies, or in the opinion of a physician is incapable of giving a consent by reason of injury or disease and his death is imminent,

(a) his spouse of any age; or

(b) if none or if his spouse is not readily available, any one of his children who has attained the age of majority; or

(c) if none or if none is readily available, either of his parents; or

(d) if none or if neither is readily available, any one of his brothers or sisters who has attained the age of majority; or

(e) if none or if none is readily available, any other of his next-of-kin who has attained the age of majority; or

(f) if none or if none is readily available, the person lawfully in possession of the body other than where he died in hospital, the administrative head of the hospital, may consent,

(g) in a writing signed by the spouse, relative or other person, or

(h) orally by the spouse, relative or other person in the presence of at least two witnesses; or

(i) by the telegraphic, recorded telephonic, or other recorded message of the spouse, relative or other person, to the body or the part or parts thereof specified in the consent being used after death for therapeutic purposes, medical education or scientific research.

(2) No person shall give a consent under this section if he has reason to believe that the person who died or whose death is imminent would have objected thereto.

(3) Upon the death of a person in respect of whom a consent was given under this section the consent is binding and is, subject to section 6, full authority for the use of the body or for the removal and use of the specified part or parts for the purpose specified except that no person shall act on a consent given under this section if he has actual knowledge of an objection thereto by the person in respect of whom the consent was given or by the person of the same or closer relationship to person in respect of whom the consent was given than the person who gave the consent.

(4) In subsection 1, "person lawfully in possession of the body" does not include,

(a) the supervising coroner or a coroner in possession of the body for the purposes of the Coroners Act;

(b) the Public Trustee in possession of the body for the purpose of its burial under The Crown Administration of Estates Act;

(c) an embalmer or funeral director in possession of the body for the purpose of its burial, cremation or other disposition; or

(d) the superintendent of a crematorium in possession of the body for the purpose of its cremation.

6. Where in the opinion of a physician, the death of a person is imminent by reason of injury or disease and the physician has reason to believe that section 7, 21 or 22 of The Coroners Act may apply when death does occur and a consent under this part has been obtained for a post-mortem transplant of tissue from the body, a coroner having jurisdiction, notwithstanding that death has not yet occurred, may give such directions as he thinks proper respecting the removal of such tissue after the death of the person, and every such direction has the same force and effect as if it had been made after death under section 8 of The Coroners Act.

7.

    (1) For the purposes of a post-mortem transplant, the fact of death shall be determined by at least two physicians in accordance with accepted medical practice.

    (2) No physician who has had any association with the proposed recipient that might influence his judgment shall take any part in the determination of the fact of death of the donor.

    (3) No physician who took any part in the determination of the fact of death of the donor shall participate in any way in the transplant procedures.

    (4) Nothing in this section in any way affects a physician in the removal of eyes for cornea transplants.

8. Where a gift under this Part cannot for any reasons be used for any of the purposes specified in the consent, the subject matter of the gift and the body to which it belongs shall be dealt with and disposed of as if no consent had been given.

PART III GENERAL

9. No action or other proceeding for damages lies against any person for any act done in good faith and without negligence in the exercise or intended exercise of any authority conferred by this Act.

10. No person shall buy, sell or otherwise deal in, directly or indirectly, for a valuable consideration, any tissue for a transplant, or any body or part or parts thereof other than blood constituent, for therapeutic purposes, medical education or scientific research, and any such dealing is invalid as being contrary to public policy.

11.

    (1) Except where legally required, no person shall disclose or give to any other person any information or document whereby the identity of any person,

        (a) who has given or refused to give a consent;

        (b) with respect to whom a consent has been given; or

        (c) into whose body tissue has been, is being or may be transplanted, may become known publicly.

    (2) Where the information or document disclosed or given pertains only to the person who disclosed or gave the information or document, subsection 1 does not apply.

12. Any dealing with a body or part or parts thereof that was lawful before this Act came into force shall, except as provided in this Act, continue to be

lawful.

13. Every person who knowingly contravenes any provision of this Act is guilty of an offence and on summary conviction is liable to a fine of no more than $1,000 or to imprisonment for a term of not more than six months, or to both.

14. Except as provided in section 6, nothing in this Act affects the operation of The Coroners Act.

15. A request made or an authorization given under The Human Tissue Act (Canada), 1962-63 before this Act came into force may be acted upon in accordance with that Act notwithstanding the repeal of that Act.

PART IV MISCELLANEOUS

16. The Human Tissue Act, 1962-63 and the Human Tissue Amendment Act, 1967 are repealed.

17. This Act comes into force on the day it receives Royal Assent.

18. This Act may be cited as The Human Tissue Gift Act, 1971.

## G. EMBALMERS CLASSIFICATION: TYPES OF CORPSES

(Developed by Ray E. Slocum of the Dodge Chemical Company in the late 1950s and published in *Pre-embalmimg Considerations* (pamphlet) Boston, MA: The Dodge Company. Cited in Mayer RG: *Embalming—History, Theory, and Practice*. Norwalk, CT: Appleton & Lange, 1990. p 192-3. This is a very small portion of the Slocum text. Note that these are older techniques. Reprinted by permission of The Dodge Company.)

This classification is used by embalmers to generally note the degree of difficulty they will have embalming the corpse. Fees may be related to this classification.

TYPE I: Generally require mild to moderate strength embalming solutions. Note: All bodies in this classification (the "average body") still retain some body heat.

1. Bodies dead of heart disease that have not undergone a lingering illness preceding death.
2. Bodies dead of vascular diseases that have not been bedridden prior to death.
3. Stout (obese) bodies in which there is no bloodstream or coccal infection.
4. All bodies that suddenly expired, not dead over 12 hours, except those requiring restorative treatments.
5. Bodies dead of childbirth.
6. Bodies not later specified that appear to have a normal or abnormally large protein content (as usually exists in fleshy bodies or where skin is dry)

TYPE II: Generally require moderate to strong embalming fluid.

1. Bodies not dead more than 24 hours that have low albumin content as indicated by moist or clammy tissue, usually with angular faces and still retaining body heat.
2. Bodies not dead more than 12 hours from coccal infections.
3. Bodies not dead more than 12 hours from uremic poisoning (uremia), diabetes, nephritis, dropsy, or any disease wherein the organs of elimination have not functioned properly for some time prior to death.
4. Bodies not dead more than 12 hours where death occurred in a public institution.

5. Bodies not dead more than 24 hours from wasting diseases such as tuberculosis and cancer.

6. Bodies not dead more than 12 hours that require major restorative treatments.

7. Bodies not dead more than 12 hours that may have been administered large quantities of drugs preceding death.

8. Bodies that might have been classified as Type I but that have been dead long enough (but not over 24 hours) to have lost body heat.

9. Bodies not dead over 12 hours that show evidence of considerable senile changes, such as extreme flabbiness of tissue.

10. Bodies drowned but not in the water more than 24 hours in cold weather or 12 hours in warm weather.

11. Bodies originally classified as Type I, in which the treatment recommended for that type was begun but difficulty is encountered in securing desired circulation, drainage, or tissue firming.

12. Autopsied bodies not subjected to refrigeration that have not been dead more than 24 hours.

Bodies placed in this classification are undoubtedly those that most frequently could cause embalming difficulties unless some consideration is given to the individual conditions present and plans are made to circumvent these conditions with specific treatments.

**TYPE III**: Generally require strong embalming solutions.

1. All bodies dead more than 24 hours that do not show evidence of advanced putrefaction.

2. Bodies that have been frozen improperly and do not show advanced stages for putrefaction.

3. Bodies that fail to respond to Type II treatment.

4. Bodies in which the initial embalming:reinjection; arterial injection was insufficient to the extent that reinjection became necessary for proper preservation, but wherein the advanced stages of putrefaction have not occurred.

5. Autopsied bodies dead more than 24 hours.

Bodies in this classification undoubtedly present a more serious problem to the embalmer than do Type I and II bodies. It is likely that the number of bodies in this classification will continually increase because of the ever-growing demands of medical science for more autopsies. In many instances, even though permission for autopsy is not secured from nearest kin, the bodies are held at hospitals pending attempts to secure such permission.

**TYPE IV**: Generally require strong embalming solutions.

1. Bodies dead of diseases affecting the biliary tract as evidenced by a jaundice discoloration, but still retaining body heat or dead not more than 12 hours prior to embalming.

2. Bodies dead of asphyxiation or from any cause for which methylene blue had been used intravenously as a resuscitory measure, but which have not been dead more than 12 hours.

3. Bodies not dead more than 12 hours from Addison's disease.

**TYPE V**: Generally require strong embalming solutions.

1. All bodies showing advanced stages of putrefaction.

2. Bodies wherein "tissue gas" (gas bacillus, Bacillus aerogenes capsulatus, or B. welchii) or gas gangrene is present.

3. Bodies that develop putrefaction after arterial injection.

4. Bodies that require distal injection of gangrenous limbs.

5. Bodies that require treatment for advanced stages of ascites wherein the limbs have become ulcerated.

## H. THE U.S. CODE OF FEDERAL REGULATIONS FOR THE RETURN OF REMAINS TO THE U.S.
(Revised, April 1, 1982)

§72.11 Cremation.

1. *Arrangements.* When cremation is desired, and the facilities are available, the consular officer should see that all necessary arrangements are made if compatible with the requirements of the country in which the death occurred, having in mind particularly such local laws as may prohibit cremation unless specific request for such disposition was made in writing by the individual prior to death.

2. *Disposition of ashes.* Disposition of the ashes should be made in accordance with the expressed wishes of the deceased or the next of kin, or other interested person. If shipment to the United States is desired, only local health requirements must be met, as there are no sanitary requirements for entry of ashes into the United States. A marking should be made on, or a marker firmly affixed to, the container in which the ashes are shipped. The latter should be accompanied by:

(1) An official death certificate;

(2) Cremation certificate;

(3) Certificate from the crematorium stating that the container holds only the cremated remains of the deceased; and

(4) A permit to export (if required locally).

§72.12 Shipment of remains to the United States.

(a) *Arrangements.* Whenever the remains of persons who have died abroad, regardless of the nationality of the deceased, are to be shipped to the United States, the consular officer should assure himself that they are properly encased and accompanied by all necessary papers pertaining to the death, exhumation (if applicable) and preparation for shipment. The requirements of the country where the death occurred must be met at all times.

(b) *Local documents accompanying remains.* The following documents should accompany the remains for shipment, attached to the consular mortuary certificate (see paragraph (d) of this section):

(1) A certificate of death issued by the local registrar of deaths, or similar authority, identifying the remains, showing the place, date and cause of death as certified by the attending physician, with a listing of the cause of death conforming as far as practicable with the terminology of the

627

International List of Causes of Death (needed to comply with United States Quarantine and interstate requirements);

(2) The affidavit described in paragraph (c) of this section (for United States Customs), which also would generally include evidence of embalming, when applicable (needed to comply with the requirements for interstate shipment);

(3) A "transmit permit" authorizing export of the body out of the country, issued by the health authority at the port of embarkation, stating the date of its issuance, name of deceased, sex, race, age, cause and date of death (needed to comply with interstate requirements)

(c) *Packing and labeling of casket.* In order to facilitate clearance through United States Customs at the port of entry, the funeral director, or whatever person is responsible for packing the body for shipment, should be required to make a sworn declaration—to be attached to the consular mortuary certificate (see paragraph (d) of this section)—that the casket or box contains only the body of the deceased and the necessary clothing and packing. The sworn declaration should be made, if practicable, before the consular officer; if not, it should be made before a qualified local official, whose signature and seal can be authenticated by the consular officer. The outer box should be labeled in conformity with port of entry health requirements.

(d) *Consular mortuary certificate.* A consular mortuary certificate should be prepared indicating how the case is marked and addressed, means of transportation to the United States, name of carrier, date and place of shipment, port of entry and scheduled time of arrival. The documents listed in paragraph (b) of this section should be ribboned to the consular mortuary certificate, which should be signed by the consular officer and sealed with the consular press seal.

## I. FEDERAL TRADE COMMISSION'S "FUNERAL RULE,"
### 16 C.F.R. §453, Effective April, 1984.

The following excerpts are reprinted from Part III: Federal Trade Commission—Funeral Industry Practices; Trade Regulation rule. *Federal Register*, 1982;47:186:42260-304:

### §453.2 Price disclosures

The funeral provider must:...

(4) General price list. (i) Give a printed or typewritten price list for retention to persons who inquire in person about funeral arrangements or the prices of funeral goods or funeral services. When people inquire in person about funeral arrangements or the prices of funeral goods or funeral services, the funeral provider must offer them the list upon beginning discussion either of funeral arrangements or of the selection of any funeral goods or funeral services. This list must contain at least the following information:

(A) the name, address, and telephone number of the funeral provider's place of business;

(B) A caption describing the list as a "general price list";

(C) The effective date for the price list; and

(D) In immediate conjunction with the price disclosures required by paragraph (b)(4)(ii) of this section, the statement: "This list does not include prices for certain items that you may ask us to buy for you, such as cemetery or crematory services, flowers, and newspaper notices. The prices for those items will be shown on your bill or the statement describing the funeral goods and services you selected."

(ii) Include on the price list, in any order, the retail prices (expressed either as the flat fee, or as the price per hour, mile or other unit of computation) and the other information specified below for at least each of the following items, if offered for sale:

(A) Forwarding of remains to another funeral home, together with a list of the services provided for any quoted price;

(B) Receiving remains from another funeral home, together with a list of the services provided for any quoted price;

(C) The price range for the direct cremations offered by the funeral provider, together with: (1) A separate price for a direct cremation where the purchaser provides the container; (2) separate prices for each direct cremation offered including an unfinished wood box or alternative container; and (3) a description of the services and container (where applicable), included in each price;

(D) The price range for the immediate burials offered by the funeral provider, together with: *(1)* A separate price for an immediate burial where the purchaser provides the casket; *(2)* separate prices for each immediate burial offered including a casket or alternative container; and *(3)* a description of the services and container (where applicable) included in that price;

(E) Transfer of remains to funeral home;

(F) Embalming.

(G) Other preparation of the body;

(H) Use of facilities for viewing;

(I) Use of facilities for funeral ceremony;

(J) Other use of facilities, together with a list of facilities provided for any quoted price;

(K) Hearse;

(L) Limousine;

(M) Other automotive equipment, together with a description of the automotive provided for any quoted price; and

(N) Acknowledgment cards.

(iii) Include on the price list, in any order, the following information:

(A) Either of the following:

*(1)* The price range for the caskets offered by the funeral provider, together with the statement: "A complete price list will be provided at the funeral home."; or

*(2)* The prices of individual caskets, disclosed in the manner specified by paragraph (b)(2)(i) of this section; and

(B) either of the following:

*(1)* The price range for the outer burial containers offered by the funeral provider, together with the statement: "A complete price list will be provided at the funeral home."

*(2)* The prices of individual outer burial containers, disclosed in the manner specified by paragraph (b)(3)(i) of this section; and

(C) Either of the following:

*(1)* The price for the services of the funeral director and staff, together with a list of the principal services provided for any quoted price and, if the charge cannot be declined by the purchaser, the statement: "This fee for our services will be added to the total cost of the funeral arrangements you select. (This fee is already included in our charges for direct cremations, immediate burials, and forwarding or receiving remains.)"; or

*(2)* The following statement: "Please note that a fee for the use of our services is included in the price of our caskets. Our services include (specify)." The statement must be placed on the general price list together with casket price range, required by paragraph (b)(4)(iii)(A)*(1)* of this section, or together with the prices of individual caskets, required by

(b)(4)(iii)(A)*(2)*.

### §453.3 Misrepresentations

(a) *Embalming Provisions* — (1) *Deceptive acts or practices.* In selling or offering to sell funeral goods or funeral services to the public, it is a deceptive act or practice for a funeral provider to:

(i) Represent that state or local law requires that a deceased person be embalmed when such is not the case;

(ii) Fail to disclose that embalming is not is not required by law except in certain special cases.

(2) *Preventive requirements.* To prevent these deceptive acts or practices, as well as the unfair or deceptive acts or practices defined in §§453.4(b)(1) and 453.4 (b)(1) [of these rules and regulations], funeral providers must:

(i) Not represent that a deceased person is required to be embalmed for direct cremation, immediate burial, a funeral using a sealed casket, or if refrigeration is available and the funeral is without viewing or visitation and with a closed casket when state or local law does not require embalming; and

(ii) Place for following disclosure on the general price list, required by §453.2(b)(4), in immediate conjunction with the price shown for embalming: "Except in certain special cases, embalming is not required by law. Embalming may be necessary, however, if you select certain funeral arrangements, such as a funeral with viewing. If you do not want embalming, you usually have the right to choose an arrangement which does not require you to pay for it, such as direct cremation or immediate burial."

(b) *Casket for cremation provisions.* (1) *Deceptive acts or practices.* In selling or offering to sell funeral goods or funeral services to the public, it is a deceptive act or practice for a funeral provider to:

(i) Represent that state or local law requires a casket for direct cremations;

(ii) Represent that a casket (other than an unfinished wood box) is required for direct cremations.

(2) Preventive requirements. to prevent these deceptive acts or practices, as well as the unfair or deceptive acts or practices defined in §453.4(a)(1), funeral providers must place the following disclosure in immediate conjunction with the price range shown for direct cremations: "If you want to arrange a direct cremation, you can use an unfinished wood box or an alternative container. Alternative containers can be made of materials like heavy cardboard or composition materials (with or without an outside covering), or pouches of canvas." This disclosure only has to be placed on the general price list if the funeral provider arranges direct cremations.

(e) *Provisions on preservative and protecting value claims.* In selling or offering to sell funeral goods or funeral services to the public, it is a deceptive act or practice for a funeral provider to:

(1) Represent that funeral goods or funeral services will delay the natural decomposition of human remains for a long-term or indefinite time;

(2) Represent that funeral goods have protective features or will protect the body from gravesite substances, when such is not the case.

### §453.4 Required purchase of funeral goods or funeral services.

(b) *Other required purchases of funeral goods or funeral services.* — (1) Unfair or deceptive acts or practices. In selling or offering to sell funeral goods or funeral services, it is an unfair or deceptive act or practice for a funeral provider to condition the furnishing of any funeral good or funeral service to a person arranging a funeral upon the purchase of any other funeral good or funeral service, except as required by law or as otherwise permitted by this part.

(2) Preventive requirements. (i) To prevent this unfair or deceptive act or practice, funeral providers must:

(A) Place the following disclosure in the general price list, immediately above the prices required by §453.2(b)(ii) and (iii): "The goods and services shown below are those we can provide to our customers. You may choose only the items you desire. If legal or other requirements mean you must buy any items you did not specifically ask for, we will explain the reason in writing on the statement we provide describing the funeral goods and services you selected."

*Provided, however,* That if the charge for "services of funeral director and staff" cannot be declined by the purchases, the statement shall include the sentence: "However, any funeral arrangements you select will include a charge for our services" between the second and third sentences of the statement specified above herein;

(B) Place the following disclosure on the statement of funeral goods and services selected, required by §453.2(b)(5)(ii): "Charges are only for those items that are used. If we are required by law to use any items, we will explain the reasons in writing below."

(ii) A funeral provider shall not violate this section by failing to comply with a request for a combination of goods or services which would be impossible, impractical, or excessively burdensome to provide.

### §453.5 Services Provided Without Prior Approval

(a) *Unfair or deceptive acts or practices.* In selling or offering to sell funeral goods or funeral services to the public, it is an unfair or deceptive act or practice for any provider to embalm a deceased human body for a fee unless:

(1) State or local law or regulation requires embalming in the particular circumstances regardless of any funeral choice which the family might make; or

(2) Prior approval for embalming (expressly so described) has been obtained from a family member or other authorized person; or

(3) The funeral provider is unable to contact a family member or other authorized person after exercising due diligence, has no reason to believe the family does not want embalming performed, and obtains subsequent approval for embalming already performed (expressly so described). In seeking approval, the funeral provider must disclose that a fee will be charged if the family selects a funeral which requires embalming, such as a funeral with viewing, and that no fee will be charged if the family selects a service which does not require embalming, such as direct cremation or immediate burial.

(b) *Preventive requirement.* To prevent these unfair or deceptive acts or practices, funeral providers must include on the contract, final bill, or other written evidence of the agreement or obligation given to the customer, the statement: "If you selected a funeral which requires embalming, such as a funeral with viewing, you may have to pay for embalming. You do not have to pay for embalming you did not approve if you selected arrangements such as a direct cremation or immediate burial. If we charged for embalming, we will explain why below."

## A LIST OF OTHER FUNERAL RULE REQUIREMENTS:

*Specific price information that must be provided:*

1. Disclosure of information over the telephone.
2. Casket price list.
3. Outer container price list.
4. General price list (other merchandise and service costs).
5. Written, itemized statement of goods and services.

*Prohibits misrepresentations and requires a disclosure statement about:*

1. Embalming.
2. Casket for cremation.
3. Need for outer container.
4. Legal or cemetery requirements.
5. Cash advance requirement.
6. Preservation or merchandise. (Statement not required)

*Prohibits required purchases:*

1. Casket for cremation other than unfinished wood box. Must provide an inexpensive alternative container.
2. Must disclose any other required purchases.

## J. THE NATIONAL SELECTED MORTICIANS CODE OF GOOD
## FUNERAL PRACTICE, 1987
(National Selected Morticians, Evanston, IL 60201.)

As funeral directors, our calling imposes upon us special responsibilities to those we serve and to the public at large. Chief among them is the obligation to inform the public so that everyone can make knowledgeable decisions about funerals and funeral directors.

In acceptance of our responsibilities, and as a condition of our membership in National Selected Morticians, we affirm the following standards of good funeral practice and hereby pledge:

1. To provide the public with information about funerals, including prices, and about the functions, services and responsibilities of funeral directors.

2. To afford a continuing opportunity to all persons to discuss or arrange funerals in advance.

3. To make funerals available in as wide a range of price categories as necessary to meet the need of all segments of the community, and affirmatively to extend to everyone the right of inspecting and freely considering all of them.

4. To quote conspicuously in writing the charges for every funeral offered; to identify clearly the services, facilities, equipment and merchandise included in such quotations; and to follow a policy of reasonable adjustment when less than the quoted offering is utilized.

5. To furnish to each family at the time funeral arrangements are made, a written memorandum of charges and to make no additional charge without the approval of the purchaser.

6. To make no representation, written or oral, which may be false or misleading, and to apply a standard of total honesty in all dealings.

7. To respect all faiths, creeds and customs, and to give full effect to the role of the clergy.

8. To maintain a qualified and competent staff, complete facilities and suitable equipment required for comprehensive funeral service.

9. To assure those we serve the right of personal choice and decision in making funeral arrangements.

10. To be responsive to the needs of the poor, serving them within their means.

11. To comply fully with the requirements of the FTC Trade Regulation Rule on funeral practices.

We pledge to conduct ourselves in every way and at all times in such a manner as to deserve the public trust, and to place a copy of this Code of Good Funeral Practice in the possession of a representative of all parties with whom we arrange funerals.

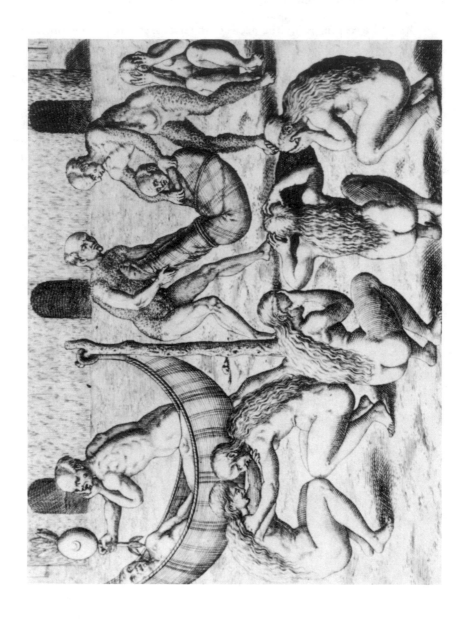

Explorers' view of New World burial in Brazil. Originally published by Jean de Lery: *[Great and small voyages]*, (Reproduced with permission. National Library of Medicine.)

# INDEX

British Columbia
  leased graves 528
*British Medical Journal* 33
Britons
  prehistoric burials 516
Brittany
  crude coffins 474
  graves reused 526
Bronze Age
  burials 516
  cremation 239, 240
Brooklyn
  horse-drawn hearse 488
Bruce, Robert 434
Buddhism
  cremation 240, 274
  skulls as musical instruments 398
Buddhist
  reliquaries 434
Buddhists
  autopsies 161
  cremation 273
  embalming 228
  funerals 447
  organ/tissue donation 67, 68
Bulgarian Revolt
  corpses 461
Bull's hide shrouds 392, 454
Burial cases 466
Burial chests 466, 594
Burial clothing 451-6
  Amish 454
  cerecloth 454
  Chinese 454
  clown costume 450
  commercially made 454
  cross-dressers 455
  Cypriots 452
  Edward I 514
  effect decomposition 309
  Gypsies 454
  Jewish 446
  laws 452
  Mormons 454

  prehistoric 451
  reuse 456
  Romans 445, 451
  U.S. 454
  unusual 455
Burial container
  misrepresentation 633
Burial ground 584
Burial insurance 482
Burial of an ass 509
Burial societies. *See* Memorial societies
Burial vault 570, 594. *See also* Vaults
Burial-transit permit 594
Burials 507-54, 578-86
  after
    cremation 506
    dismemberment 392
  air 391
    description of 391
    Mongolia 391
  allowance
    stealing corpses for
      U.S. 345
    veteran 520
  alternative containers 474
  American Revolution 502
  articulate 500
  as atonement 499
  at crossroads 410, 502
  at night 502
  authorized locations 501
  based on religious custom 445
  begun by gods 499
  Bermuda 501
  biblical 499-501
  body parts 508
  Britain, early 500
  catacombs 501, 538
  cave 499, 501
  cemetery product 522
  choices 500-3
  Christian, early 517
  churchyards 517
  city names & 498

650

# Index

679

# Index

Permissions

707

## ABOUT THE AUTHOR

Kenneth V. Iserson, M.D., MBA, FACEP, is a Professor of Surgery and Director of the Arizona Bioethics Program at the University of Arizona Health Sciences Center, Tucson, AZ. He practices emergency medicine and is the medical director of southern Arizona's major search and rescue operation. Although Dr. Iserson treats dying patients, counsels professionals and families about sudden death, and has been in medicine for more than twenty years, he found that he had large gaps in his knowledge about what happened to dead bodies—and was initially stymied in his attempt to get more information. This book is the result of his investigations.


## CODA

Some readers may ask what I plan as the final disposition of my body when I no longer need it. Given the importance of organ and tissue donation and the trade-offs with other forms of corpse disposition I discussed in this book, I plan to donate all useable organs and tissues for transplant or research, with the remainder being cremated. My hope is that the ashes will be scattered on Finger Rock, overlooking Tucson, in the majestic Santa Catalina Mountains.


## GALEN

Galen of Pergamum (A.D. 130-201), the Greek physician whose writings guided medicine for more than a millennium after his death, inspired the name, Galen Press. As the father of modern anatomy and physiology, Galen wrote more than one hundred treatises while attempting to change medicine from an art form into a science. As practicing physician, Galen first ministered to gladiators and then to Roman Emperor Marcus Aurelius. Far more than Hippocrates, Galen's work influenced Western physicians, and was the "truth" until the late Middle Ages when physicians and scientists challenged his teachings. Galen Press, publishing non-clinical, health-related books will follow Galen's advice that "the chief merit of language is clearness...nothing detracts so much from this as unfamiliar terms."

5/96. 4 12/95
9/00  14 3/00
4/01  14  3/00
4/02  15  5/01
4/03  20 1/03